BASIC ANESTHESIOLOGY EXAMINATION REVIEW

BASIC ANESTHESIOLOGY EXAMINATION REVIEW

EDITED BY

George W. Williams, MD, FCCP

CHIEF OF CRITICAL CARE MEDICINE
DEPARTMENT OF ANESTHESIOLOGY
ASSOCIATE PROFESSOR OF ANESTHESIOLOGY
AND NEUROSURGERY
UNIVERSITY OF TEXAS MEDICAL SCHOOL
AT HOUSTON
HOUSTON, TEXAS

EDITED BY

Erin S. Williams, MD, FAAP

ASSISTANT PROFESSOR OF PEDIATRICS
AND ANESTHESIOLOGY
BAYLOR COLLEGE OF MEDICINE
TEXAS CHILDREN'S HOSPITAL
HOUSTON, TEXAS

OXFORD
UNIVERSITY PRESS

OXFORD
UNIVERSITY PRESS

Oxford University Press is a department of the University of Oxford. It furthers the University's objective of excellence in research, scholarship, and education by publishing worldwide.Oxford is a registered trade mark of Oxford University Press in the UK and certain other countries.

Published in the United States of America by Oxford University Press
198 Madison Avenue, New York, NY 10016, United States of America.

First Edition published in 2016

Library of Congress Cataloging-in-Publication Data
Basic anesthesiology examination review / edited by George Williams, Erin Williams.
p.; cm.
Includes bibliographical references and index.
ISBN 978–0–19–938162–3 (alk. paper)
I. Williams, George (George W.), editor. II. Williams, Erin (Erin Scott), editor.
[DNLM: 1. Anesthesia—Examination Questions. 2. Anesthetics—Examination Questions. WO 218.2]
RD82.3
617.9′6076—dc23
2015022387

9 8 7 6 5 4 3 2 1

Printed by Sheridan, USA

This book is dedicated to our wonderful children, Eden, Emeri and Gabriel, our gifts from the Lord who bring out the best in us.

CONTENTS

PREFACE

With the resident's education comes a multitude of opportunities and demands of learning. Clinical competencies and academic competencies are valued, emphasized, and confirmed via a series of exams that encompass the certification process for an anesthesiologist. It is this intense and vigorous process that works to ensure the production of skilled, knowledgeable, competent, compassionate, safe consultants in the field of anesthesiology. Given the significant volume of material the resident physician must master, *Basic Anesthesiology Examination Review* (BAER) provides the Clinical Anesthesia–1 (CA-1) resident with a single, complete source constructed to cover the content of the American Board of Anesthesiology (ABA) Basic Science of Anesthesia.

Basic Anesthesiology Examination Review not only strategically takes the resident through all of the content encompassed by the "Basic Exam" but also allows the physician-in-training to exercise and confirm mastery of each topic with a series of questions followed by solutions and suggested reading after each chapter. This style of information followed by review with questions and answers will serve as a guide for the resident during preparation not just for the exam but also as a roadmap for the mastery of the basic science concepts in the field of anesthesiology with specific attention to pharmacology, anatomy, and physiology as well as anesthesia equipment and monitoring. Having read many medical texts over the years, experience has informed us that finding focused resources to prepare for a specific examination may be difficult. With each new examination, new question types and objectives are generated. Being mindful of the ABA's description of the Basic Examination, we have aimed to stay true to the needs of an individual preparing for this examination in this book.

It is with sincere thanks that we honor and acknowledge all of the contributing authors for their exceptional dedication to this task and their tireless efforts and timely submissions for the success of this review book. We wouldn't be the physicians we are today without the love and support of our parents, who always encouraged us to be the best we could be. Furthermore, we are grateful to the educators of Case Western Reserve University School of Medicine and the Cleveland Clinic Foundation who instilled in us the art and science of anesthesiology. We also thank Dr. Shilpa Dabhade, Dr. Shruti Deshpandhe, Dr. Salma El Marjiya-Villarreal, Dr. Sabeen Mujtaba, and Dr. Andrea Rojas for their hard work in providing illustrations and support for this project. Furthermore, we sincerely thank our department chairs, Dr. Dean Andropoulos and Dr. Carin Hagberg, respectively, without whose mentorship we could not have initiated or completed BAER. Finally, we thank Oxford University Press for giving us the opportunity to help facilitate resident physicians' success in the education and examination process. It has been the utmost pleasure to work with Andrea Knobloch and Rebecca Suzan in creating this book. We are forever grateful for this opportunity that we have been blessed with. It is our hope that all who read BAER will be better prepared for the rigorous resident education process, and better anesthesiologists, after doing so.

Erin S. Williams
George W. Williams, II

CONTRIBUTORS

Varsha D. Allampalli, MBBS, MD
Senior Resident
Department of Anesthesiology and Critical Care
Jawaharlal Institute of Postgraduate Medical Education and Research
Pondicherry, India

Andrew Allison, MD
Assistant Professor of Anesthesiology
University of Texas Health Science Center at Houston
Houston, Texas

Carlos A. Artime, MD
Associate Professor of Anesthesiology
University of Texas at Houston Medical School
Houston, Texas

Sudha A. Bidani, MD
Assistant Professor of Pediatrics and Anesthesiology
Baylor College of Medicine
Staff Anesthesiologist
Texas Children's Hospital
Houston, Texas

Alina Bodas, MD
Staff Pediatric Anesthesiologist
The Cleveland Clinic Children's Hospital
Cleveland, Ohio

Yefim W. Bogomolny, MD
Director of Orthopedic Anesthesia, Regional Anesthesia, and Acute Pain Medicine
Assistant Professor of Anesthesiology
University of Texas Health Science Center at Houston
Houston, Texas

Vera Borzova, MD
Department of Pediatric Anesthesiology
Cleveland Clinic
Cleveland, Ohio

Katya H. Chiong, MD
Assistant Professor of Anesthesiology
Case Western Reserve University School of Medicine
Associate Program Director of Anesthesiology and Perioperative Medicine
Attending Anesthesiologist
University Hospitals Case Medical Center
Cleveland, Ohio

Tolutope Coker, MD
Staff Anesthesiologist and Intensivist
Greater Houston Anesthesiology
Houston, Texas

Shilpa Dabhade, MD
Fellow in Neuroanesthesiology
Department of Anesthesiology
University of Texas Health Science Center at Houston
Houston, Texas

Shruti Deshpande, MD
Department of Anesthesiology
University of Texas Health Science Center at Houston
Houston, Texas

Harold Doerr, MD
Director of Anesthesia Simulation
Assistant Professor of Anesthesiology
University of Texas Health Science Center at Houston
Houston, Texas

Marie-Francoise Doursout, PhD
Professor of Anesthesiology
University of Texas Health Science Center at Houston
Houston, Texas

Rhashedah A. Ekeoduru, MD
Assistant Professor of Anesthesiology
University of Texas Health Science Center at Houston
Children's Memorial Hospital
Houston, Texas

Salma El Marjiya-Villarreal, MD
Professional Trainee,
Department of Anesthesiology
University of Texas Medical School at Houston

Priscilla J. Garcia, MD, MHA
Assistant Professor of Anesthesiology and Pediatrics
Texas Children's Hospital
Houston, Texas

Chris D. Glover, MD, FAAP, MBA
Director of Anesthesia Services for Community Hospitals
Associate Professor of Anesthesiology
Baylor College of Medicine
Texas Children's Hospital
Houston, Texas

Cheryl Gore, MD
Assistant Professor of Pediatrics and Anesthesiology
Baylor College of Medicine
Staff Anesthesiologist
Texas Children's Hospital
Houston, Texas

Erin A. Gottlieb, MD
Associate Professor of Anesthesiology
Division of Pediatric Cardiovascular Anesthesiology
Baylor College of Medicine
Texas Children's Hospital
Houston, Texas

Kaylani Govindan, MD
Assistant Professor of Pediatric Anesthesiology
Baylor College of Medicine
Texas Children's Hospital
Houston, Texas

Sam Gumbert, MD
Assistant Professor of Anesthesiology
Residency Program Director
University of Texas at Houston
Houston, Texas

Sarah Guzman-Reyes, MD
Associate Professor of Anesthesiology
University of Texas Health Science Center at Houston
Houston, Texas

Mark Harbott, MD, MHA
Assistant Professor and Program Director of Anesthesiology
Baylor College of Medicine
Houston, Texas

Kenneth N. Hiller, MD
Assistant Professor of Anesthesiology
University of Texas at Houston Medical School
Houston, Texas

Timothy Hollenbeck, MD
Assistant Professor of Anesthesiology
University of Texas at Houston Medical School
Houston, Texas

Olakunle Idowu, MD
Staff Anesthesiologist and Intensivist
Greater Houston Anethesiology
Houston, Texas

Vadim Ioselevich, MD
Assistant Professor of Anesthesiology
University of Texas at Houston Medical School
Houston, Texas

Ranu R. Jain, MD
Assistant Professor of Anesthesiology
University of Texas at Houston Medical School
Houston, Texas

Matthew D. James, MD
Assistant Professor of Anesthesiology
Baylor College of Medicine
Texas Children's Hospital
Houston, Texas

Jibin Sam Mathew, MBBS, MD
Resident Physician
Department of Intensive Care Medicine
Alexandra Hospital
Singapore

James W. Jones, MD
Valley Anesthesiology Consultants
Phoenix, Arizona

David O. Joseph, MS, MD
Diplomate of the American Board of Anesthesiology
Attending Anesthesiologist and Intensivist
US Anesthesia Partners/Greater Houston Anesthesiology
Houston, Texas

Aimee Gretchen Kakascik, DO
Assistant Professor of Anesthesiology and Pediatrics
Baylor College of Medicine
Texas Children's Hospital
Houston, Texas

Yang Liu, MD
Assistant Professor of Anesthesiology and Pediatrics
Baylor College of Medicine
Houston, Texas

Heather McFarland, DO
Anesthesia Residency Program Director
Critical Care Anesthesiologist
Assistant Professor of Anesthesia and Perioperative Medicine
University Hospitals Case Medical Center
Cleveland, Ohio

Maria Matuszczak, MD
Professor of Anesthesiology
Division Chief, Pediatric Anesthesia
University of Texas at Houston Medical School
Houston, Texas

Kim-Phuong Nguyen, MD
Assistant Professor of Pediatrics and Anesthesiology
Baylor College of Medicine
Texas Children's Hospital
Houston, Texas

Omonele Ohen Nwokolo, MD
Assistant Professor of Anesthesiology
Assistant Residency Program Director, Anesthesiology
University of Texas at Houston Medical School
Assistant Chief of Anesthesiology
Lyndon B. Johnson Hospital
Houston, Texas

Timothy Pawelek, MD
Assistant Professor of Anesthesiology
University of Texas at Houston Medical School
Houston, Texas

Muhammad B. Rafique, MD
Pediatric Cardiac Anesthesiologist
Assistant Professor of Anesthesiology
University of Texas Medical School at Houston
Houston, Texas

Bilal Rana, DO
Anesthesiologist and Intensivist
Houston, Texas

Esi M. Rhett, MD
Assistant Professor of Anesthesiology
University of Texas Medical School at Houston
Houston, Texas

Karel Riha, MD
Assistant Professor of Anesthesiology
University of Texas at Houston Medical School
Houston, Texas

Ricardo Riveros, MD
Congenital Cardiac Anesthesia Staff
Department of Outcomes Research
Cleveland Clinic Children's Hospital
Cleveland Clinic
Cleveland, Ohio

Shelly-Anne Rodriguez, MD
Staff, Department of Pediatric Anesthesiology
Cleveland Clinic Children's Hospital
Cleveland, Ohio

Arianna Rojas, MD
Professional Trainee
Department of Anesthesiology
University of Texas Medical School at Houston
Houston, Texas

Madhumani Rupasinghe, MBBS, FRCA
Assistant Professor of Anesthesiology
University of Texas Health Science Center at Houston
Medical Director for Obstetric Anesthesia
Lyndon B. Johnson Hospital
Houston, Texas

Catherine P. Seipel, MD
Assistant Professor Anesthesiology and Pediatrics
Baylor College of Medicine
Staff Anesthesiologist
Texas Children's Hospital
Houston, Texas

Joanne Spaliaras, MD
Pediatric Anesthesiologist
New York, New York

Stephen Stayer, MD
Professor of Anesthesiology and Pediatrics
Baylor College of Medicine
Associate Chief of Pediatric Anesthesiology
Texas Children's Hospital
Houston, Texas

Imelda Tjia, MD
Assistant Professor of Pediatrics and Anesthesiology
Baylor College of Medicine
Texas Children's Hospital
Houston, Texas

Young Su, MD
Anesthesiologist and Intensivist
Houston, Texas

Erikka L. Washington, MD
Assistant Professor of Anesthesiology
University of Texas Health Science Center at Houston
Lyndon B. Johnson Hospital
Houston, Texas

Mehernoor F. Watcha, MD
Associate Professor of Anesthesiology and Pediatrics
Baylor College of Medicine
Texas Children's Hospital
Houston, Texas

Naveen Vanga, MD
Assistant Professor of Neuro-Anesthesiology
University of Texas Health Science Center at Houston
Houston, Texas

Jennifer D. Wu, MD, MBA
Assistant Professor of Anesthesiology
University of Texas Health Science Center at Houston
Houston, Texas

Sherif Zaafran, MD
Greater Houston Anesthesiology
Houston, Texas

SECTION I

ANATOMY

1.

BASIC ANATOMY

Salma El Marjiya-Villarreal, Yang Liu, and George W. Williams

CRICOTHYROID MEMBRANE

The pharynx is the region posterior to the nasal and oral cavity and superior to the larynx. It extends from the base of the skull inferiorly until it becomes continuous with the esophagus. The pharynx is divided into three regions: nasopharynx, oropharynx, and laryngopharynx. The maxillary nerve, glossopharyngeal nerve, and vagus nerve provide the nerve supply.

The larynx is the organ that connects the lower part of the pharynx with the trachea. The larynx consists of three single cartilages (thyroid, cricoid, and epiglottic) and three paired cartilages (arytenoid, corniculate, and cuneiform). The thyroid cartilage comprises two laminae, which are fused anteriorly to form a median elevation termed the laryngeal prominence (Adam's apple). The laryngeal prominence is larger in adult men, in whom it is usually clearly visible and palpable (Figure 1.1).

The larynx is innervated bilaterally by the superior laryngeal nerve and the recurrent laryngeal nerve. The recurrent laryngeal nerve supplies all of the intrinsic muscles of the larynx, with the exception of the cricothyroid muscles. Injury to one side of the nerves can paralyze the ipsilateral posterior cricoarytenoid muscle, causing vocal cord dysfunction. The mucosa of the larynx is supplied by the internal laryngeal branch of the superior laryngeal nerve. The recurrent laryngeal nerve supplies sensation to the larynx below the vocal cords.

The cricoid cartilage is shaped like a signet ring and sits just inferior to the thyroid cartilage in the neck. The cricoid cartilage is at the level of the C6 vertebra, and its arch is palpable. The inferior border of the cricoid cartilage marks the end of the pharynx and larynx. During a rapid sequence induction for a patient at high risk of aspiration, the cricoid cartilage can be pressed to compress the esophagus behind it, which is known as the Sellick maneuver.

The cartilages of the larynx are connected to each other by muscles and/or ligaments. The thyrohyoid membrane connects the thyroid cartilage with the superior border of the hyoid bone. The vocal ligaments are enclosed within the vocal folds. Each side of a vocal ligament attaches to the angle of the thyroid cartilage anteriorly and the vocal process of the arytenoid cartilage posteriorly. The cricothyroid membrane consists of a median (anterior) and twin lateral ligaments. It connects the arch of the cricoid cartilage with the thyroid cartilage. In the event of a life-threatening airway obstruction, cricothyrotomy should be performed to provide an airway. Again, this is performed only when a patient is unable to be mask ventilated and a tracheal intubation is deemed impossible. A cricothyrotomy is an incision made through the skin and cricothyroid membrane between the thyroid cartilage and cricoid cartilage to provide an open airway in the larynx. It is easier and quicker to perform than tracheotomy and provides a temporary airway before a definitive airway can be established (Figure 1.1).

INTERNAL AND EXTERNAL JUGULAR VEINS

The jugular veins collect deoxygenated blood from the head and neck and return it to the heart. There are three main jugular veins—external, internal, and anterior (Figure 1.2).

The external jugular vein and its tributaries return the blood from the majority of the external face. It is formed by the union of the posterior auricular vein and retromandibular vein. It has a relatively superficial course and runs anteriorly to the sternocleidomastoid muscle, crossing it in an oblique, posterior, and inferior direction. At the root of the neck, the vein passes underneath the clavicle and terminates by draining into the subclavian vein.

The anterior jugular veins are paired veins draining the submaxillary region. They descend down the midline of the neck, emptying into the subclavian vein.

The internal jugular vein drains the brain, neck, and face. It is formed by the anastomosis of the sigmoid sinus

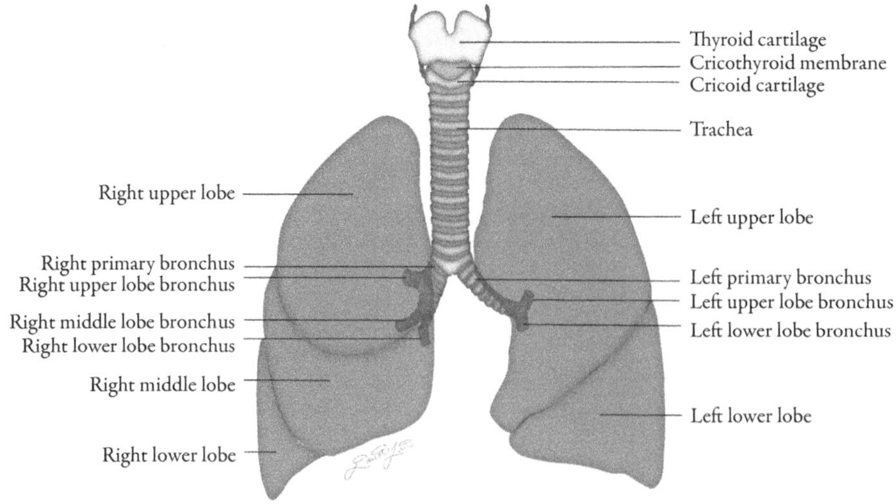

Figure 1.1 Cricothyroid membrane, trachea, bronchi, and lungs.

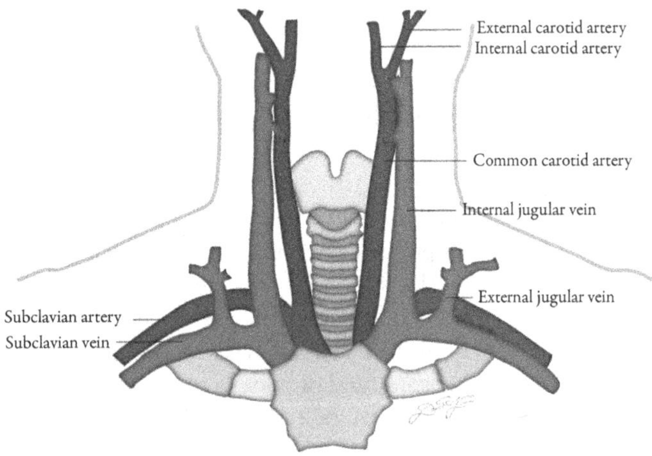

Figure 1.2 Carotid artery and jugular vein.

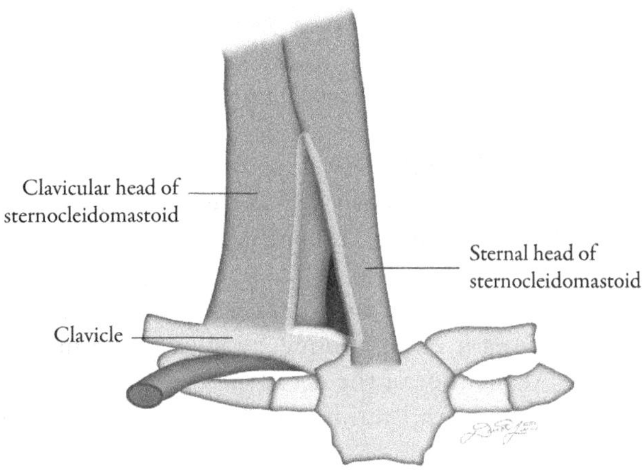

Figure 1.3 Sedillot's triangle. Sedillot's triangle (yellow triangle) is composed of the borders of the clavicular head of the sternocleidomastoid, the sternal head of the sternocleidomastoid, and the superior border of the medial third of the clavicle. Cannulation begins with cutaneous puncture at the superior apex of this triangle.

of the dura mater and the common facial vein. The internal jugular runs laterally to the common carotid artery and vagus nerve within the carotid sheath, which is hidden by the sternocleidomastoid muscle. At the bottom of the neck, posteriorly to the sternal end of the clavicle, the internal jugular vein unites with the subclavian vein to form the brachiocephalic vein.

The internal jugular vein, especially the right internal jugular vein, is often a reliable access site for central venous cannulation to support hemodynamic monitoring, fluid and medication administration, and parenteral nutrition. The internal jugular vein lies immediately posterior to the apex of Sedillot's triangle, which is formed by the sternal head of the sternocleidomastoid, the clavicular head of the sternocleidomastoid, and the clavicle (Figure 1.3). Advantages of the right side internal jugular vein approach include a superficial location, easy ultrasonic visualization, and a straight course to the superior vena cava.

THORACIC DUCT

Most of the lymph in the body reaches the venous system by way of the thoracic duct. The lymphatic duct originates in the abdomen from the confluence of the right and left lumbar trunks and the intestinal trunk. It extends vertically between the descending thoracic aorta and the azygos vein and empties into the junction of the left subclavian vein and left jugular vein. Variations are common. There are two valves at the junction of the duct with the left subclavian vein to prevent the flow of venous blood into the duct. The thoracic duct can be damaged during thoracic surgery and cause a large amount of lymph to accumulate in the pleural cavity. This situation is called chylothorax, which may require surgical ligation of the thoracic duct. Of note, the anastomoses of lymphatic vessels are so extensive that no serious effects result if the thoracic duct is ligated.

CAROTID AND VERTEBRAL ARTERIES

The left and right common carotid arteries supply oxygenated blood to the head and neck (Figure 1.2). The right common carotid originates in the neck from the brachiocephalic trunk, while the left arises from the aortic arch in the thoracic region. The common carotid artery is contained in a carotid sheath with the internal jugular vein and vagus nerve. The internal jugular vein lies lateral to the carotid artery with the vagus nerve situated between the artery and vein posteriorly. The common carotid artery divides into the external and internal carotid arteries at the upper border of the lamina of the thyroid cartilage (approximately the level of the fourth cervical vertebra). The common carotid artery and the internal carotid artery usually ascend along a line from the sternoclavicular joint, along the anterior border of the sternocleidomastoid muscle, to a point medial to the lobule of the auricle without giving off branches. The internal carotid artery enters the skull through the carotid canal of the temporal bone and divides into the anterior and middle cerebral arteries in the middle cranial fossa. The external carotid divides into the superficial temporal and maxillary arteries within the parotid gland. The carotid sinus is a dilated area superior to the bifurcation of the common carotid. Its wall contains numerous baroreceptors sensitive to changes in blood pressure. The carotid body lies in the angle of bifurcation of the common carotid artery and is sensitive to hypoxemia.

The common carotid artery is often used in measuring the pulse, especially in patients who are in shock and who lack a detectable pulse in the peripheral arteries of the body. The pulsation of the common carotid arteries can be felt along the anterior border of the sternocleidomastoid muscle. The common carotid arteries can also be compressed against the anterior tubercle of the sixth cervical vertebra (Chassaignac's tubercle) (Figure 1.4).

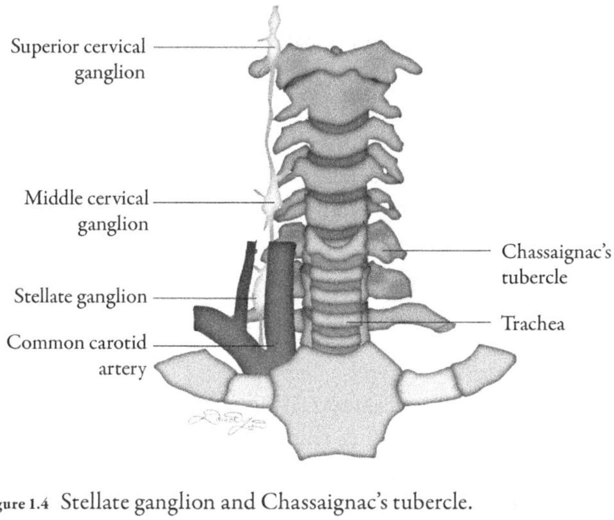

Figure 1.4 Stellate ganglion and Chassaignac's tubercle.

The vertebral arteries branch from the subclavian arteries, pass through the foramina of the transverse processes of vertebrae C6–C1, and merge to form the single midline basilar artery, which supplies blood to the posterior part of the circle of Willis.

STELLATE GANGLION

The sympathetic nerve supply to the head and neck arises from spinal cord segments T1 and T2. Their axons exit by way of spinal nerves and lead to three paravertebral ganglia: superior, middle, and inferior cervical ganglion. The inferior cervical ganglion is frequently fused with the first thoracic ganglion forming the stellate ganglion, which is located at the level of the sixth and seventh cervical vertebrae, anterior to the transverse process of C7 (Figure 1.4). Stellate ganglion block can be used to alleviate the sympathetically mediated symptoms such as complex regional pain syndrome type I and to relieve vascular spasm involving the brain or an upper limb. Injection is often given near the Chassaignac's tubercle. Nerves emerging from cervical sympathetic ganglia also contribute to the cardiac plexus.

CERVICAL SPINE LANDMARKS (VERTEBRA PROMINENS, CHASSAIGNAC'S TUBERCLE)

Vertebra prominens is the name of the seventh cervical vertebra. The vertebra prominens is characterized by a prominent spinous process, which is palpable from the skin surface. The vertebra prominens has the most prominent spinous process in about 70% of people. In the remaining population, either the spinous process of the sixth cervical vertebra or the first thoracic vertebra is the most prominent. The spinous process of the vertebra prominens is an important conspicuous bony landmark to identify vertebral level for thoracic epidural placement.

Chassaignac's tubercle is the name of the anterior tubercle of the transverse process of the sixth cervical vertebra. It can be felt on deep pressure opposite cricoid cartilage, in the course of the carotid artery. It is also called the carotid tubercle, because the carotid artery can be easily compressed against it. In case of supraventricular tachycardia, the carotid artery can be massaged against the Chassaignac's tubercle to relieve the symptoms. Chassaignac's tubercle is an important landmark for performing brachial plexus block and cervical plexus block.

CHEST

The thorax or chest is a region of the body between the neck and the abdomen. It is mostly protected and supported by the rib cage, spine, and shoulder girdle. The thorax includes the thorax cavity and the thorax wall. The former contains vital organs such as the heart and lungs as well as important vessels such as the aorta, the superior and inferior vena cava and the pulmonary artery and the latter provides rigid protection to the content of the thorax cavity and flexibility to aid in the functional respiration process.

PULMONARY LOBES

The lungs are located within the thoracic cavity, on either side of the heart. The right lung is divided into three lobes—superior, middle, and inferior— by the minor horizontal fissure and the major oblique fissure. The left lung consists of only two lobes, upper and lower, divided by the oblique fissure. The central region of each lung has a triangular depression called the hilum of the lung, which is the entry point for the root of the lung. The bronchi, pulmonary vessels, bronchial vessels, and lymphatic vessels form the root of the lung.

The trachea connects the pharynx and larynx to the lungs. The cricoid cartilage forms the inferior wall of the larynx and is the only complete ring of cartilage in the trachea. The trachea descends inferiorly from the larynx for about 10 to 16 cm and lies immediately anterior to the esophagus. Then, the trachea bifurcates into a right main bronchus and a left main bronchus, usually at the level of the fifth thoracic vertebra. At the site of the tracheal bifurcation, a cartilaginous ridge presents itself in the tracheal lumen, the carina. The carina lies to the left of the midline of the trachea. The right main bronchus is wider, shorter, and more vertical than the left main bronchus. Therefore, foreign bodies that fall down the trachea are more likely to enter the right bronchus. The mucous membrane of the carina is the most sensitive area of the trachea and is intimately involved in the cough reflex. The lumen of the trachea is maintained by incomplete c-shaped cartilaginous rings on the anterior and lateral aspects of the tracheal wall. The posterior wall of the trachea is a flattened membrane. The right main bronchus subdivides into three lobar bronchi, and the left main bronchus divides into two lobar bronchi to deliver air to the specific lung segments (Figure 1.1).

CARDIAC LANDMARKS

The heart has four chambers. The right atrium receives deoxygenated blood from the vena cava and pumps it through the tricuspid valve into the right ventricle. The right ventricle then pumps the blood through the pulmonary valve into the pulmonary arteries leading to the lungs. The left atrium receives oxygenated blood from the lungs through the pulmonary veins and pumps it through the mitral valve into the left ventricle. The left ventricle pumps the blood out through the aortic valve to the aorta leading to the systemic circulation. Heart sounds are generated when the heart valves slam shut during the cycle of the contractions. Heart murmurs are generated by turbulent flow of blood. The heart sounds and murmurs can be best heard from particular regions of the chest. The anatomical landmarks are (1) aortic valve—second right intercostal space at the sternal border, (2) pulmonic valve—second left intercostal space at the sternal border, (3) tricuspid valve—fourth left intercostal space at the sternal border, and (4) mitral valve—fifth left intercostal space at the sternal border (Figure 1.5).

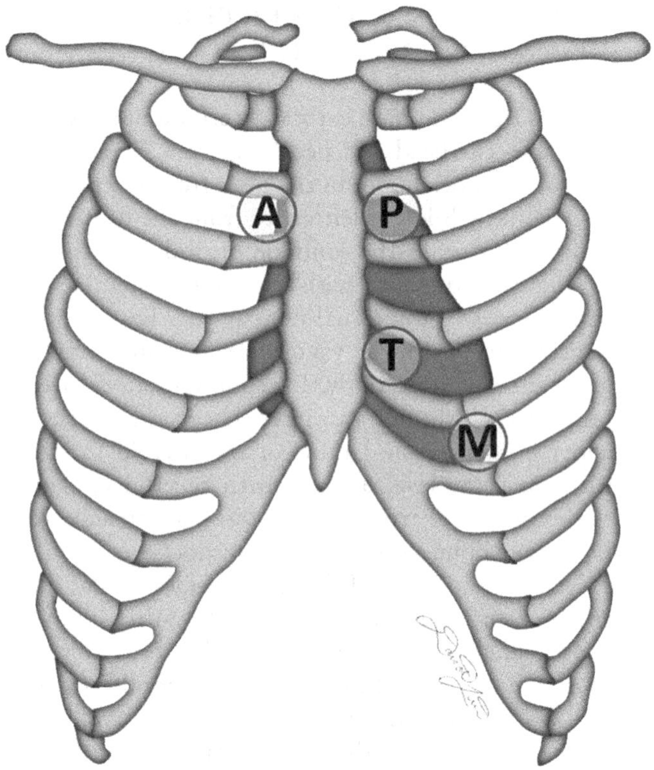

Figure 1.5 The surface relations of bones and heart. The locations for best auscultation of each heart valve are labeled: "A" for aortic valve, "P" for pulmonary valve, "M" for mitral valve, and "T" for tricuspid valve.

Subclavian Vein

The subclavian vein is a major vein that drains blood from the upper extremities and returns it to the heart. It is the continuation of the axillary vein at the outer border of the first rib. There are two of these veins, the right and the left subclavian veins. The subclavian vein runs under the clavicle, where it passes anterior to the anterior scalene muscle and unites with the internal jugular vein to form brachiocephalic veins (innominate veins) draining blood into the superior vena cava. The left vein also connects with the thoracic duct. The subclavian veins are commonly used for central line placement (Figure 1.2).

VERTEBRAL COLUMN ANATOMY

One of the distinctive characteristics of human development compared with animals is the achievement of erect posture and the maintenance of equilibrium. This task is performed by the vertebral column, also known as the rachis.

Two fundamental requirements of the rachis are rigidity, required for static efficiency and structural support/protection of important organs contained/enclosed in it (spinal cord and nerves), and flexibility.

In a normal adult, there are four curvatures of the rachis—acquired lordosis (posteriorly concave) in the cervical and lumbar segments and congenital kyphosis (posteriorly convex) in the thoracic and sacral segments. These physiologic curves confer more capacity to cushion/dampen strains and solicitations during movement.

The vertebral column is composed of overlying bone/vertebra segments, 33 vertebrae with interposed fibrocartilaginous intervertebral discs (cushion-like pads, each composed of a nucleus pulposus surrounded by the annulus fibrosus). Each vertebra shares an analogous fundamental structure with peculiar and different characteristics depending on the segment to which it belongs. For such differences we distinguish the different segments, which are discussed in Chapter 23.

During the first 3 months of intrauterine development, the vertebral column and spinal cord grow at the same velocity, so the spinal nerves emerge perpendicularly to the spine (right angle). Thenceforth, the thoracic and lumbar vertebral column develops more rapidly than the correspondent spinal cord and the latter apparently seems to reascend (spinal cord ascension). In the adult, the first cervical spinal nerves emerge from their correspondent neuromere perpendicularly to the spine (the first cervical spinal nerve emerges above C1 and the eighth cervical spinal nerve emerges below C7) while the thoracic and lumbar spinal nerves need to run obliquely downward to reach their respective intervertebral foramen (e.g., spinal nerve L3 emerges through the intervertebral foramen formed between L3 and L4) (Table 1.1).

The vertebral bodies are stabilized by five ligaments that increase in size between the cervical and lumbar vertebrae:

1. The **nuchal** ligament is an interspinous ligament in the cervical spine (C1–C6).
2. The **supraspinous** ligament extends from C7 to the sacrum along the tips of the spinous processes.
3. The **interspinous** ligament attaches successive spinous processes.
4. The **ligamentum flavum** attaches adjacent laminae on the anterior vertebral surface.
5. The **anterior longitudinal** ligament attaches to the anterior surface of vertebral bodies and prevents excessive extension.
6. The **posterior longitudinal** ligament attaches to the posterior surface of the vertebral bodies and prevents excessive flexion.
7. The **denticulate** ligaments are an extension of pia mater on each side of the spinal cord. They connect pia mater to arachnoid and dura mater for better stability.

THE SACRAL SPACE

The **sacrum** is a triangular-shaped bone formed by the fusion of the five sacral vertebrae, articulating above with the fifth lumbar vertebra and below with the coccyx. The posterior surface is convex and has a middle ridge; the extent of this ridge varies, usually from S1 to S3 or S4. The laminae of the fifth and sometimes of the fourth sacral vertebrae fail to fuse in the midline; the deficiency thus formed is known as the *sacral hiatus*. The sacral hiatus is covered by the sacrococcygeal ligament (a functional counterpart of ligamentum flavum).

The tubercles representing the inferior articular processes of the fifth sacral vertebra are prolonged downward as the *sacral cornua*. These cornua with the rudimentary spine of the fourth vertebra above, bond the sacral hiatus. There are four posterior sacral foramina that correspond with the anterior foramina, and each transmits a sacral nerve posterior ramus and communicates with the sacral canal. The **sacral canal** is a prismatic cavity running through the length of the bone and following its curves from the lumbar canal to the sacral hiatus. Fibrous strands sometimes occur in the canal

Table 1.1 SURFACE LANDMARKS OF THE SPINE

LEVEL	CORRESPONDING STRUCTURE
C2-3	Mandible
C3	Hyoid bone
C4-5	Thyroid cartilage
C6	Cricoid cartilage
C7	Vertebra prominens of spinous process
T3	Spine of scapula
T7	Inferior angle of the scapulae
T8	Point of inferior vena cava pierces diaphragm
T10	Xiphisternal junction; Point where esophagus enters stomach
T12	Point where aorta enters abdomen
L1	End of spinal cord
L3	Subcostal plane
L3-4	Umbilicus
L4	Bifurcation of aorta; Iliac crests
S2	End of dural sac; Line between posterior and superior iliac spine

and divide the extradural space into compartments: The posterior wall is the fused dorsal laminae of S1 through S4; the superior border is the end of the dura, the inferior edge is the sacrococcygeal ligament, and laterally four laminae are present. The contents of the sacral canal include:

1. The dural sac, which ends at the border of the second sacral vertebra on a line joining the posterior iliac spines. The pia mater is continued as the filum terminale.
2. Sacral nerves and the coccygeal nerve, with their dorsal root ganglia.
3. The venous plexus, formed by the lower end of the internal vertebral plexus. These vessels are more numerous anteriorly than posteriorly, and so the needle point should be kept as far posteriorly as possible.
4. Fatty tissue—more dense in males than in females.

Sacral Surface Anatomy

The caudal tip of the triangle will rest near the sacral cornua, which can be useful in confirming palpation of the sacral hiatus. The sacrum is distinctly different in men and women: In males the cavity of the sacrum has a smooth curve from S1 to S5, while in females the sacrum is quite flat from S1 to S3 with a more pronounced curve in the S4 and S5 region.

Radiological Landmarks of the Caudal Canal

Laterally, the caudal canal appears as a slight step-off on the most posterior part of the sacrum. The median sacral crest is seen as an opaque line posterior to the caudal canal.

The sacral hiatus is usually visible as a translucent opening at the base of the caudal canal.

Anteroposteriorly, the intermediate sacral crests are seen as opaque vertical lines on either side of the midline. The sacral foramina are seen as translucent, nearly circular areas lateral to the intermediate sacral crests.

UPPER EXTREMITY ANATOMY

Each upper extremity is composed of two parts: the shoulder and the arm. The shoulder connects the upper extremity to the trunk. Its skeleton is composed of the scapula and clavicle, which together are called the thoracic girdle. It has five total joints: three anatomical joints—(1) glenohumeral, (2) acromioclavicular, and (3) sternocostoclavicular— and two physiological joints—(1) subdeltoid and (2) scapulothoracic. Furthermore, it has extrinsic and intrinsic musculature that allows function.

The free part of the upper extremity consists of arm (humerus), forearm (radius and ulna), and hand (wrist or carpus, metacarpus, and phalanges or phalanxes). The elbow connects the arm with the forearm, and it has three joints—humeroulnar, humeroradial, and radioulnar. For reference, the carpus consists of, in proximal to distal and lateral to medial order, the *scaphoid, lunate, triquetrum, pisiform, hamate, capitate, trapezoid*, and *trapezium*. These bones are not commonly tested but are useful to recall when planning an orthopedic anesthetic.

The muscles of the arm are most easily separated into anterior and posterior. Anteriorly there are the biceps brachii, coracobrachialis, and brachialis (three). Posteriorly there is only the triceps brachii.

BONE MARROW

There are two types bone marrow—red marrow and yellow marrow. Red marrow contains hematopoietic tissue (red blood cells, white blood cells, and platelets) and is found mainly in the flat bones (hip, sternum, skull, ribs, vertebrae, and shoulder blades). Red marrow is also found in the spongy metaphyseal and epiphyseal ends of the long bones (i.e., femur, tibia, and humerus). Yellow marrow contains fat cells (adipose tissue) and is found in the hollow interior of the diaphyseal portion (or the shaft) of long bones. At a young age, almost all the bone marrow is red marrow, but as humans age, nearly all of the red marrow is replaced by yellow marrow. However, the yellow marrow can revert to red if there is increased demand for red blood cells (e.g., hemorrhage with great blood loss) (Table 1.2).

Aspiration of bone marrow, for various diagnostic purposes, is usually from the iliac crest or sternum. In children, the upper tibia can provide a good sample, because it still contains good amount of red bone marrow. Fat embolism, 12 to 72 hours following long-bone fracture (especially femur or tibia), represents disruption of the adipose architecture of bone marrow. The pathophysiology relates to obstruction

Table 1.2 **HEMORRHAGE THAT MAY CAUSE DEMAND FOR RED BLOOD CELLS**

FRACTURE	APPROXIMATED BLOOD LOSS (ML)
Foot	500
Ankle	1000
Tibia	1000
Femur	1000–2500
Pelvis bones (hip, sacrum, and coccyx)	1000–5000
Upper extremity	1000–1500
Open fractures with bone exposure	500–1000
Multiple fractures	1000–5000

of blood vessels by fat particles and to the deleterious/toxic effects of free fatty acids released from the fat particles (by lipase activity) on pneumocytes and the pulmonary capillary endothelium.

VASCULARIZATION OF THE UPPER EXTREMITY

The vital role of the upper extremity circulation in maintaining homeostasis depends on the continuous and controlled movement of blood through arteries, veins and capillaries. Nutrients and other essential materials pass from arterial blood into fluids surrounding the cells as waste products are removed through veins.

ARTERIES

The arterial supply to the upper limb begins in the chest as the **subclavian artery**; on the right, it originates from the brachiocephalic trunk behind the right sternoclavicular joint, and on the left, it arises from the arch of the aorta. It first runs medially to the scalenus anterior muscle, then behind it, and continues as the **axillary artery** after crossing the *lateral edge of the first rib*, behind the subclavius muscle and the subclavian vein. The axillary artery passes the axilla, underneath the pectoralis minor muscle, and at the level of the humeral surgical neck, it gives rise to the anterior and posterior **circumflex humeral** arteries and the subscapular artery (supply to the shoulder region) and finally, at the level of inferior edge of the teres major muscle, becomes the **brachial artery**, which descends down the arm posteriorly to the median nerve, giving rise to the profunda brachii artery (travels along the posterior surface of the humerus, running in the **radial groove**, and supplies structures in the posterior aspect of the arm, e.g., the triceps brachii). It then crosses the cubital fossa, below the brachialis muscle, it terminates by dividing into the **radial** (supplies the posterior aspect of the forearm) and **ulnar** (supplies the anterior aspect) **arteries.** The ulnar artery gives rise to the **common interosseous artery** that in turn divides into the anterior and posterior interosseous arteries.

VEINS

The major **superficial** veins that drain the upper limb are the **cephalic** and **basilic** veins that are located within the subcutaneous tissue of the upper limb. The **basilic vein** originates from the dorsal venous network of the hand. It ascends medially along the upper limb then deep into arm at the border of the **teres major**, where it conjoins with the **brachial vein** to form the axillary vein. The **cephalic vein** arises from the dorsal venous network of the hand, ascends anterolaterally the upper limb, and passes anteriorly to the elbow, where it connects with the basilica vein via the median cubital vein. At the shoulder it travels between the deltoid and pectoralis major muscles (known as the deltopectoral groove) and enters the axilla region via the clavipectoral triangle, where it terminates by joining the axillary vein.

The **deep** veins of the upper limb are situated underneath the deep fascia. They are paired veins that accompany and lay on either side of an artery. The brachial veins are the largest in size, and are situated on either side of the brachial artery. The pulsations of the brachial artery aid in venous return. Veins that are structured in this way are known as vena comitantes. Perforating veins run between the deep and superficial veins of the upper limb, connecting the two systems.

INNERVATION OF THE UPPER EXTREMITY

The motor and sensory supply of the upper limb is provided by the brachial plexus.

Brachial Plexus

The brachial plexus arises from the ventral (anterior) branches of spinal nerves C5-C8 and T1. These anterior branches connect in the following pattern:

1. Anterior branches of C5-C6 form the primary superior trunk.
2. Anterior branch of C7 forms the primary middle trunk.
3. Anterior branches C8 and T1 form primary inferior trunk.

Each primary trunk divides into anterior and posterior divisions:

1. Posterior divisions of the three primary trunks form the posterior cord.
2. Anterior divisions of the superior and middle primary trunks form the lateral cord.
3. Anterior division of primary inferior trunk forms the medial cord.

The upper portion of the brachial plexus (consists of the anterior branches of spinal nerves and the primary trunks) is found in the neck at the supraclavicular region, then it continues posteriorly to the clavicle and the subclavius muscle, reaches the axillary cavity (the cords and first terminal branches), and continues along the arm via terminal branches.

The brachial plexus has collateral and terminal branches:

a. Dorsal collateral branches: dorsal nerve of scapula (levator of scapula and rhomboid muscle), long thoracic nerve (anterior serratus muscle), superior and inferior subscapular nerves (subscapular and teres major muscles) and thoracodorsal nerve (latissimus dorsi)

b. Ventral collateral branches: branches for scalene muscles, subclavian nerve for subclavius muscle, pectoralis minor and major nerves for correspondent muscles and suprascapular nerve (infraspinatus and supraspinatos)

c. Dorsal terminal branches: axillary and radial nerve

d. Ventral terminal branches: ulnar, median, and musculocutaneous nerves and medial cutaneous nerve of arm and forearm

The shoulder is innervated anteroposteriorly by supraclavicular (upper ¾) and intercostobrachial (lower ¼) nerves. The arm is innervated by the lateral and medial cutaneous nerves of the arm, which innervate the anterior lateral and medial part of the arm, respectively. Lateral, medial, and posterior cutaneous nerves innervate the posterior lateral, medial, and middle part of the arm, respectively. The forearm is innervated by the lateral and medial cutaneous nerves of the forearm, which innervate the anterior and posterior lateral and medial sides of the forearm, respectively.

LOWER EXTREMITY ANATOMY

The lower extremity refers to the part of the body from the hip to the toes. The skeleton of the lower extremity consists of femur, tibia, fibula, tarsal and metatarsal bones, and phalanges.

VASCULARIZATION OF LOWER EXTREMITY

The blood circulation through the lower extremities is important to maintain their homeostasis, functionality, viability and vitality. The blood vessels of the lower extremities include arteries that supply oxygenated blood to the lower extremities and veins that drain the deoxygenated blood and remove waste products from the lower extremities.

Arteries

The internal iliac artery gives rise to gluteal superior and inferior arteries that supply the gluteal region, to the internal pudendal artery, and to the obturator artery. The external iliac gives rise to the femoral artery that supplies the lower extremity, which then gives the profunda femoris artery that supplies adductor muscles and the quadriceps femoris muscle and finally the popliteal artery (an extension of the femoral artery) that in return gives rise to the subsequent branches: the articular branches that supply the knee, the anterior tibiale artery that supplies the muscles of the foot/anterior leg, and the posterior tibiale artery that supplies the flexor muscles, the plantar arch of the foot, and the toes

Veins

The veins of the lower extremity are organized in two groups: (1) deep veins, which lie below the deep fascia and accompany the arteries that supply the lower extremity; and (2) superficial veins, which lie in the superficial fascia and are not accompanied by arteries.

Veins called perforating veins pierce the deep fascia and connect the two systems of veins.

INNERVATION OF THE LOWER EXTREMITY

The nerves of lower limb arise from **lumbar** and **sacral** plexuses (most of which are mixed).

Cutaneous nerves can arise directly from the lumbar or sacral plexuses—for example, the ilioinguinal nerve arises directly from the lumbar plexus—or, as cutaneous branches of the **mixed nerves** that arise from the lumbar or sacral plexuses (e.g., the saphenous nerve arises from the femoral nerve), travel into the **subcutaneous tissue** of the limb to innervate the overlying skin.

The **lumbar plexus** is located anterior to the transverse processes of the lumbar spine and consists of spinal roots of L1 to L4, with a contribution from the last thoracic nerve T12. In general, the nerves arising from the lumbar plexus supply the anterior and medial **thigh**. The most important nerves that derive from the lumbar plexus are the **femoral nerve** (L2-L4), and the **obturator nerve** (L2-L4). The **femoral**, **tibial**, and **common fibular** nerves are the major cutaneous nerves of the lower limb that give rise to cutaneous branches.

The **femoral** nerve (L2-L4) is a mixed nerve (i.e., contains sensory and motor fibers), that arises from the **lumbar plexus**. It descends through the psoas major muscle and enters the lower limb on the anterior aspect of the thigh, innervating the anteromedial thigh and the medial leg and foot. The femoral nerve divides into the **anterior cutaneous branches** and the **saphenous nerve**.

1. The **saphenous nerve** (sensory) arises in the femoral triangle and descends down the thigh, via the adductor canal. It exits the canal just before the adductor hiatus, crossing the medial aspect of the knee and passing deep to the **sartorius** tendon. It innervates the medial cutaneous aspect of the leg and foot.

2. The **anterior cutaneous branches** also arise in the femoral triangle. These nerves innervate the skin of the anterior and medial aspects of the thigh.

The **tibial** nerve is one of the terminal branches of the **sciatic nerve**; it arises at the apex of the popliteal fossa and descends down the posterior compartment of the leg to innervate the skin of posterolateral leg, the sole, and the heel. It has several cutaneous branches:

- **Sural nerve**—Formed by branches of the tibial and common fibular nerves. It supplies the skin of the posterolateral leg and the lateral margin of the foot.
- **Medial plantar nerve**—Supplies the skin of the medial sole of the foot, and the plantar aspect, nails, and sides of the medial three and a half toes.
- **Lateral plantar nerve**—Supplies the skin of the lateral sole and the plantar aspect, nails, and sides of the lateral one and a half toes.
- **Calcaneal nerves**—Supplies the skin of the heel.

The **common fibular** nerve is one of the terminal branches of the **sciatic nerve**; it arises at the apex of the popliteal fossa and enters the lateral compartment to innervate the skin of the *anterolateral leg, posterolateral leg*, and the *dorsal surface of the foot*. Its cutaneous branches are:

- **Superficial fibular nerve** (a mixed nerve)—Moves through the lateral compartment of the leg and perforates the deep fascia of the leg. It innervates the skin of the anterolateral leg and dorsum of the foot (apart from the skin between the big and second toes).
- **Deep fibular nerve** (a mixed nerve)—Innervates the web of skin between the big and second toes.
- **Sural nerve**—Formed by branches of the tibial and common fibular nerves. It innervates the skin of the posterolateral leg and the lateral margin of the foot.
- **Lateral sural nerve**—Innervates part of the anterolateral leg.

In addition to the major cutaneous nerves, smaller areas of skin are innervated by minor nerves that arise directly from the lumbar or sacral plexuses.

The Lumbar Plexus

- **Iliohypogastric**—Parallels iliac crest, generally divides into anterior and lateral branches.
- **Ilioinguinal**—Moves through the inguinal canal.
- **Genitofemoral**—Moves down anterior surface of psoas major, where it divides into genital and femoral branches.
- **Lateral cutaneous nerve of thigh**—Passes 2–3 cm medial to anterior superior iliac spine (deep to inguinal ligament).
- **Cutaneous branch of obturator nerve** (via obturator nerve)—Descends between adductors longus and brevis and splits into branches.

From the **sacral plexus** arises the **posterior cutaneous nerve of thigh**, which enters the gluteal region via greater sciatic foramen then passes deep to fascia lata. This plexus is composed of the anastomosis of the anterior branches of first three sacral nerves S1-S3 conjoined to the lumbosacral trunk (formed by the anterior branches of L4-L5). It gives rise to nerves that supply the posterior thigh, leg, and foot. The main branch of the sacral plexus is the **sciatic nerve**. Almost all its branches emerge from the small pelvis.

The **pudendal plexus** is composed of anterior branches of S2-S4, below the sacral plexus. Almost all its branches combine to form the pudendal nerve (terminal branch), which leaves the small pelvis after pairing with the internal pudendal artery, runs through the subpiriform canal of the greater sciatic foramen, passes around the ischial spine, and finally runs through the pudendal canal and supplies the external genitalia and the posterior region of the perineum (ischiorectal fossa).

The **coccygeal plexus** is composed of anterior branches of S4-Coccyx.

BIBLIOGRAPHY

1. Bernards C. Epidural and spinal anesthesia. In: Barash P, et al. *Clinical Anesthesia*. 6th ed. Philadelphia, PA: Lippincott Williams and Wilkins; 2009.
2. Tsui B, Rosenquist R. Peripheral nerve blockade. In: Barash P, et al. *Clinical Anesthesia*. 6th ed. Philadelphia, PA: Lippincott Williams and Wilkins; 2009.
3. Gray's Anatomy of the Human Body. Yahoo Education website. https://education.yahoo.com/reference/gray/. Accessed November 10, 2014.
4. Brown D. Spinal, epidural and caudal anesthesia. In: Miller R. *Miller's Anesthesia*. 7th ed. Philadelphia, PA: Elsevier; 2010.
5. Wedel D, Horlocker T. Nerve blocks. In: Miller R. *Miller's Anesthesia*. 7th ed. Philadelphia, PA: Elsevier; 2010.
6. Gilroy AM, MacPherson BR, Ross LM. *Atlas of Anatomy*. 2nd ed. Stuttgart, Germany: Thieme; 2008.
7. Newfield P, Cottrell J. *Handbook of Neuroanesthesia*. 4th ed. Philadelphia, PA: Lippincott Williams and Wilkins; 2007.
8. Morgan G, Mikhail M, Murray M. *Clinical Anesthesiology*. 4th ed. New York, NY: McGraw Hill; 2005.

FURTHER READING

Collins A, Gray A. Peripheral nerve blocks. In: Miller R, ed. *Basics of Anesthesia*. 6th ed. Philadelphia, PA: Elsevier Saunders; 2011.

Drasner K, Larson M. Spinal and epidural anesthesia. In: Miller R, ed. *Basics of Anesthesia*. 6th ed. Philadelphia, PA: Elsevier Saunders; 2011.

Stackhouse R, Infosino A. Airway management. In: Miller R, ed. *Basics of Anesthesia*, 6th ed. Philadelphia, PA: Elsevier Saunders; 2011.

QUESTIONS

QUESTION 1. When intubating a patient with full stomach during a rapid sequence induction, which structure is pressed in to prevent aspiration?

A. Hyoid bone
B. Thyroid cartilage
C. Cricoid cartilage
D. Trachea

QUESTION 2. Chassaignac's tubercle is located at:

A. The spinous process of C6
B. The spinous process of C7
C. The anterior tubercle of the transverse process of C6
D. The sternoclavicular articulation

QUESTION 3. Which of the following is NOT a border of Sedillot's triangle?

A. The sternal head of sternocleidomastoid
B. The sternal notch
C. The clavicular head of sternocleidomastoid
D. The clavicle

QUESTION 4. The recurrent laryngeal nerve supplies all of the following muscles, EXCEPT:

A. The interarytenoid muscle
B. The lateral cricoarytenoid muscle
C. The posterior cricoarytenoid muscle
D. The cricothyroid muscle

QUESTION 5: Which of the following **MOST** accurately reflects bone marrow physiology?

A. Yellow marrow predominates in younger patients
B. Red marrow is found in the shaft of long bones
C. Red marrow is not found in flat bones
D. Yellow marrow can revert to red marrow
E. Free fatty acids from marrow are protective

QUESTION 6: Which of the following **DOES NOT** accurately reflect anatomical landmarks?

A. C3—Mandible
B. T3—Spine of scapula
C. L1—Aortic bifurcation
D. L3—Subcostal plane
E. S1—Termination of dural sac

ANSWERS

1. C. The cricoid cartilage is the only complete ring-like cartilage at the base of the larynx and forms the uppermost part of the trachea. Applying pressure on the cricoid cartilage will compress the esophagus lying behind the cartilage, thereby preventing any gastric influx from occurring. This procedure is known as the Sellick maneuver.
2. C. Chassaignac's tubercle is the name of the anterior tubercle of the transverse process of the sixth cervical vertebra, against which the carotid artery may be compressed by the finger. Chassaignac's tubercle is also used as landmark for the stellate ganglion nerve block, deep cervical plexus block, and supraclavicular brachial plexus block.
3. B. Sedillot's triangle is formed by the sternal head of sternocleidomastoid, clavicular head of sternocleidomastoid, and clavicle. The apex of the triangle is the position of appropriate cutaneous puncture for anterior approach for the placement of internal jugular venous catheter.
4. D. The recurrent laryngeal nerve supplies all of the intrinsic muscles of the larynx, with the exception of the cricothyroid muscles. Injury to one side of the nerves can paralyze the ipsilateral posterior cricoarytenoid muscle, causing vocal cord dysfunction.
5. D. Yellow marrow predominates in older patients and is found in the shaft of long bones. Red marrow is primarily found in flat bones. Recall that in times of stress or increased demand, bone marrow can convert from yellow to red in order to meet need for RBCs. Free fatty acids released from the bone have deleterious effects and are not protective.
6. C. The aortic bifurcation takes place at L4. The remaining options are correct. Recall that the mandible can correlate with C2 or C3.

2.

RADIOLOGICAL ANATOMY

James W. Jones

INTRODUCTION

Rapid advancements in radiographic technology have enhanced the skillsets of anesthesiologists and improved patient safety. Within the last decade, our ability to diagnose and treat patients has grown alongside advancements in CT, MRI, and ultrasound. Today, there is a growing demand for anesthesiologists to comprehend and utilize these imaging modalities, both as a preoperative predictor of anesthetic complications, and at the bedside to treat. While the use of physical landmarks to guide the placement of central lines and nerve blocks remains an important fundamental of practice, there is a growing demand for anesthesiologists to understand and utilize these newer tools. The expectation of the American Board of Anesthesiology is that every new trainee be competent in his or her ability to read and understand chest radiographs, evaluate CT and MRI for specific disease states, and utilize ultrasound for all invasive procedures including central venous lines and the placement of neuraxial and regional nerve blocks. These fundamentals and their practice is now the standard of care. The goal of this chapter is to review the various radiologic modalities, with specific emphasis on the anatomic and pathologic information pertinent to the practice of anesthesia.

CHEST RADIOGRAPH

The chest radiograph (CXR) is the most commonly encountered source of radiographic information. Although the American Society of Anesthesiology does not recommend routine preoperative CXRs for healthy patients, the CXR is an invaluable diagnostic tool for those with preoperative indicators of cardiopulmonary disease. The CXR is a projection radiograph used to identify bony and soft tissue pathology of the chest. There are three basic forms of the CXR based on the projection of the x-ray beam. For ambulatory patients, the posteroanterior, or PA, radiograph is the standard and preferred view, produced by projecting an x-ray beam through the patient's back toward a film plate immediately anterior to the chest. This type of projection produces a higher quality image and more accurately represents the size of the heart secondary to its close proximation to the exposed plate[1] (see Figure 2.1a). For hospitalized patients, specifically for those who are bedridden, the anteroposterior, or AP, radiograph is generally obtained (see Figure 2.1b). The AP film can also be acquired in the supine or upright position based on which disease process is being evaluated. Supine films are generally adequate for evaluation of most bony and pulmonary abnormalities, for example rib fractures and parenchymal lung diseases, as well as for the identification and positioning of implanted medical devices. Supine films, however, are inferior to upright films for the evaluation of disease processes where the pooling of air or fluid is required. When evaluating for pneumothorax, pneumoperitoneum, or pleural effusions, the upright radiograph is preferred.

A common approach for reading a CXR is via the ABCDEFGHI mnemonic:

- Assessment of quality
- Bones and Soft Tissues
- Cardiac
- Diaphragm
- Effusions
- Fields and Fissures
- Great Vessels
- Hila and Mediastinum
- Impression

ASSESSMENT OF A CHEST RADIOGRAPH

A proper assessment of a CXR first requires identifying the patient, date, type of film (AP, PA, portable, supine,

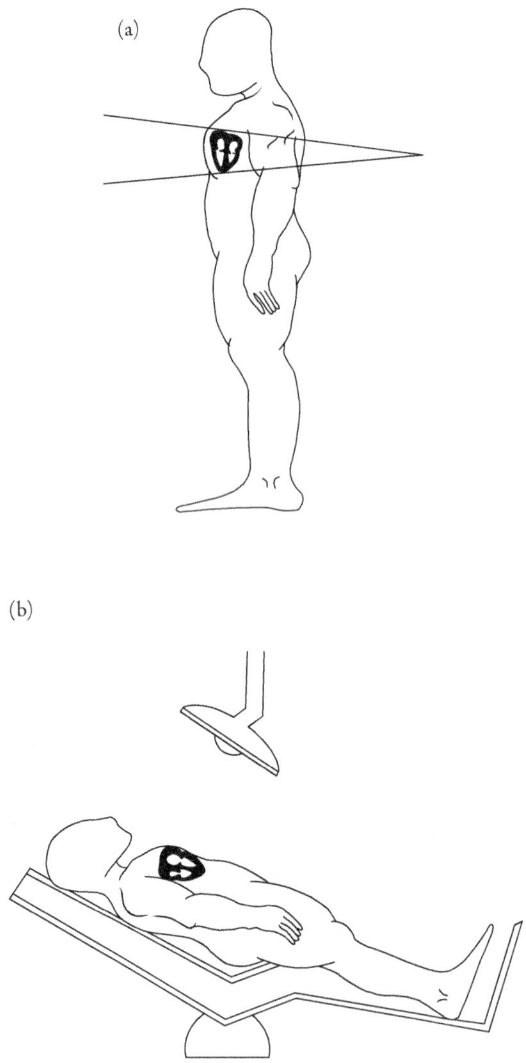

Figure 2.1 Patient positioning in an AP vs. PA film. A PA film is more commonly acquired on an outpatient basis, whereas an AP film is more commonly acquired on patients who are in bed (i.e., the ICU).

upright), and orientation (anatomical position and rotation). Although computerized representations have supplanted traditional film and lightbox stations, orientation errors still occur, and the interpreter must ensure the image is displayed in the proper anatomical position. Second, the interpreter must note the quality of the exposure, which is a fixed, inalterable quality of the radiograph determined at the time the film is produced. Newer software may compensate for improper exposure, however it cannot create uncaptured detail. Proper exposure requires that x-rays properly penetrate the soft and bony tissues in order to provide contrasting details on the negative. Overexposed radiographs tend to appear very dark, whereas underexposed radiographs tend to appear too white. Both extremes, however, lose critical details required to facilitate an appropriate diagnosis. A properly exposed film should demarcate both distinct spinal disc spaces and bronchovascular structures within the borders of the heart (Figure 2.2a); improper exposure makes interpretation difficult, regardless of the examiner (Figure 2.2b).

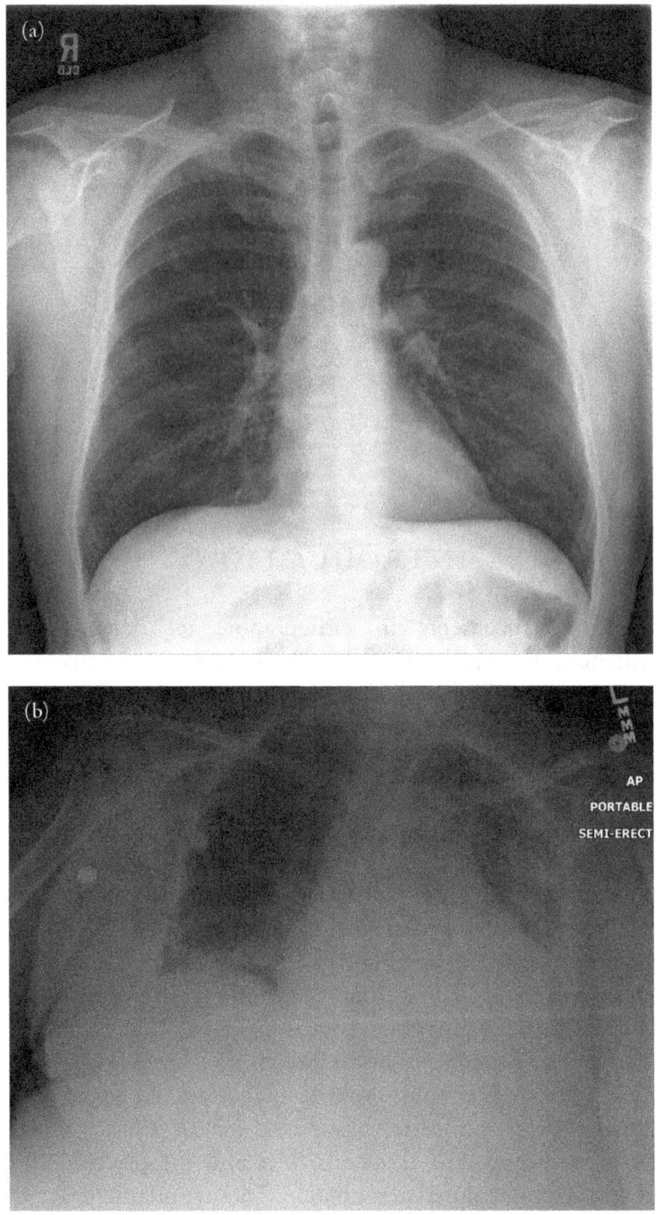

Figure 2.2 (A) Upright PA CXR. (B) Supine AP CXR.

The film should also demonstrate proper rotation and inspiration of the patient. X-rays should precisely follow the AP plane of axis in a properly rotated film, positioning thoracic spinous processes directly between the medial borders of the clavicles. Spinous processes closer to the right clavicle signify a patient that is "rotated left," whereas spinous processes closer to the left clavicle signify a patient "rotated right." Failure to properly note the rotation will lead to an inaccurate interpretation of cardiac size and tracheal position (Figure 2.3). Determining the inspiratory level of the film is also important. Cooperative patients are asked to inspire and hold their breath during exposure. A proper inspiratory film should demonstrate the anterior portion of the sixth or seventh rib passing through the midclavicular

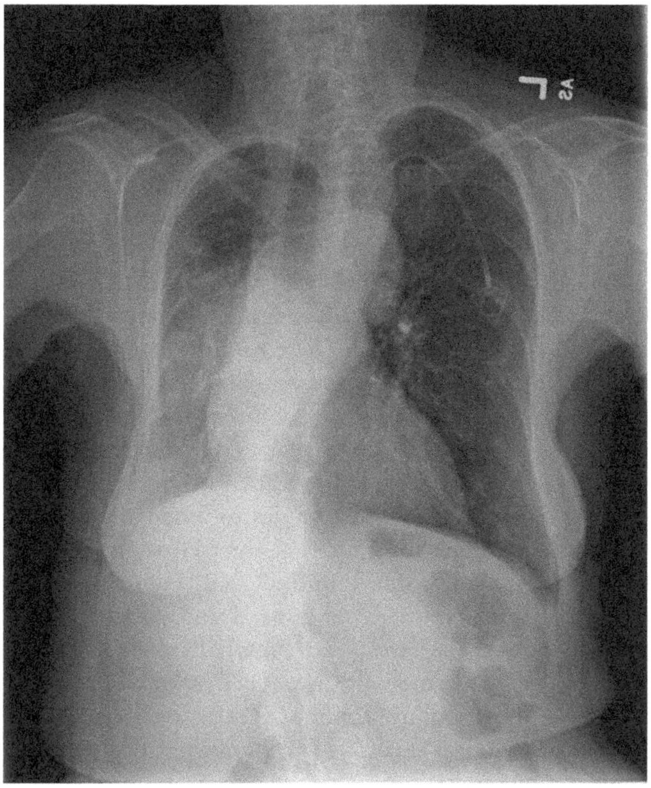

Figure 2.3 CXR showing left or right rotation with false deviation and COPD.

line of each hemidiaphragm. Both the intersection of the diaphragm by a superior rib (≤4) and an inferior rib (≥8) represents hypoinflation and hyperinflation respectively, and may signify disease.

Tracheal deviation is an important finding for the anesthesiologist, signifying a mass effect within the neck and chest. Cancers, postsurgical hematomas, and goiters can all compress the trachea, resulting in airway compromise that may predict a difficult intubation. Deviations of the trachea

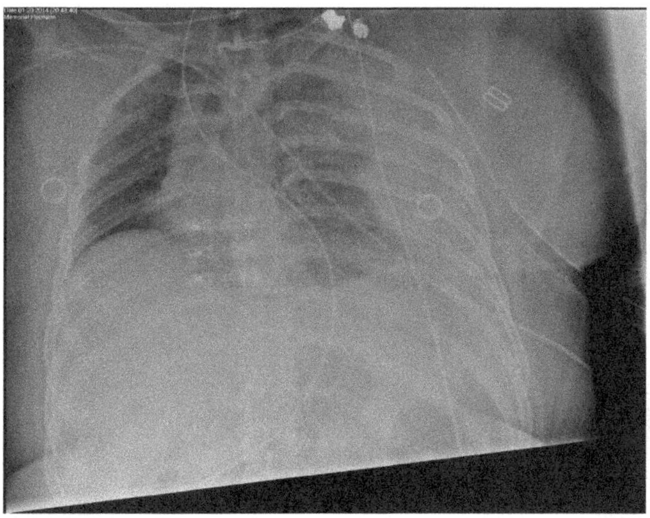

Figure 2.4 A and B. CXR with tracheal deviation due to hemothorax (push).

may also point to the presence of a pneumothorax or consolidation of lung tissue. A tension pneumothorax tends to push the trachea in the opposite direction (Figure 2.4), whereas atelectasis or lobar collapse tends to pull the trachea toward it (Figure 2.5a and b).

Cardiac size is best estimated on a PA film due to less distortion of the lateral heart borders. A relative width greater than 50% of the surrounding thoracic cavity signifies cardiomegaly for PA views only (Figure 2.6). For the more commonly acquired AP films of supine patients, the cardiac borders can be falsely widened and cardiomegaly cannot be diagnosed. A heart width less than 50% on an AP projection however, can rule out cardiomegaly.

A normal diaphragm appears slightly elevated on the right compared with the left secondary to the liver, and

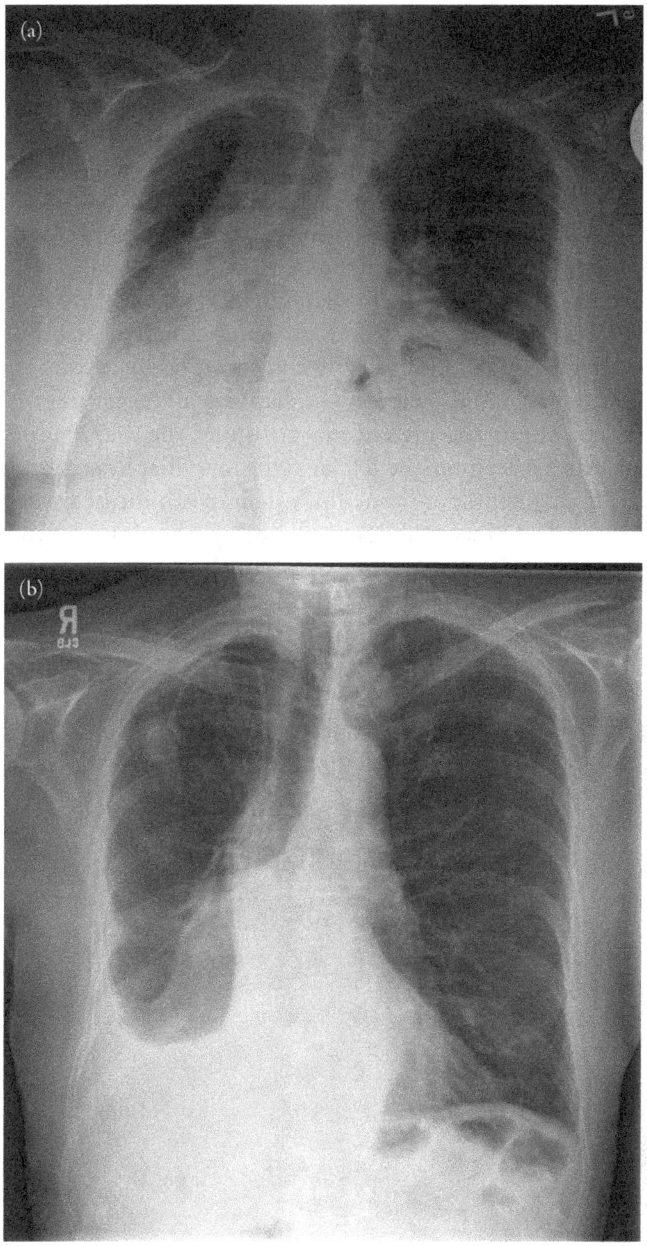

Figure 2.5 CXR with tracheal deviation due to lung collapse (pull).

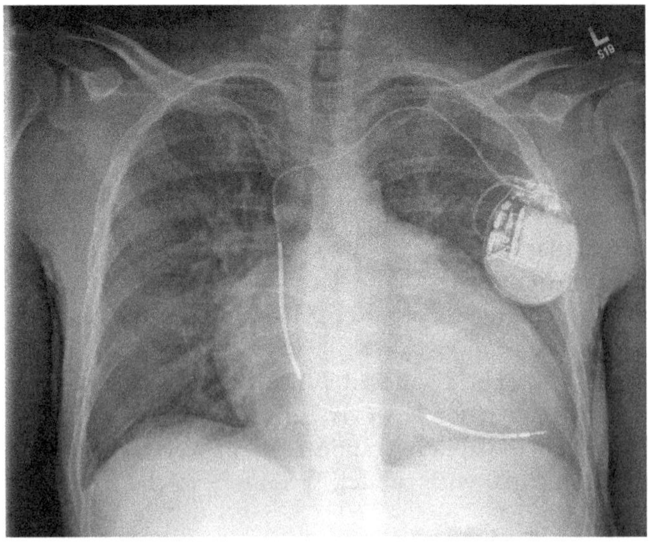

Figure 2.6 PA CXR showing cardiomegaly

deviations from this are pathological clues. An elevated hemidiaphragm (Figure 2.7) can indicate pathology above, within, or below the diaphragm. Contraction of a lung may falsely elevate the diaphragm on that side. Phrenic nerve paralysis, secondary to either cancer or a previously placed nerve block (interscaline block) will produce an elevated hemidiaphragm on the ipsilateral side, and may complicate the patient's ability to breathe. Intraabdominal conditions such as abscesses, hematomas, and tumors may also elevate the diaphragm. A very important finding is the presence of air under the diaphragm. This can be seen on the left or right hemidiaphragm and signifies a pneumoperitoneum, which may indicate bowel perforation or recent abdominal surgery. The air under the left hemidiaphragm must be distinguished from a normal gastric bubble by the demarcation of tissue planes. A large gastric bubble may result from prolonged mask ventilation or bowel obstruction. This information can assist in the decision to perform a rapid sequence intubation, or suggest the need for a nasogastric tube.

Localized consolidation of parenchymal lung tissue on CXR may signify pneumonia, pulmonary hemorrhage, or partial collapse secondary to mucus plugging. It is important to locate the denser, whiter areas that follow the characteristic lobar shape of the lung and note the less dense, darker bronchi that travel within. This relatively dense area of lung tissue with maintained patent bronchi is termed a "bronchogram." These findings may indicate a need for infection workup or bronchoscopy, and can herald episodes of desaturation under anesthesia secondary to the loss of functional residual capacity. Pleural effusions, in comparison, are best seen on upright CXRs and range from blunting of the costophrenic angles to broader, smoother opacification of the lung fields. Larger effusions tend to appear as a graded haziness on the CXR (Figure 2.8). The pooling of fluid between the visceral and parietal pleura appears whiter at the bases, which gradually darkens toward the apex. Bilateral effusions on CXR may be the systemic effect of left heart failure, volume overload, or liver and kidney disease, whereas unilateral effusions may denote carcinoma or previous lung surgery.

The fields and fissures also provide valuable information. A common and very serious complication of trauma or central line placement is a pneumothorax (Figure 2.9). The accumulation of air within the chest cavity will often collect at the highest point, therefore, supine films may miss a small or moderate pneumothorax as the air pools anteriorly over the lung field. On an upright film, however, one should note a smooth area, devoid of bronchovascular structures between the outer lung border

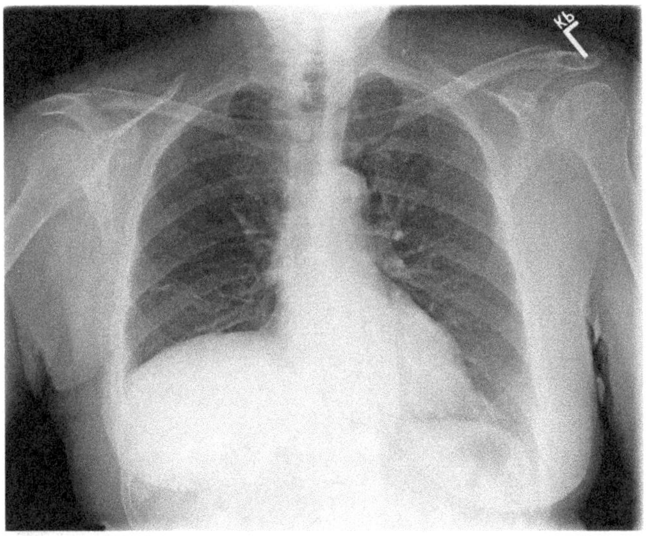

Figure 2.7 CXR showing elevated hemidiaphragm.

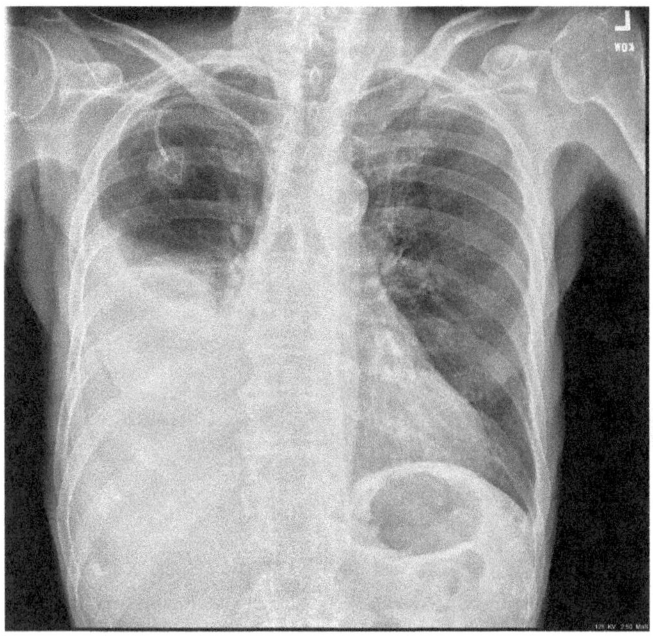

Figure 2.8 CXR showing pleural effusions with graded haziness.

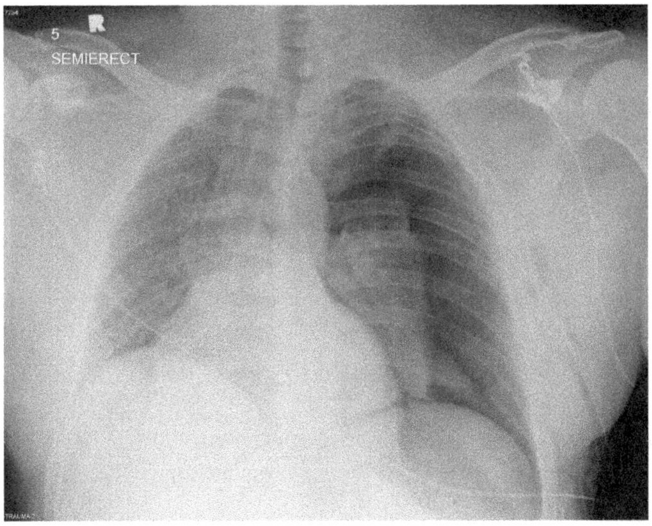

Figure 2.9 CXR pneumothorax.

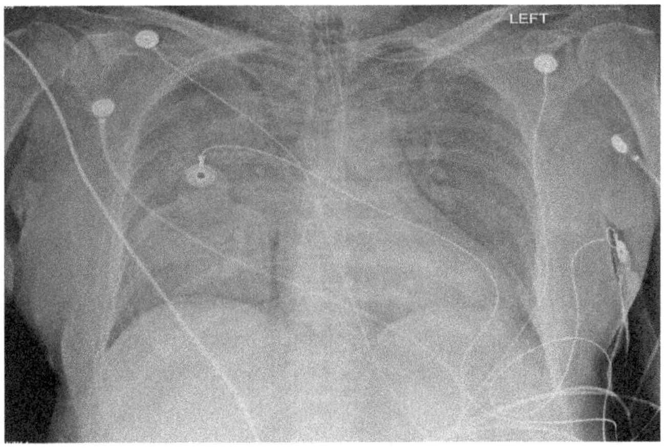

Figure 2.11 CXR acute respiratory distress syndrome (ARDS).

and the internal chest wall. Many times a pneumothorax may appear as a small sliver above the apex, however this collection may expand over subsequent hours possibly leading to cardiovascular compromise. The anesthesiologist must recognize and monitor this complication, and weigh the therapeutic benefits of chest tube placement. As an aside, a thickened pleura in the area of reduced lung volume that is not affected by gravity may represent an empyema.

More commonly, evaluation of CXR in the preoperative area will provide clues to the presence of chronic pulmonary disease. Hyperinflated lungs with flattening of the diaphragm are characteristic of chronic obstructive pulmonary disease, including emphysema (Figure 2.10) and acute respiratory distress syndrome (ARDS) (Figure 2.11). The presence of bullae may also be seen as rounded areas of hypodense lung. Opacifications or densities spread evenly throughout the lung fields may indicate either metastatic disease, or, based on the patient's clinical condition, parenchymal lung edema or the presence of acute respiratory distress syndrome. These findings will help to guide proper ventilatory management in the operating room and the post anesthesia care unit.

The area of the hilum, which contains the pulmonary vessels, bronchi, and lymph nodes should be inspected. Bilateral enlargement and opacification of the hilum may indicate sarcoidosis, pulmonary hypertension or lymphoma, whereas unilateral change may indicate carcinoma. Change in position of the hilum may also indicate a push or pulling effect of the surrounding lung tissue; a tension pneumothorax may push the hilum away from midline, whereas radiation fibrosis may pull it toward the affected side. In addition to assessment of the hilum, estimation of the width of the mediastinum provides clues to potentially life-threatening conditions, most importantly, a dissecting thoracic aortic aneurism (Figure 2.12). The mediastinum may be falsely enlarged on

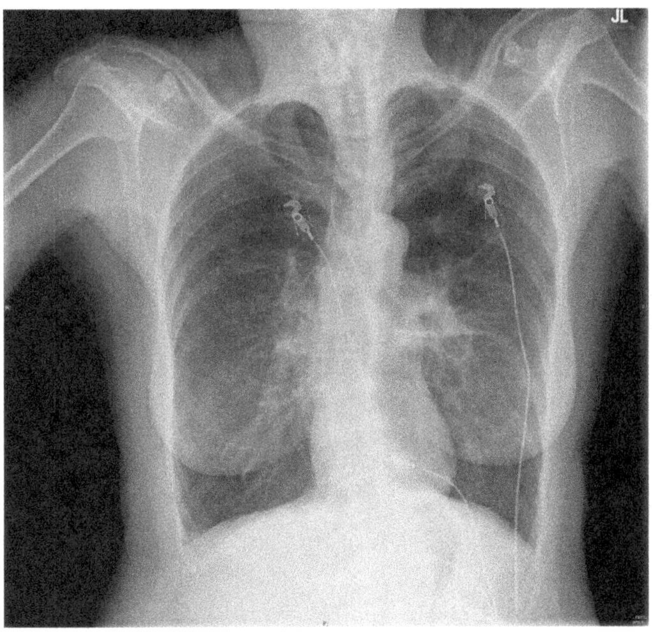

Figure 2.10 CXR emphysema.

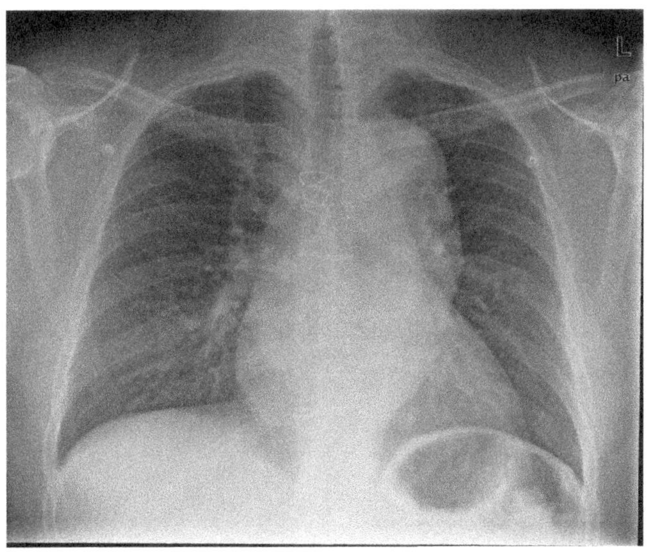

Figure 2.12 CXR dissecting thoracic aortic aneurism.

AP views, therefore follow-up studies should be obtained based on the patient's clinical condition (see Figure 2.1).

APPEARANCE OF DEVICES ON CHEST RADIOGRAPH

Finally, the anesthesiologist must be familiar with the plethora of devices and their characteristic appearance on CXR, providing an enormous amount of information regarding the patient's prior history and current disposition. The most common device evaluated by the anesthesiologist is the endotracheal tube and its position. The tube, with its characteristic Murphy's eye at the tip, should be noted running inferiorly within the trachea. The ideal position of the tube is halfway between the level of the carina and the clavicles, or commonly, 4 centimeters above the carina in adults. An endotracheal tube displaced inferiorly may enter one of the main bronchi, leading to lung collapse on the contralateral side. This tube should be retracted to its ideal position. In contrast, a tube ending at the level of the clavicles may need advancement or may already be dislodged. Overinflated cuffs can also be seen as outwardly compressing the mucosal walls of the trachea.

Vascular access lines come in many shapes and sizes and the anesthesiologist must identify these and ensure their proper positioning. All upper extremity lines that deliver medications and fluids, entering from either the internal jugular or subclavian veins should terminate in the lower superior vena cava outside the right atrium and above the pericardial reflection (Figure 2.13).[2] The pericardial reflection correlates well with the level of the carina, which is generally accepted as the ideal tip depth in adults. Introducers, on the other hand, appear larger and may terminate higher in the superior vena cava, whereas pulmonary artery catheters follow a course through the right atrium and ventricle to terminate in the pulmonary artery. The pulmonary artery catheter should be properly advanced to curl slightly at the tip with a terminal distance no further than one-third the width of the ipsilateral lung field (Figure 2.14). A pulmonary artery catheter crossing over itself on CXR is likely advanced too far and needs to be retracted.

Anesthesiologists should familiarize themselves with the numerous and variable appearance of implantable devices on CXR. Nasogastric and orogastric tubes may coil within the esophagus or appropriately terminate below the diaphragm. Chest tubes commonly enter laterally above the diaphragm and terminate in the apex (Figure 2.15). Mechanical cardiac valves are located in their respective

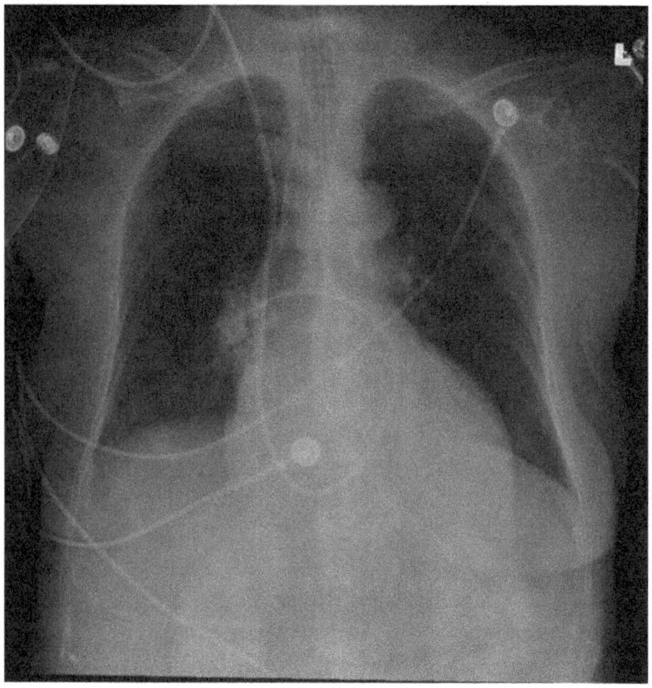

Figure 2.14 CXR of PA catheter.

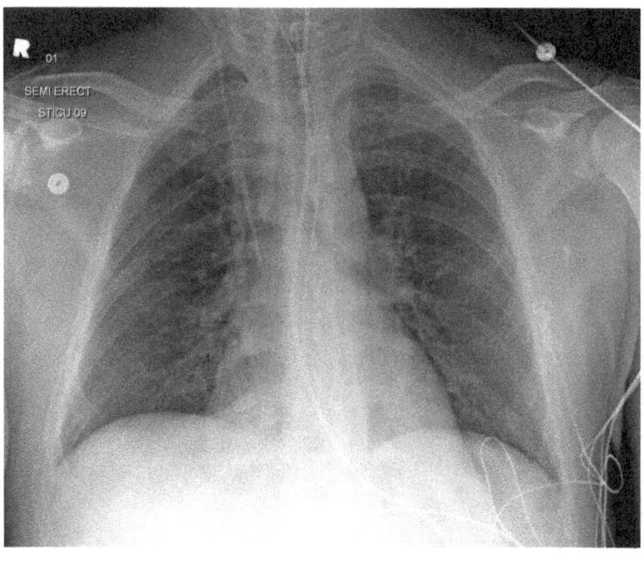

Figure 2.13 CXR of CVC at proper depth.

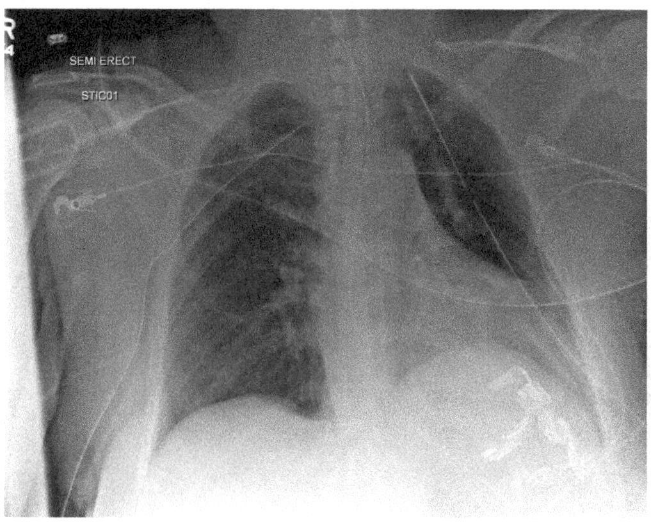

Figure 2.15 CXR with bilateral chest tubes.

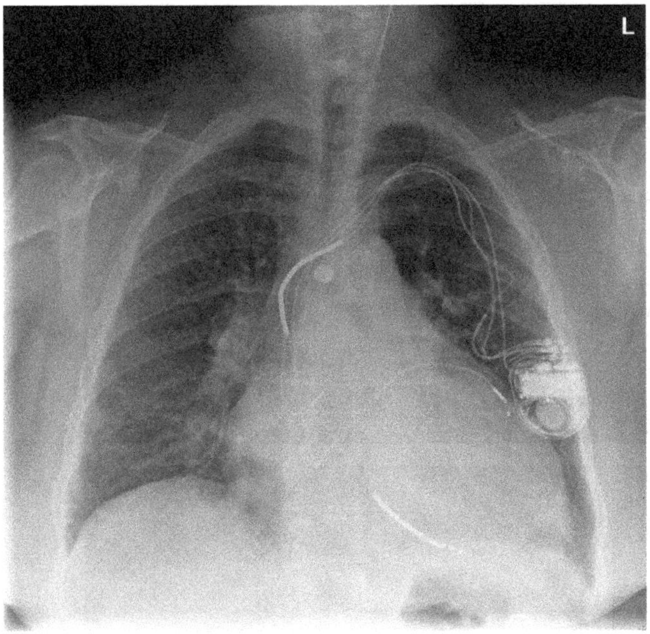

Figure 2.16 CXR permanent pacemaker (PPM)/automatic implantable cardioverter defibrillator (AICD).

anatomical positions. Sternal wires may point to prior open chest procedures such as coronary artery bypass grafting and valve repair. Pacemaker generators typically appear in the upper left chest and may give off single or multiple leads terminating in the atrium, right ventricle, or through the coronary sinus into the left ventricle (biventricular) (Figure 2.16). Some pacemakers may have lead coils and a generator typical of implantable cardioverter defibrillators. Most implantable devices are radiopaque to help identify their position, information that is critically important to developing and carrying out a safe and effective anesthetic plan.

CHEST (CT AND MRI)

The widespread use of computed tomography (CT) and magnetic resonance imaging (MRI) as a first-line diagnostic tool is increasing.[3] Whereas the CXR provides a two-dimensional view of the chest, CT and MRI eliminates the superimposition of structures at the area of interest, and offers greater detailed information to help guide appropriate care.[1] The expectation from the American Board of Anesthesiology is that practitioners be familiar with CT and MRI representations of anatomical structures and their relative locations, especially in regard to issues involving the airway, pulmonary, and cardiac status of the patient, as well as structures pertinent to the safe placement of neuraxial catheters and regional blocks. References to CT scans in this section will imply the more commonly used x-ray based CT (as compared to perfusion, etc.), but for MRI, the anesthesiologist must distinguish between T1 and T2 weighted images. T1 and T2 weighting, a measurement of how protons return to equilibrium over time, displays water differently; water appears black on T1 and white on T2. In general, T1 weighted MRI is most useful for contrasting adjacent tissue such as gray and white matter of the brain, whereas T2 images present abnormal fluid collections, such as abscesses and effusions, as bright white against the darker surrounding tissue. The remainder of this section is dedicated to exploring the anatomic structures and pathologies most pertinent to the practice of anesthesia as seen on CT and MRI.

A basic understanding of normal anatomy and its abnormal variants is important to predicting anesthetic complications (see Figure 2.17a–c for examples of normal chest CT with contrast images). Air on CT appears black. The path and patency of the trachea can therefore be assessed, and proper placement of an endotracheal tube confirmed. It is important to rule out "mainstemming" of the endotracheal tube into the right (and less commonly the left) mainstem. In addition, knowing a patient's bronchial anatomy prior to placement of a double lumen tube or bronchial blocker can greatly enhance success. Parenchymal lung diseases are also well defined on CT, revealing areas of atelectasis, pneumonia, and blebs. A pneumothorax has the characteristic appearance of a smooth black void surrounding a compressed lung, which may, in turn, deviate the trachea to the opposing side. Effusions, however, are homogenous gray, and frequently pool into the posterior portions of the thorax. Traditionally, CTs can help evaluate suspected effusions amenable to drainage for size and location. The size of the heart and its border should also be inspected. Always note the pathological presence of fluid within the pericardial sac, a finding that may suggest tamponade. Vascular structures surrounding the heart also give clues to proper placement of central lines and chest tubes.

BRAIN (CT AND MRI)

Many patients coming to the hospital following trauma or stroke will have a brain CT (Figure 2.18). Evaluating the CT for any midline shift suggestive of either brain edema or compressive hematoma is a must. The parenchyma and ventricles should always be symmetrical and any appearance of blood will appear white.[4] The ventricles also tend to grow smaller and may obliterate with severe increases in intracranial pressure, suggesting a benefit to emergent hyperventilation, mannitol, or hypertonic saline. Signs of increased intracranial pressure may also contraindicate any lumbar puncture, including spinal anesthetics. The skull and facial bones must also be evaluated for the presence of fractures and bleeding—potentially important contraindications to implantable devices such as nasogastric tubes.

Evaluation of the CT also provides clues to the need for maintaining inline stabilization of the cervical, thoracic, and lumbar spine, which can complicate intubation and

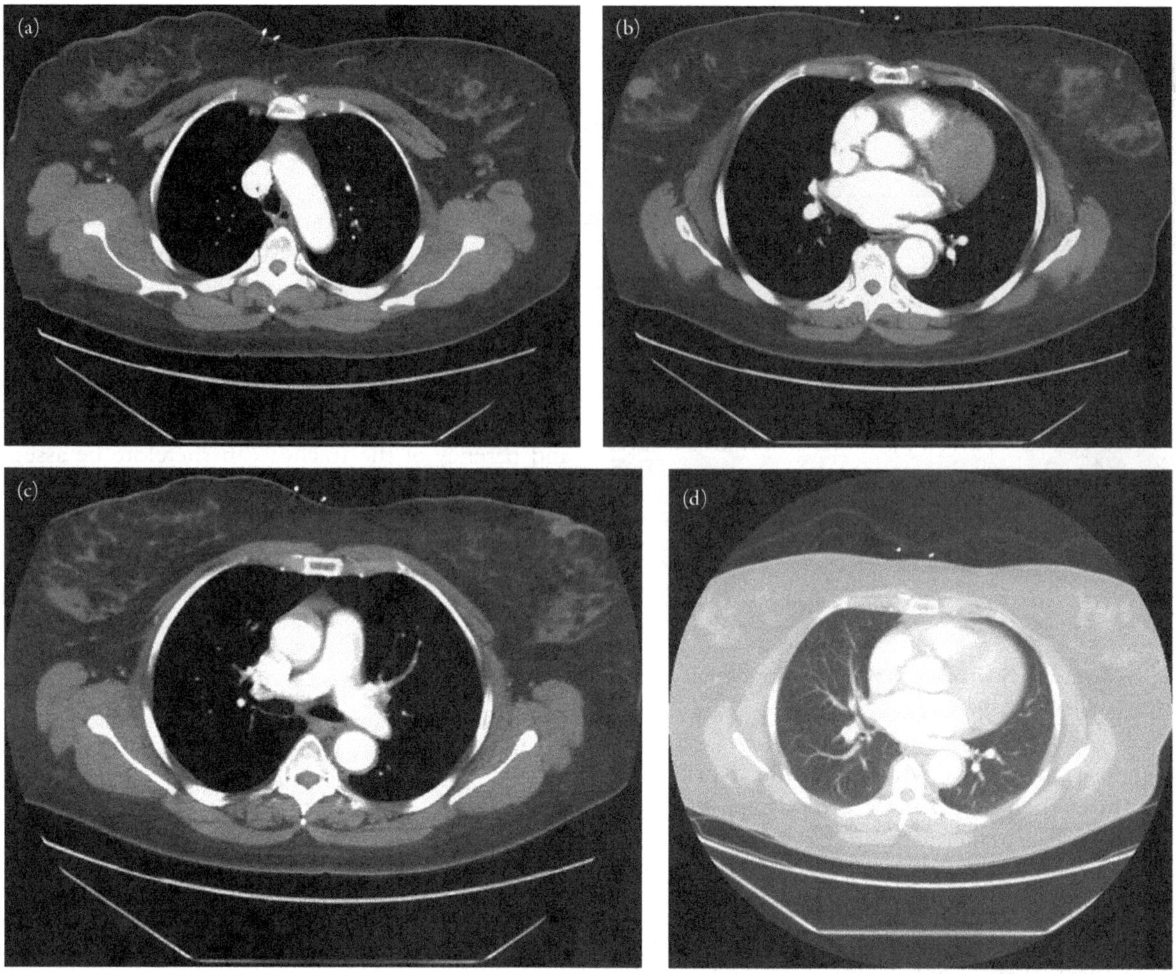

Figure 2.17 CT of the chest showing normal anatomy.

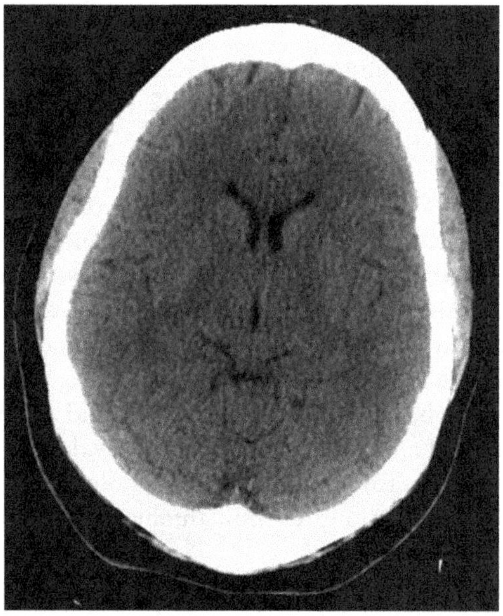

Figure 2.18 CT of normal brain.

body positioning. While only a radiologist and a thorough physical exam can exclude disease, visible cervical spine subluxation (Figure 2.19), especially atlantoaxial subluxation, are important indicators of the need to maintain stabilization in the neutral position during intubation.

An MRI of the brain takes longer and is rarely obtained in emergent situations. An MRI is superior for evaluating less detectable brain pathologies that may be obscured by the skull on head CT. Cerebrospinal fluid (CSF), blood, edema, and infarction will appear dark on T1 weighted images (Figure 2.20) and white on T2 weighted images (Figure 2.21).

For the anesthesiologist, MRI evaluation of the thoracic and lumbar spine is the gold standard for diagnosing epidural hematoma, a complication of spinal and epidural catheter placement and a true medical emergency. The classic presentation is a painful nonradiating back pain that progresses to lower extremity motor weakness with bowel and bladder dysfunction. Any patient with signs of spinal cord compression either during or following catheter placement or removal should be evaluated for epidural hematoma by MRI with the involvement of a neurosurgeon.

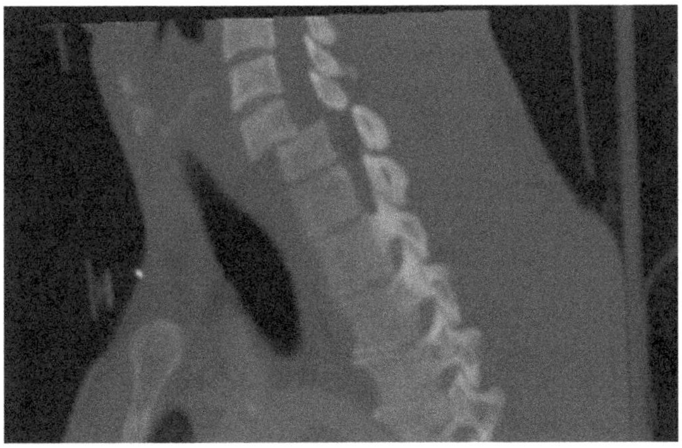

Figure 2.19 CT of Cervical Spine showing subluxation.

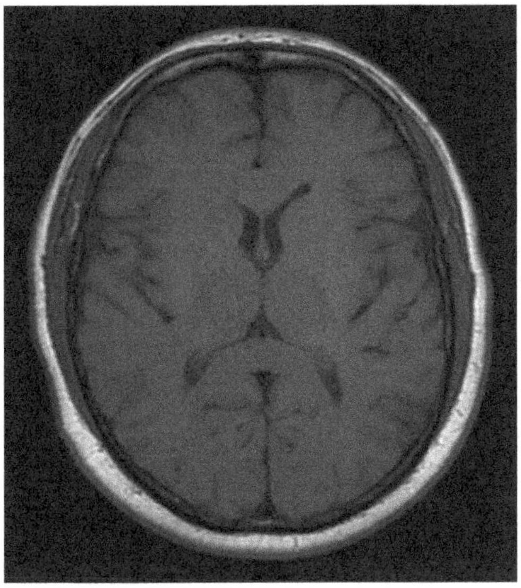

Figure 2.20 MRI T1 normal brain.

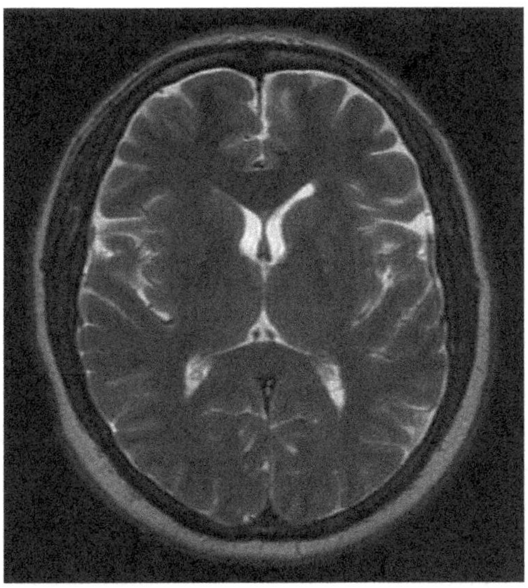

Figure 2.21 MRI T2 normal brain.

NECK (ULTRASOUND FOR CENTRAL VENOUS CATHETER)

Ultrasound is the most recent and clinically significant advancement in the practice of anesthesiology. Within the last decade, the use of bedside ultrasound imaging has drastically improved quality of care and reduced complications from the placement of central lines and regional anesthetic blocks. Before the mainstream availability of ultrasound, anesthesiologists relied on physical landmarks for the placement of internal jugular and femoral vein catheters. Certain access points in dangerous proximity to vital structures were considered too risky to target routinely. Through the development of ultrasound guided techniques, anesthesiologists not only are able to reduce the risk of pneumothorax and intraarterial catheterization for central line placement but also are now able to safely perform supra- and infraclavicular nerve blocks and catheter placements.[5] As such, in many centers ultrasound-assisted line insertion is considered standard of care.[6] Anesthesiologists tend to maintain access to the patient's head during surgery, therefore the internal jugular vein continues to remain the most common site for obtaining central vein access. Before ultrasound, the relative distance of the internal jugular vein from the lung was inherently protective against causing a pneumothorax. The use of ultrasound, however, is thought to have reduced this complication further by resolving the larger, thinner walled vein from the smaller, thicker walled carotid artery.

While access of the femoral vein has increased risk of catheter line infection, its placement is considered relatively safe especially in emergent situations. Ultrasound guidance can enhance this placement by reducing unintentional needle injuries to the femoral artery and nerve.

The ultrasonic view of the subclavian vein is impeded by the overlying clavicle, and the use of landmarks to guide placement remains the most commonly used approach.

REFERENCES

1. Morris A, Kanne J, Stern E. Imaging of the chest. In: Vincent JL, et al. *Textbook of Critical Care*. 6th ed. Philadelphia, PA: Elsevier Saunders; 2011:378–387.
2. Hill JR, Horner PE, Primack SL. ICU imaging. *Clin Chest Med*. 2008;29(1):59–76, vi.
3. Rubinowitz AN, Siegel MD, Tocino I. Thoracic imaging in the ICU. *Crit Care Clin*. 2007;23(3):539–573.
4. Broder JS. Head computed tomography interpretation in trauma: a primer. *Psychiatr Clin North Am*. 2010;33(4):821–854.
5. Gardelli G, Feletti F, Nanni A, Mughetti M, Piraccini A, Zompatori M. Chest ultrasonography in the ICU. *Respir Care*. 2012;57(5):773–781.
6. Lennon M, Zaw NN, Pöpping DM, Wenk M. Procedural complications of central venous catheter insertion. *Minerva Anestesiol*. 2012;78(11):1234–1240.

FURTHER READING

Broder JS. Head computed tomography interpretation in trauma: a primer. *Psychiatr Clin North Am.* 2010;33(4):821–854.

Hill JR, Horner PE, Primack SL. ICU imaging. *Clin Chest Med.* 2008;29(1):59–76, vi.

Morris A, Kanne J, Stern E. Imaging of the chest. In: Vincent JL, et al. *Textbook of Critical Care.* 6th ed. Philadelphia, PA: Elsevier Saunders; 2011:378–387.

QUESTIONS

1. A right internal jugular central line was placed following induction for a Whipple procedure. In PACU, the patient shows signs of respiratory distress. SpO2 is 88% and the respiratory rate is 32. Auscultation of the lung fields reveals reduced breath sounds over the right lung. Which of the following BEST describes what a stat chest x-ray would most likely show:
   A. A right-sided pleural effusion
   B. Tracheal deviation to the right
   C. A right tension pneumothorax
   D. Hematoma in the neck

2. When visualizing the neck under ultrasound, the most likely effect of Trendelenberg (head down) positioning during central line placement is:
   A. Improved identification of the carotid artery
   B. Improved identification of the lung pleura
   C. Increased size of the internal jugular vein
   D. Improved needle visualization

3. In a patient with suspected cardiomegaly, the best CXR projection for proper diagnosis is:
   A. Supine anteroposterior (AP)
   B. Lateral decubitus
   C. Upright anteroposterior (AP)
   D. Upright posteroanterior (PA)

4. Despite adequate sedation, an intubated patient is noted to be "bucking" the ventilator excessively. The MOST likely explanation on CXR is:
   A. Mucus plugging with atelectasis of the right upper lobe
   B. Pneumoperitoneum with elevated left hemidiaphragm
   C. An endotracheal tube tip at the level of the carina
   D. Bilateral hypoinflated lungs

5. An obese patient is scheduled for an exploratory laparotomy for an incarcerated hernia with small bowel obstruction. The patient last ate 3 hours ago, and an abdominal x-ray reveals a large quantity of fluid in the stomach. The MOST appropriate management by the anesthesiologist would be:
   A. Delay the case for a total of 8 hours from the last meal
   B. Insert a nasogastric tube and suction the stomach prior to anesthetic induction
   C. Urgently transport the patient to the OR and induce, utilizing a modified rapid sequence technique
   D. Administer preoperative metoclopramide to enhance gastric emptying

6. Twelve hours after a difficult lumbar epidural placement for a radical prostatectomy, a patient reports severe lower back pain with slight weakness of the lower extremities. An epidural hematoma is suspected. The FIRST radiologic exam for evaluation should be:
   A. Contrast enhanced lumbar CT
   B. Noncontrast lumbar CT
   C. Lumbar MRI
   D. Ultrasound of the posterior lumbar spine

7. Following induction of anesthesia for a laparoscopic cholecystectomy, a 24-year-old patient vomits and aspirates approximately 50 mL of clear gastric fluid in the supine position. The patient is intubated, suctioned, and taken immediately to the surgical ICU. The patient is soon extubated and maintains good oxygenation on room air, however is tachypneic and febrile on day 3. The MOST likely finding on CXR would be:
   A. Diffuse patchy infiltrates throughout both lung fields
   B. Atelectasis of the bilateral lower lobes
   C. Infiltrates of the right upper lobe
   D. Empyema of the right lower lung

8. The use of ultrasound for placement of internal jugular central venous catheters is indicated for:
   A. Obese patients with poor landmarks
   B. Hypovolemic patients
   C. Anticoagulated patients
   D. All patients

9. During placement of a right femoral artery line, the screen on the ultrasound machine reveals the femoral vein to be on the right side of the artery. The MOST likely explanation for this finding is:
   A. Aberrant anatomy of the patient
   B. Incorrect orientation of the ultrasound probe
   C. This is its proper anatomical position
   D. Previous vascular surgery

ANSWERS

1. C. The patient has just had a procedure with known risk for causing a pneumothorax, namely the central line insertion. The drop in saturation is indicative of a pneumothorax. Usage of ultrasound does not preclude the occurrence of a pneumothorax but arguably reduces the risk of a pneumothorax. A right-sided effusion is certainly possible, but it is not the likely cause of the rapidly progressed presentation described and therefore is not the

best choice. If there were a tension pneumothorax, the tracheal deviation would be away from the side of the pneumothorax, not toward it. Furthermore, while tracheal deviation may seem like an equally appropriate choice as tension pneumothorax, recall that tracheal deviation may occur under many circumstances (mass, hematoma, radiation therapy) and does not necessarily correlate with loss of breath sounds on the affected side. A neck hematoma would not explain the reduced breath sounds on the right. Tension pneumothorax is the best answer.

2. C. Increased size of the internal jugular vein is the most likely effect of Trendelenberg positioning. The carotid artery, lung pleura, and needle visualization are not primarily affected by positioning changes. It should be noted that the primary reason for Trendelenberg during central line placement is not venous engorgement but reduced risk of an air embolism traveling to the head. When a 14-gauge needle is in the vein and exposed to air, inspiration from the patient may result in air entrainment of up to 100 mL/sec.
3. D. Recall that AP films (commonly used in the ICU population) tend to overestimate the size of the heart. Therefore an upright PA film is best for determining the presence of cardiomegaly. A lateral decubitus film is not useful for assessing cardiomegaly, but is more helpful in determining posterior lung field status.
4. C. Mucous plugging does not generally result in "bucking" (patient-ventilator dysynchrony), but more likely results in increased airway pressures detected by the ventilator. Pneumoperitoneum would globally increase peak and plateau airway pressures. In patients with hypoinflated lungs from inadequate ventilation, one may expect to see increased patient effort or tachypnea on the ventilator, but not necessarily increased "bucking." Carinal contact is a powerful noxious stimulus and therefore is a common cause of "bucking."
5. B. An incarcerated hernia is an emergent surgical case, as the bowel viability may be lost. Furthermore, waiting for 8 hours cannot be expected to result in reduction of gastric volume in a patient with bowel obstruction and incarceration. Therefore, insertion of an NGT should be initiated by the anesthesiologist if not already done by the surgeon. The stomach produces 1.5–2 liters or more of secretions per day; definitive decompression of the stomach is needed. This case has indications for a full rapid sequence intubation given the full stomach found on CXR. Metoclopramide is useful for facilitating gastric emptying, but cannot be expected to be efficacious in the setting of a bowel obstruction.
6. C. When a lumbar epidural hematoma is suspected, an MRI is the most definitive way to assess the spinal cord. Contrast versus nonconstrast CT scans of the spine are useful for locating malignancies or bony lesions, but not ideal for assessing the integrity of the spinal cord. Ultrasound of the spine has been studied for the purposes of catheter placement but is not reliable for diagnosis of epidural hematoma.
7. C. The right upper lobe takeoff has a directly posterior direction and is the likely location for fluid aspiration in the supine position. This is the most likely area affected to be found on chest x-ray, and this would correlate with having a pneumonia (clinical findings as described). Diffuse patchy lesions would be consistent with ARDS, however, ARDS patients normally cannot be weaned off of the ventilator until their clinical course improves following several days. While atelectasis could be found on this chest x-ray, the clinical picture is more consistent with mild pneumonia (fever, hypoxemia). An empyema is a thoracic abscess and would generally result in a systemic inflammatory response syndrome (SIRS) response. In this case, there is not a mechanism mentioned that would explain an intrathoracic abscess.
8. D. While this answer may be considered controversial at the time of book publication, the use of ultrasound is becoming more accepted as standard of care, and should be utilized whenever available considering the wide variability in patient anatomy.
9. B. Inversion of the ultrasound probe is a commonly noted occurrence in vascular access procedures. Care should be taken to ensure that the probe is oriented correctly to avoid flipped anatomical views. While aberrant anatomy and previous vascular surgery are possible, they are not MOST likely. Normal anatomy has the vein medial to the artery on proper probe positioning.

SECTION II

PHYSICS, MONITORING, AND ANESTHESIA DELIVERY DEVICES

3.

GENERAL PHYSICS AND MECHANICS

David O. Joseph and George W. Williams

INTRODUCTION

This chapter explains certain basic scientific concepts of gases and liquids in order to understand how carrier gases are stored and used on our modern anesthesia machines. It reviews vapor pressure and gas pressure measurements as applied to anesthesia delivery. Other topics covered include viscosity, density, laminar versus turbulent flow, and flow meters. There is further discussion on concepts relating to gas delivery systems, pressure regulation systems, and transducers that are used for invasive measurements of blood pressure, central venous pressure, and pulmonary arterial pressure. Pipeline gas supply and cylinder gas supply are also reviewed. In addition, certain safety features incorporated into anesthesia machines to prevent an accidental delivery of the wrong gas are reviewed as well. The final topic is Doppler ultrasound.

BASIC SCIENTIFIC CONCEPTS

Understanding equipment requires knowledge of certain physical principles.

PRESSURE

Pressure is defined as the amount of force that is applied over a certain area and it is expressed with the following equation:

$$\text{Pressure} = \text{Force} / \text{Area}$$

When one studies units of pressure, it is not uncommon to see units expressed as pounds per square inch (psi) or Newtons-per-square-meter. We also sometimes refer to pounds per square inch gauge (psig). The psig unit refers to pressure above atmospheric pressure when the pressure gauge is zeroed to atmospheric pressure. When referring to atmospheric or contained gas (i.e., partial pressure), pressure units are expressed in terms of millimeters of mercury (mmHg) and centimeters of water (cmH_2O). These are units used in a barometer, and they are different in that they express the degree of displacement of a certain liquid in a column when a force is applied by a particular gas. The liquid displaced can be either mercury (Hg) or water (H_2O), but it is important to understand that it is still a force applied over an area (the cross-sectional area of a column). Whether one is using the unit "mmHg" or "cmH_2O," each expresses the same idea. An expression of this concept is tire pressure for an automobile (commonly 35 psi, for example). This pressure could easily be expressed in 35 psi, 2461 cmH_2O, or 1810 mmHg; we simply use psi by convention because the numbers are too large for practical application. The unit "mmHg" is also as synonymous with "Torr," which was named after Evangelista Torricelli, the 18th-century Italian physicist who invented the barometer.[1] Pascals are the SI units that represent pressure. A Pascal (Pa) is equivalent to a Newton-per-square-meter. When referring to atmospheric pressure, 1 atm is equivalent to 760 mmHg. It is possible to mathematically convert from one of these units to another. The following expression summarizes the relationship all of these units have to each other and therefore provides a conversion factor[2]:

$$1 \text{ atm} = 101.3 \text{ kPA} = 760 \text{ mmHg} = 14.7\text{psi} = 1033 \text{ cmH}_2\text{O}$$

As mentioned, pressure is a force applied to a specific area. When molecules of a gas are moving about in a closed container, they exert a force along the inside surface of the container. Remember that we generally use the units "mmHg" or "Torr" and sometimes cmH_2O when talking about gases in the supply cylinders.

Dalton's Law of partial pressures states that the total pressure of a mixture of gases in a container is simply the sum of the partial pressures of each gas within the container. It is expressed in the following equation[1]:

$$P_{total} = P_1 + P_2 + P_3 + \cdots + P_n$$

When looking at room air, we know that it is composed mostly of nitrogen, oxygen, water vapor, and argon (hence, we live in a nitrogen/oxygen atmosphere). At sea level, atmospheric pressure due to the presence of air is 760 mmHg. To calculate each individual component's contribution of partial pressure, we first subtract the vapor pressure of water from the total pressure:

$$760\ \text{mmHg} - 47\ \text{mmHg} = 713\ \text{mmHg}$$

Then, the fraction of each component is multiplied by this difference.

$$\text{Oxygen } (21\%) = 713\ \text{mmHg} \times 0.21 = 149.73\ \text{mmHg}$$

$$\text{Nitrogen } (78\%) = 713\ \text{mmHg} \times 0.78 = 556.14\ \text{mmHg}$$

$$\text{Argon } (\sim 1\%) = 713\ \text{mmHg} \times 0.01 = 7.13\ \text{mmHg}$$

This, in turn, gives the partial pressure of each gas. There are actually several other trace gases in our atmosphere, but for demonstrative purposes we have included only the main gases in the calculations.

GAS CONCENTRATION

Two methods used to express concentration of a gas are partial pressure and volumes percent. Partial pressure is typically expressed in mmHg. Volumes percent is simply the partial pressure of a gas over the total pressure of the mixture of gases present. It is expressed this way:

$$\text{Partial pressure} / \text{Total pressure} = \text{volumes percent}$$

The importance of understanding volumes percent is evident when one looks at the vaporizers used in the anesthesia workstations, where all concentrations are dialed in as a percentage.[3]

VAPOR PRESSURE AND EVAPORATION

Liquids have a tendency to vaporize at room temperature and pressure. When air moves over liquid in a dish, the liquid evaporates over time. Vapor pressure is related to a liquid's ability to turn into vapor. Think about a closed jug of a liquid. When the air in a closed container of liquid becomes saturated with the vapor of that liquid, the pressure exerted on the walls of the container is defined as the vapor pressure. Remember that the higher the vapor pressure of a liquid, the faster it evaporates. The more energy applied to the liquid, the higher the vapor pressure (e.g., when you heat water it evaporates faster).[3,4] Temperature added to a liquid increases its vapor pressure. At one point, the vapor pressure of the liquid will equal the surrounding atmospheric pressure, and the temperature at which this occurs is called the boiling point. If atmospheric pressure decreases for some reason (e.g., climbing Pike's Peak), then the vapor pressure necessary to reach the boiling point is lowered and therefore the temperature to reach this equilibrium is lowered. Put simply, lower atmospheric pressure found at higher altitudes lowers the boiling point.[3,4]

FLOW

Understanding the physical principle of flow is important. Flow (whether it be for liquids or gases) is defined as the volume of substance that moves past a point per unit time. Resistance is that which impedes flow: as resistance increases, flow decreases, and conversely as resistance decreases, flow increases. Viscosity is simply the ability of a liquid or gas to resist flow. Consider a bottle of water that tips over on a table and the water flows quickly over the table onto the floor. Now think of a bottle of syrup that tips over on a table; the syrup flows much slower over the table to the floor. This is because syrup has a higher viscosity. Factors that increase resistance include decreased diameter of the conduit through which liquid or gas flows, length of the conduit and viscosity of the gas or fluid in question. These factors can be summarized in Poiseuille's equation:

$$Q = \frac{\Delta V}{\Delta t} = \frac{\pi r^4 \Delta p}{8 \eta L}$$

Where r is the radius of the conduit, L is the length, η is the viscosity of the gas, and Δp is the pressure difference between the ends of the conduit.

With respect to anesthesia gas flow, the units commonly used are L/min. With reference to gas flow through a tube (e.g., a flow meter), there are two types of flow: laminar and turbulent. Normally in clinical settings both occur simultaneously.

I. Laminar flow is orderly, and particles move in parallel layers. The sides of the tube cause a frictional drag on the adjacent particles, causing them to move slower, whereas the central particles move faster, as they are further away from the sides of the tube.

II. Turbulent flow is a nonparallel movement of gas particles. It is not orderly. It occurs when a certain threshold velocity of the particles is exceeded. This velocity is called the critical flow rate. What is seen are eddies that move across or against the general direction of flow.

Viscosity of a liquid or gas has been defined above. Density of a gas or liquid is the mass of the substance divided by the volume in which it is contained. The importance of these concepts will be made clear when discussing flow meters.[5]

GAS DELIVERY AND INVASIVE MONITORING IN THE OPERATING ROOM

Understanding how equipment works in the operating room is essential particularly for patient safety.

GAS DELIVERY

In order to deliver anesthetics to patients in the operating room, we require carrier gases, which flow through our anesthesia machines, pick up a volatile anesthetic agent from a vaporizer and carry it to the patient's body. The two main systems we have are the pipeline system and the cylinder system. The pipeline system is our primary source of carrier gas. Typically there is a central storage of the gases in the hospital or surgery center that runs through a network of pipes in the facility to patient floor rooms, ICU rooms, operating rooms and procedure rooms. There are shut off valves placed in these networks to stop gas flow in case of an emergency. The gases available are oxygen, nitrous oxide, and air. A standard oxygen pipeline is normally pressurized to 50–54 psi. While readily available, it should be noted that pipeline systems are not infallible. Problems with inadequate pressure have been reported. Problems have occurred with hypoxic deaths particularly in newly constructed hospitals with newly laid pipeline systems. This is an issue of the nitrous oxide and oxygen lines having been accidently crossed during construction.[6] As such, pipeline systems are color coded by type of gas with the same color coding as seen on an anesthesia machine (green—oxygen, yellow—air, blue—nitrous oxide).

The second type of delivery system is the cylinder system. These are portable containers that hold pressurized gas to be used for patient transport or emergencies. They can be free standing or mounted to the back of an anesthesia machine for the purpose of an emergency backup supply. Also, if one is working in a procedure area that does not have a pipeline supply of a particular gas, a cylinder is necessary. In the event of a pipeline crossover or failure, the cylinder should be turned on and the wall pipeline supply disconnected.[6]

Oxygen for medical use is produce by a two-phase process: (1) liquefication of air and (2) fractional distillation of liquid air into its components. Air is first filtered to remove impurities and then cooled to −200°C (Carbon dioxide freezes at −79°C and is discarded. Oxygen liquefies at −183°C). Once at −200°C, the liquefied air is passed through a fractionating column, which has a differential temperature at its top and bottom. Because of the temperatures involved and the different boiling points of the individual components, liquid nitrogen boils, becomes a gas, and exits the column, with liquid oxygen and argon remaining. Another fractionation with a different column is required to separate the argon from the liquid oxygen. The purified oxygen that results is delivered as a cryogenic liquid.

Alternatives to liquid oxygen in cylinders for small-scale use include oxygen concentrators, which are commercially available, and oxygen candles (sodium chlorate and iron powder).[7]

I. Connections for Gas Delivery

Once again, safety must be maximized with gas delivery systems. The connections to the supplies are designed specifically for that.

A. Diameter Index Safety System

This system is a connector system used in our operating rooms to ensure that pipeline gas systems are connected properly to the anesthesia machine (see Figure 3.1). The three main gases that are supplied to the machine are oxygen, nitrous oxide, and air. These are the gases we use as carriers for the volatile agents that serve as our anesthetics. A pipeline supply of a particular carrier comes from a large central tank in the hospital and is carried to each operating room and hospital bed. The diameter index safety system uses different diameter notch connectors on color-coded

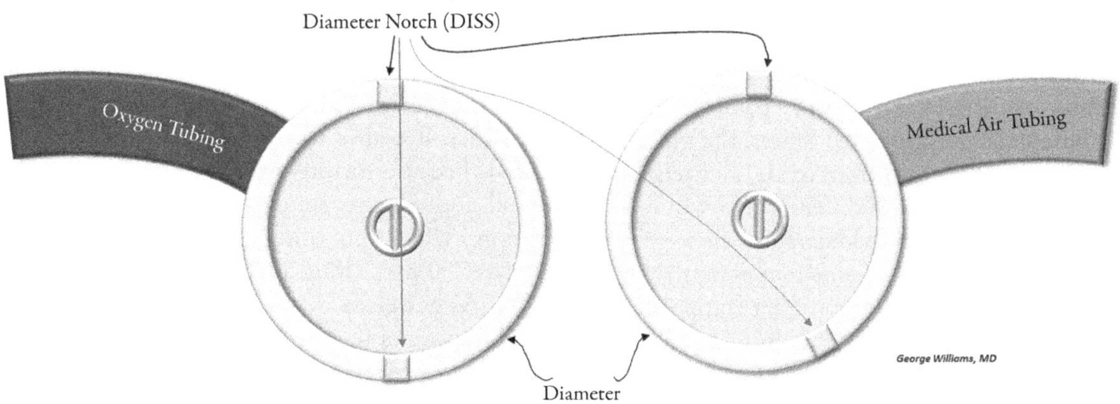

Figure 3.1 Diameter index safety system (DISS). The connection nozzle for oxygen and medical air appear identical with the exception of the notches on the "diameter" of the connection, hence the term DISS. This example shows how the air nozzle diameter notch is slightly different in angle than the oxygen notch.

hoses to hook up gas supply to the anesthesia machine. In the United States, green hoses are meant for oxygen and have a particular diameter notch for the connector on the machine. Yellow hoses are used for air and have a different diameter notch, and finally nitrous oxide has blue hoses that have their own diameter notch. This prevents one from hooking up the wrong gas to the wrong hose. It is clear how hazardous it could be if you need to hook up oxygen and accidently connect your nitrous supply to the oxygen inlet on the machine. This system can be used for connection of a hose to the machine and connection of a hose to the wall.

B. Pin Index Safety System

This is a system that is used to connect gas cylinders to an anesthesia machine. Each machine has what is called a hanging yoke mount on the back each for an oxygen cylinder, nitrous oxide cylinder, and air cylinder. As mentioned, these cylinders serve as backup carrier gas supplies for the machine. Part of a standard machine check every day is to check the pressure of gas in each cylinder to determine how much of a supply you have. Most of the time, they do not get used unless there is a need for a gas that the pipeline supply cannot provide. The pin index system is a unique configuration of metal pins on the hanging yoke mount, depending on the gas. A yoke mount for a particular gas cylinder has a certain pin configuration that will connect to that type of cylinder only. The pins fit into receiving ports on the cylinder, which allows its proper attachment to the machine. In addition to this the cylinders are color coded. This is discussed later in this chapter.

C. Quick Connectors

These are connectors from the wall outlet of the pipeline supply to the hose that attaches to the machine. They allow a single action using one or two hands without any special tools. They are more convenient compared with diameter index safety system connectors but have a great chance of leaking.[3]

All of these different connections and color codes are there for safety. They provide some redundancy to prevent the improper delivery of a gas to a patient. It goes without saying that improper carrier gas delivery could result in a catastrophic outcome. In the United States, the green cylinders are for oxygen, blue for nitrous oxide, and yellow for air (international color coding is different and will be discussed later). Most traditional cylinders are made of steel with some various alloys added. Some manufacturers have moved to producing steel with carbon fiber composite cylinders. Others have gone to making aluminum cylinders. Each has a pressure gauge giving the pressure inside each container to indicate how "full" the cylinder is. For oxygen and air tanks, the amount of gas contained is proportional to the pressure of the gas within the cylinder.[3,8]

II. Cylinders

A. Size A–E cylinders: These are the smaller portable cylinders that are used on the anesthesia machines and used as backup in case of a pipeline gas failure in the operating room. The most used cylinders in the operating room on the anesthesia machine are the "E" size cylinders.

B. Size G–H cylinders: These are the bigger cylinders used in banks to supply or backup the pipeline system. Sometimes they can be used to supply the anesthesia machine.

C. Size M cylinders: These are the biggest cylinders used for the storage of oxygen.[8]

III. Nonliquefied Compressed Gas Versus Liquefied Compressed Gas

Certain gases do not liquefy in a closed container at regular ambient temperature no matter how high the pressure gets. These are known as nonliquefied gases. Examples of this would include oxygen, nitrogen, air, and helium. Liquefied compressed gases become liquid in closed containers at ambient temperatures and at pressures ranging from 25 to 1500 psig. Nitrous oxide and carbon dioxide fall into this category.[3] Liquefied gases are also called nonideal gases.

IV. Calculation of Cylinder Contents

Oxygen and air cylinders contain nonliquefied compressed gas at ambient temperature, and therefore we can determine how much gas is in a container based on the pressure of the gas within the container. There is a direct relationship between volume of the gas and the pressure it exerts on the cylinder. A full E cylinder of oxygen contains approximately 625 L of gas, and the pressure exerted on the inner walls of the cylinder is about 2000 psi. If the pressure inside the cylinder were 1000 psi, it would indicate a volume of 312.5 L. In other words, when the volume is decreased by 50%, the pressure of the gas inside the container also decreases by 50%. An easier way to remember this information would be to set a full tank at 600L (in many textbooks), half tank at 300, and so on, in order to make the math easier to perform in your head.

When it comes to nitrous oxide, things are different. This is because nitrous oxide within a container exists in liquid and gaseous states at ambient temperature. A full nitrous cylinder contains 1590 L of gas. The pressure will read as 750 psi as long as there is any liquid left in the cylinder. As gas escapes, the liquefied portion of the nitrous oxide vaporizes to form more gas. As long as there is liquid to vaporize into gas, the pressure will stay at 750 psi. After all the liquid nitrous oxide is gone, the pressure will decrease. When this happens one can assume that the cylinder is 75% depleted. This would correspond to a volume of

Table 3.1 GAS TANK CHARACTERISTICS

	OXYGEN	NITROUS OXIDE	AIR
Cylinder color	Green	Blue	Yellow
Phase of contents	Gas	Gas/Liquid	Gas
Content vol (L)	625	1590	625
Weight empty (kg)	5.90	5.90	5.90
Weight full (kg)	6.76	8.80	
Psi when full	2000	750	1800

Adapted from Stoelting RK, Miller RD. *Basics of Anesthesia*. 5th ed. Philadelphia, PA: Churchill Livingstone Elsevier; 2007:187–188, 308–309.

about 400 L remaining. When there is liquid nitrous oxide remaining in the tank, rather than utilizing the pressure gauge (which will say 750 psi), the cylinder can be weighed to determine how much gas remains (1.87 g/L of gas). See the table below for physical characteristics of cylinders and their contents (E Size Cylinders).

Table 3.1 reviews these concepts in detail and includes the color designations used in the United States (different from international color designations). For example, the World Health Organization specifies that medical oxygen cylinders should be painted white, however manufacturers in the United States use green to designate oxygen. Likewise, the international color standard for medical air cylinders is a combination of black and white, but in the United States air cylinders are color coded yellow.[8,9]

IV. Pressure Regulators

Gas cylinder pressure starts out high and decreases as the contents are depleted from use. The pressure regulator, also known as the reducing valve, converts the high-pressure and variable gas supply to a constant, low-pressure gas supply of around 400 kPa or 50 psi. Without this device the anesthesia provider would have to adjust the gas flow continually to keep a constant flow through the machine as the pressure from the cylinder decreases. Aside from regulating the flow, other advantages of a pressure regulator include:

1. Prevention of damage to the flow control valves from the high pressures.
2. Prevention of barotrauma to the patient's lungs from high pressures.
3. Fine adjustments to the flow are possible.

Some machines employ a two-stage pressure regulation system. There are two regulators in series along a gas supply. If there is a secondary regulator, it receives gas from the pipeline or the cylinder and reduces pressure further to 177 kPa.[10] In summary, remember that the pressure in full gas tanks is very high (much higher than pipeline pressure), and if the nozzle were damaged (dropped), the tank would have pressure release similar to that of a missile. Be very careful when moving these tanks.

FLOW METERS/ROTAMETERS

Flow meters or rotameters are devices on the anesthesia machine that allow the operator to know exactly how much fresh gas flow is going through the machine. For this chapter, only mechanical flow meters will be discussed (and not the electronic kind). Each carrier gas (air, nitrous oxide, and oxygen) has a separate flow meter. A flow meter consists of a glass tube (known as a Thorpe tube) that has markings on the outside to indicate the flow rate and a flow control valve that regulates the amount of flow going through it. The Thorpe tubes have a tapered design to where the top of the tube is widest in diameter. Each tube has a mobile indicator float that is smaller in diameter than even the narrowest part of the tube. The amount of space between the float and the sides of the tube changes, and therefore the term *variable orifice* is used to describe that space. The float hovers in a position that represents the equilibrium between the downward force of its weight and the upward force exerted on it from gas flow, which comes from the bottom of the tube. With each carrier gas, the physical properties of viscosity and density exert their influence on flow. Specifically, at low flow rates, laminar flow of the gas predominates and moves the float upward. Laminar flow is dependent on the viscosity of the gas. As flow rates increase, turbulent flow is more prevalent and that is what gives the float its upward force. Turbulent flow is dependent on the density of a gas. The position of the float based on flow rates is used as a measure and corresponds to the markings on the tube. The way a float's position is read depends on what type of float it is. There are plumb-bob floats, rotating skirted floats, and ball floats. When reading the ball float, one looks at the center of the ball. In contrast, with plumb-bob and rotating skirted floats, one looks at the top of the float. Problems can occur with the accuracy of the flow meter if there is damage to the tube or the float. Dirt in the tube or on the float can cause problems with accuracy and can cause the float to stick. A dial at the bottom of each tube is used as a control to increase or decrease the amount of flow. The dials on the flow meters are designed to prevent a hypoxic mixture of gases from being delivered to the patient. Nitrous oxide and oxygen dials are linked mechanically and/or pneumatically to ensure that nothing less than an oxygen concentration of 23% is given to the patient.[3,6]

INVASIVE BLOOD PRESSURE MONITORING

Invasive blood pressure (BP) monitors provide a continuous display of information numerically and graphically. Continuous monitoring is demonstrated with the use of arterial catheters, central venous catheters, and pulmonary arterial catheters. Through a catheter pressure fluctuations are transmitted along a column of liquid. Recall that any pressure exerted on one part of a liquid is equally exerted everywhere else in the liquid. This property is what makes hydraulics possible. In monitoring blood pressure, the column of liquid connects the arterial blood to a pressure transducer. In order to do this, the following are needed:

1. An intra-arterial cannula
2. Special pressure tubing
3. A transducer
4. A microprocessor and display screen
5. A mechanism for zeroing and calibration.

The intra-arterial catheter is placed in an artery that has a collateral circulation. The reason is that there is always risk of thrombosis in the catheter or the artery. With good collateral flow, perfusion to the distal tissues continues even if thrombosis occurs in the cannulated artery. The pressure tubing should be stiff, and the liquid in the tubing should contain no bubbles. Both bubbles and compliant tubing can dampen the pressure fluctuations, resulting in erroneous readings. The tubing is attached to a saline (or heparinized saline) bag. It is worth mentioning that while in the past heparinized saline was used to help maintain arterial patency, this is no longer a common practice.[2,11] There have been different studies over the years done to determine whether the added heparin provides any benefit. A Cochrane database systematic review was done by Robertson et al regarding this issue. They reviewed seven studies with 606 total participants. They could not make a definitive conclusion about using heparinized saline due to the poor quality of the available evidence and the risk of bias.[12]

In the tubing, the liquid is compressed with a pressure bag to ensure that there is a very low flow of liquid through it. This small flow helps prevent thrombosis in the catheter. The flow also prevents the backflow of blood into the tubing. This flow is typically about 3 mL/hr. The liquid in the tubing is in contact with a diaphragm in the transducer. The diaphragm moves with the transmitted pressure fluctuations. The transducer converts the pressure fluctuations into electrical signals. The signals then are displayed on the display screen and provide a constant measurement of the pressure in question. The transducer apparatus usually has a stopcock that can be closed to the patients and opened to the atmosphere. When opened, a control on the monitor display allows zeroing. When the transducer is exposed to atmospheric pressure and zeroed, it is important to realize that this is the "zero point" on which all other pressures are being based.[2,11]

Zeroing the transducer is very important in order to have accurate information regarding the pressure measurements in the heart. The level at which the transducer should sit to have the most useful readings is referred to as the phlebostatic axis. The phlebostatic axis corresponds to the position of the right atrium. With the head of the bed at 60° or less, the axis is located at the fourth intercostal space at the mid-anterior-posterior diameter of the chest wall. If the patient is in the right lateral position at 90°, it is located at the fourth intercostal space at the level of the midline sternum. In the left lateral position at 90°, it is located at the fourth intercostal space at the level of the left sternal border.[13,14]

The transducer employs a device called a strain gauge. A strain gauge relies on the concept that resistance in a wire increases when it is stretched. A series of four strain gauges together form what is called a Wheatstone bridge. Current passes constantly through the Wheatstone bridge, and when the structure of the bridge is distorted by the pressure of the column of water, the resistance change results in a voltage change. This then is converted to a signal that can be visualized on a display.[2,11] This technology is not only applicable to arterial blood pressure measurement, but central venous, intracerebral, or any other type of pressure measurement.

PRINCIPLES OF DOPPLER ULTRASOUND

Ultrasound is a commonly used tool in medicine. It is of particular importance and interest among anesthesiologists because it is used for central line placement, echocardiography, and placement of nerve blocks. Ultrasound refers to frequency of the sound waves. Specifically anything above 20,000 Hz is considered "ultra." Audible sound for humans is between 20 Hz and 20,000 Hz.

A moving object vibrates and creates sound waves. Sound waves travel through a medium. The wave carries energy and not matter from place to place. Sound waves are composed of compressions (increases in pressure or density of the medium) and rarefractions (decreases in pressure or density of the medium). Sound travels in a straight line, and the waves travel in a longitudinal fashion.

With ultrasound machines in clinical practice used for imaging, sound waves are sent in short bursts into the body. A number of individual waves are in a burst or pulse. The number of pulses per minute is referred to as the pulse frequency. As ultrasound pulses travel through biological tissues, some of them are reflected back to their source. The pulses that get reflected back are detected by a transducer and interpreted as an image on a screen based on distance traveled by the reflected pulse. For a stationary object, the speed at which a pulse travels in tissue as well as travel time to and from the object provides distance information.

For moving objects (e.g., red blood cells in an artery) the measurement of distance depends on a phenomenon known as the Doppler effect. The Doppler effect refers to a moving sound source. It is the perceived increase in sound frequency as a source approaches and the perceived decrease in sound frequency as a source moves away.

There are two different types of Doppler ultrasound that are used: pulse wave Doppler and continuous wave Doppler. With pulse wave Doppler, the transducer serves as both transmitter and receiver. The transducer sends out a signal and has to "listen" for the signal to come back in order to determine distance to the object in question. Also the perceived increase in frequency that occurs (described by the Doppler effect) will give information regarding the speed of the moving object off which the pulse signal bounced (e.g., red blood cells in a vessel).[15] With such a system, the pulse frequency has to be relatively low, so that there is enough time for a single pulse reflection to be detected. If the emitted pulse frequency is too high, a second pulse generated before the first one is reflected back can cause problems in perceived range to the object in question (if the first pulse reflection is detected soon after the generation of the second, one might perceive the reflection of the first pulse to be the reflection of the second). This phenomenon is known as *range ambiguity*.[16,17] Continuous wave Doppler has a separate receiver. It detects the Doppler shift frequency for objects that move faster (e.g., red blood cells moving through a stenotic valve). It cannot be used to generate an image. Both pulse wave and continuous Doppler can be used to determine a range of velocities and plot them on a graph over time. The curves generated can be integrated (velocity time integral), and that figure can be used in a continuity equation to determine area of stenotic vessels.[15]

REFERENCES

1. Kotz J, Treichel P, Townsend J. *Chemistry and Chemical Reactivity*. 7th ed. Belmont, CA: Brooks/Cole, Cengage Learning; 2010:516–517, 530, 534.
2. Miller R, ed. *Miller's Anesthesia*. 6th ed. Philadelphia, PA: Churchill Livingstone Elsevier; 2005:1198–1199, 1220, 1279–1280.
3. Dorsch J, Dorsch S. *A Practical Approach to Anesthesia Equipment*. Philadelphia, PA: Lippincott Williams & Wilkins; 2011:4–10, 21–25, 53–54, 57, 59, 67–74, 110–111.
4. Moore J. *Chemistry Made Simple*. Rev. ed. New York, NY: Broadway; 2004:66, 81–82, 146.
5. Wilson J, Buffa A, Lou B. *Physics*. 6th ed. Upper Saddle Hall, NJ: Pearson Prentice Hall; 2007:319–327.
6. Barash P, Cullen B, Stoelting R. *Clinical Anesthesia*. 5th ed. Philadelphia, PA: Lippincott Williams & Wilkins; 2006:563–568.
7. Das S, Chattopadhyay S, Bose P. The anaesthesia gas supply system. *Indian J Anaesth*. 2013;57(5):489–499.
8. Srivasta U. Anaesthesia gas supply: cylinders. *Indian J Anaesth*. 2013;57(5):500–506.
9. Stoelting R, Miller R. *Basics of Anesthesia*. 5th ed. Philadelphia, PA: Churchill Livingstone Elsevier; 2007:187–188, 308–309.
10. Gurudatt C. The basic anaesthesia machine. *Indian J Anaesth*. 2013;57(5):438–445.
11. Ward M, Langton J. Blood pressure measurement. *Cont Edu Anaesth Crit Care and Pain*. 2007;7(4):122–126.
12. Robertson-Malt S, Malt G, Farquhar V, Greer W. Heparin versus normal saline for patency of arterial lines. *Cochrane Database Syst Review*. 2014;13(5):CD007364.
13. Iverson C. Understanding the phlebostatic axis. *Nursing Made Incredibly Easy!* 2011;9(5):56.
14. Sole M, Goldenberg-Klein D, Moseley M. *Introduction to Critical Care Nursing*. 6th ed. St. Louis, MO: Elsevier Saunders; 2013:152.
15. Sidebotham D, Merry A, Legget M, Edwards M. *Practical Perioperative Transesophageal Echocardiography with Critical Echocardiography*. 2nd ed. Philadelphia, PA: Elsevier Saunders; 2011:2, 23–24.
16. Huang J, Triedman J, Vasilyev N, Suematsu Y, Cleveland R, Dupont P. Imaging artifacts of medical instruments in ultrasound-guided interventions. *J Ultrasound Med*. 2007;26:1303–1322.
17. Mathew J, Swaminathan M, Ayoub C. *Clinical Manual and Review of Transesophageal Echocardiography*. 2nd ed. New York, NY: McGraw Hill Medical; 2010:7–8.

FURTHER READING

Dorsch J, Dorsch S. *A Practical Approach to Anesthesia Equipment*. Philadelphia, PA: Lippincott Williams & Wilkins; 2011.

Roth P. Anesthesia delivery systems. In: Miller R, ed. *Basics of Anesthesia*. 6th ed. Philadelphia, PA: Elsevier Saunders; 2011.

Sidebotham D, Merry A, Legget M, Edwards M. *Practical Perioperative Transesophageal Echocardiography with Critical Echocardiography*. 2nd ed. Philadelphia, PA: Elsevier Saunders; 2011.

QUESTIONS

1. Doubling which of the following would have the greatest effect on flow through a tube?
   A. Viscosity of a gas
   B. Length of tubing
   C. Radius of the tube
   D. Pressure differential

2. If the pressure gauge on a green E-cylinder reads 500 mmHg, how long will one be able to supply oxygen to a patient requiring a flow through a facemask of 6 L/min?
   A. 45 minutes
   B. 165 minutes
   C. 25 minutes
   D. 120 minutes

3. Continuous wave Doppler is a modality of ultrasound that is best used for:
   A. Generating high-resolution images
   B. Measuring distances of far-away objects
   C. Measuring velocities of objects in motion
   D. Resolving issues with range ambiguity

4. Which of the following BEST describes the physical property measured by a Wheatstone bridge:
   A. Oscillation

B. Strain
C. Temperature
D. Density

5. An extraventricular drain is alarming, indicating intracranial hypertension with a pressure of 30 cmH20. Which of the follow BEST reflects the patient's intracranial pressure in mmHg?
A. 11 mmHg
B. 22 mmHg
C. 40 mmHg
D. More information required in order to determine

ANSWERS

1. C. In order to solve this problem, consider the principles of the Poiseuille equation, within which one can see that the single largest contributor to resistance to gas flow is tube radius, followed by tube length and gas viscosity.
2. C. Recall, a full oxygen tank contains 600L of volume at full pressure (2000 psi). As such, half a tank (1,000 psi) has 300L volume, and one-quarter of a tank (500 psi) has 150 L volume. At 6 L/min, it would take 25 minutes to exhaust the oxygen supply.
3. C. Continuous wave Doppler is the best modality for measuring speed of objects in fluid (e.g., red blood cells moving through a valve). Tw-dimensional ultrasound with higher frequency is utilized to generate high-resolution images. Doppler is used to measure distances of faraway objects. Range ambiguity would not be resolved with continuous wave Doppler; it is a phenomenon associated with the computer/ultrasound unit attempting to determine the distance (not speed) of objects that are moving.
4. B. The Wheatstone bridge is a strain gauge, and is the primary mechanism by which pressure is measured in the operating room in arterial lines, central lines, and extraventricular drains. It functions by correlating changes in conductance with changes in strain in a circuit. If resistance is known everywhere in a circuit, the change in resistance can be correlated with the strain, or pressure, exerted on a system, thereby giving pressure. Oscillimetry is the mechanism by which noninvasive blood pressure cuffs function and is not applicable in this instance. While extremes of temperature may change conductance of the materials used in a Wheatstone bridge, temperature is not the responsible mechanism for pressure measurement. Density is not related to the Wheatstone bridge.
5. B. Recall that each unit of Torr (or mmHg) equals 1.34 units of cmH_2O. In effect, in order to calculate this value, the examinee would need to divide 30 by 1.34, to yield 22. This type of calculation can be done mentally without a notepad to a nongranular degree of accuracy. But keep in mind, most questions are not there to test your math prowess, but your understanding of the concept. Thirty divided by 2 is 15, so any number less than 15 would obviously be too small, thereby eliminating A. The number would have to be smaller than 30, so C can be eliminated. You already have enough information to answer the question, thereby eliminating D. One could have second-grade mathematical proficiency and still answer the question correctly once the concept being asked is understood.

4.

PROPERTIES OF LIQUIDS, GASES, AND VAPORS

Sudha A. Bidani and Stephen Stayer

BRIEF HISTORICAL PERSPECTIVE

See Table 4.1 for an overview of anesthetic agents.

FUNDAMENTAL TERMINOLOGY

Common terms describing inhaled anesthetics and their definitions:

Diffusion of Gases: Oxygen and carbon dioxide diffuse between alveoli and blood, and between blood and tissues, following a concentration gradient. Similarly, anesthetic gases follow the same gas laws.

Relative and Absolute Humidity: Humidity is the amount of water vapor in air. Absolute humidity is the water content of air; and relative humidity, expressed as a percent, is the measurement of absolute humidity relative to the maximum for a given temperature and pressure.

Critical Temperature: A temperature above which a vapor/gas cannot be liquefied no matter how much pressure is applied. As a substance approaches critical temperature, the properties of its gas and liquid phases converge, producing a single phase.

Critical Pressure: A pressure required to liquefy a vapor/gas at its critical temperature.

Gas Laws: Developed at the end of the 18th century, these laws show the relationship between pressure, volume, and the temperature of any given gas. The following are some of the important laws applicable to anesthesia:

$$\text{Boyle's law: } P_1V_1 = P_2V_2$$

At constant temperature, the product of an ideal gas's pressure and volume is always constant.

$$\text{Charles' law: } V_1 / T_1 = V_2 / T_2$$

The law of volumes: for an ideal gas at constant pressure, volume is directly proportional to its temperature.

$$\text{Gay-Lussac's law: } P_1 / T_1 = P_2 / T_2$$

The pressure exerted by an ideal gas of fixed volume is proportional to its temperature.

Vaporizers: There are several different types of vaporizers. Simple open drop administration involves using layers of gauze placed on a wire mask, which increases the surface area for vaporization as the liquid agent is dropped onto the gauze. Adding too much liquid on the gauze leads to blockage of air passages and hinders its vaporization, delaying induction time. The draw over vaporizer uses ether, with air or oxygen as a carrier gas. The bubble through vaporizer, or Copper Kettle, allows the carrier gas to be bubbled through the anesthetic agent, which will increase the surface area of contact. Modern vaporizers are temperature compensated, which means they work in a variety of temperatures and produce a constant concentration even with altering carrier gas flows. They are calibrated for individual anesthetics and are NOT interchangeable. Since the boiling point of desflurane is within the range of room temperature, a severe overdose of anesthetic could be produced if desflurane is administered through a sevoflurane vaporizer. Such an error is prevented with the use of mechanical filling devices that do not allow filling of the wrong agent.

Vapor: The gaseous state of a liquid or solid at a temperature below its boiling point

Vapor Pressure: The pressure of vapor when it is in equilibrium with its condensed form (liquid or solid) in a closed space.

Table 4.1 A HISTORICAL PERSPECTIVE OF ANESTHETIC AGENTS

YEAR	INTRODUCED BY	ANESTHETIC AGENT	BOILING POINT	VAPOR PRESSURE	BLOOD/GAS SOLUBILITY COEFFICIENT	MAC
1844	Colton or Wells*	Nitrous oxide	−88.48	5150	0.47	105
1846	WTG Morton or Crawford Long*	Diethyl ether	34.6	425	12.1	1.92
1847	Simpson	Chloroform	61.2		8	0.77
1956	Johnstone	Halothane	50	244	2.04	0.74
1960	Artusio	Methoxyflurane	104.8	22.5	12	0.2
1963	Terrel	Enflurane	56.5	172	1.9	1.68
		Isoflurane	48.5	238	1.4	1.15
1990	In Japan via Maruishi Company	Sevoflurane	58.6	157	0.68	2.1
1992		Desflurane	23	88	0.42	6

*There is controversy over who initially introduced these agents into clinical practice.

Boiling Point: The temperature when vapor pressure is equal to 1 atmosphere.

Partition Coefficient: At equal pressures, it is an indicator of quantitative ratio between two compartments.

Time Constant: Denotes speed of equilibrium.

Second Gas Effect: The influence of one gas on uptake of the companion gas. In the alveoli, a large volume uptake of the first gas leads to an increased concentration of the second gas. A large difference in uptake of two gases is necessary for this effect to come into play.

Concentration Effect: In order to achieve a more rapid equilibrium, inhaled gases are commonly delivered at a high concentration, as they are rapidly removed from the blood into the tissues during induction. This is sometimes referred to as over pressure.

Guedel Classification: This system was originally designed to determine the depth of anesthesia when diethyl ether was used as a sole anesthetic. Even though this classification does not exactly apply to newer insoluble anesthetic agents and usage of adjuvants (opioids, hypnotics, regional blocks, and muscle relaxants), the terms of stage of anesthesia are still commonly used. Stage I is a state of analgesia, Stage II is a state of excitement, Stage III is a surgical plane of anesthesia, and Stage IV is a state of respiratory and hemodynamic instability.

Anesthesia: There is no single definition.

Operational Definition of Anesthesia: A state where the subject has:

- Amnesia
- Analgesia—a lack of response to painful stimulus.
- Suppression of protective reflexes, namely swallowing, coughing, eyelash
- Muscle relaxation

Mechanism of Action of Anesthetics:

- Inhibit the excitatory ion channel function and/or enhance the inhibitory ion channel function.
- May affect neurotransmitter release.
- May cause hyperpolarization of neurons by increasing efflux of K+ – K+ channels, influx of Cl- through GABA receptors, and/or influx of Na+ through NMDA Na+ channels.

Minimal Alveolar Concentration (MAC): The concentration/partial pressure of anesthetic agent in the alveoli that prevents a response in 50% of patients/animals to painful stimuli, when measured at steady state. It is used to compare potency of different anesthetic agents. MAC-BAR is concentration required to block autonomic response to painful stimuli. MAC-awake is the concentration required to control perceptive awareness, on an average about one-third to one-fourth the MAC value for a given agent.

Table 4.2 GAS PARTITION COEFFICIENTS OF VARIOUS GASES USED IN ANESTHESIA

ANESTHETIC AGENT	BLOOD/ GAS	BLOOD/ BRAIN	MUSCLE/ BLOOD	FAT/ BLOOD
Nitrous Oxide	0.47	1.1	1.2	2.3
Halothane	2.5	1.9	3.4	51
Isoflurane	1.46	1.6	2.9	45
Sevoflurane	0.65	1.7	3.1	48
Desflurane	0.45	1.3	2.0	27
Nitrogen	0.015			

Vessel Rich Group (VRG) (heart, lung, liver, and kidneys): constitutes about 10% of the body mass and receives about 75% of the cardiac output. These tissues equilibrate rapidly with inhaled anesthetics, usually in three time constants or 6–12 minutes.

Vessel Poor Group (VPG) (skin, muscle, and fat): constitutes about 70% of the body mass and receives < 25% of the cardiac output. These tissues equilibrate slowly with inhaled anesthetics, and during the elimination of anesthetics they act as a reservoir.

Solubility/Partition Coefficient: determines distribution ratio of gases at equilibrium. It remains constant at body temperature for any given anesthetic agent. A high blood/gas partition coefficient, as with diethyl ether, means that a large amount of the agent dissolves before PA-Pa (pressure in alveolar gas and pressure in arterial blood) equilibrium is reached. Using sevoflurane, with a low blood/gas partition coefficient, the PA-Pa equilibrium develops faster, resulting in a faster anesthetic induction. Even though nitrous oxide has a very low blood/gas partition coefficient, it is 30 times more soluble than nitrogen (see Table 4.2). When nitrous oxide is delivered to a patient with a closed air space (bowel, pneumothorax, and air embolus) it will be transferred into this space much faster than nitrogen is transferred out, and therefore this air space will expand. The volumetric expansion of a closed air space is dependent on PA—at 50% it may double, and at 75% may quadruple the size of the space.

PHARMACOKINETICS

Pharmacokinetics of inhaled anesthetics describes the uptake of gases from alveoli into the systemic circulation, distribution to the tissues, and elimination.

INDUCTION

The primary objective is the delivery of inhaled anesthetics to the brain (the target organ). Many things affect the pharmacokinetics of inhaled anesthetics.

Fresh gas flow (FGF) from the flow meter affects the time constant for equilibrium of gases in the system. Higher flow rates shorten the time constant, and higher concentrations of gases, over pressure, are used during the induction phase to offset the impact of higher uptake into the blood. As the VRG reaches equilibrium, uptake is reduced, and the anesthetic concentration can be decreased to maintain the desired brain concentration.

The type and gas volume of the anesthesia circuit is also an important variable. A circle system with high volume takes a longer time to equilibrate when compared with a non-rebreathing and low-volume circuit such as the T-piece with Jackson Rees modification. Depending on the solubility of the gases used, the rubber and plastic components of the system may absorb them and act as a reservoir especially during the elimination phase.

When considering alveolar ventilation, the higher the alveolar ventilation (VA), the faster the speed of induction. Hyperventilation will speed the rate of induction, and hypoventilation will slow the rate of induction. A spontaneously breathing patient will reduce VA as the depth of anesthesia increases, slowing the rate of induction. At equilibrium, PA ≈ Pa ≈ Pbrain, therefore PA can be used to guide the depth of anesthesia.

Cardiac output is also important. Decreased cardiac output leads to a faster induction because partial pressure equilibrium is reached faster. The slower passage of blood in the lungs allows more time for alveolar to arterial concentrations to equilibrate. Increased cardiac output will slow the induction time. The pharmacokinetics of more soluble agents is more significantly affected by changes in cardiac output.

The blood/gas partition coefficient affects the rate of transfer of anesthetics from the alveoli to arterial blood. A high blood/gas partition coefficient will slow the PA-Pa equilibrium as opposed to anesthetics with a low blood/gas coefficient.

The tissue/blood partition coefficient will affect the time required to equilibrate Pa (arterial partial pressure) with tissue (brain, muscle, fat, etc.) The brain has a much lower partition coefficient compared with fat. The brain will equilibrate much more rapidly than fat, and once saturated, fat will very slowly release anesthetic agent back into the blood, which is then eliminated in the lungs.

An intracardiac shunt can affect anesthetic uptake of more soluble gases. A right-to-left shunt produces cyanosis as a portion of the blood is shunted past the lungs. This also will slow the speed of induction, but is only clinically relevant when using more soluble agents like halothane.

The concentration effect is also important to consider. In order to achieve a more rapid equilibrium, inhaled gases are commonly delivered at a high concentration as they are rapidly removed from the blood into the tissues during induction. This is sometimes referred to as over pressure.

When using gases with differing solubilities, the second gas effect may be of clinical importance. The second gas effect is defined as the influence of one gas on uptake of the companion gas. In the alveoli, a large volume uptake of the first gas leads to an increased concentration of the second gas. Again, a large difference in uptake of two gases is necessary for this effect to come in play.

RECOVERY FROM ANESTHESIA

The pharmacokinetics of recovery is more or less the inverse of induction. The least inspired concentration (PI) can only be zero. Therefore a higher concentration effect cannot be used in order to maintain PI close to zero. A high FGF will help wash the agent out of the anesthesia circuit.

Depending on the duration and solubility of the anesthetic, saturation of VPG may act as a reservoir, redistribution to VRG, and eventually to alveoli for washout. Hypoventilation and decreased cardiac output will delay the anesthetic washout and the recovery.

Currently used inhaled anesthetics have less than 5% metabolism, and this route does not significantly contribute to elimination. Halothane undergoes approximately 20% metabolism, which speeds elimination. The composition of circuit material may become a reservoir depending on its capacity to adsorb the anesthetic gas. Diffusion hypoxia can occur when patient is allowed to breathe room air at the conclusion of an anesthetic before nitrous oxide is washed out.

SPECIFIC TOXICITIES

Methoxyflurane is no longer in use because extensive metabolism produces fluoride ions and dichloroacetic acid, which leads to dose-dependent high-output renal failure.

Sevoflurane can be metabolized to compound A (trifluoroethyl vinyl ether), and prolonged exposure from the use of dry baralyme and FGF contribute to compound A accumulation, which is associated with proteinuria, glucosuria, and enzymeuria. Full desiccation of soda lime can lead to carbon monoxide production after any volatile anesthetic agent regardless of temperature. The degradation is an exothermic process that leads to sudden increase in soda lime temperature and carbon monoxide production. Newer preparations of CO_2 absorbents have very small amounts or no NaOH or KOH, reducing the carbon monoxide production. Desflurane leads to the least amount of carbon monoxide production.

FURTHER READING

Miller R, Pardo M. *Basics of Anesthesia*. 6th ed. Philadelphia, PA: Elsevier; 2011.

Sdrales L, Miller R. *Miller's Anesthesia Review*. 2nd ed. Philadelphia, PA: Elsevier; 2012.

QUESTIONS

1. Which of the following factors may cause a modern vaporizer to deliver a different concentration of anesthetic than the dialed concentration?
   A. Reducing the fresh gas flow to less than 1 L/min
   B. Heating the room, and vaporizer to 35°C (95°F)
   C. Converting from positive pressure ventilation to spontaneous ventilation
   D. Filling the sevoflurane vaporizer with isoflurane
   E. Changing the carrier gas mix from oxygen/air to oxygen/nitrous oxide

2. Which combination of factors would produce the highest alveolar concentration of anesthetic agent?
   A. High blood/gas solubility, low cardiac output, low alveolar ventilation
   B. Low blood/gas solubility, low cardiac output, high alveolar ventilation
   C. Low blood/gas solubility, low cardiac output, low alveolar ventilation
   D. Low blood/gas solubility, high cardiac output, low alveolar ventilation
   E. High blood/gas solubility, high cardiac output, high alveolar ventilation

3. In which of the following situations is nitrous oxide absolutely contraindicated?
   A. A patient undergoing hysterectomy
   B. A patient with a history of transient ischemic events
   C. A patient with a pneumothorax
   D. A patient undergoing open gastrostomy
   E. A patient with ischemic heart disease

4. Which of the following factors will speed the elimination of anesthetic agent, that is, speed recovery?
   A. High fresh gas flows in the anesthesia circuit
   B. Use of an anesthetic agent with a low blood/gas solubility coefficient
   C. Combining nitrous oxide with oxygen as a second gas
   D. Reducing minute ventilation
   E. Increasing cardiac output

ANSWERS

1. D. Unlike the old vaporizers, namely draw over, the modern vaporizer is a plenum vaporizer that works with compressed gases. They are designed for a specific anesthetic liquid, which means they are not interchangeable. The vaporizer design takes into account the physical properties of the specific anesthetic. Performance of the vaporizer remains unaltered regardless of whether the patient breathes spontaneously or is ventilated mechanically. The aim is to get a desired concentration of vapor mixed with the carrier gas (usually compressed gases, i.e., oxygen and/or nitrous oxide) for delivery to the lungs/alveoli.

   Temperature compensation is the crux of the vaporizer design.

   1. The metallic container of the vaporizer acts as a heat reservoir. As the liquid vaporizes it cools and in turn draws heat from the container.
   2. A temperature-compensating bypass valve controls the flow of gases through the vaporizing chamber. Usually the valve is a bimetallic strip that expands or contracts depending on the temperature of the liquid anesthetic. A cooler liquid will not vaporize as well as a warm one, so there is a need for higher flow to maintain the quantity of vapor needed for a constant concentration. The contracted bimetallic strip allows higher flow through the vaporizing chamber. The opposite happens when the temperature of the liquid is warm.
   3. In the vaporizing chamber, there are series of wicks that are saturated with liquid anesthetic. Their presence leads to an increase in the surface area of vaporization of the liquid. As the carrier gas passes over the wicks, it becomes saturated with anesthetic vapor. The mixture enters the mixing chamber and mixes with the bypassed carrier gas.
   4. At room temperature, that is, 20°C, desflurane vapor pressure is near atmospheric (669 mm). Because of this, a dangerously high concentration could be delivered if using a conventional variable bypass vaporizer. Easy vaporization would lead to quick cooling of the liquid and a reduction of vaporization. Since desflurane is not as potent as sevoflurane and isoflurane, the need for a higher concentration would not be easily met because of cooling of the liquid.

      A heated vaporizer was developed for desflurane. The liquid is heated to 39°C. The gas in the vaporizer is usually at 200 kPa or approximately 2 atm. The bypass valve senses the FGF and injects small quantities of vapor in the mixing chamber.

2. B. A balance between input and output of anesthetic to the lungs determines the alveolar partial pressure. The input is dependent on a combination of vaporizer output, that is, inspired concentration (PI), alveolar ventilation (VA), and characteristic of the breathing circuit. The output or uptake of the anesthetic is dependent on the blood/gas solubility, cardiac output, and alveolar to venous partial pressure gradient. Higher VA will deliver more gas to the alveolus, a low blood/gas solubility coefficient will maintain a high alveolar concentration because less anesthetic is taken up by the blood. Finally a low cardiac output will allow adequate time for anesthetic gas equilibration between the alveolus and blood, again producing a higher alveolar concentration.
3. C. The blood/gas solubility coefficients for nitrogen and nitrous oxide are 0.015 and 0.47 respectively. A larger volume of nitrous oxide will diffuse into air-filled compartments than the rate of nitrogen leaving the air compartment. This imbalance results in a rapid increase in the volume of gas in a closed air-filled space. If the walls of the space are compliant (air embolus, bowel, pneumothorax), the size of the space increases. If the walls are noncompliant (middle ear, eye, cerebral ventricles) then pressure in the air-filled space increases. Therefore, nitrous oxide is to be avoided in these situations.
4. A. Using high fresh gas flows in a circle system will wash exhaled gas out of the system and avoid rebreathing of anesthetic agent, therefore speeding elimination. Anesthetics with low blood/gas solubility will be more rapidly eliminated from the blood as the blood and alveolar gas equilibrate. There is no second gas effect that affects elimination; however, if nitrous oxide is eliminated and the patient breathes air, a hypoxic gas concentration can develop, and patients should be given oxygen during the washout of nitrous oxide from the blood. Similar to the uptake of anesthetic, low minute ventilation will slow equilibration between blood and alveolar gas, as will a high cardiac output. Therefore these conditions will slow the elimination of anesthetic agents.

5.

PHYSICS OF ANESTHESIA MACHINE BREATHING SYSTEMS

Rhashedah A. Ekeoduru and Harold Doerr

PORTABLE VENTILATION DEVICES (SELF-REINFLATING, NON-SELF-REINFLATING), NON-REBREATHING VALVES

Supplemental oxygen may be required in the perioperative period to treat an arterial oxygen saturation (PaO_2) of less than 60 mmHg or a hemoglobin oxygen saturation (SaO_2) of less than 90%. The provision of oxygen therapy can be accomplished using several delivery devices, depending on the amount of supplementation required (see Table 5.1). The least invasive mode of providing supplemental oxygen is via nasal cannula (see Figure 5.1 and Figure 5.2). This method is ideal for patients who require long-term oxygen therapy, because it does not interfere with movement of the mouth and is relatively lightweight and small. The nasal cannula consists of two soft, plastic nasal prongs that are connected to a flow meter. Oxygen is then delivered through the flow meter at a rate varying from 1 to 6 liters per minute. The higher the flow, the more oxygen is expelled during expiration.[1] An inspired oxygen concentration (FiO_2) of up to 0.44 can be delivered via nasal cannula when a rate of 6 L/min is used. Flow rates higher than 4 liters can be associated with epistaxis if not properly humidified. A potential solution is to use a reservoir nasal cannula. These cannulas can store approximately 20 mL of oxygen in the reservoir, increasing the amount of oxygen available to the patient at inspiration, but at a decreased required flow rate.[2] The reservoir decreases the dilution of oxygen by decreasing mixing with room air during inhalation. Lower flow rates are needed, and humidification is not necessary secondary to retention of exhaled moisture.

Another common device used to deliver supplemental oxygen is a simple face mask (see Figure 5.3). These masks allow a mixture of oxygen and entrained room air to be inhaled by the patient. Simple face masks are prone to rebreathing. In order to decrease the amount of rebreathing, it is advisable to deliver a minimum of 5 L/min of oxygen. One can expect to deliver an FiO_2 of 0.3–0.6 via a simple face mask when delivered oxygen flow ranges from 5 to 10 L/min.[1] The delivered amount of oxygen decreases during high tidal volume states or during tachypnea because the ratio of fresh oxygen delivery to oxygen consumption and CO_2 production within the mask favors rebreathing. Simple face masks are designed to provide higher levels of supplemental oxygen therapy short-term to stable patients who are capable of protecting their airways.

By attaching a reservoir bag to a simple face mask and installing a one-way valve, the administered FiO_2 can be increased (see Figure 5.4). These masks are referred to as partial rebreathing masks. These are disposable plastic masks that are attached to an oxygen source that fills the sealed reservoir bag. A partial rebreathing mask allows some of the patient's exhaled gas, usually dead space gas, to fill the reservoir, in addition to fresh oxygen. This differs from a non-rebreather mask that directs exhaled gas through a one-way valve to prevent rebreathing and room air entrainment. Both reservoirs are designed to accept 10–15 L/min of fresh gas flow that can accomplish an FiO_2 of 0.4–1.00 (see Figure 5.4). Proper function of reservoir bags relies on a proper seal between the mask and the patient's face. In addition, the operator should ensure an adequate source of oxygen is constantly supplied to the reservoir or risk delivering a reduced FiO_2, potentially leading to worsened hypoxia.

CO_2 ABSORPTION: PRINCIPLES, CANISTERS, EFFICIENCY

The principle disadvantage of portable ventilation devices and semiclosed and closed ventilation circuits is the rebreathing of CO_2[3]. Over time patients can become acidotic, hypertensive, tachycardic, and tachyarrythmic and can develop coagulopathy. Modern circuits include

Table 5.1 OXYGEN LEVELS ACHIEVED WITH VARIOUS DELIVERY DEVICES

DEVICE	FLOW IN L/MIN	RESULTING FIO_2
Nasal cannula	1	0.23
	2	0.23–0.28
	3	0.27–0.34
	4	0.31–0.38
	5–6	0.32–0.44
Simple face mask	5–8	0.3–0.6
Partial rebreather mask	7	0.35–0.75
	15	0.65–1.00
Non-rebreather mask	7–15	0.4–1.00

removable CO_2 absorbents to counter these problems. The most common types of absorbents are soda lime (sodium hydroxide), Baralyme (calcium hydroxide and barium hydroxide, though not available in the United States), and Amsorb (calcium hydroxide). These absorbents combine with exhaled CO_2 to first form carbonic acid and then water plus hydroxides:

$$CO_2 + H_2O \rightarrow H_2CO_3$$

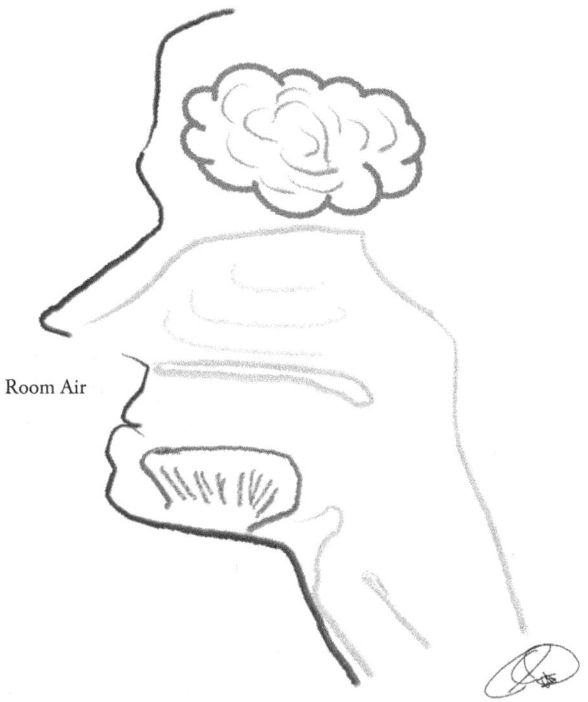

Figure 5.1 Overview of nasal and oral cavity anatomy while breathing room air. Image courtesy of George Williams, MD.

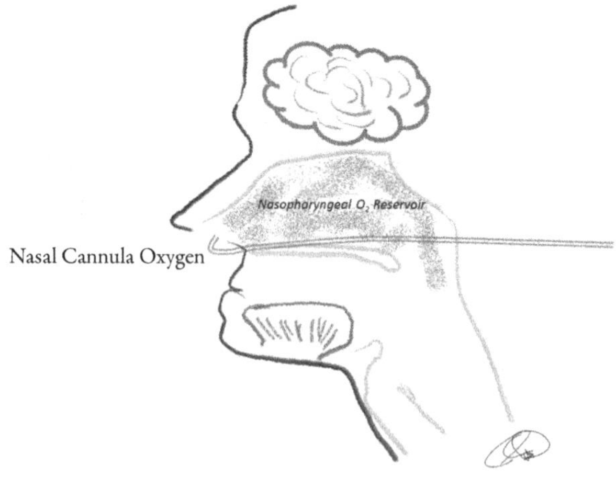

Figure 5.2 Overview of nasal and oral cavity while breathing nasal cannula oxygen, which allows for the "reservoir" effect. Image courtesy of George Williams, MD.

$$H_2CO_3 + 2NaOH \rightarrow Na_2CO_3 + 2H_2O + \text{Heat}$$
$$Na_2CO_3 + Ca(OH)_2 \rightarrow CaCO_2 + 2NaOH$$

This formula is highly testable by the American Board of Anesthesiology and should be mastered. The principle differences between soda lime, Baralyme, and Amsorb are the potentially toxic byproducts and adverse events secondary to variable heat production (see Table 5.2). A desiccated Baralyme absorber can combine with desflurane to produce significant amounts of carbon monoxide that can poison a patient. Compound A (trifluoromethyl vinyl ether) is another toxic byproduct that is created when sevoflurane is

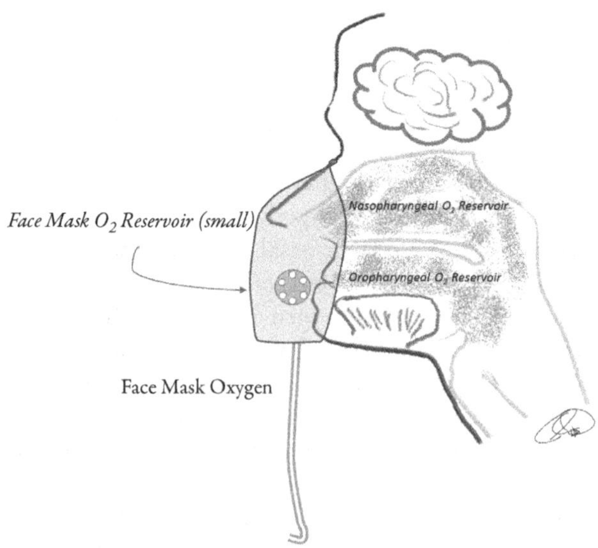

Figure 5.3 Overview of nasal and oral cavity while breathing facemask oxygen. The "reservoir" effect is more prominent given the internal and external reservoir provided by the mask. Image courtesy of George Williams, MD.

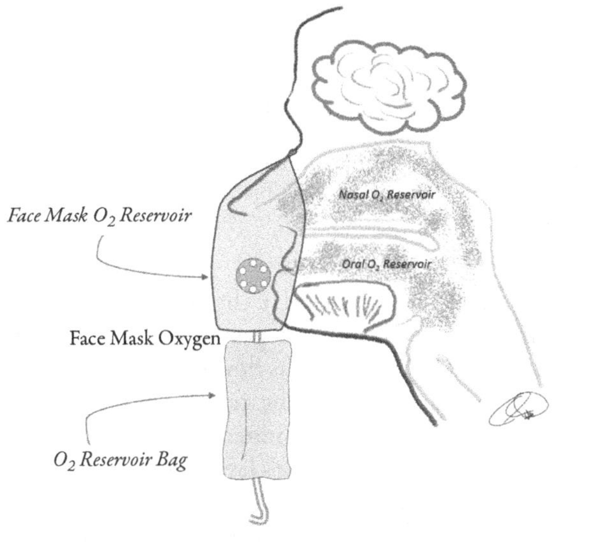

Figure 5.4 Overview of nasal and oral cavity while breathing oxygen with a partial rebreather mask. The "reservoir" is maximized by the large bag attached the mask. Ideally the bag empties freely enough for the patient to obtain the reserve oxygen during a portion of the inspiratory cycle. Image courtesy of George Williams, MD.

Table 5.2 BYPRODUCTS ASSOCIATED WITH VARIOUS CO_2 ABSORBERS

AGENT	TOXIC BYPRODUCT
Baralyme	Fires Carbon monoxide (mnemonic, "Fires can make carbon monoxide")
Sevoflurane	Compound A (@ < 2 L flow)

administered at high concentrations in the presence of low gas flow. Compound A can cause renal damage, though significant effects in humans is inconclusive.[3]

Given the potential toxic compound formation that can occur in the presence of desiccated CO_2 absorbents, it is important to have a visual indicator that signifies limited residual absorptive capacity. Ethyl violet is a pH indicator that changes from colorless to violet when sufficient CO_2 has been absorbed to decrease the pH below 10.3.

In addition, desiccated Baralyme can result in significant heat loss sufficient to ignite a fire, when used in the presence of sevoflurane.

WASTE GAS EVACUATION SYSTEMS

Though conclusive research is still needed to determine the precise effects of prolonged exposure to anesthetic waste gases, the consensus is that high levels of continuous exposure pose health hazards to operating room personnel. The National Institute for Occupational Safety and Health (NIOSH) has suggested limiting exposure to 2 parts per million (ppm) of halogenated anesthetics when used alone, and 0.5 ppm when used in combination, with no more than 25 ppm of nitrous oxide.[3] This data was published in 1977 and primarily referred to halothane and enflurane exposure. New data has not been published with specific recommendations for sevoflurane, desflurane, or isoflurane.

Modern ventilators are equipped with scavenger systems to reduce the levels of anesthetic gas in the operating room and surrounding areas. Scavenger systems consist of an adjustable pressure-limiting (APL) valve and a ventilator spill valve (part of the gas-collecting assembly), transfer tubing, a scavenging interface that can either be open or closed, disposal tubing, and a disposal assembly that uses either a vacuum or passive disposal.[3] The collecting assembly is designed to collect excess gas and then direct it through the transfer tubing to the scavenging interface. Of note, any waste anesthetic gas that fails to pass through the gas-collecting assembly, via leaking around the endotracheal tube or around the mask, will contaminate the operating room environment.

Gas leaving the collection assembly is then transferred to the scavenging interface via tubing. Inefficient scavenging can occur if the tubing becomes kinked or is too small to enable the appropriate gas flow. In addition, occlusion of the transfer tubing not only can prevent adequate gas scavenging but also can allow pressure to build in the breathing system, leading to barotrauma.

Gas leaving the tubing then enters the scavenging interface, which can be open or closed. Open interfaces require no pressure relief valves because they are open to the environment. This system requires a reservoir to collect the gas between breaths and is typically designed as a part of a central evacuation system. The interface is connected to an active vacuum disposal system that shuttles the gas to a safe evacuation area, which can be directly outside. The vacuum flow rate must be greater than the minute volume of gas entering the open interface or it will overwhelm the system and allow OR contamination.[3]

Closed interfaces have relief valves to release excess gas, protecting from barotrauma and excessive vacuum pressure. There are two types of closed interfaces: Positive pressure relief interfaces and interfaces that contain both positive and negative pressure relief valves. Interfaces containing only positive pressure relief valves can only be combined with passive disposal systems or risk overpressurizing the system. These interfaces do not contain reservoir bags and are designed to release waste when the pressure of the waste exceeds the calibrated positive pressure relief setting of the system. Interfaces that incorporate both positive and negative pressure relief valves utilize a reservoir bag to store excess waste until the vacuum evacuation system can release it. This system relies on the operator to adjust the vacuum to ensure proper reservoir bag inflation, allowing gas to escape through the positive pressure valve at pressures greater than 5 cmH_2O and retaining environment air if the system has negative pressure within it. The effectiveness of this system relies on proper interface gas flow and proper reservoir bag volume.

In addition to using scavenger systems, other ways that an anesthesia provider may limit anesthetic gas exposure is by using cuffed endotracheal tubes, turning off gas flow at the conclusion of an anesthetic, using circle systems, turning off the vaporizer when disconnecting the circuit, and checking the vaporizers and scavenger systems for leaks daily.

ERGONOMICS OF ANESTHESIA MACHINES AND SAFETY FEATURES (PROPORTIONING DEVICES, ROTAMETER CONFIGURATION, PRESSURE FAIL-SAFE)

Equipment-related morbidity is a common occurrence, in association with misuse of anesthesia machines and lack of familiarity with safety features. Thus, it is important that all anesthesia providers be knowledgeable of the basic design ergonomics of anesthesia machines and be familiar with the protective safety features designed to reduce anesthetic risk.

The anesthesia machine is designed to receive pipeline gases, cylinder gases, and anesthetic gases, then to deliver these safely to the patient, without risk of hypoxia or concentration-related toxicity. This is accomplished via a series of checks and valves. The first safety check is a color-coded, diameter index safety system that ensures the correct pipeline hose is connected to the correct gas source (i.e., green hose to the oxygen inlet). Second, the pin index safety system involves different-sized pins, specifically calibrated for gas cylinder type, to prevent accidental placement of a gas cylinder in the wrong position on the machine, thus preventing the delivery of a hypoxic gas mixture to the patient.

Another mechanism used to prevent delivery of a hypoxic gas mixture is the pressure regulator valve. It is designed to reduce cylinder pressure to 45 psig (less than pipeline supply), to encourage preferential use of the pipeline supply. This is a safety mechanism to prevent depletion of oxygen cylinders that would be used in case of pipeline failure. In case of oxygen supply failure, modern machines reduce the flow of other gases when oxygen pressure within the system is not adequate. This is accomplished by using oxygen to power the ventilator, to supply the flush valve, and to pressurize the safety devices. Thus, if the oxygen pressure falls below 20 psig, the fail-safe valve shuts off the flow of all other gases.

Gas then travels from the pressure-regulating system to the flow meters. Flow meters are vertical, glass, tapered tubes that regulate the gas flow rate within the tubes. Gas enters through the bottom of the flow meter, traveling up

$$\text{Resistance} = \frac{8 \cdot \mu \cdot L}{\pi \cdot r^4}$$

Figure 5.5 Poiseuille's law, indicating that resistance is proportional to tube length and fluid viscosity. Given that the radius is in the denominator and amplified to the fourth power, even a small increase in radius greatly reduces resistance. This formula is applicable for both gases and fluids (endotracheal tubes or venous access).

the tube and causing rotation of the bobbin (indicator float) equal to the upward force of gas flow and the downward force of gravity. The rate of gas flow through the flow meter is altered by gas viscosity, the friction between the bobbin and the glass, and the annular opening circumference around the bobbin. Poiseuille's law governs gas flow within the rotameter, because the volume in the tube is directly proportional to the pressure decrease across the length of the tube and to the fourth power of the tube radius and inversely proportional to the viscosity and length of the tube. See Figure 5.5 for Poiseuille's law.

Flow meters are arranged in series, with gas flowing from the bottom to the top and from left to right. Oxygen is usually found furthest to the right (furthest downstream) to prevent delivery of a hypoxic mixture if there is a leak in the system permitting gas escape. Newer machines also pneumatically link oxygen to nitrous oxide to mandate minimum oxygen concentration. The *oxygen analyzer* monitors the oxygen concentration in the system and sounds an alarm when a hypoxic mixture of gas is delivered. The oxygen analyzer differs from the fail-safe valve, the proportioning system, and the oxygen failure alarm in that it is the only one to detect a low-pressure leak upstream from the flow control valves (this is discussed more in Chapter 7, on ventilators).

Every anesthesia machine should be checked for leaks in the gas supply lines between the flow meters and the common gas outlet, prior to use. This is done by performing a low-pressure circuit leak test. The most common sources of leaks are from loose filler caps on the vaporizers, from cracked flow tubes, and from leaks between the gas flow tubes and the manifold (Figure 5.6). Each manufacturer has specific instructions on how to perform a low-pressure leak

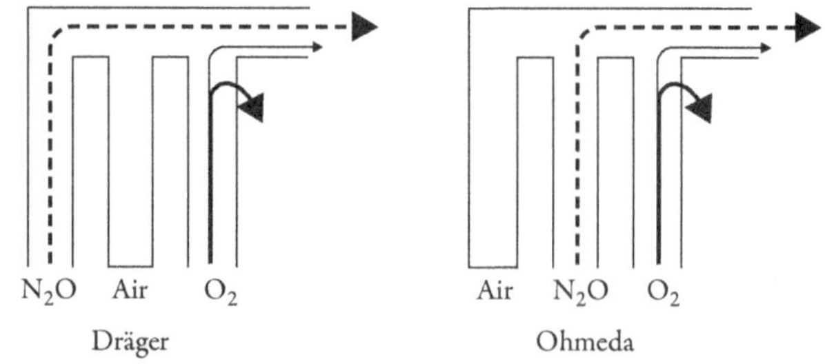

Figure 5.6 Diagram demonstrating different gas flow designs based on anesthesia machine manufacturer. The oxygen is always closest to the patient in order to minimize dilution. Image courtesy of George Williams, MD.

test for individual models. A leak test should be performed daily, at a minimum, and after a vaporizer is changed on the machine.

PHYSICS AND PHYSIOLOGY

Certain mechanical and physiologic principles will affect the breathing system in multiple ways. These include both laminar and turbulent flow to the lungs. We always consider what types of resistance the airway presents. There are multiple factors determining how we ventilate a patient. Elastic recoil, chest wall compliance, and pulmonary resistance must be determined. This can be considered as frictional resistance of the airways as well as the resistance of the chest wall tissue. Pulmonary resistance is the friction created as the lung tissues move against each other during inspiration. In normal patients this would account for only 20% of resistance, and the airway resistance would account for the majority of the resistance we encounter. There are comorbid illnesses that can greatly change resistance to air flow. Asthma, COPD, and bronchitis can change the airway resistance greatly, while diseases such as pulmonary fibrosis and asbestosis severely affect pulmonary resistance and not the airway. Although the net effect to the patient is similar in terms of overall resistance, the mechanism of these diseases varies greatly.

The natural tendency of the lungs is to collapse due to elastic recoil, therefore expiration is generally passive as gas is expelled out of the lungs. There is an opposite force created: As the thoracic cage moves outward, the lungs pose an inward force. The functional residual capacity (FRC) is determined when the inward and outward forces are equal. As mentioned above, when patients have decreased lung compliance their FRC is reduced. In this scenario this results in smaller tidal volumes. The result is the chest wall has to work harder to maintain adequate lung volumes. The end result is the patient's respiratory rate increases significantly. In cases where lung compliance is increased, due to disease, just the opposite happens. The increase in compliance makes filling the lungs easier, however there is a decrease in elastic recoil, resulting in air trapping, as seen in chronic obstructive lung disease.

The next consideration is the type of flow patterns; here we explore laminar, turbulent, and transitional flow. Laminar flow can be described as unobstructed flow through a single unbranched tube. This can be calculated by

$$\text{Pressure difference} = \text{flow} \times \text{resistance}.$$

So we can look at

$$\text{Resistance} = \text{pressure difference } (cmH_2O) / \text{flow (liters)}.$$

What this describes is at low flows the flow of air is typically laminar in certain areas of the pulmonary system; however, as flow increases, so does the turbulent flow. At low flows, the gas goes through a straight tube as a series of concentric cylinders that connect to each other. Fully developed flow has a parabolic profile with a velocity of zero at the wall and maximum velocity at the center. This provides a situation where some of the fresh gas will reach the end of the tube before the tube is filled with gas. Therefore the advantage to this type of flow is the alveolar ventilation can occur before tidal volume has become greater than the alveolar dead space.

$$R = 8 \times \text{length} \times \text{viscosity}/\pi \times (\text{radius})^4 = Pb - P_A/\text{flow}$$

Pb = barometric pressure
P_A = alveolar pressure.

Turbulent flow can be described as flow through branched or nonuniform tubes or high-flow delivery.

Much of the turbulent flow is seen in the upper airway. This refers to the nasal passages, nasal turbinates, and the nasal pharynx, oropharynx, and larynx. The highest resistance to airway flow resides in the upper airway and the medium-sized bronchi. The lowest resistance to air flow is actually in the smallest airways, because they are small uniform tubes arranged in parallel, thereby reducing resistance during normal respiration.

Transitional flow is described as a mixture of both laminar and turbulent air flow. This type of flow is seen in highly branched tubes distal to a partial obstruction. It is frequently in the highly branched upper bronchi. These factors affect our attempt to deliver anesthetics. In general, we are trying to adequately deliver the correct volume and pressure to arrive at a state where the alveolar pressure equilibrates with atmospheric pressure.

Humidity is described as the amount of water vapor present in the air. A fundamental to humidity is to understand how gaseous water is affected by both temperature and pressure. *Saturated vapor pressure* is a term describing the amount of water that can be held in a gaseous state for a given temperature and pressure. It is actually the temperature of the water, not the air, that is the important factor. Therefore, evaporation occurs when the water component of the gas is elevated in temperature and the water molecules gain more energy, allowing the evaporation. The converse occurs when the water temperature is decreased. The molecules have less energy and begin to attach to each other because condensation exceeds evaporation. This shift is known as the dew point.

Humidification of air in normal respiration happens by way of the inferior nasal turbinates. As cold air passes the turbinates, the air is warmed and water vapor is added. Moisture in the respiratory tract is necessary for ciliary function and mucus transport. Anesthetic gases have multiple effects on ciliary function and mucus production. There is a cooling effect of the dry gases used in anesthesia; this in turn leads to diminished ciliary function. The gases have a drying effect on the endothelial lining of the airway. This can lead to increased mucus production that becomes thicker and more difficult to expel. We can see this effect when an endotracheal tube or laryngeal mask airway is used. We are essentially bypassing the effect of warming and humidification from the nasal turbinates.

Heat and moisture exchange filters can be used to minimize the aforementioned effects of anesthetics even in longer cases or in patients with known reactive airway disease. The advantages of these devices are to both warm and humidify the airway. This is a sealed unit placed close to the patient end of the circuit. The units utilize a hygroscopic material. This effectively gathers moisture from the first breath, and then as the next delivery of cold dry gas passes the filter it is warmed and humidified via latent heat condensation. This is described as the energy required to transform matter from one state to another. This should be a consideration for all cases that will last for an extended period of time.

BREATHING SYSTEMS

This section discusses Mapleson breathing systems and the circle system.

MAPLESON SYSTEMS

The Mapleson breathing systems were first introduced in 1954 in the *British Journal of Anesthesia*. At that time the British physicist described five semiclosed circuits (A, B, C, D, and E). In 1974, Willis described the F system that was later added to the Mapleson systems.

The Mapleson A, or Magill circuit, is primarily used for gas inductions. This variant has fresh gas flow flowing past the reservoir bag through the breathing tube. The APL valve is next to the mask. During inspiration, fresh gas flows through the tubing and the APL valve closes due to negative pressure from the lungs. The circuit is primed from the reservoir. During expiration, the first 150 mL of expired gas (dead space gas) is expired down the circuit. The resistance from the bag and the patient overcomes the APL, and the CO_2-containing alveolar gas is then vented. For this flow pattern to occur, regular respiration and fresh gas flow equal to minute ventilation must occur to prevent rebreathing. In controlled ventilation, positive pressure is added. Thus, the APL is opened during inspiration and fresh gas is vented. During expiration alveolar gas is rebreathed before APL venting. High flows can overcome this effect. The high flow makes this circuit a bad choice for controlled ventilation. A variant of this circuit, the coaxial (Lack) version, places the APL at the machine, offering the ability to scavenge off the waste gas.

The Mapleson B circuit is a variant that places the reservoir bag at the distal end of the breathing tube and introduces the fresh gas flow just distal to the APL. This effectively doubles the minute ventilation. This variant is not used as often because of the increased demand on gas flows.

The Mapleson C circuit is a shortened version of the Mapleson B circuit. Once again, this variant demands high flows, two times the minute ventilation. The Water's circuit is more common for this circuit, and is used more often for resuscitation rather than anesthesia delivery.

The Mapleson D circuit is known as an efferent circuit, where the reservoir bag is on the expiratory limb of the circuit. The fresh gas flow is next to the mask. The gas flow starts from negative pressure from the patient. During exhalation the gas begins to refill the bag, as simultaneously fresh gas fills the tube. At this time the fresh, alveolar, and dead space gas are mixed. Exhaled gases are vented when the pressure exceeds the APL valve settings. In this setting, to avoid rebreathing, 150 mg/kg/min of fresh gas flow is required. Therefore this system is more effective in a controlled ventilation setting. A common variant of the Mapleson D circuit is a coaxial version, Bain (1972). In this circuit, fresh gas flows through the inner tube and exhaled gas through the outer hose. As with the Lack breathing system, care must be taken to assure good connection to the machine. Inadvertent disconnection of the inspiratory tube is not readily apparent and can result in a large dead space.

The Mapleson E, or the Ayre's T-piece, was specifically designed for infant HEENT surgery in 1937. This variant has the fresh gas flow delivered to the T-piece next to the mask. High gas flows are necessary to prevent rebreathing at three times the minute ventilation.

The Mapleson F, or the Jackson-Reese modification, adds a reservoir bag to the circuit. This allows for controlled ventilation as well as scavenging of waste gases.

CIRCLE SYSTEM

The circle system is so named because of the circular arrangement of its components. This is the most popular breathing system in United States.

It has seven components (very important): (1) a fresh gas inflow source; (2) inspiratory and expiratory unidirectional valves; (3) inspiratory and expiratory corrugated tubes; (4) a Y-piece connector; (5) an overflow or pop-off valve, referred to as the APL valve; (6) a reservoir bag; and (7) a canister containing a CO_2 absorbent. The most important component is the CO_2 absorbent in the canister, as it removes all the exhaled CO_2 by a chemical reaction with soda lime or its equivalent. It allows partial rebreathing of the remaining gases in the exhaled air; this feature makes it unique.

Depending on the position of the components and the fresh gas flow rate, the circle system has different variations. The circle system can also be divided into semiopen, semiclosed, and closed systems. The semiopen system does not allow any rebreathing but requires very high fresh gas flow. The semiclosed system, which is the most commonly used system in the United States, allows rebreathing of the gases. The closed circle system requires a fresh gas flow rate that is almost equal to the rate at which the gases are being taken up or consumed by the patient. The advantage of rebreathing is that it conserves airway moisture and body heat. It also prevents pollution of the surrounding area by the exhaled anesthetic gases when the fresh gas flow rate is set at less than the patient's minute ventilation.

Disadvantages of circle system include the increased resistance from the unidirectional valves and the CO_2 absorber. These circuits are bulky and lack portability. The circuit is very complex with lots of connections, which increases the chances for its malfunctioning or disconnection. During induction of anesthesia, there in increased uptake of volatile anesthetic by the patient until the minimum alveolar concentration (MAC) of the volatile anesthetic is reached. During this phase, dilution of the volatile anesthetic occurs as a result of the rebreathing of exhaled gases, which are depleted in volatile anesthetics. The dilutional effect of gases can be counterbalanced by increasing the delivered concentration of the volatile anesthetic. This is more commonly seen in a semiclosed circle system.

Components of the Circle System

Fresh gas inlet and unidirectional valves: The fresh gas in the circle system is delivered by the common gas outlet on the anesthesia machine.

There are two unidirectional valves—one each in the inspiratory and the expiratory system. The function of these valves is to provide positive pressure ventilation and to prevent rebreathing of exhaled gases until they have passed through the CO_2 absorber canister and have been replenished with O_2. The valves in most of the circle systems are of Turret's type. As the pressure in the system increases, the disc in the valve is lifted up to allow the gas to flow.

If the unidirectional valve is stuck in the open position, rebreathing and hypercapnia can occur. If the valve is stuck in the closed position, complete obstruction of the breathing system occurs. Breath stacking and barotrauma can happen when the unidirectional valve in the expiratory limb is stuck in the closed position. When it functions properly, the dead space in the system is the air present between the Y-piece and the patient.

Corrugated rubber tubing: This acts as a carrier of the gases to and from the patient. They are made corrugated to prevent kinking, provide flexibility, and make gas flow turbulent instead of laminar. The large bore of the tubing decreases resistance to gas flow.

Y-piece connector: It has an outer diameter of 22 mm and inner diameter of 15 mm to fit into the face mask and endotracheal tube respectively. It is present at the patient end of the circuit.

Adjustable pressure-limiting (APL) valve: This valve is also called the "pop-off" valve, as pressure "pops off" the resistor in the valve and allows outward flow. The APL valve is adjusted when the patient is being ventilated manually on bag mode to provide assisted or controlled breaths. The excess gas is vented out through it into the anesthetic waste gas scavenging system. A fully opened APL valve helps reduce the resistance in the breathing system while patient is spontaneously breathing.

Reservoir bag: The spontaneous inspiratory flow rate is far greater than the fresh gas flows (3–5 L/min) from the anesthesia machine. The gas reservoir bag maintains sufficient volume of reserve gas to fulfill the patient's spontaneous inspiratory flow rate up to 60 L/min. It maintains the pressure in the circuit below 60 cmH_2O due to its distensibility even when the APL valve is closed. This is one of the safety features in the circle system when the bag/vent selector switch is set on bag mode. Bags are available in different sizes. The American Society for Testing and Materials (ASTM) standard for the reservoir bag requires that the pressure shall not be less than 30 cmH_2O or more than 50 cmH_2O for a bag of 1.5 liters or less when the bag is inflated to four times its size. Furthermore, the pressure should not be less than 35 cmH_2O or more than 60 cmH_2O when a bag larger than 1.5 liters is inflated to four times its size. The standard size reservoir bag for adults is 3 liters.

The most efficient arrangement of components in the circle system to achieve the highest conservation of fresh gases is to have with the unidirectional valves near the patient and the pop-off valve just downstream from the expiratory valve. This increases the efficiency by eliminating the alveolar gases and preserving the dead space gases in the system. But the practical arrangement allows mixing of alveolar and dead space gases before venting.

Three rules must be followed to prevent CO_2 rebreathing: (1) A unidirectional valve must be located between the patient and the reservoir bag on both the inspiratory and the expiratory limbs of the circuit, (2) the fresh gas inflow cannot enter the circuit between the expiratory valve and the patient, and (3) the overflow (pop-off) valve cannot be located between the patient and the inspiratory valve. If these rules are followed, any arrangement of the other components prevents rebreathing of CO_2.

The fresh gas coming from the anesthesia machine flows as following:

Fresh gas inlet → corrugated breathing tube → inspiratory valve → inspiratory limb of Y-piece → patient's airway → expiratory limb of Y-piece → corrugated breathing tube → expiratory valve → reservoir bag and

APL valve or ventilator → CO_2 absorber → gas after the CO_2 absorption mixes with fresh gas flowing from anesthesia machine → patient's airway through corrugated breathing tube.

There are various diagrams displaying the above items, but understanding the flow pattern as described above can minimize confusion regarding this important concept.

Circle System for Pediatric Patients

Previously there were special pediatric circle systems with smaller CO_2 absorber canisters. Now there is no difference in the size of the canister, but the system may have smaller-diameter corrugated breathing tubes and a smaller reservoir bag. Studies have shown that the adult circle system can be used for pediatric anesthesia with low fresh gas flows.

Various authors have described the classification of breathing systems, often on the basis of functions like rebreathing and non-rebreathing. A breathing system can also be classified—on the basis of presence and absence of (1) a reservoir bag, (2) rebreathing, (3) a CO_2 absorber canister, (4) directional valves—into the following types according to Dripps, Ekenhoff, and Vandam, but this seemingly more complex and confusing classification is avoided these days:

1. Insufflation System: When the gases are directly delivered to the patient's airway without any directional valve or a reservoir bag and without passing them through a CO_2 absorber canister. Ventilation cannot be controlled by this technique, and inspired gas contains unpredictable amounts of entrained atmospheric air. This is an open breathing system, also called a noncircle breathing system.
2. Open System: This system has a unidirectional valve that directs exhaled air into atmosphere, with minimal rebreathing. Patient receives only the mixture of air that is delivered by the anesthesia machine. There is no CO_2 absorber, and a reservoir bag may or may not be present.
3. Semiopen System: In this system, rebreathing occurs depending on the fresh gas flow rate. The exhaled gases from the patient flow out of the system and into the inspiratory line to be rebreathed. In this system, the directional valves and the reservoir bag are optional. No chemical absorption of the CO_2 occurs in this system.
4. Semiclosed System: in this system, minimal rebreathing happens, because some of the exhaled gas exits out of the system but some gets mixed with the fresh gas flow. Unidirectional valves, a reservoir bag, and a CO_2 absorber all are present in the system.
5. Closed System: In this system, complete rebreathing occurs, as the exhaled gases mix with the fresh gas flow after complete absorption of CO_2 from the expired gas. The system uses a reservoir bag and unidirectional valves.

REFERENCES

1. Butterworth I, Mackey D, Wasnick J. *Clinical Anesthesiology*. 5th ed. Philadelphia, PA: McGraw-Hill; 2013.
2. Dumont C, Tiep B. Using a reservoir nasal cannula in acute care. *Crit Care Nurse*. 2002;22(4):41–46.
3. Barash P, Cullen B, Stoelting R, Cahalan M, Stock M. *Clinical Anesthesia*. 6th ed. Philadelphia, PA: Lippincott Williams & Wilkins; 2009.

FURTHER READING

Dorsch JA, Dorsch SE. *Understanding Anesthesia Equipment*. 5th ed. Philadelphia, PA: Lippincott Williams & Wilkins; 2008.

Miller R, Pardo M. *Basics of Anesthesia*. 6th ed. Philadelphia, PA: Elsevier; 2011.

QUESTIONS

1. What is the highest FiO2 that can be delivered via nasal cannula?
   A. 0.21
   B. 0.30
   C. 0.44
   D. 0.65

2. How much oxygen can be stored in the reservoir of a reservoir-containing nasal cannula?
   A. 10 mL
   B. 20 mL
   C. 30 mL
   D. 40 mL

3. A desiccated Baralyme absorber can combine with desflurane to form what toxic byproduct?
   A. Compound A
   B. Barium hydroxide
   C. Carbon monoxide
   D. Sodium hydroxide

4. The National Institute for Occupational Safety and Health has suggested limiting the exposure to a halogenated agent, when it is the sole anesthetic, to what amount?
   A. 0.5 ppm
   B. 0.8 ppm
   C. 1.3 ppm
   D. 2.0 ppm

5. The pin-index safety system is designed to prevent the incorrect connection of what to the anesthesia machine?
   A. Pipeline supply
   B. Flow meter
   C. Scavenger unit
   D. Gas cylinder

6. Which of the following components is NOT included in a circle system?
   A. Expiratory corrugated tube
   B. Inspiratory bidirectional valve
   C. Reservoir bag
   D. CO_2 absorbent
   E. Fresh gas inflow source

7. Which of the following BEST describes respiratory tract physiology?
   A. Air humidification occurs in the trachea.
   B. Turbulent flow occurs in the nasal passages.
   C. Air flow resistance is lowest in small airways.
   D. Tachypnea increases the dew point.
   E. Mucociliary clearance is inhibited by volatile anesthetics.

8. Which of the following is NOT a safety feature in the circle system?
   A. Y-piece connector
   B. Reservoir bag
   C. Corrugated tubing
   D. APL valve
   E. Common gas outlet

ANSWERS

1. C. An FiO2 of up to 0.44 can be delivered via nasal cannula when a rate of 6 L/min is used.
2. B. Flow rates higher than 4 liters can be associated with epistaxis if not properly humidified. A potential solution is to use a reservoir nasal cannula. These cannulas can store approximately 20 mL of oxygen in the reservoir, increasing the amount of oxygen available to the patient at inspiration, but at a decreased required flow rate.
3. C. A desiccated Baralyme absorber can combine with desflurane to produce significant amounts of carbon monoxide that can poison a patient.
4. D. The National Institute for Occupational Safety and Health (NIOSH) has suggested limiting exposure to 2 parts per million (ppm) of halogenated anesthetics when used alone, and 0.5 ppm when used in combination, with no more than 25 ppm of nitrous oxide.
5. D. The pin index safety system involves different-sized pins, specifically calibrated for gas cylinder type, to prevent accidental placement of a gas cylinder in the wrong position on the machine, thus preventing the delivery of a hypoxic gas mixture to the patient.
6. B. Recall that a circle system has seven components (very important): (1) a fresh gas inflow source; (2) inspiratory and expiratory unidirectional valves; (3) inspiratory and expiratory corrugated tubes; (4) a Y-piece connector; (5) an overflow or pop-off valve, referred to as the APL valve; (6) a reservoir bag; and (7) a canister containing a CO_2 absorbent. Unidirectional valves are required to prevent backflow of gas to the patient and therefore CO_2 rebreathing. The other components are included in a circle system.
7. E. Recall that there is a cooling effect from the dry anesthetic gases administered on the normal cilia in the patient, and this drying effect results in reduced mucociliary clearance. This leads to a buildup of mucus that is thicker and more difficult to expel. Air humidification occurs in the upper airway, namely the nasal turbinates. Turbulent flow occurs in the nasal passages, nasal pharynx, oropharynx, and larynx (occurs in order of high-flow delivery or branched/nonuniform tubes. Tachypnea is not directly related to the dew point; this answer is a distracter.
8. E. While the common gas outlet is necessary to keep the patient alive, it is not in itself a safety feature. The APL valve allows for reduction in pressure administered to the patient during manual ventilation. The reservoir bag is designed to prevent barotrauma by expanding up to four times its standard volume without exceeding 60 cmH_2O. Corrugated tubes are used in order to prevent kinking of the circuit. The Y-piece connector has a set diameter at the patient end in order to prevent incorrect connection to other system components (i.e., scavenger, etc.).

6.

MONITORING METHODS

Shelly-Anne Rodriguez and Joanne Spaliaras

NEUROMUSCULAR FUNCTION

NERVE SIMULATORS

In the clinical practice of anesthesia where paralytic agents are needed, an objective means to evaluate the return of muscle strength is important to ensure patient safety during emergence and the removal of airway devices. A nerve stimulator is useful when it is easy to operate and has the ability to deliver current effectively by way of single twitch, train of four (TOF), tetanic, and double burst impulses (Table 6.1).[1,2]

Assessment of impulse response is more accurately determined by touch (tactile) than visual observation. Peripheral sites frequently chosen for stimulation are more easily blocked or require less non-depolarizing blocker (NDB) agent than the more resistant diaphragm and laryngeal muscles. This is at odds with the fact that the diaphragm has a more rapid onset of block (brisk perfusion).[3] It is advantageous to monitor recovery from paralysis in more NDB-sensitive sites like the adductor pollicis, as the diaphragm is the first muscle to recover prior to the monitored hand. Thus, when strong tactile TOF stimulus is noted in the thumb, the diaphragm and respiratory muscles have likely recovered.[1,2]

Nerve stimulators are battery powered and are capable of creating a monophasic 0.1–0.3 msec pulse with a constant 25–80 mA current. This impulse is approximately 20% greater than what is needed to depolarize a peripheral nerve. It should have safety parameters to monitor current output, leaks, and battery life. Surface gel silver-silver electrodes are used to create contact with a clean site over the nerve of interest. Depolarization is maximized when the electrodes are separated by 3–6 cm with the negative electrode in a distal position on dry and normothermic skin. This ensures that current transmission will not be impeded by elevated skin resistance.[1–3] Frequent sites for assessment are the ulnar nerve (adductor pollicis), facial nerve (orbicularis oculi), temporal branch of the facial nerve (corrugator supercilli; eyebrow movement), and posterior tibial nerve sites.[2]

In combination with traditional clinical signs of returning muscle strength, nerve stimulators are put to practical use during the perioperative period. Initiation of TOF or single twitch stimulus prior to administration of a paralytic agent can help gauge readiness for endotracheal intubation. Eyebrow movement from corrugator supercilli stimulation best predicts relaxation of the vocal cords.[3] This is particularly helpful given the interpatient variability in neuromuscular block sensitivity. Maintenance of good surgical conditions can be monitored intraoperatively with periodic TOF stimulus. If a strong block is required with zero TOF response, post-tetanic count (PTC) is a very useful monitoring tool in the unconscious patient. Adductor pollicis correlates well with upper airway geniohyoid muscle recovery during emergence.[3] Typically, safe reversal of NDB can be accomplished in the presence of two or greater TOF contractions.[1–3] However, despite four TOF response and full double burst stimulation (DBS) response, residual blockade may exist.[4]

ELECTROMYOGRAPHY

Controversy has been waning regarding the use of nerve stimulators to assess return of neuromuscular receptor site activity. However, when a nerve stimulator is used, very rarely is quantified data obtained or documented. Electromyography (EMG) is one of several recording modalities used to note muscle response to stimulated peripheral nerves. Electromyography allows for graphic visualization of measured action potentials (amplitude) generated along the ulnar or median nerves during contraction of thenar or hypothenar muscle groups.[2,3] This information regarding muscle group electrical activity is presented as a TOF ration or a percentage of baseline strength. The setup is complex, with precise placement of surface or needle electrodes. Expense and lack of product availability have made use of EMG impractical in anesthetizing locations. Laryngeal and

Table 6.1 MODES OF ELECTRICAL PERIPHERAL NERVE STIMULATION

STIMULUS	CHARACTER	MEASUREMENT
Double Burst Stimulation (DBS)	Two 50-Hz bursts; three 0.2 ms impulses per burst; 750 ms between the two bursts	2nd DBS amplitude/1st DBS amplitude No paralysis—2 equal contractions Paralysis—weaker 2nd contraction
Train of Four (TOF)	Four bursts; 0.5 s between each burst; TOF repeated every 10–20 s	4th TOF amplitude/1st TOF amplitude No paralysis—4 equal contractions NDB—fade DB—no fade DB—fade present = Phase II Block
Single Twitch Stimulation (STS)	One burst every 1 s (1.0Hz) to 10 s (0.1Hz)	NDB, DB—decreased amplitude of contraction to absence of contraction
Tetanic Stimulation*	50 Hz burst given over 5 s Wait 6 minutes between bursts to avoid prolonged antagonism (15, 18miller)	No paralysis, DB—unweakened contraction for 5 s NDB, Phase II DB—fade; post-tetanic facilitation
Post-Tetanic Count Stimulation (PTC)*	50Hz burst given over 5 s, then 1.0 Hz bursts	Deep NDB—no TOF, post-tetanic facilitation count of 1–16 twitches present

*Painful; not appropriate in the conscious patient.

Adapted from Miller RD, ed. *Miller's Anesthesia*. 7th ed. Philadelphia, PA: Churchill Livingstone, Elsevier; 2010.

diaphragmatic monitoring is possible, but it is used almost exclusively for research purposes.

VENTILATION

The American Society of Anesthesiologists Standard II, 3.2.3, dictates that "when ventilation is controlled by a mechanical ventilator, there shall be in continuous use a device that is capable of detecting disconnection of components of the breathing system. The device must give an audible signal when its alarm threshold is exceeded." Disconnect properties are associated with pressure, volume, and oxygen and carbon dioxide levels.

RESPIROMETERS

Inspiratory and expiratory gas can be monitored by direct airflow sensors (i.e., gas sampling, thermocouples, pinwheels) or indirectly from thoracic movements (i.e., ECG analysis, impedance, strain gauges).[2] Respirometers measure respiratory rate and gas volumes and can calculate minute ventilation. The force applied to the wheel or vane of the respirometer is driven by the gas flow. This gas flow generates the momentum that turns the vane. How fast or slow each rotation occurs is directly impacted by how heavy the vane is, the density and temperature of the gas, and the amount of resistance the vane must overcome.[3] A transducer counts the number of respirations and quantifies the gas volume by mechanical or optic means.

Respirometers are rotating (i.e., Wright's respirometer model) or stationary (i.e., sealed Drager Spiromed respirometer). The 1955 design of Wright's respirometer[2] is represented by a more up-to-date version in the Ohmeda 5400 volume monitor (optical transducer). Unlike the original design, which faced accuracy challenges at low flow rates (<2L/min) and small tidal volumes (i.e., spontaneously breathing infants), this model compensates for both low and high flow states. The Drager Spiromed electronically measures gas flow across rotating dumbbells within a sealed chamber. Flow is still impacted by gas density and temperature, however, reversal of flow can now be detected and a mechanical gauge is no longer needed to measure volume.[3]

SPIROMETRY

Spirometry allows for the comparison of flow, volume, and pressure (y-axis) against time (x-axis) (Figure 6.1). Graphic representations highlight changes in resistance and compliance and the traits of different modes of ventilation. These relationships can be viewed as quantitative values or as real-time "loops" to aid with clinical decision-making. Volume-control ventilation begins by briskly reaching peak

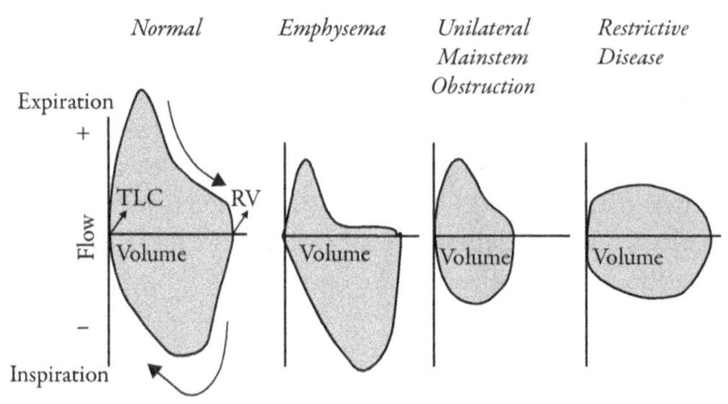

Figure 6.1 Flow-volume loops.

inspiratory pressure (PIP) with a "box-like" plateau and a short inspiratory period. In contrast, pressure control ventilation reaches PIP as a "peak" then gradually slopes down over a longer inspiratory period.

Spirograms can be performed in the awake or anesthetized patient and demonstrate the size and speed of an exhaled tidal volume expressed as FEV1, FIV1, and FVC. Airway function can best be evaluated without the bias of patient effort by comparing the volume expired after 25% of the FVC has been exhaled with the volume when 25% of the FVC remains.[2,3,5]

Resistance during breathing and mechanical ventilation is the sum of resistances contributed by the thorax and the lung, where R = driving pressure/flow rate (Ohm's law)[2] with flow rate determinants varying for turbulent (Bernoulli's equation) and laminar (Hagen-Poiseuille law) flow.[3] *Compliance* (change in volume/change in pressure) is the slope of the pressure-volume loop. An increase in compliance produces an increase in the slope of the loop (steeper, moving toward the y-axis) and larger tidal volumes.[2,3,5] By monitoring these patterns in combination with pressure alarms and continuous end-tidal carbon dioxide ($ETCO_2$) monitoring,[3] ventilator and cardiopulmonary problems (Table 6.2) can be more succinctly managed.

GAS CONCENTRATIONS

Over the past 50 years or so, there has been a rapid acceleration in the development of technology to monitor gas concentrations. Since the first beginnings, when White and Wardley-Smith used silicone strips to capture gas particles,[6] sophisticated devices have been artfully engineered to take advantage of several electromagnetic principles. There are many clinical clues that can be exploited from monitoring inspired and expired gases (Table 6.3).[1-3] The provision of continuous data affords time sensitive information regarding potentially ominous cardiovascular and respiratory changes. This is supported by the American Society of Anesthesiologists Standards for Basic Anesthetic Monitoring, in that the "continual monitoring for the presence of expired carbon dioxide shall be performed unless invalidated by the nature of the patient, procedure or equipment—Quantitative monitoring of the volume of expired gas is strongly encouraged."[7]

OXYGEN

Gas analyzers are built on the principles described by the Lambert-Beer law of absorption, which subscribes determination of inspired and expired gas sample fractions.[2] There are three models for scrutinizing inspired oxygen content: (1) paramagnetic oxygen sensors, (2) polargraphic oxygen sensors and (3) galvanic cell oxygen sensors. These analyzers are typically placed within the inspiratory limb of the anesthesia machine. They function by monitoring current changes that occur as a result of electron movement. Expired oxygen may be measured by (1) mass spectrometry, (2) Raman scattering, or (3) infrared absorption spectrophotometry (IRAS).[1]

Mass spectrometry showers a gas sample with electrons, breaking the gas up into ion fragments. Each particle has a given weight and charge that allows each element to be identified and quantified when it lands on a detector plate.[1,2] *Raman scattering* uses an argon laser to direct photons at a gas. When the photons hit the gas samples, scattered photons constitute a characteristic spectrum for molecule identification.

CARBON DIOXIDE

Advanced gas analysis allows for the monitoring and quantification of oxygen, carbon dioxide, and nitrogen in inspired and expired volumes. Gas analyzers are built on the principles described by the Beer-Lambert law allowing for the determination of inspired and expired gas sample fractions.[3] Perhaps the gas with the greatest diversity of clinical applications in disease interpretation is carbon dioxide (CO_2), which exists in a continuum between the gas and liquid phases in human tissues:

$$CO_2 + H_2O <\cdot> H_2CO_3^- + H^+ <\cdot> CO_3^{2-} + H^+$$

Table 6.2 ENDOTRACHEAL TUBE PLACEMENT CONFIRMATION AND TROUBLE SHOOTING

	VOLUME	PRESSURE	COMPLIANCE	FLOW	LOOP SHIFT
Disconnect/Apnea	Decreased	Decreased	Increased	Unimpeded	No loop observed
Esophageal Intubation	Decreased	Increased	Decreased	Decreased/none	Right; reduced globally
Endobronchial Intubation	Decreased	Increased (Paw)	Decreased	Decreased (expiratory)	Down, right; narrower; decreased loop area
Obstructed ETT	Decreased	Increased (Paw and inspiratory pressure)	Decreased	Decreased	Down, right; wider; increased loop area

Adapted from references 1,2,4

Table 6.3 GAS MONITORING CAN AUGMENT CLINICAL DECISION MAKING DURING THE PERIANESTHETIC PERIOD

Oxygen	**Errors in gas delivery, machine malfunction, disconnect, hypoxic gas delivery**
Carbon Dioxide	**Errors in gas delivery, machine malfunction, disconnect, systems leaks, endotracheal tube/laryngeal mask/mask conform, ventilation, malignant hyperthermia, obstruction, bronchospasm, venous air embolism, adequate CPR**
Nitrogen	**Errors in gas delivery, machine malfunction, system leaks, venous air embolism, preoxygenation effectivity**
Inhaled Agents, N_2O	**Errors in gas delivery, machine malfunction, disconnect, vaporizer malfunction**

Adapted from references 2,3,4

Carbon dioxide shifts through tissue, plasma, and erythrocyte compartments, eventually creating an arterial to alveolar gradient in the lung. During visualization of the respiratory cycle on the capnogram, the point of maximal expiratory CO_2 flow is the end-tidal value ($ETCO_2$), before inspiration begins.[1–3,8] In the awake patient, capnometers can best estimate alveolar and thus arterial CO_2 partial pressure ($PaCO_2$). This assumes the absence of ventilation–perfusion mismatch and no problems with diffusion of CO_2 in the capillary bed.[2] Under anesthesia, a 5–10 mmHg difference exists. This is a noninvasive technique of sampling compared with arterial blood gas measurements and is a recommended standard of monitoring ventilation.[7] Much can be inferred from changes in $ETCO_2$ (Figure 6.2).[1]

Carbon dioxide is sampled by (1) mainstream sampling, with a device situated within the breathing circuit, or with (2) sidestream sampling. Mainstream sampling gives accurate real time digital or pH sensitive chemical output (color change), but has the disadvantage of being a bulky device within the airway. More frequently, gas is removed at a rate of 200–400 mL/min from the tidal volume and sent to a separate chamber for measurement and output after a brief time delay.[2] Moisture and kinking of the sample line can affect values, but are easily overcome with vigilant inspection.

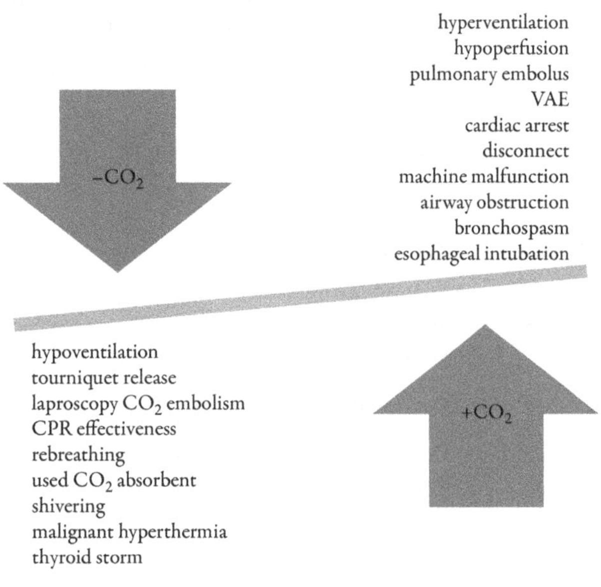

Figure 6.2 Alterations in end-tidal CO_2 tracing provide information during patient management.

The most commonly used method for all gas analysis is IRAS, although mass spectrometry and Raman scattering can also appraise CO_2 levels. In IRAS, a gas sample is exposed to infrared light while temperature, pressure, and acoustic conditions are manipulated. The resulting generated currents are compared with known gas signatures predicted by the Beer-Lambert law. This analysis requires a series of complex algorithms and calculations, as gases are in constant motion and tend to interact with each other.[1,2,8] Xenon gas cannot be distinguished by this method.[1]

NITROGEN, ANESTHETIC GASES, NITROUS OXIDE

Scrutiny of nitrogen gas from a mixed expired sample can be calculated directly by Raman scattering and with indirect inference via IRAS monitoring.[1] Continuous monitoring during preoxygenation prior to induction of anesthesia can report information regarding denitrogenation of the functional residual capacity of the lung and in exchange for oxygen. A sudden increase in nitrogen gas levels may indicate the occurrence of air emboli or leaks in the breathing system. As described in Table 6.3, monitoring of inhaled volatile agents and nitrous oxide can intercept problems with the breathing circuit, disconnect problems, or vaporizer malfunction.[1,2]

TEMPERATURE

INTRODUCTION

General and regional anesthesia blunt adaptive behavioral and physiologic thermoregulatory mechanisms designed to maintain body temperature.[1] Derailed transmissions between afferent C fibers (heat) and A delta fibers (cold) via the spinothalamic tract and hypothalamus, necessitate active warming via blankets, forced air devices (gold standard),[1,9] warmed intravenous solutions, and/or heating lamps in the absence of behavioral changes. The majority of the 0.5 to 1.5 degrees centigrade of body heat lost during the first 30 minutes of sedation is as a result of heat movement from the central to peripheral tissues.[2] Radiative (major), convective, evaporative, and conductive heat losses are not without consequences. Mild body temperature reductions can triple the risk for myocardial infarction and wound infections and increase the risks for coagulopathy, blood loss, and length of stay.[1,2] In order to offset these risks, quick and reliable temperature monitoring modalities need to be in place.

DESIGN

The molecules of a given substance are in constant motion. The velocity at which these molecules move, expand, and interact is a function of the elemental electrostatic forces and changes in temperature at a constant pressure.[3] Temperature monitoring utilizes several engineering and electrical principles to transduce the kinetic ($KE = mv^2$) and volume changes of one or more substances adjacent to the body. This information is amplified and expressed as a reproducible signal for intermittent or continuous monitoring.[2] Table 6.4 outlines different types of monitoring devices and their challenges.

PERIOPERATIVE APPLICATIONS

Temperature can be monitored at central or peripheral sites. Core sites such as the pulmonary artery, distal third of the esophagus, tympanic membrane, and nasopharynx produce accurate values with proper probe positioning and insulation.[3] The axillary site in pediatric patients is an acceptable core measurement. Rectal and bladder temperature sites are less reliable due to stool and low urine flow confounders. Accurate core temperature values are especially vital during periods of rapid body temperature fluctuation (i.e., massive blood transfusion, cardiopulmonary bypass, malignant hyperthermia).[1–3]

Once a monitoring modality is chosen, continuous observation during initial heat redistribution and exposure to potential malignant hyperthermia triggers will allow for early intervention and diagnosis (Table 6.5).

OXYGEN

OXIMETRY

Three designs of oxygen analyzer systems exist to ensure that hypoxic gases are not delivered to patients (Table 6.6). Per the ASA Standards for Basic Anesthetic Monitoring, "assessment of color and oxygenation via pulse oximetry is necessary during each anesthetic" as well as "an anesthesia breathing system measured by an oxygen analyzer with alarms for low oxygen concentration limits."[7] To minimize the chance of hypoxia, oxygen sensors are placed within the inspiratory limb of the breathing circuit. Oximeters must quickly and accurately quantify oxygen concentration and be easily calibrated.[2]

Table 6.4 TEMPERATURE MONITORING DEVICES

DEVICE	ENGINEERING	ADVANTAGES	DISADVANTAGES
Thermistors	Metal-oxide semiconductors; decrease in resistance when heated	Low cost, small size, reliable quick readings. (Examples: pulmonary artery catheter, esophageal probes)	Probe positioning; damage to components may increase resistance & false low temperature readings
Resistance Thermometers	Increase in resistance when heated; platinum		
Thermocouples	Copper-nickel differential heating properties; Seeback Effect; voltage produced from temperature difference between two metals.	Low cost, small size, reliable	More complex design
Infrared Thermopile	Radiant heat intercepted at detector site that translates an electrical signal for temperature measurement	Reliable, noninvasive. (Examples: external auditory meatus probe, temporal artery forehead scanner)	Cost, probe positioning; cerumen
Mercury	Liquid mercury in glass	Cost; ease of use; large range of measurement (−39 to 250 degrees centigrade)	Toxic; 3 minutes for measurement; glass fragility
Liquid Crystal	Matrix sensitive to temperature and pressure; changes in matrix symmetry > changes in plane of polarized light	Low cost, small size (Example: skin temperature monitor; increased temperature with good neural blockade—AE)	Positioning, decreased reliability; no core temperature measure.

Adapted from references 1,2,3

Table 6.5 OVERVIEW OF TEMPERATURE-MONITORING RECOMMENDATIONS

GOVERNING BODY	RECOMMENDED PRACTICE GUIDELINES
1. American Society of Anesthesiologists, Standards for Basic Anesthetic Monitoring (effective July 1, 2011)	Standard 5, 5.2 Methods—"Every patient receiving anesthesia shall have temperature monitored when clinically significant changes in body temperature are intended, anticipated or suspected."[7]
2. Surgical Care Improvement Project, Centers for Medicare and Medicaid Services.	"patients undergoing general or neuraxial anesthesia > 60 minutes should have at least one body temperature equal to or greater than 36 degrees centigrade 30 minutes prior to or the 15 minutes immediately after anesthesia end time"[2]
3. US Malignant Hyperthermia Association (*Anesthesiology* 1998;89:1298–1300). A proposal for new temperature monitoring and thermal management guidelines.)	"core temperature measurement when under GA for > 30 minutes ... temperature measurement during regional anesthesia ... maintain intraoperative core temperature >36 degrees centigrade."[3]

Adapted from references 1,2,3

CO-OXIMETRY

Laboratory co-oximetry is the basis from which pulse oximetry R ratio calibration data was calculated from human volunteers.[10] This in vitro analysis incorporated the Lambert-Beer law to calculate extinction coefficient constants for hemoglobin species exposed to various wavelengths of light.[1,2] It is this data that has allowed for the determination of the oxygen-hemoglobin dissociation curve and estimations of arterial oxyhemoglobin saturation (SaO_2) from pulse oximetry saturation measurements (SpO_2).[3,10]

Co-oximetry measures the *fractional saturation* of hemoglobin moieties (Equation 1)[1–3] utilizing multiple wavelengths and spectrophotometry; the application of the Lambert-Beer law (Equation 2).[1–3] In short, the quantity of hemoglobin in a blood sample can be determined by how each species absorbs wavelengths of light (Table 6.7). This is helpful when elevation of methemoglobin (MetHb) or carboxyhemoglobin (COHb) is suspected. Pulse oximetry uses *functional saturation* (Equation 3)[1–3] and cannot determine true fractional saturation of each hemoglobin species. Clinical use of the co-oximeter is often seen in facilities engaged in the management of inhalation and poisoning injuries.[1,3]

Equation 1. Fractional Saturation

$$SaO_2 = \frac{HbO_2}{HbO_2 + Hb + COHb + MetHb} \times 100\%$$

Equation 2. Lambert-Beer Law

Transmitted light
= Incident light × (-optical path length
× solution concentration × extinction coefficient)

Equation 3. Functional Saturation

$$SpO_2 = HbO_2 / HbO_2 + Hb \times 100\%$$

PULSE OXIMETRY

It was only in 1986 that pulse oximetry became a monitoring standard for anesthetized patients.[7] This was made possible by the development of easy to use and accurate continuous estimation[1] of hemoglobin oxygen saturation and pulse rate. Spectrophotometry uses red light (660 nm) and near infrared light (940 nm) from light-emitting

Table 6.6 OXYGEN ANALYZER SYSTEMS

ANALYZERS	ENGINEERING	IN VIVO USE
Galvanic Cell	• A current is created when O_2 diffuses across a membrane and undergoes reduction • PP O_2 = measured current	• Can be removed easily • Narkomed, Drager Fabius • When the reactants are consumed for the reduction of oxygen, the galvanic cell needs to be exchanged. • Daily calibration with FiO_2 0.2, 1.0 FiO_2
Polargraphic	• A current is created when O_2 diffuses through a membrane and is converted to $4OH^-$ ($O_2 + 2H_2O + 4e^- > 4OH^-$) • # of O_2 molecules = degree of change in current	• Many monitoring applications. • Gas machine • Blood gas • transcutaneous
Paramagnetic	• When the unpaired electrons of O_2 are attracted to a magnetic field, a signal is generated	

Adapted from references 1,2,3

Table 6.7 RELATIVE ABSORBANCE FOR VARIOUS SOLUTES AS EXPRESSED BY MEASURED SPO_2

SOLUTE	RED (660NM)	NEAR INFRARED (940NM)	SPO_2 VALUE	COLOR OF BLOOD
Hb	Yes		Decreased	Dark
O_2Hb		Yes	Increased (PaO_2 20mmHg = SaO_2 of 30%) (PaO_2 27mmHg = SaO_2 of 50%; P_{50} value) (PaO_2 40mmHg = SaO_2 of 75%)	Bright red
MetHb	Yes	Yes	Decreased (i.e., R = 1, SpO_2 of 85%)	Brown
COHb		Yes	Increased (i.e., SpO_2 = 90% in presence of 70% COHb)	Bright cherry red
Methylene blue dye			Large decrease (SpO_2 = 1%)	
Indigo carmine dye			Small decrease (SpO_2 = 92%)	
Indocyanine green dye			Decreased (SpO_2 = 84%)	
Motion Artifact			Decreased (SpO_2 = 85%)	
Nail polish, acrylic nails			Decreased to no pulsatile absorbance (sensor positioning lateral to nail bed)	

diodes (LEDs) to capture oxygenated hemoglobin signals on a photodetector. Plethysmography incorporates pulsatile (AC—alternating current; arterial) and nonpulsatile elements (DC—direct current; venous; tissue; constant) at the monitoring site. When the Lambert-Beer law is applied, a ratio, R (Equation 4),[3] can be generated that estimates the SaO_2 to PaO_2 relationship along the steep aspect of the oxyhemoglobin dissociation curve.[1–3] However, pulse oximetry (SpO_2) does not account for COHb or MetHb and therefore expresses functional saturation only (Equation 4).[1–3]

Equation 4.

$$\text{R ratio of two pulse-added absorbances} = [\text{AC } 660 / \text{DC } 660]/[\text{AC } 940 / \text{DC } 940]$$

Where, R ranges from 0.4 (100% SpO_2 saturation) to 3.4 (0% SpO_2 saturation).

Over time, biomedical engineers have taken strides to overcome some of the limitations created by the inherent assumptions of pulse oximetry—that is, that (1) arterial blood is the only pulsatile component; (2) the R ratio is the same for the entire human race; (3) blood color is directly related to the amount of oxygen bound to hemoglobin; and (4) there is no shift of the oxygen-hemoglobin dissociated curve (i.e., right shift in sepsis). Room lighting interference, low arterial blood flow or pulsatile venous blood flow, patient movement, electrocautery,[2,3] and other "solutes" (i.e., dyes, dyshemoglobins)[2,3] impact accuracy. Pulse oximeters overcome some of these challenges by using multiple wavelengths and/or complex signal-processing algorithms.[2]

REFERENCES

1. Barash PG, et al. *Clinical Anesthesia*. Philadelphia, PA: Lippincott Williams & Wilkins; 2013.
2. Miller RD, ed. *Miller's Anesthesia*. 7th ed. Philadelphia, PA: Churchill Livingstone, Elsevier; 2010.
3. Ehrenwerth J, et al. *Anesthesia Equipment: Principles and Applications*. 2nd ed. Philadelphia, PA: Saunders, Elsevier; 2013.
4. Kopman AF, et al. Relationship of the train-of-four ratio to clinical signs and symptoms of residual paralysis in awake volunteers. *Anesthesiology*. 1997;86:765–771.
5. Lumb AB, et al. *Nunn's Respiratory Physiology*. 7th ed. Philadelphia, PA: Churchill Livingstone, Elsevier; 2010.
6. White DC, Wardley-Smith B. The "narkotest" anaesthetic gas meter. *Br J Anaesth*. 1972; 44:1100–1104.
7. American Society of Anesthesiologists: Standards for basic anesthetic monitoring. Committee of origin: standards and practice parameters. October 20, 2010, amendment.
8. Srinivasa V, Kodali BS. Caution when using colorimetry to confirm endotracheal intubation. *Anesth Analg*. 2007;104:738.
9. Sessler DI, et al. Perioperative thermal insulation. *Anesthesiology*. 1991;74:875–879.
10. Severinghaus JW, et al. History of blood gas analysis. *Int Anesthesiol Clin*. 1987;25:1–224.
11. Gravenstein JS, et al. *Capnography in Clinical Practice*. Boston, MA: Butterworths; 1989.

QUESTIONS

1. In the pH-stat approach to managing pH in hypothermic patients undergoing cardiopulmonary bypass:

A. The pH is allowed to rise naturally into the alkalotic range as the patient is cooled
B. Normal pH is not maintained
C. Cerebral perfusion is thought to be maintained by adding CO_2
D. Heating the blood sample does not have any effect on pH and gas solubility
E. Is a more clinically useful correction

2. The measurement of gas tensions in exhaled air is most commonly obtained by:
A. Mass spectrometry, whereby a gas sample is passed through an ionizer allowing for separation of particles based on mass
B. Analysis of the behavior of gas molecules in a magnetic field
C. Clark type electrodes and galvanic cells, allowing for electrochemical determination of gas
D. Infrared absorption, whereby gas tensions are calculated based on the intensity of transmitted light
E. Scattered radiation, which contains information about the energies of molecular vibrations and rotations

3. To minimize the potential of amplification or overshooting of dynamic pressure measurements, the transducer system should include:
A. Stiff, noncompliant tubing
B. Large-diameter tubing, to maximize the total mass of liquid in the system
C. Long tubing
D. Several stopcocks in series to produce higher natural frequencies

4. In the oscillometry method of noninvasive blood pressure monitoring,
A. Too small or too large a cuff would not have an effect on the pressure reading
B. The pressure at which the oscillating pressure signal first appears is noted as the mean pressure
C. Pressure is recorded by a Doppler device over the radial artery
D. The point at which the signal is at maximal amplitude is interpreted as mean arterial pressure
E. Pressure measurements are more accurate and precise than manual auscultation of Korotkoff sounds

5. Different types of autologous transfusion techniques can be employed to avoid complications associated with allogenic transfusions and for the conservation of blood resources. In intraoperative blood collection:
A. Microaggregate filters do not need to be used
B. The oxygen transport properties of recovered RBCs are equivalent to stored allogenic RBCs
C. The hematocrit of the washed RBCs is 20% to 30%
D. There are no published adverse events of reinfusion of recovered blood
E. Intraoperative collection is not contraindicated when procoagulant materials are applied to the surgical field, as these are filtered and washed out

6. Which of the following is the most effective measure to avoid intraoperative hypothermia?
A. The heating and humidification of inspiratory gases
B. The administration of heated intravenous fluids
C. Circulating water mattresses placed under the patient
D. Cutaneous warming devices, such as forced air warming devices
E. Avoidance of neuraxial anesthesia, which can decrease the thresholds triggering vasoconstriction and shivering

ANSWERS

1. C. Modern blood gas analyzers measure blood gas tensions at 37° C, and blood samples must be heated or cooled to 37°C for analysis. Heating a blood sample decreases gas solubility, pH, and Hb affinity for O_2 and CO_2. As the blood from a hypothermic patient (as in cardiopulmonary bypass) is heated and analyzed at 37° C, more gas becomes dissolved in solution and the measured PO_2 and PCO_2 will be higher than at 35° C.

   pH-stat and alpha-stat are two approaches that have been used to manage pH in hypothermic patients undergoing cardiopulmonary bypass. The alpha-stat approach lets pH rise naturally into the alkalotic range as the patient is cooled, while pH-stat maintains normal pH and cerebral perfusion by adding CO_2. There is limited data to suggest that one approach is more clinically useful than the other.
2. D. The ability to measure concentrations of inspired and expired gas concentrations is crucial in anesthesia practice. Several systems such as mass spectrometry, infrared absorption, electrochemical analysis, and paramagnetic analysis are available for the measurement of gas tensions in exhaled air.

   Most expired gas analyzers currently used in anesthesia involve infrared absorption. Infrared light is passed through a gas sample, and gas tensions are derived based on the intensity of the transmitted light. All anesthetic agents as well as CO_2 and N_2O are able to be measured with the exception of oxygen, which does not absorb infrared light.
3. A. Pressure measured in an invasive arterial catheter can overshoot or amplify the actual blood pressure, a phenomenon referred to as the dynamic frequency response of the fluid-filled arterial line and transducer system. To minimize the potential of real arterial pressure amplification, the system should have stiff, noncompliant tubing and a minimal total mass of liquid accomplished by small-diameter tubing of short length.

4. D. Automated noninvasive blood pressure monitoring devices commonly used in operating rooms monitor the oscillating signal generated in the cuff by the arterial pressure changes. The cuff inflates to above systolic pressure and the oscillations are abolished. This is followed by slow cuff deflation in a stepwise fashion. Systolic pressure is recorded as the pressure at which the oscillating pressure signal first appears. The signal then increases in amplitude as cuff pressure decreases. Mean arterial pressure is interpreted as the point at which the signal is at maximal amplitude. Diastolic pressure is inferred from the systolic and mean pressures.
5. B. Intraoperative blood collection or recovery refers to the technique of collection and reinfusion of blood lost during surgery. The oxygen transport properties of recovered RBCs are equivalent to those of stored allogenic RBCs. The blood is collected, washed, and concentrated with a resultant hematocrit of 50% to 60%.

   Intraoperative collection is contraindicated when procoagulant materials are applied on the surgical field, because of the risk of systemic coagulation. Microaggregate filters are often used for the removal of small blood clots and tissue debris.
6. D. Anesthetic-induced impairment of thermoregulatory control and a cool operating room environment makes most patients hypothermic. Even mild hypothermia causes adverse perioperative outcomes. Because nearly 90% of metabolic heat is lost via the skin surface, cutaneous warming is essential. Forced air and increased operating room temperature are two major systems that require consideration to maintain normothermia.

   Little heat is lost via respiration, thus active airway heating and humidification minimally influence core temperature. Patients also cannot be warmed by administering heated fluids, because fluids cannot exceed body temperature.

7.

VENTILATORS

Maria Matuszczak and Madhumani Rupasinghe

The role of a ventilator is to substitute for the ventilation of a patient. Ventilators are used in different scenarios: in the operating room, in the intensive care unit, in the emergency room, in transport, and at home.

CLASSIFICATION

There are many different classifications of ventilators; they can be historical or they can depend on the preference of different textbooks and authors. For the purpose of this book ventilators are divided into groups of different mechanism.

NEGATIVE VERSUS POSITIVE PRESSURE VENTILATION

A negative pressure ventilator reproduces most closely the physiological breath by creating a negative intrathoracic pressure that allows the air to flow into the lung. This activity can be seen in Figure 7.1. This negative pressure physiology is why incentive spirometry is more effective in recruiting alveoli when compared with other techniques.

The "iron lung" developed during a poliomyelitis epidemic last century is an example. See Figure 7.2. The patient lies in an air-tide cylindrical tube with head and neck being free. Since the introduction of the endotracheal tube this type of negative pressure ventilator is rarely used today. Positive pressure ventilation (PPV), invasive or noninvasive, is today's standard.[1]

THE POWERING MECHANISM

Ventilators can be different powering mechanism.

Flow Versus Pressure Generation

A flow generator is a ventilator generating a high pressure; the inspiratory flow is unaffected by patient lung changes. There may be a constant or a nonconstant flow pattern. A pressure generator generates a lower pressure; the inspiratory flow can be influenced by lung changes. The pressure waveform remains the same even if the flow varies. The pressure may be constant or nonconstant. Modern ventilators combine flow and pressure generation, changing from one to the other depending on the patient's impedance and alveolar pressures.

Other Classifications of Powering Mechanism

Some older-generation ventilators are pneumatically powered by compressed gas. The wall gas supply provided to the ventilator is at high pressure, around 50–54 psi. (For comparison, the pressure in your car tire is normally around 35–40 psi.) The energy in the gas supply provided in a hospital can be captured to do various things, like run a ventilator.

Other ventilators are also pneumatically powered but with an electronic control, and are used to operate most anesthesia machines. Electrically powered and controlled ventilators are more frequently found in the intensive care unit (ICU). These ventilators have historically supported many more features than the average anesthesia ventilator, because there is no need to use and conserve anesthetic gas. Today's anesthesia workstations incorporate many features of an ICU ventilator and allow proper ventilation of all age groups.

THE CYCLING MECHANISM

Most ventilators are time cycled. The initiation of inspiration and expiration can be different depending on the ventilator and on the chosen ventilation setting. The cycle can depend on reaching a set time (time cycled), a set volume (volume cycled), a set pressure (pressure cycled), a change in flow (flow cycled), a set trigger (manually cycled), or a combination of the above. Modern ventilators can also electronically adjust the cycle from a set inspiratory:expiratory phase time ratio (I:E ratio) and respiratory rate. Flow

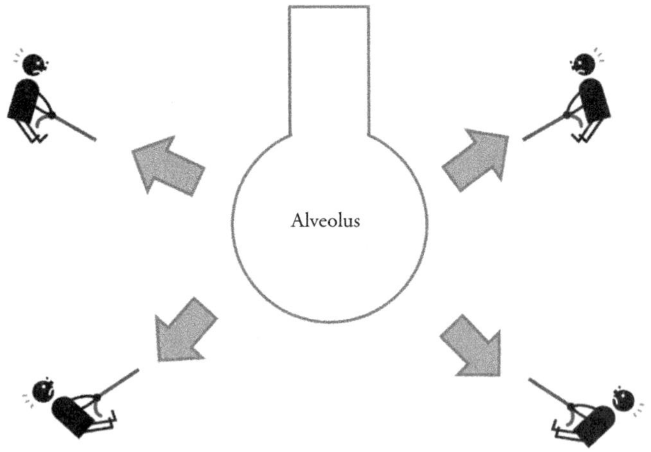

Figure 7.1 Normal alveolar physiology.

control valves in modern ICU ventilators have a rapid response time and great flexibility in controlling the flow.

THE DRIVING MECHANISM

The way the tidal volume is generated depends on the driving mechanism, which is another way to classify ventilators.[2]

Minute Volume Dividers

The fresh gas flow (FGF) is divided into a set tidal volume, and this determines the respiratory rate. That is, the delivered fresh gas is the minute volume, and by setting a tidal volume the respiratory rate is set as well.

Example: FGF is 6 L/min, the tidal volume is set at 600 mL, the respiratory rate will be 10 BPM.

Bellows

Bellows are pneumatically powered but electronically controlled ventilators, mostly used in the operating room. They are also called bag squeezers, bag-in-bottle ventilators, or double circuit ventilators. A collapsible bag or bellow sits in a gas-tight transparent chamber. See Figure 7.3. There are ascending and descending bellows. The "ascending" bellow is standing and ascends during expiration while being filled with the next tidal volume. During inspiration, the bag is "squeezed" by the gas inside the chamber and air flows into the patients lungs. The "descending" bellow is hanging and descends during expiration. The two circuits, one being connected to the patient lung, the other being used to "squeeze" the bellow, do not communicate. The newer ventilators have a descending bellows because it allows for decoupling of fresh gas during controlled ventilation. Some anesthesia machines have a horizontal bellow.[3]

JET VENTILATORS

Jet ventilators can be low frequency or high frequency, and are either pneumatically powered and manually controlled or pneumatically powered and electronically controlled. See Figure 7.4. They use a high-pressure oxygen source to ventilate through a small orifice, which can be a needle or a small, long catheter. These ventilators are used in the operating room for airway surgery, thoracic surgery, or in can't-ventilate-can't-intubate situations. Jet ventilation operates via controlled inspiration and passive expiration.[2] During jet ventilation, gas is entrained like a second stream of gas and results in a larger tidal volume than the delivered jet volume alone.

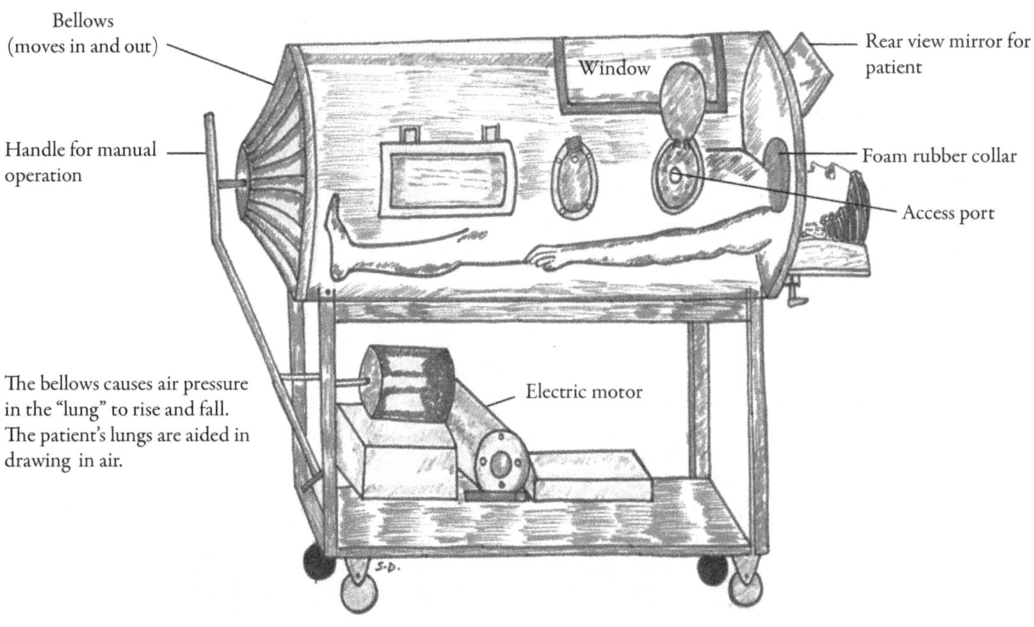

Figure 7.2 An iron lung maintains breathing by artificial means.

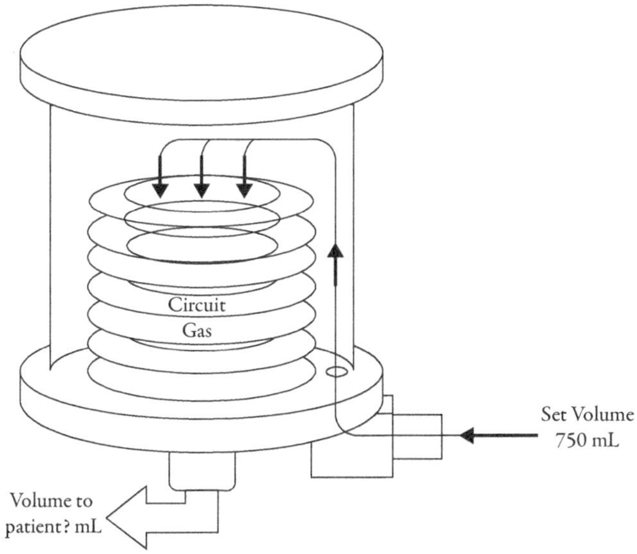

Figure 7.3 Bag in bottle ventilator. To deliver a tidal volume to the patient, that volume is delivered into the bellows compartment, displacing the bellows and pushing circuit gas to the patient. If the peak inflating pressure increases, pressure increases within the bellows and the same gas delivered to the bellows chamber will produce a smaller tidal volume. Stayer S, Olutoye O. Anesthesia ventilators: better options for children. *Anesthesiol Clin North America*. 2005;23(4):677–691.

OSCILLATORS

Oscillators are high-frequency ventilators used to ventilate patients with a severe lung injury when oxygenation with conventional ventilation cannot be achieved. See Figure 7.5. In contrast to jet ventilation, both inspiration and expiration are active. [2]

High-frequency oscillation ventilation uses small tidal volumes (1–3 mL/kg) and significantly higher levels of positive end expiratory pressure (PEEP). This allows a continuous pressure, equal to the mean airway pressure (MAP). The risk of cyclical alveolar collapse and overdistention is

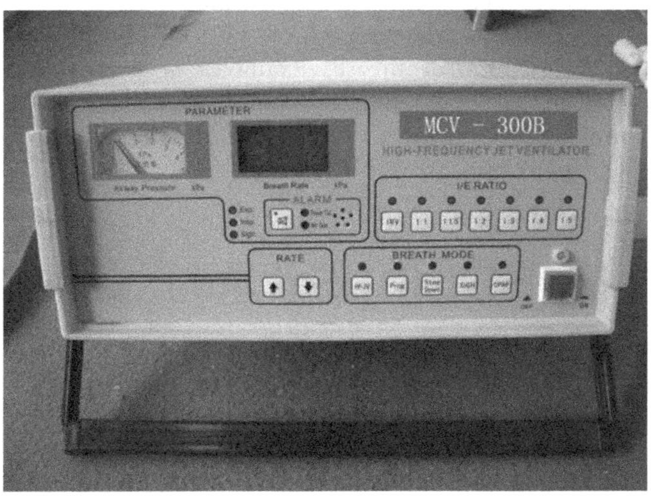

Figure 7.4 High-frequency ventilator.

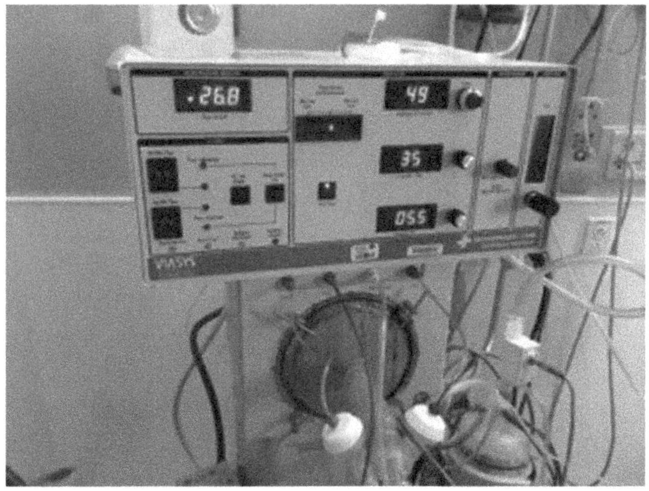

Figure 7.5 High-frequency oscillator. Image courtesy of George Williams, MD.

reduced. If you recall the hysteresis curve, which is the curve that demonstrates lung volumes at different pressures, the overall function of the oscillator is to sustain a MAP that is "just right" (Figure 7.6). Furthermore, the design of the oscillator provides fresh gas via a different mechanism than traditional ventilators (Figure 7.7).

Elimination of CO_2 is obtained even at high frequencies; the improved gas exchange is partially due to the Pendelluft principal (interregional gas mixing between units with different time constants) and to Taylor's dispersion (longitudinal dispersion due to interaction between the axial velocity profile and radial concentration gradient).

PRINCIPLES OF ACTION

The mode of ventilation decides on how the tidal volume is delivered to the patient.

Modern ventilators and anesthesia workstations allow for a multitude of ventilation settings via computerized control and the use of a solid-state electronic timing device.

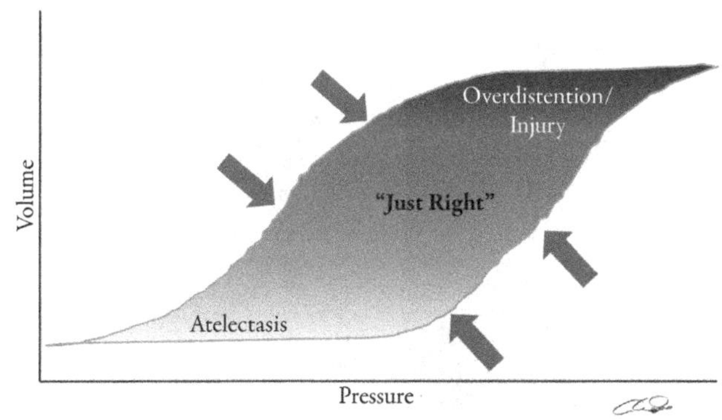

Figure 7.6 The oscillator sustains a mean airway pressure and theoretically can reduce injury from overdistention and improve oxygenation by avoiding atelectasis (low volumes).

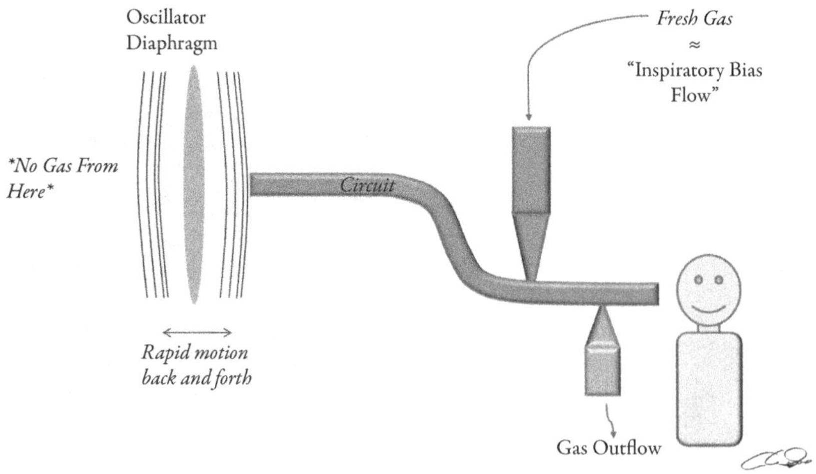

Figure 7.7 Simplified diagram of the physical principles and gas supply describing the oxcillator-based ventilation.

See Figure 7.8. Ventilation settings can control many of the patient's respiratory parameters like respiratory rate, I:E ratio, tidal volume, inspiratory pressure, end expiratory pressure, trigger, inspired oxygen concentration (FiO_2), and others.[3]

CONTROLLERS

Controlled positive pressure ventilation (C-PPV) is mostly invasive positive pressure ventilation (PPV) via an endotracheal tube. The ventilator works independently of the patient. This mode of ventilation is used for patients with no respiratory drive. The patient may be paralyzed by anesthesia, muscle relaxants, spinal injury, central nervous system injury, or other means. The ventilation mode can be volume or pressure controlled. In the volume-controlled mode (also called volume-targeted ventilation, or VTV), a predetermined volume is set to be delivered to the patient's lungs (Figure 7.9). The tidal volume is a function of flow and time and is constant; the flow is high until the set tidal volume is reached. The inspiratory pressure varies depending on lung compliance. Peak inspiratory pressure (PIP) needs to be closely monitored, because barotrauma is possible if pressure is not limited. In the pressure-controlled mode (also called pressure-targeted ventilation, or PTV), the PIP is set and constant, the tidal volume depends on the respiratory rate, the I:E ratio and changes depending on lung compliance. The flow is decelerating, which improves the distribution of ventilation, and is better tolerated by the patient. There is decreased risk of barotrauma. Pressure-targeted ventilation achieves a given tidal volume with less airway pressure compared with VTV. If lung compliance decreases significantly, the tidal volume may become insufficient. Depending on the reason for respiratory failure additional settings like high positive end expiratory pressure (PEEP), and/or inversed I:E ratio may be needed. Newer ventilators are capable of switching between VTV and PTV; they operate in dual-control modes. Two different modes exist: one switches from breath to breath, one switches within the breath. Examples of dual-control modes are pressure-regulated volume control (PRVC), volume-assured pressure support ventilation (VAPSV), and adaptive pressure ventilation (APV).

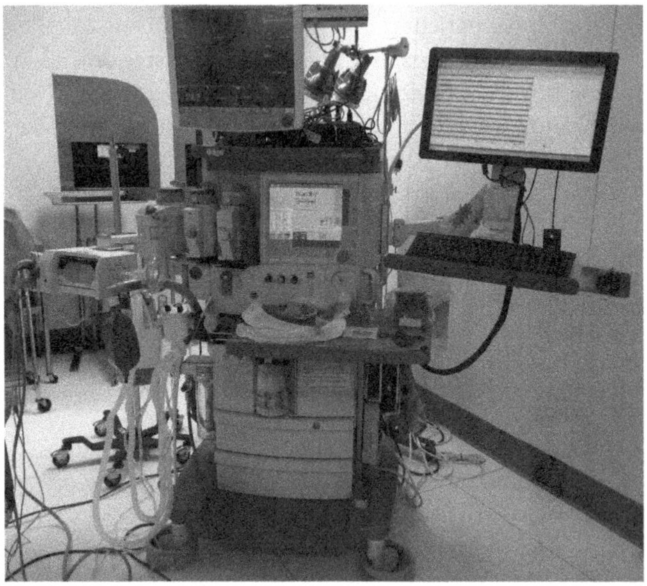

Figure 7.8 Modern anesthesia workstation. Image courtesy Erin Williams, MD

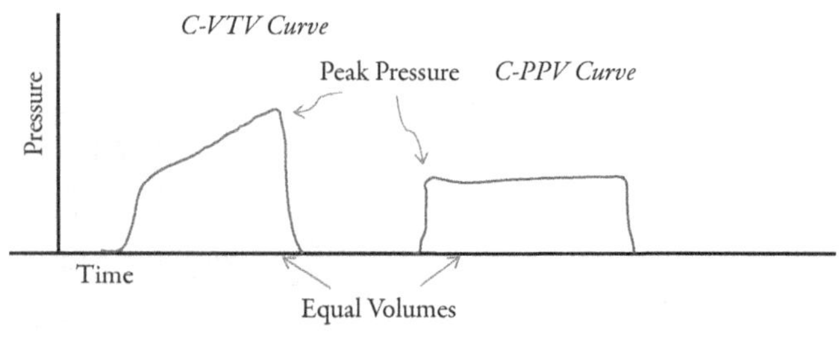

Figure 7.9 Controlled positive pressure ventilation.

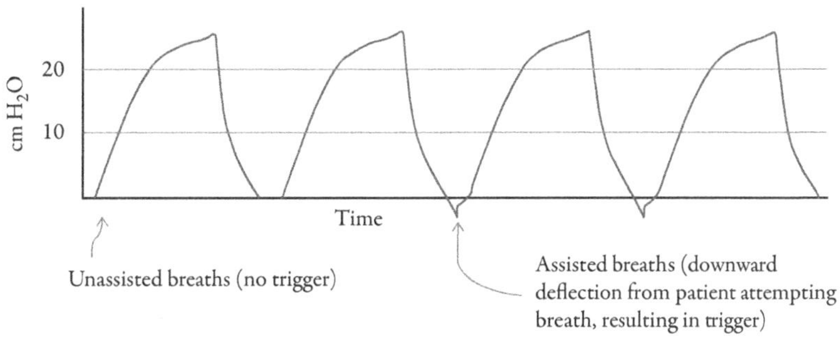

Figure 7.10 Negative pressure, which triggers a response from a ventilator in assisted mode.

ASSISTORS

Assisted PPV is used for patients who have a limited respiratory drive—not strong enough to produce a normal tidal volume or not strong enough to sustain the breathing work over a longer period of time. Examples are patients under anesthesia but nonparalyzed or patients exhausted by a disease process or trauma. In the assisted mode, the ventilator recognizes the patient's effort to breath. The patient's breathing effort creates a negative pressure that triggers the ventilator's response (Figure 7.10). Several assisted ventilation modes can be used; assisted VTV and PTV are similar to controlled VTV and PTV.

ASSIST-CONTROL

Assist-control ventilation (ACV) combines both the controlled and the assisted ventilation modes. The control mode kicks in when the patient is unable to trigger the machine. Assist-controlled ventilation is particularly useful for long-term ventilation, where it has been shown to prevent muscle atrophy. It facilitates the weaning process and is now also more frequently used for patients under general anesthesia who do not need to be paralyzed. It has been shown to decrease the work of breathing as compared with other ventilation modes. Continuous mandatory ventilation (CMV), synchronized intermittent mandatory ventilation (SIMV), intermittent mandatory ventilation (IMV), intermittent demand ventilation, and pressure support ventilation (PSV) are all assist-control ventilation modes. The most frequently used are SIMV and PSV.

Pressure-Limited, Volume-Limited

Pressure-regulated volume control is a dual-control ventilation mode that combines pressure-controlled and volume-controlled ventilation by setting a constant tidal volume but limiting it to a set pressure. Pressure-regulated volume control will compensate for the decrease in tidal volume when lung compliance increases. The ventilator's microprocessor analyzes the tidal volume of each breath and adjusts pressure from breath to breath.

Volume-assured pressure support ventilation PSV is also a dual-control ventilation mode. It is a pressure support mode that allows spontaneous ventilation and changes control within the breath. Two flow sources are triggered by the patient's respiratory effort. The first flow is constant, the second changes depending on the achieved pressure and tidal volume.

Intermittent Mandatory Ventilation

Also called intermittent demand ventilation, in IMV a mandatory respiratory frequency is set on the ventilator and the patient is allowed to breathe in between. There is no synchronization between the patient breath and the mandatory preset frequency. This ventilation mode was used to wean patients but it demands significant work of breathing. All modern ventilators have changed from IMV to SIMV.[3]

Synchronized Intermittent Mandatory Ventilation

As compared with IMV, the SIMV mode synchronizes the mandatory breath with the spontaneous breath of the patient. When the patient tries to take a breath and a mandatory breath is about to be delivered, the ventilator synchronizes to the patient's breath. Synchronized intermittent mandatory ventilation can be volume controlled or pressure controlled. In opposition to pressure support ventilation (PSV), the patient's own spontaneous breath is unsupported. This ventilation mode is frequently used to wean a patient when emerging from anesthesia or in the ICU if more sophisticated ventilators are not available.[1–3] Modern ventilators automatically include a PSV function with SIMV, thereby combining both modes.

Pressure Support

During PSV, the patient is allowed to breathe spontaneously, with every breath being supported by the ventilator. A respiratory rescue rate can be set and is only activated if the patient stops triggering the ventilator. In PSV, the set inspiratory pressure support level is kept constant and there is a decelerating flow. As for pressure-controlled ventilation, if lung compliance changes, the tidal volume will change and support will need to be adjusted. At initiation of a weaning process, the pressure support is higher and can be decreased as the patient's spontaneous ventilation gets stronger. The patient's effort to initiate a response from the ventilator depends on the trigger sensitivity setting. To initiate a breath the patient has to create the negative pressure that is set as trigger sensitivity. The higher the negative trigger pressure is set on the ventilator, the more work of breathing the patient must perform. The trigger sensitivity should be set as sensitive as possible without causing self-triggering—autotriggering. Pressure-support ventilation is widely used in the operating room and in the ICU setting for all ages.[3,4]

Periodic Sigh

Periodic sigh superposed to PSV seems to improve oxygenation during the weaning phase and may prevent atelectasis. One sigh breath can be set at 1–2 times the patient's tidal volume and is administered every 6 to 10 minutes. Most ventilators can set a sigh breath several times per hour. Contraindications are an already high tidal volume, PIP pressures >30 mmHg, and spontaneous breathing patients on noninvasive continuous positive airway pressure (CPAP).

Inverse Ratio

The normal I:E ratio for a healthy adult is 1:2, meaning that if the respiratory rate is 10 breaths per minute, an inspiration/expiration cycle is 6 seconds long with 2 s for inspiration and 4 seconds for expiration. Inversed ratio 2:1 ventilation (IRV) is used to improve oxygenation in patients with already maximized ventilation settings (Figure 7.11). Inversed I:E ratio ventilation may increase functional residual capacity (FRC). Benefits and protocols on when to use IRV are not clearly defined at this point.[5] This mode of ventilation is functionally similar to "bagging" a patient in order to bring up their oxygen saturation. It can also be compared with a recruitment maneuver.

AIRWAY PRESSURE RELEASE VENTILATION

Airway pressure release ventilation (APRV) is a proprietary name (Drager Medical, Evita 4). Conceptually, APRV is IRV combined with PTV (*jokingly*, reverse I:E ratio ventilation "on steroids"). A high pressure and a low pressure are set on the ventilator with limited time. Ventilation occurs during the release time from high to low pressure (Figure 7.12). Times are set depending on patient pathology: 0.2 to 0.8 seconds for restrictive lung disease and 0.8 to 1.5 seconds for obstructive lung disease. The low pressure time is also called the release phase. As the patient spends about 4–6 seconds in the high pressure phase, APRV is similar to pressure-targeted IRV. The BiLevel ventilation (BiLevel) is also a proprietary name (Covidien, Puritan Bennett 840), and functions essentially in the same way. APRV/BiLevel is indicated in patients with hypoxemic respiratory failure because this ventilation mode has been shown to improve oxygenation by optimizing alveolar recruitment and ventilation/perfusion (V/Q) matching.[1]

HIGH-FREQUENCY VENTILATION

Two modes of high-frequency ventilation exist. It has been shown that adequate alveolar ventilation is achieved with tidal volumes much smaller than dead space if respiratory rates are very high.[2,6,7]

Automated high-frequency jet ventilation (HFJV) is mostly used for airway surgery. High-pressured gas is broken up into small pulses; frequency, inspiratory time, and driving pressure can be adjusted to achieve a sufficient airflow. It creates a nearly motionless surgical field, as opposed to the oscillator. Also, HFJV reduces alveolar distention and produces less cardiac instability as compared with conventional ventilation. High-frequency jet ventilation needs a jet airway device to deliver the tidal volume, and ambient air entrainment is present. It cannot be used if there is an

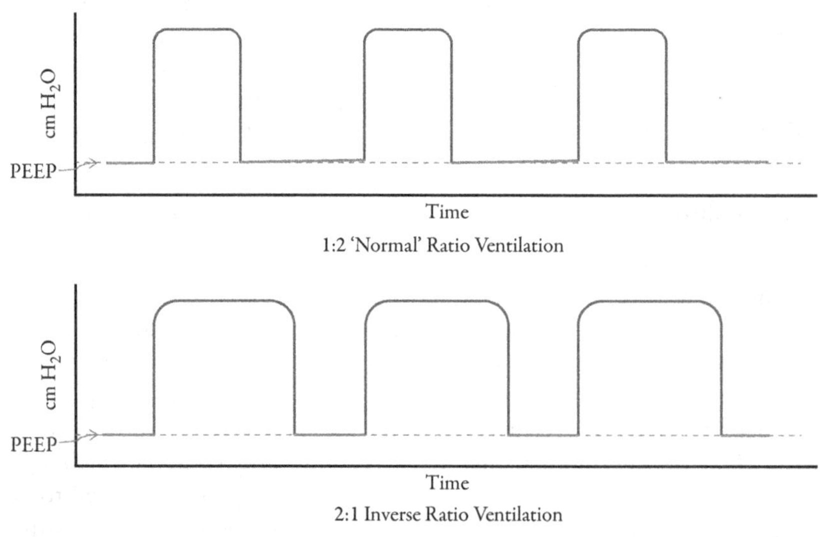

Figure 7.11 Normal I:E ratio vs. inversed I:E ratio. Image courtesy George Williams, MD

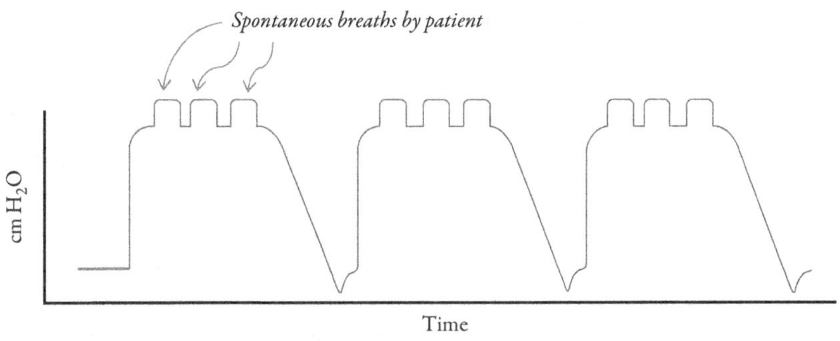

Figure 7.12 APRV ventilation.

airway obstruction, because it relies on passive return of air. Over time, CO_2 accumulates, end-tidal CO_2 cannot be correctly measured, and volatile gas cannot be delivered.

High-frequency oscillator ventilators are significantly different from HFJVs. The oscillator is connected to an endotracheal tube or a tracheostomy tube. Both inspiration and expiration are active. There is no ambient air entrainment. High-frequency oscillator ventilation is used in the early stage of acute respiratory distress syndrome (ARDS). The primary setting consists of a pressure set 3–5 cmHg over the MAPs used during conventional ventilation. The mean pulmonary airway wedge pressure (mPaw) can be compared to PEEP. The fresh gas flow, also called bias flow, is delivered using a flow meter set at 25–40 L/min. Changes in bias flow will produce changes of the mPaw. Also, CO_2 removal depends on the bias flow. The delta P of the oscillation is controlled by the power dial. Auscultation of the lungs is not possible because of the noise created by the oscillation. Symmetric and adequate "wiggle" of the body from shoulder to abdomen is the clinical sign to observe, and if a sudden change is seen, an issue with the endotracheal tube (ETT) should be suspected. The frequency is measured in Hertz; an adult setting starts with 3–7 Hz, which equals 180–420 breaths per minute. The I:E ratio is close to 1:2. In the pediatric population, the oscillator is used in newborns with meconium aspiration, with congenital diaphragmatic hernia, and with respiratory failure associated with Respiratory Syncytial Virus (RSV) infection. The benefits of this mode of ventilation over conventional ventilation modes are not established.

NONINVASIVE TECHNIQUES

Noninvasive positive pressure ventilation (NIPPV) is widely used today. Historically the "iron lung" is also a form of NIPPV and is rarely used today. Use of NIPPV via a face mask has been shown to reduce intubation rates and its complications. NIPPV is delivered via a continuous positive airway pressure (CPAP) or BiLevel positive airway pressure (BIPAP) device or a standard ICU ventilator.

CPAP is delivered at a predetermined level. It prevents airway collapse due to sleep apnea, and prevents alveolar collapse in patients with neuromuscular disease, COPD, and other respiratory problems. In infants, the use of nasal CPAP has significantly reduced intubation time for premature babies.

BIPAP delivers two levels of pressure: a high inspiratory pressure (IPAP) and a low expiratory pressure (EPAP). It is used to treat central sleep apnea, severe obstructive sleep apnea, and patients with respiratory distress due to cardiac and pulmonary diseases. No naso-gastric-tube (NGT) is needed if pressures used are below esophageal opening pressures (20–25 cmHg).

There is frequently confusion about CPAP and PEEP. Positive end expiratory pressure is pressure applied only during expiration, while CPAP is continuous and constant pressure applied during inspiration and expiration. The term PEEP should be used when other inspiratory support is provided, while CPAP should be used for noninvasive respiratory support. Both CPAP and PEEP reduce alveolar atelectasis and edema.[2,6]

PEDIATRIC ADAPTATION

Most modern ventilators can be used for adults and children with the exception of the very low birth weight (VLBW) babies. A few very sophisticated ventilators can be used for all age groups, including VLBW babies. It must be mentioned that as complexity increases, the potential for error increases too. Ventilators used for VLBW babies are pressure-, volume-, or time cycling. For all three types of ventilators, the baby's lung compliance determines the tidal volume, unless a pressure-limiting device is added. Synchronized intermittent mandatory ventilation and pressure support are incorporated in modern neonatal ventilators. The trigger mechanism has to be very sensitive to the minimal inspiratory effort a VLBW child can produce. Proportional assist ventilation, a fairly new ventilation mode, will regulate inspiratory pressure "proportionally" to patient effort. Infants with poor lung compliance and high airway resistance have been shown to benefit from this type of ventilation. When conventional ventilation fails, high-frequency ventilation is used.[8]

Noninvasive respiratory support (NRS) has gained an increasing place in the treatment of respiratory failure of the neonate. The terminology of NRS is confusing, and a multitude of acronyms exist. Continuous distended pressure (CDP) is used to prevent alveolar collapse at the end of expiration; CPAP and BIPAP are forms of CDP. Several CDP devices also allow assisting inspiratory effort in order to facilitate CO_2 elimination.[9] A commonly used device is nasal CDP or NCPAP. Continuous distended pressure is often used to transition from PPV to unassisted breathing after extubation and to manage apnea of prematurity. There are other indications such as atelectasis, thoracic wall instability, decreased FRC, and so forth. Although its use has been widespread and has been shown to reduce the use of PPV in premature babies, NCPAP as compared with intubation has not been shown to decrease bronchopulmonary dysplasia or chronic lung disease in premature babies.[8–12] Studies have shown an increased incidence in pneumothorax. Several non-respiratory-related contraindications to CDP exist: gastroschisis, choanal atresia, tracheoesophageal fistula, cleft palate, congenital heart disease, and cardiovascular instability.

INSPIRED OXYGEN CONCENTRATION CONTROL

In all ventilation modes the FiO_2 can be set between 21% and 100%, and oxygen is delivered during inspiratory time.

STANDARDS FOR BASIC INTRAOPERATIVE MONITORING

Standards for basic intraoperative monitoring have been adopted by the American Society of Anesthesiologists. Standard I requires that qualified anesthesia personnel shall be present at all times during the procedure. Standard II requires that the patient's oxygenation, ventilation, circulation, and temperature shall be under continuous evaluation. The anesthesiologist must ensure adequate ventilation of the patient during all anesthetics, and every patient must have the adequacy of ventilation continually evaluated. While qualitative clinical signs such as chest expansion, observation of the reservoir breathing bag, and auscultation of breath sounds may be adequate, when ventilation is controlled by a mechanical ventilator, there must be a device which is in continuous use, capable of detecting abnormalities.

PRESSURE

PLATEAU PRESSURE

The static or "plateau" pressure is normally defined as the end-inspiratory pressure during a period of at least 0.5 seconds of zero gas flow. It is measured during an inspiratory pause on the ventilator. It is representative of the compliance or elasticity of the respiratory system (lung, chest wall, and abdomen). It is an indication of how much pressure is necessary to inflate the small airways and alveoli with each breath. The goal plateau pressure is <30–35 cmH_2O. Higher plateau pressures will lead to volutrauma or ventilator-induced lung injury secondary to overdistention of alveoli.[13,14]

Any problem that causes a fall in the compliance of the respiratory system will cause static pressures to rise. Examples of such problems include the onset of ARDS or pulmonary edema, large pleural effusions, pneumothorax, abdominal distention, or circumferential chest wall burns. With a rigid chest.

- Pressure on manometer after inspiration has ended
- Represents pressure needed to overcome elastic resistance
- Used to calculate static compliance
- Static compliance = /Tidal Volume/plateau pressure

PEAK PRESSURE

Peak inspiratory pressure (PIP) or peak airway pressure (PAP) is the maximum pressure obtainable during active gas delivery (Figure 7.13). In VTV, peak pressure is dependent on both compliance and airway resistance as well as tidal volume, peak flow, and flow pattern. For a given compliance and airway resistance, higher peak flow results in higher PAP. The peak pressure is representative of the resistance in the system from the ventilator tubing all the way down to the segmental bronchi. Anything that affects the resistance of these tubes (mucus plugging, bronchospasm, and kinked endotracheal tube) and/or increased elastic pressure from decreased lung or chest wall compliance will cause the peak pressure to rise. The machine displays the peak pressure with every breath. It is important to know that, while some of the same factors contribute to both peak and static airway pressures, a number of things that affect peak pressure are external to the patient and do not necessarily reflect a change in the compliance of the patient's lungs.[13,14] Peak airway pressure greater than 50 cmH_2O is generally discouraged, because high values of peak pressure carry increased risk of barotrauma and hypotension due to decreased venous return.

- Pressure on manometer immediately at end of inspiratory phase
- Represents pressure needed to overcome both elastic and airway resistance
- Used to calculate dynamic compliance
- Dynamic compliance = VT/Peak pressure

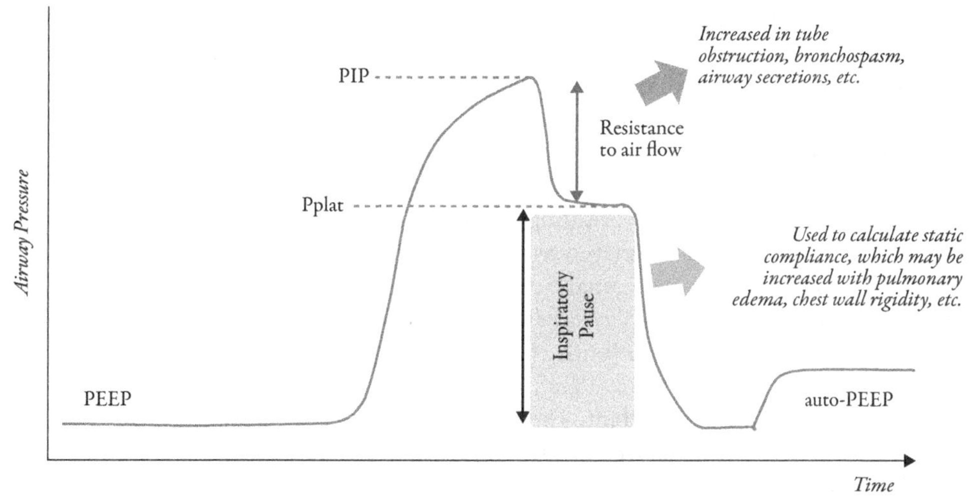

Figure 7.13 Peak inspiratory pressure (PIP) = plateau pressure (Pplat) + pressure required to overcome airway resistance. Note the various factors that can affect each described pressure. Static compliance is most clinically useful, as it reflects lung compliance once lungs are inflated. Dynamic compliance is not calculated at plateau pressures, and therefore normal values are highly variable and less clinically useful. Image by George Williams, MD.

Airway pressure monitoring in most anesthesia machines is electronic, using flow transducers, with the results displayed as waveforms on the machine monitors. Some older machines still use a mechanical pressure gauge, the Bourdon gauge. Newer electronic sensors use the principle of piezoelectricity, the property of certain crystals, usually quartz, to produce a small electric current when compressed. This output may be calibrated and amplified into a usable signal. The purpose of airway pressure monitors is to prevent pressure from either going too high (to prevent barotrauma) or dropping too low (to detect leaks or disconnection).

OXYGEN

Anesthesia machines have a number of safety features and monitors that protect against administration of a hypoxic mixture, which is defined as an FiO_2 less than 25%. For example, hypoxia can be caused by an excessive concentration of nitrous oxide. Modern machines have interlocked oxygen and nitrous oxide flow controls in order to prevent inadvertent delivery of a hypoxic inspired gas mixture, as the ratio of oxygen to nitrous oxide concentrations can never decrease below 0.25. This can be achieved by a mechanical, pneumatic, or electronic mechanism.

Mechanical devices use a chain to link flow control valves for oxygen and nitrous oxide. This system may fail to account for other gases, such as air, which could reduce the oxygen concentration to <25%. A stop fitted to the oxygen flow meter control valve ensures a minimum flow of oxygen at 175–250 mL/min, even with the valve apparently closed. This type of device is utilized in Datex-Ohmeda anesthesia machines.

Pneumatic devices use a ratio mixer valve. Oxygen supplied to this valve exerts a pressure on one side of the diaphragm, which is opposed by the pressure of nitrous oxide on the opposite side. The diaphragm construction ensures an increase in oxygen flow rate by a ratio of 25% of any increase in the nitrous oxide flow rate. This type of device is utilized in Dräger anesthesia machines.

Electronic devices use a paramagnetic oxygen analyzer to continuously sample the gas mixtures from the flow meters. If the FiO_2 decreases below 25%, nitrous oxide is temporarily cut off, whereas an increase in FiO_2 will temporarily restore nitrous oxide flow.

The oxygen analyzer is one of the most important monitors on the anesthesia workstation. It is the only machine safety device that evaluates the integrity of the circuit in an ongoing fashion. It is the only machine monitor that detects problems downstream from the flow control valves. In effect, by the time the gas has reached the oxygen sensor, there is nothing else the machine can "do" to change the concentration of the oxygen flowing to the circuit. The paramagnetic method is currently the most widely used in modern anesthetic machines; galvanic fuel cells and the polarographic electrode are still found in older machines.

PARAMAGNETIC OXYGEN ANALYZER

Paramagnetic gases are attracted to magnetic energy because of unpaired electrons in their outer shell orbits. An oxygen molecule has unpaired electrons in its outer electron ring, which makes it paramagnetic and thus attracted to the magnetic field. Older paramagnetic analyzers used dumbbell and torsion wire systems, but the newer analyzers use switched electromagnetic fields. The analyzers comprise two chambers (sampling and reference chambers) with a sensitive pressure transducer in between. The sampling chamber receives sample gas via a sampling tube, while the reference chamber receives room air. The changing magnetic field is created by an electromagnet that rapidly switches on and off, causing oxygen molecules to be attracted and agitated. This in turn results in pressure on either side of the pressure transducer, and the pressure difference across the transducer is proportional to the oxygen partial pressure difference between the sample gas and the reference gas. Although the measurement is in partial pressure, it is displayed as a percentage. Modern miniaturized paramagnetic analyzers incorporate a rapidly oscillating magnetic chamber and are capable of breath-to-breath analysis of oxygen in both the inspired and expired limbs of the circuit. They are affected by water vapor and have a water trap incorporated into their design.[15] There are two types of electrochemical oxygen analyzers. The polarographic cell analyzer and the galvanic cell.

ELECTROCHEMICAL OXYGEN ANALYZERS

Galvanic Cell (Hersch/Fuel Cell)

The galvanic cell measures the current produced when oxygen diffuses across a membrane and is reduced to molecular oxygen at the anode of an electrical circuit. It is similar to a polarographic cell analyzer except that it contains a lead anode and a gold mesh cathode in potassium hydroxide solution and no polarizing voltage is applied. The chemical reaction involves: $Pb + 2OH^- \rightarrow PbO + H_2O + 2e^-$ (Figure 7.14). The electron flow (current) is proportional to the partial pressure of oxygen in the fuel cell. In effect, the galvanic fuel cell is a battery activated by oxygen; as such, in order to maximize sensor life, the sensor should be exposed to room air when not in use (i.e., overnight). When a galvanic fuel cell is exhausted, the whole sensor cartridge must be replaced.

POLAROGRAPHIC OXYGEN ANALYZER (CLARK ELECTRODE)

In a polarographic oxygen analyzer, the analyzer sensor is placed in the inspiratory limb of the circuit. The sensor consists of a silver/silver chloride anode and a platinum cathode in a potassium chloride electrolyte solution with a polarizing voltage. Oxygen diffuses through an oxygen-permeable polymeric Teflon membrane and participates in the following reaction: $O_2 + 2H_2O + 4e^- \rightarrow 4OH^-$. The current generated is proportional to the oxygen concentration of the samples gas. Sensors have a limited life span and should be placed in an upright position to avoid accumulation of moisture. Polarographic oxygen sensors are versatile and are important components of gas machine oxygen analyzers, blood gas analyzers, and transcutaneous oxygen analyzers.

Generally, the oxygen-concentration-sensing element (usually a fuel cell on traditional machines) must be exposed to room air (at sea level) for calibration to 21%. This may require temporary removal of the sensor, selecting and then confirming (from a set of menus on the workstation's display screen) that the oxygen calibration is to be performed, and finally reinstalling the sensor. Newer workstations have automatic oxygen sensor calibration.

APNEA

Breathing circuit disconnections and misconnections leading to apnea are the leading causes of critical events in anesthesia. Occlusion (obstruction) of the breathing circuit may occur. Tracheal tubes can become kinked. Hoses throughout the breathing circuit are subject to occlusion by internal obstruction or external mechanical forces, which can impinge on flow and have severe consequences. Monitors for disconnection (apnea alarms) can be based on gas flow (tidal volume), circuit pressure (if PIP is below threshold, an alarm rings), chemistry (CO_2 or oxygen), or acoustic (precordial sounds or normal sounds of the ventilator cycle).

Mechanical ventilation is achieved by generating positive pressure in the breathing circuit. A low-pressure alarm, also referred to as a disconnect alarm, sounds when sufficient pressure is not generated in order to reach normal inspiratory peak pressures or standing bellows fail to fill. Some machines also offer an alarm that warns if insufficient expired gas is returned. A low-pressure alarm is not intended to be a specific disconnection alarm but, when used in conjunction with other monitors/alarms, it may be of help in warning of disconnections.

Capnographs (CO_2 monitors) are probably the best devices for revealing patient disconnection. Concentration of CO_2 is measured near the Y-piece either directly (mainstream) or by continuous aspiration of a gas sample to the analyzer instrument (sidestream). Either a sudden change in the differences between the inspiratory and end-tidal CO_2 concentrations or the acute absence of measured CO_2 indicates a disconnection, a nonventilated patient, or other problems like low (or no) cardiac output.[3,15]

Gas volume and flow monitoring is performed with spirometers and flow sensors. The Wright respirometer or the electronic Spiromed uses a rotating vane. The Fleisch pneumotach measures flow by measuring the pressure difference across a flow resistor (capillary tube) in a tube. In the heated-wire anemometer (thermal dissipation device) heat is dissipated when gas flows past a wire. The ultrasonic flow sensor measures the influence of gas flow on the transmission times of pulses between two crystals. Fixed and variable orifice flow sensors are also used to generate pressure- and flow-volume loops. Thus, absent readings on the spirometer or pressure trace, can also be an indication of a disconnection.

In the presence of disconnection, during spontaneous ventilation the reservoir bag will fail to inflate and the patient may show signs of insufficient depth of anesthesia. Clinical signs of apnea include loss of breath sounds during auscultation or failure of the chest to rise. Hypoxemia as measured by a reduction in SpO_2 with pulse oximetry is a

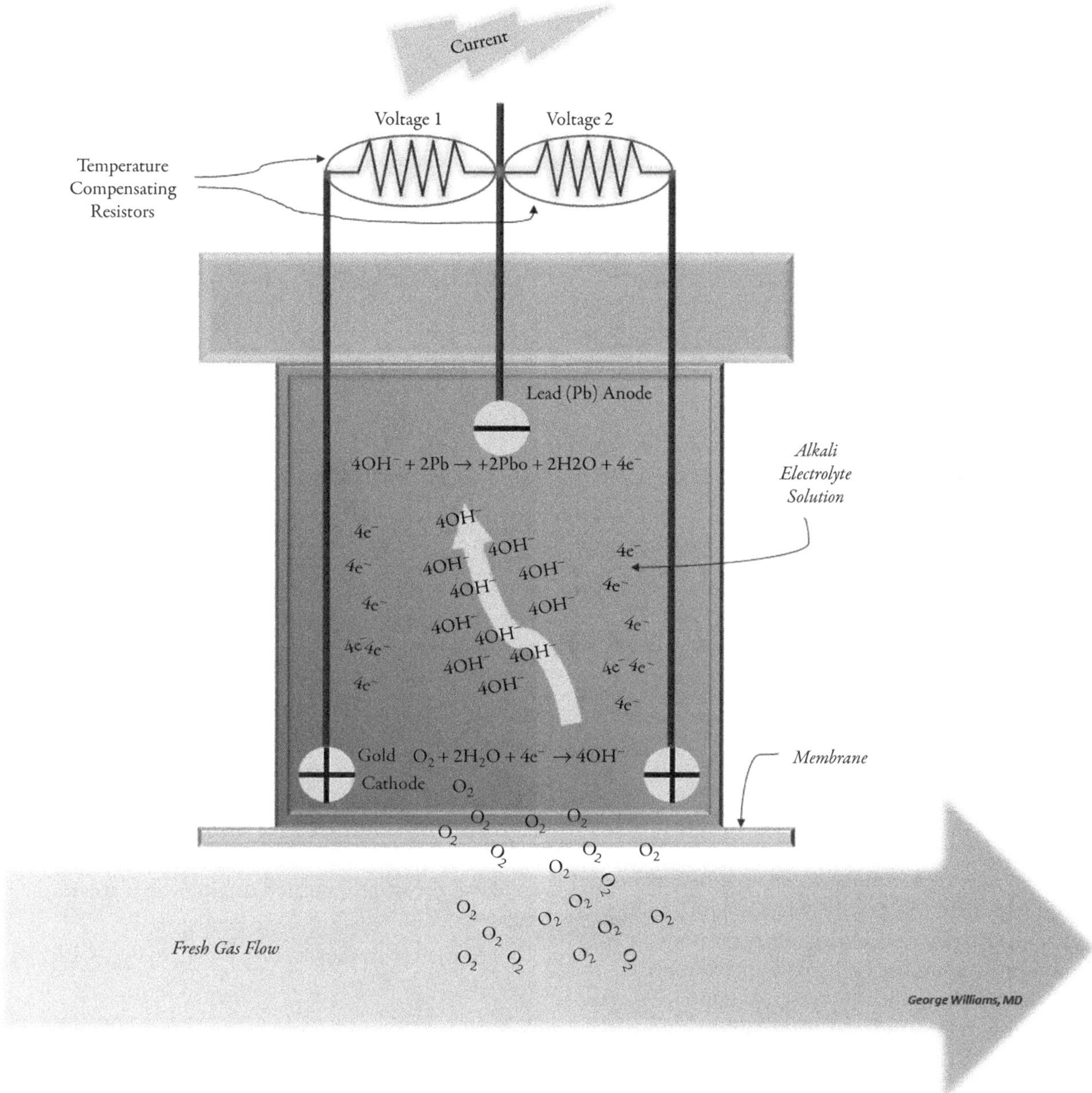

Figure 7.14 A galvanic oxygen sensor cell reaction flow diagram. Fresh gas with a set concentration of oxygen flows past the semipermeable membrane. Once the oxygen then diffuses into the solution, which is rich in electrons (an alkali solution), the initial reduction reaction occurs. Recall that gain of an electron is reduction; loss of an electron is oxygenation (LEO says GER). Following reduction, the hydroxide molecules diffuse through the solution to the anode, which is composed of lead where oxidation occurs, releasing the recently bound electrons. The lead anode is gradually consumed in this reaction. On the converse, the gold anode, water, and electrolyte solution are not consumed. Current is generated and measured with temperature-compensating resistors. If the voltage difference between each lead is significantly different, the machine produces an alarm to check the oxygen sensor.

late sign. In general, the use of multiple monitors enhances the level of vigilance and diagnostic utility.

INSPIRATORY:EXPIRATORY RATIO

The I:E ratio is the ratio of the inspiratory phase time to the expiratory phase time.

Inspiratory phase time is the time between the start of inspiratory flow and the beginning of expiratory flow. It is the sum of the inspiratory flow and inspiratory pause times. *Inspiratory pause time* is the time during which the lungs are held inflated at a fixed pressure or volume (i.e., the time during which the inspiratory phase has zero flow). It is also called the inspiratory hold, inflation hold, or inspiratory plateau. The *expiratory phase time* is the time between the start of expiratory flow and the start of inspiratory flow. It is the sum of the expiratory flow and expiratory pause times.

The selection of a specific I:E ratio is generally based on hemodynamic response to ventilation, oxygenation status, and level of spontaneous breathing. In spontaneously breathing patients, gas delivery should be coordinated with the patient's inspiratory effort to ensure synchrony. During controlled mechanical ventilation I:E ratios may be lengthened in order to elevate MAP and enhance oxygenation. When lengthening I:E ratios, the impact of these alterations on the cardiovascular system must be carefully monitored. The primary factors limiting increases in I:E ratios are patient discomfort, the need for sedation, the development of auto-PEEP, and hemodynamic compromise.[14,16]

- During spontaneous breathing, the normal I:E ratio is 1:2, indicating that for normal patients the exhalation time is about twice as long as the inhalation time.
- If exhalation time is too short, "breath stacking" occurs, resulting in an increase in end-expiratory pressure also called auto-PEEP.
- Depending on the disease process, such as in ARDS, oxygenation may be improved by increasing the inspiratory time (see earlier sections regarding "sigh" and recruitment breaths).
- Patients with obstructive airway disease, that is, bronchial asthma, would require a prolonged expiratory time to allow time for alveolar emptying.

COMPLIANCE

Compliance refers to the ability of the lung to expand and is a measure of distensibility. It is the volume change in the lung achieved per unit change in pressure: $C = V/P$. Most commonly, compliance is used in reference to the lungs and chest wall. Breathing system components, especially breathing tubes and the reservoir bag, also have compliance.

In a spontaneously breathing patient, the total compliance is about 0.1 L/cmH_2O. Compliance varies depending on a person's posture, position, and active breathing. For an intubated, mechanically ventilated patient with normal lungs and a normal chest wall, compliance varies from 40 to 50 mL/cmH_2O in males and from 35 to 45 mL/cmH_2O in females. In either gender, normal compliance can range from 50 to 80 mL/cmH_2O.

- change in volume in liters (ΔV)/change in pressure in cmH_2O (ΔP)
- can be static (when there is no air flow) or dynamic (during breathing—where airflow resistance becomes a factor)

DYNAMIC COMPLIANCE

Dynamic compliance is a measure of both elastic and airway resistance. Dynamic compliance is the total impedance to inflation and includes the extra pressure needed to overcome resistance to airflow, inertia of chest wall, and viscoelasticity of tissues. Dynamic compliance is calculated when there is no gas flowing, usually at end inspiration and end expiration. Pressure gradient and respired volume in the pressure volume loop are used for calculation. When no gas is flowing, the airway pressure equals alveolar pressure.

$$\text{Dynamic Compliance}\left(C_{dyn}\right) = V_T / \left(\text{PIP} - \text{PEEP}\right)$$

Where VT = tidal volume in liters, PIP = peak inspiratory pressure, and PEEP = positive end-expiratory pressure in cmH_2O.

Dynamic compliance is always less than or equal to static lung compliance.

STATIC COMPLIANCE

Static compliance is a measure of the "stiffness" of lung and chest wall and represents pulmonary compliance measured during periods without gas flow, such as during an inspiratory pause. It is usually attributable due equally to lung and chest wall compliances (100 mL/cmH_2O each). The lung is inflated with normal tidal volume and then paused at end inspiration (inspiratory pause) for between 0.5 and 2 seconds to eliminate the effects of airway resistance. Static compliance is calculated from the volume delivered and pressure recorded during the plateau.

$$\text{Static Compliance}\left(C_{stat}\right) = V_T / \left(P_{plat} - \text{PEEP}\right)$$

Where VT = tidal volume in liters, PPlat = plateau pressure, and PEEP = positive end-expiratory pressure in cmH_2O.

Total compliance reflects the elastic properties of the lungs, thorax, abdomen, and the breathing system. Using muscle relaxants will increase chest wall compliance but will not affect lung compliance, so in paralyzed patients, changes in compliance reflect mainly alterations in lung compliance.

Many ventilators and anesthetic monitoring systems now routinely measure airway pressure and tidal volume. This enables a pressure volume loop to be displayed from which the dynamic compliance of the respiratory system may be calculated on a continuous breath-by-breath basis. Some ventilators also measure static compliance. Monitoring of changes in compliance is a valuable means of assessing changes in a patient's condition during mechanical ventilatory support. There is decreased lung compliance, both dynamic and static, in pulmonary fibrosis, consolidation, edema, and ARDS. Emphysema is the only condition in which static compliance is increased.[3,16]

REFERENCES

1. Brockwell R, Andrews J. Inhaled anesthetic delivery systems. In: Miller R, ed. *Miller's Anesthesia*. 6th ed. Philadelphia, PA: Elsevier; 2005:273.
2. Aston D, Rivers A, Dharmadasa A. *Equipment in Anesthesia and Critical Care*. 1st ed. Banbury, UK: Scion; 2014:100.
3. Dorsch J, Dorsch S. *Anesthesia Equipment*. 5th ed. Philadelphia, PA: Wolters Kluwer, Lippincott Williams & Wilkins; 2008.
4. Sassoon C. Triggering of the ventilator in patient-ventilator interactions. *Respir Care*. 2011;56(1):39–51.
5. Santanilla J, Daniel B, Yeow M. Mechanical ventilation. *Emerg Med Clin N Am*. 2008;26:849–862.
6. Eisenkraft J, Cohen E, Neustein S. Anesthesia for thoracic surgery. In Barash P, Cullen B, Stoelting R, eds. *Clinical Anesthesia*. 3rd ed. Philadelphia PA: Lippincott-Raven; 1997:769.
7. Wilson W, Benumof J. Anesthesia for thoracic surgery. In: Miller R, ed. *Miller's Anesthesia*. 6th ed. Philadelphia, PA: Elsevier; 2005:1847.
8. Goldmith J, Karotkin E. Introduction to assisted ventilation. In: Goldmith J, Karotkin E, eds. *Assisted Ventilation of the Neonate*. 5th ed. St. Louis, MO: Saunders Elsevier; 2011.
9. Blum R, Cote C. Pediatric equipment. In: Cote C, Lerman J, Anderson B, eds. *A Practice of Anesthesia for Infants and Children*. 4th ed. Philadelphia, PA: Elsevier Saunders; 2013:1053.
10. Wiswell T, Courtney S. Noninvasive respiratory support. In: Goldmith J, Karotkin E, eds. *Assisted Ventilation of the Neonate*. 5th ed. St. Louis, MO: Saunders Elsevier; 2011.
11. Cochrane Neonatal Review. Health and Human Services website. http://www.nichd.nih.gov/cochrane_data/spencek_01/spencek_01.html. Published November 15, 2006. Accessed March 26, 2015.
12. Kovaric W. Pediatric and neonatal intensive care. In: Miller R, ed. *Miller's Anesthesia*. 6th ed. Philadelphia, PA: Elsevier; 2005:2831.
13. Morgan M, Edward G, Mikhail M, Murry M. *Clinical Anesthesiology*. 4th ed. Philadelphia, PA: McGraw-Hill; 2006.
14. Moon R, Camporesi E. Respiratory monitoring. In: Miller R, ed. *Miller's Anesthesia*. 6th ed. New York, NY: Elsevier; 2005.
15. Al-Shaikh B, Stacey S. *Essentials of Anesthetic Equipment*. 4th ed. New York, NY: Elsevier; 2013.
16. Dorsch J, Dorsch S. *Understanding Anesthesia Equipment*. 5th ed. Philadelphia, PA: Lippincott Williams & Wilkins, 2008.

FURTHER READING

Dorsch J, Dorsch S. *Anesthesia Equipment*. 5th ed. Philadelphia, PA: Lippincott Williams & Wilkins; 2008.

QUESTIONS

1. By definition, compliance is a measurement of:
   A. Change in volume divided by change in pressure.
   B. Change in dead space divided by tidal volume.
   C. Change in pressure divided by change in volume.
   D. Tidal volume times respiratory rate.
   E. None of the above.

2. A 76-year-old patient with a history of idiopathic pulmonary fibrosis develops pneumonia and has to be intubated and placed on mechanical ventilation. What lung mechanics do you expect to find in this patient?
   A. Increased peak pressure, normal plateau pressure
   B. Increased peak pressure with decreased plateau pressure
   C. Increased peak and plateau pressure with decreased compliance
   D. Decreased peak pressure
   E. Decreased peak pressure with no change in plateau pressure or compliance

3. Which monitor is not a reliable detector of breathing system disconnection?
   A. Oxygen analyzer
   B. End-tidal CO_2 monitor
   C. Ultrasonic flow sensor
   D. Spirometer pressure trace
   E. Sound of bellows

4. In a patient with ARDS, the following are reasonable components of ventilation strategy:
   A. Tidal volume of 12 mL/kg
   B. Prolonged inspiratory time
   C. Peak inspiratory pressure of >40 cmH_2O
   D. Low values of PEEP
   E. Low FiO_2

5. The following are true of oxygen analysis:
   A. Oxygen is a diamagnetic molecule.
   B. Oxygen has paired electrons in its outer ring.
   C. N_2O is paramagnetic.
   D. Paramagnetic analyzers are not affected by water vapor.
   E. Paramagnetic analyzers can provide breath-to-breath measurement.

6. The safety features found in an anesthesia machine include all of the following except:
   A. Oxygen supply failure alarm.
   B. Color-coded flow meters.
   C. Ventilator disconnection alarm.
   D. Hypoxic mixture prevention device.
   E. Ability to use two vaporizers at the same time.

7. Which of the following is not a powering mechanism used by ventilators?
   A. Flow generator
   B. Pneumatic power
   C. Controlled pressure
   D. Dual electric-pneumatic
   E. Electrical power

8. Which of the following ventilators does not require an endotracheal tube?
   A. Oscillator
   B. Jet ventilator
   C. "Bag-in-the-bottle" ventilators
   D. Pressure-cycled ventilator
   E. ICU ventilators

9. The ventilation mode that allows the patient to breathe spontaneously within a time-triggered mandatory breath mode is called?

A. CPAP
B. BIPAP
C. PS
D. SIMV
E. PRVC

10. Patients suffering from sleep apnea are often treated with?
A. PPV
B. CPAP
C. Inversed I:E
D. PRVC
E. PEEP

11. What is a crucial feature of a ventilator suitable for VLBW newborns?
A. Pressure control
B. Volume control
C. Sensitive trigger
D. Time cycled
E. Constant flow

12. Which of the following is an advantage of NRS in neonates?
A. Decrease in incidence of bronchopulmonary dysplasia
B. Decrease in incidence pneumothorax
C. Decrease in number of intubation days
D. Decrease in gastric distention
E. Decrease in incidence of chronic lung disease

ANSWERS

1. A. Compliance is calculated by dividing the patient's exhaled tidal volume by the pressure needed to provide that same tidal volume. If the measured exhaled tidal volume is 500 mL and the pressure observed is 10 cmH_2O, one divides 500 by 10. This gives a compliance of 50 mL per cmH_2O. Normal compliance in a spontaneously breathing healthy adult, measured via esophageal balloon, is approximately 200 mL/cmH_2O. Intubation reduces this number to approximately 100 mL/cm H_2O. Answers B and C are fictional equations. Answer D is the formula for minute ventilation.
2. C. The patient has an underlying lung disorder (pulmonary fibrosis) that is associated with decreased compliance. The presence of pneumonia will worsen the compliance further. The peak and plateau pressures will be elevated, reflecting the altered compliance.

   Increased peak pressure with normal or low plateau pressure indicates an increase in airway resistance, as in an obstructed endotracheal tube due to mucus plugging, kinking, or biting or acute bronchospasm. Peak pressure will be decreased if there is an air leak or in the presence of hyperventilation. Decreased peak pressure with no change in plateau pressure or compliance indicates a favorable bronchodilator response.
3. A. An oxygen analyzer will indicate the concentration of oxygen in a gas mixture at the common gas outlet. Manufacturers customarily place them on the inspiratory limb to ensure that a hypoxic mixture is not being delivered. If they were placed on the expiratory limb they could be useful as a disconnect alarm, but moisture in the expiratory circuit adversely affects the functioning of oxygen analyzers. Hence, a decrease in pressure (attributable to a leak) will be more reliably indicated by either an ultrasonic flow sensor, loss of end-tidal CO_2, a spirometer pressure trace, or the sound of ventilator bellows.
4. B. Varying the inspiratory time without increasing the peak or plateau pressure facilitates maintaining oxygenation within a pressure limit without overstretching the alveoli.

   Two modern approaches to ventilating patients with acute lung injury are the open lung approach and the low tidal volume approach. *Low tidal volume ventilation* reduces the damaging, excessive stretch of lung tissue and alveoli (volutrauma), and a tidal volume of 6 mL/kg is recommended. The open lung approach employs higher PEEP along with low tidal volume ventilation, where PEEP should be kept just above the lower point of inflection on the lung compliance curve (Pflex). Hence, the patients receive a higher than conventional PEEP level, with lower tidal volumes.
5. E. An oxygen molecule has unpaired electrons in its outer electron ring, which makes it paramagnetic. Nitrous oxide and CO_2 do not have paramagnetic properties. Oxygen analyzers are affected by water vapor and have a water trap incorporated into their design. Modern paramagnetic analyzers have a rapid response time, allowing them to provide breath-to-breath measurement.
6. D. Oxygen supply failure alarm is an essential safety feature in the anesthetic machine. The ideal design should operate under the pressure of oxygen itself, give a characteristic audible signal, be capable of warning of impending failure and give a further alarm when failure has occurred, and be capable of interrupting the flow of other gases. The flow meters are color coded, and the shape and size of the oxygen flow meter knob is different from that of the nitrous oxide knob. A ventilator disconnection alarm is essential when a ventilator is used. Alarms are also used to monitor leaks, obstruction, and malfunction. They can be pressure- and/or volume-monitoring alarms. In addition, clinical observation, end-tidal CO_2 concentration, and airway pressure are also "disconnection alarms." Only one vaporizer can be used at any one time due to an interlocking system where extension rods prevent more than one vaporizer being used.

7. C. Controlled pressure is a ventilation mode, not a power mechanism.[1–4]
8. B. Jet ventilators are used in clinical situations where an endotracheal tube is impossible to place or where it is in the way of the surgical procedure. All other listed ventilator modes would require an endotracheal tube for their safe application to the patient.[1–4]
9. D. Synchronized intermittent mandatory ventilation mode is synchronizing the patient's spontaneous breath with the mandatory delivered mechanical breath.[1,4,5]
10. B. Continuous PAP keeps the patient's airway open during sleep.[5,10]
11. C. The trigger must be able to respond to the minimal respiratory effort a VLBW newborn is able to generate.[9,10,12]
12. C. It has been shown in multiple studies that the use of NRS decreases the number of PPV days for neonates in respiratory failure.[10–12]

8.

SAFETY

Timothy Hollenbeck and Erikka L. Washington

ALARMS AND SAFETY FEATURES

There are many possible dangers in operating rooms. One of the anesthesiologist's primary goals is to protect their unconscious patient from all of these possible dangers. Adequate monitoring with and manipulation of sensors used in the delivery of an anesthetic are essential to the safe care of patients. Some dangers include possible malfunctioning of the anesthesia machine, electrical incidents such as shock, ventilator malfunction, and patient-monitoring devices malfunctioning.

ELECTRICAL SAFETY FEATURES

All operating rooms use some sort of electrical equipment to perform procedures and surgeries in an effective manner. Line isolation monitors (LIMs) are used in an attempt to decrease the chances of patients getting shocked. For safety reasons, electricity is isolated from the main power source by isolation transformers. The isolation transformer's secondary wiring is not grounded. It provides live ungrounded voltage lines for operating room equipment. Therefore, if a grounded patient has contact with one of the live wires, the patient is safe from a shock because there is no completed circuit that would allow the current to flow through the patient. The circuit is incomplete and therefore unable to cause a shock. Both lines would have to come into contact with the patient or become grounded in order to complete the circuit and result in a shock.

Line isolation monitors are used in operating rooms to monitor the isolation of the transformer. The LIM reads 0A (no leakage current) when the current is not able to make a complete loop. However, there are small leaks present all the time that slightly degrade the isolation of the system. If the ungrounded side of the circuit becomes grounded due to a short, then touching the circuit allows the current to make a complete loop and could therefore shock the patient. Line isolation monitors are present to measure the potential for current flow from the isolated power source to the ground. It measures the degree of isolation between the ungrounded live wires and the ground. It also predicts the amount of current that could potentially flow if a second short circuit developed.

The sounding of the isolation monitor alarm means that one side of the secondary circuit has been grounded. At this time, the electrical equipment that triggered the alarm should be repaired or disconnected. If the source of the alarm in unknown, then one should disconnect electrical equipment in the operating room, starting with the last item that was plugged in.[1(3044–3048)]

ANESTHESIA MACHINES

Anesthesia machines allow the anesthesiologist to deliver oxygen and inhalation anesthetics to patients in order to keep them under a general anesthetic. Anesthesia machines enable us to oxygenate and ventilate our patients while minimizing waste of the anesthetic agents that are used. In order to help prevent disasters and to keep our patients safe, many safety features have been incorporated into modern anesthetic machines.

GAS SUPPLY

Oxygen, nitrous oxide (nitrous), and air are delivered through a piping system. The tubing is color coded and connects to the anesthesia machines through a unique and specific diameter-index safety system. In the United States, oxygen is green, air is yellow, and nitrous is blue. The system prevents the unintentional connection of the wrong gas to a particular attachment. For example, the oxygen connection will not connect to the nitrous connection. It can only connect to the oxygen connection.

Similarly, oxygen, nitrous, and air cylinders also attach to the anesthesia machines via hanger-yoke assemblies that use the pin index safety system. This system prevents the connection of the incorrect gas cylinder to the yoke of an anesthesia machine.[2(48)] This reduces the possibility of administering a hypoxic gas mixture.

Pressure regulators are used by anesthesia machines to reduce the high gas pressure in the cylinders to 45–47 psig, before it enters the flow valve. Because this pressure is slightly less than the pressure in the pipeline, it allows the pipeline gas to be preferentially used instead of the cylinder gas, even if the cylinder valve is accidently left open. Because microscopic leaks can occur at any joints connecting the tank to the machine, it is generally advisable not to leave gas tanks open in order to prevent waste.

OXYGEN SUPPLY FAILURE PROTECTION DEVICES

Today's anesthesia machines are all designed to prevent the administration of hypoxic gas mixtures to patients (Box 8.1). Oxygen flow meters are routinely placed downstream from all other gases. This alleviates the possibility of an upstream oxygen flow meter with a leak producing a hypoxic gas mixture. Oxygen flow meters should always occupy the right-hand location nearest the common gas outlet. Anesthesia machines also require a mandatory minimum oxygen flow/pressure. If the oxygen pressure falls below a preset pressure, the flow of the nitrous gas will be turned completely off. This safety feature decreases the likelihood that a patient will receive a hypoxic gas mixture.

VENTILATOR SAFETY FEATURES

All modern day anesthesia machines are equipped with ventilators. These ventilators have become more complex over

Box 8.1 ESSENTIAL FEATURES OF THE MODERN-DAY ANESTHESIA MACHINE

1. Noninterchangeable gas-specific connections to pipeline inlets prevent the connection of the wrong pipeline attachments.
2. Pin index safety system prevents the incorrect attachment of cylinders to the anesthesia machine and provides backup gas supply if pipeline supply is depleted.
3. Low pressure oxygen alarm detects inadequate oxygen supply at the common gas outlet.
4. Minimum oxygen/nitrous oxide ratio controller device prevents hypoxic gas mixture delivery to the patient.
5. Oxygen must enter the common manifold downstream from all other gases. This prevents oxygen delivery failure if there is a leak or of there is high pressure upstream.
6. Oxygen concentration monitor and alarm allows the anesthesia provider to regulate the oxygen concentration and alerts provider in the event of a hypoxic gas mixture.
7. Essential alarms are automatically active. This disallows the anesthesia machine to be in use without these alarms being activated.
8. Vaporizer interlock device prevents the use of more than one inhalation anesthetic at a time. If a vaporizer is in use, then the others cannot be turned on.
9. Capnograph and anesthetic gas measurement informs the anesthesia provider of the concentration of the anesthetic. This helps to prevent overdosing of the gas. The capnograph provides key information about the ventilation of the patient.
10. Oxygen flush mechanism allows the anesthesia provider to flush the breathing circuit.
11. Breathing circuit pressure monitor and alarm informs the anesthesia provider of high breathing pressures, which allows provider to make adjustments to reduce peak pressures in order to prevent barotrauma.
12. Exhaled volume monitor provides key information regarding tidal volumes to help guide appropriate ventilation and oxygenation for the patient.
13. Basic monitoring of vital signs is provided by the pulse oximeter (which is required to have sound output), noninvasive blood pressure cuff, and the EKG cables.
14. Mechanical ventilator is present to provide ventilation for the patient who is paralyzed or who needs additional respiratory support.
15. Backup battery is a backup energy source in the case of a power outage.
16. Scavenger system prevents anesthetic waste from contaminating the operating room.

Adapted from Chapter 4. The Anesthesia Machine, Table 4Morgan M, Edward G, Mikhail M, Murry M. Clinical Anesthesiology, 4th ed. Philadelphia, PA: McGraw-Hill; 2006.

the years and are now able to provide ventilatory support to some of the most critically ill patients in the hospital. Therefore, it is imperative that these machines have many safety features present, to help avoid potential adverse events from occurring.

Ventilator Alarms

Disconnect alarms must be activated when a ventilator is in use. There should be a low peak inspiratory pressure alarm and monitor built into the ventilator. There should also be a low exhaled tidal volume alarm and a low exhaled CO_2 monitor and alarm. These two alarms may be in a separate module. Other built in ventilator alarms include high peak inspiratory pressure (PIP), high positive end expiratory pressure (PEEP), sustained high airway pressures, negative pressure, and low oxygen-supply pressure.

Capnometers are either mainstream design or side-stream design. They both utilize the Beer law by analyzing the constituents of the respiratory gas stream. In mainstream capnometers, the light absorption chamber is directly in the airway, the light source shines throughout the chamber. During inspiration and expiration, CO_2 can be directly measured. Advantages of the mainstream design include fast process and lack of clogging. Disadvantages include having a heavy infrared device in the endotracheal tube and the inability to measure anesthetic agent. Sidestream capnometers are more commonly used in operating rooms today because they use a small capillary sampling tube that aspirates a sample of the respiratory stream into a chamber inside the monitor. The sidestream capnometer is lightweight and can measure CO_2 and anesthetic gas. However, there is a delayed response and it has the potential for clogging.

Oxygen Alarms

Oxygen flow valves are designed to deliver a minimum of 150 mL/min when the anesthesia machine is in use (the minimum amount of oxygen required to sustain metabolism for most patients). One method involves the use of a minimum flow resistor. This safety feature helps ensure that some oxygen enters the breathing circuit even if the operator forgets to turn on the oxygen flow.

Hemodynamic Monitors

Noninvasive blood pressure monitoring is mandatory to monitor the blood pressure of patients receiving any kind of sedation or general anesthetic. Blood pressure cuffs should be avoided in any extremity with vascular anomalies such as dialysis shunts. It is also important to maintain adequate perfusion to the limb containing the blood pressure cuff. To ensure adequate perfusion, use the appropriate size cuff and avoid too frequent cycling of the blood pressure device.

Radial artery cannulation is often used to monitor the hemodynamics of patients with uncontrolled blood pressure, patients needing multiple blood gas analyses, and patients with other conditions necessitating tight blood pressure control. However, possible complications can arise such as thrombosis, hematoma, bleeding, vasospasm, embolization of air bubbles, necrosis of overlying skin, nerve damage, infection, and loss of digits. The occurrence of these complications can be decreased by taking the following steps: Limit your attempts, use the appropriate size catheter depending on the size of the artery. Use heparinized saline (or saline) infusion through the catheter at a rate of 2–3 mL/h. Adequate perfusion can be monitored by placing a pulse oximeter on an ispilateral finger.

The electrocardiogram (ECG) is used to monitor all patients receiving any kind of sedation or anesthesia. If used properly (placed on the correct areas of the chest) the II lead can detect atrial arrhythmias, and lead V5 is effective in determining intraoperative ischemia.[1(1364)] The ECG is monitored by placing electrodes on the patient's body. Conductive gel on the electrodes works to lower the skin's electrical resistance, which can be further decreased by cleansing the site with alcohol. Once the ECG is displayed on the monitor, it must then be standardized so that a 1-mV signal results in a deflection of 10 mm on a standard strip monitor. Many newer monitors posses the capability of continuous ST segment analysis, which increases the sensitivity of ischemia detection.

Pulmonary artery catheters (PACs) are useful when a physician needs to monitor cardiac index, preload, volume status, or the degree of mixed venous blood oxygenation of the patient as well as during surgical procedures associated with a high incidence of hemodynamic complications. Pulmonary artery catheter insertion can lead to many complications such as arrhythmias, venous air embolism, catheter coiling, and pulmonary artery rupture. Transient arrhythmias occur most commonly during catheter placement from direct irritation of the heart; therefore, it is crucial to inflate the balloon as soon as the catheter tip has exited the introducer. This can be achieved by continuous ECG monitoring during PAC placement. Pulmonary artery rupture is a rare but potentially deadly complication of PAC use and insertion. In order to decrease the incidence of pulmonary artery rupture, it is imperative to always deflate the balloon before withdrawing the catheter and to avoid overinflation or continuous inflation. The balloon should be slowly inflated with a minimal amount(1.5 cc) of air. Once wedge pressure is obtained, the balloon should be deflated. The pulmonary artery tracing should reappear, when the balloon is deflated. Continuous monitoring of the pulmonary artery tracing is required to detect catheter migration into an overwedged position which can lead to pulmonary artery rupture.

Defibrillators

A defibrillator is an electrical device that provides a shock to the heart when there is a life threatening cardiac arrhythmia present, such as unstable ventricular tachycardia or ventricular fibrillation.

Automated External Defibrillator

The most common rhythm responsible for witnessed cardiac arrest in adults is ventricular fibrillation (VF). Cardiopulmonary resuscitation (CPR) has been shown to improve outcome in patients suffering from cardiac arrest, if CPR is initiated immediately in a patient with witnessed cardiac arrest. However CPR cannot convert the arrhythmia to a stable rhythm. Prompt defibrillation is needed to terminate the life-threatening arrhythmia of VF. When an automated external defibrillator (AED) is applied properly to a patient, the AED can quickly analyze a patient's cardiac rhythm and determine whether the patient is in VF or rapid ventricular tachycardia (VT). The AED can then deliver a defibrillatory shock to the patient when a button is pushed. In most cases, the heart is at the least "stunned" by defibrillation shocks. Ventricular fibrillation is a highly metabolic state that quickly uses up oxygen and metabolic substances. Chest compressions deliver the oxygen and substrates to the myocardium, which makes defibrillation more likely to be successful.[1(2977)]

The first AED was introduced in 1979. The first microprocessor-based AED was introduced in 1986. This AED used three successive, nonescalating, 180 j monophasic damped waveform shocks. If a monophasic defibrillator is available, defibrillation energy should begin at high energy (300–360).

Advances in defibrillator technology eventually led to the conversion of the monophasic defibrillator to the lighter weight biphasic defibrillator. The biphasic defibrillator functions by delivering energy in one direction, then reversing the direction of the energy in the other direction for the remaining duration of the pulse. When biphasic waveform defibrillation is used, the body weight of the patient does not influence the energy delivered because the waveforms compensate for transthoracic impedance to allow uniform delivery of the energy and thus obviate the need to vary from the recommended defibrillation energy.[1(2978)]

The biphasic defibrillator is able to compensate for impedance and is able to assess rhythms more accurately than the monophasic defibrillator. The biphasic defibrillator has proven to terminate VF more successfully than the traditional monophasic defibrillator in the controlled setting of an electrophysiology laboratory. Biphasic defibrillation waveforms and impedance compensation together allow effective defibrillation at lower energies than with monophasic, non-impedance-compensated waveforms. The technological innovation helped facilitate the miniaturization of AICDs as well. Defibrillation success is defined as termination of VF into an organized rhythm or asystole 5 seconds after shock, regardless of the hemodynamic response.

PADDLE SIZE AND POSITION Hands-free defibrillation is more commonly preferred over the handheld defibrillation paddles. Hands-free defibrillation is safer because the pads are easier to place and the pads adhere to the patient's skin more consistently, which improves the chance of a successful defibrillation attempts. Nevertheless, it is still very important that the pads be placed in the correct position. There are two ways to correctly place defibrillation pads.

Anterior–posterior positioning of the pads is the preferred placement location. One electrode is placed over the left precordium (the lower part of the chest, in front of the heart). The other electrode is placed on the back, behind the heart in the region of the scapula. This placement is preferred because it is best for noninvasive pacing and generally results in the lowest impedance. As you can imagine, it would be difficult to place handheld paddles in this position, obviating the benefit of the adhesive pads/hands-free defibrillation.

The anterior–apex scheme is another way the pads can be placed when the anterior–posterior scheme proves to be too difficult. In this scheme, the anterior electrode is placed on the right, below the clavicle. The apex electrode is applied to the left side of the patient, just below and to the left of the pectoral muscle. Other suggestions for electrode placement are to remove excess hair and moisture if possible and to roll the pads onto the skin while applying pressure. Always avoid placing defibrillation pads on implantable devices. Place the pads at least 8 cm away from the implantable device. Do not place pads over any medication patches, because this could block delivery of energy to the heart in addition to burning the skin. It is important to remove all visual patches and to wipe the patient's skin clean prior to placement of the defibrillation pads.[3]

Implantable Cardioverter-Defibrillators

The advent of an implantable, battery-powered device able to deliver sufficient energy to terminate VT or VF represents a major breakthrough for patients with a past medical history of ventricular tachyarrhythmias (Box 8.2). These devices have been shown to decrease death in the setting of VT and VF. They have also been shown to be superior to antiarrhythmic drug therapy.

Implantable cardioverter-defibrillators (ICDs) are similar to pacemakers in that they have a four-place generic code to indicate lead placement and function (Table 8.1). Newer ICDs have many programmable features, but essentially they measure each cardiac R-R interval and categorize the rate as normal, too fast (short R-R interval), or too slow (long R-R interval). When the ICD detects a certain amount of short R-R intervals within a certain time period, it will begin an antitachycardia event. Charging time is dependent on the desired output and can take up to 15 seconds for a maximum shock. When an ICD detects enough R-R intervals that are too long, it will begin pacing.[1(1402)]

The ICDs can be placed in patients who are experience hemodynamically significant VT or VF. They can

Box 8.2 INDICATIONS FOR IMPLANTABLE CARDIOVERTER-DEFIBRILLATORS

Ventricular tachycardia

Ventricular fibrillation

Brugada syndrome (right bundle branch block, ST segment elevation in V1 to V3).

Arrhythmogenic right ventricular dysplasia

Long Q-T syndrome

Hypertrophic cardiomyopathy

Prophylactic use in some cardiomyopathy patients who meet certain criteria (low ejection fraction with ischemia or ischemic congestive heart failure with unsustained ventricular tachycardia)

Adapted from Miller Ronald, Eriksson Larsed, Fleisher Lee A, et al. Miller's Anesthesia, 7th ed. Philadelphia, PA: Elsevier; 2010.

also be placed in patients awaiting heart transplantation and patients with long QT syndrome, Brugada syndrome (right bundle branch block, ST segment elevation in leads V1 and V3), and arrhythmogenic RV dysplasia. Studies suggest that ICDs could prevent sudden death in young patients with hypertrophic cardiomyopathy.

IMPLANTABLE CARDIOVERTER-DEFIBRILLATORS AND MAGNET RESPONSE In general, most ICDs will suspend antitachycardic features of the ICD, thereby disabling the device, when a magnet is appropriately placed to activate the magnet switch on an ICD. Some devices will be temporarily deactivated, while other devices will be permanently deactivated. In general magnets will not affect an ICD's antibradycardia pacing mode or rate. Because of the vast number of devices and their different programmability programming, it is best to have the device interrogated and to call and communicate with the manufacturer to determine the device's response to a magnet.[1(1403)]

Preoperative interrogation can provide very valuable information about the patient's history of arrhythmias. Battery life should be evaluated during interrogation as well. ICDs can have more than one battery cell. This makes it more difficult to accurately determine the remaining voltage. The manufacturer should be contacted regarding any device with a "charging time" in excess of 12 seconds. Most ICDs should have their antitachycardia therapy disabled before the use of any device that causes EMI (electromagnetic interference). Monopolar electrical surgical unit can produce unwarranted shocks to the patient. After a device has been inactivated, the anesthesiologist must have the ability to perform cardioversion or defibrillation if the patient develops VT or VF. Should one of these actions become necessary, the defibrillation pads should be placed so that they avoid the pulse generator as much as possible. Postoperatively, ICDs must be reinterrogated and reenabled. Failure to do so has resulted in human deaths.[1(1404–1405)]

Pacemakers

Pacemakers are commonly encountered in the clinical setting and should be familiar to the anesthesiologist. Many pacemakers have an automatic ICD (AICD) function in addition to their pacing function, though this is not universal. Pacemakers are produced/owned primarily by three manufacturers in the United States: Boston Scientific, Medtronic, and St. Jude's Medical. If you are ever uncertain

Table 8.1 NASPE/BPEG (NORTH AMERICAN SOCIETY OF PACING AND ELECTROPHYSIOLOGY/BRITISH PACING AND ELECTROPHYSIOLOGY GROUP) GENERIC DEFIBRILLATOR CODE (NBD) "N" NASPE, "B" BRITISH "D" DEFIBRILLATOR.

POSITION 1	POSITION 2	POSITION 3	POSITION 4
Shock chambers	Anti-tachycardia Pacing chambers	Tachycardia detection	Antibradycardia Pacing chambers
O = none	O = none	E = electrogram	O = none
A = atrium	A = atrium	H = hemodynamic	A = atrium
V = ventricle	V = ventricle		V = ventricle
D = dual (A + V)	D = dual (A + V)		D = dual (A + V)

Be mindful that defibrillator coding is different from pacemaker coding.

Adapted from *Miller's Anesthesia*, p. 1402 Miller Ronald, Eriksson Larsed, Fleisher Lee A, et al. Miller's Anesthesia, 7th ed. Philadelphia, PA: Elsevier; 2010 (p.1402)

about the manufacturer of a specific pacemaker, you can call each of the three manufacturers and provide the patient's name, social security number, and date of birth to obtain the list of devices along with implantation dates. It is possible, as well, to use a chest x-ray to identify the pacemaker manufacturer, though the model number and device details may be more difficult to obtain with this method, still necessitating a call to the manufacturer in any case.

The type and function of each pacemaker is outlined in a nomenclature system. A pacemaker can pace and sense depending on the make and model. Since pacemaking is the most important function of the pacemaker, the first letter in the system reflects the chamber(s) paced. The second letter represents the chamber paced, and the third represents what is done with this information (i.e., pacing is stimulated or impeded by the sensed information).[1(1392–1393)]

BASIC ELECTRICAL PROPERTIES

At its most basic level, the understanding of electricity is represented in Ohms's law:

$$E = I \times R$$

where E is electromotive force (volts), I is current (amperes), and R is resistance (ohms). Voltage is best conceptualized as the potential difference. For example, pouring water from a pitcher at standing height would produce less voltage than pouring from the top of a five-floor building to ground level. Current is a direct indicator of the number of electrons flowing; more current results in more energy (or injury in the case of industrial electrical burns). Resistance is just as the name implies, but remember that resistance usually has a consequence because something must happen to the energy. For example, a toaster generates heat because each filament in the toaster is acting as a resistor. As such, higher resistance results in potential application of the energy (electrons) in the functional use of the device. From Ohm's law other equations can be derived, including calculations for wattage:

$$W = E \times I$$

While wattage is a measure of electrical power, electrical work is a product of wattage over a unit of time. This can be measured in Joules (watt-seconds) or kilowatt-hours. This is the common measurement used to determine power consumption in a home or building.

TYPES OF CURRENT

The two types of current are *direct* (DC) and *alternating* (AC). With direct current, all the electrons are flowing in the same direction. With alternating current, the electron flow is reversing at a set rate over time (cycles per second) called *frequency*. Both types of current can be pulsed or have continuous flow.

Within the AC circuits, the forces opposing electron flow are termed *impedance*, represented by Z in the following alteration of Ohm's law:

$$E = I \times Z$$

Impedance considers not only resistance but also *inductance* and *capacitance*. The effect of inductance on an AC circuit is to increase impedance (resistance) by the generation of an opposing electromagnetic force. When electrons flow along a conductor, a magnetic field is generated around the conductor. In an electrical transformer, wire is used as a conductor and wound repeatedly around an iron core, thereby increasing the strength of the magnetic field being generated and subsequently increasing the inductance.

Capacitance can be thought of as the measured ability to store charge. A *capacitor* contains two parallel conductors divided by an insulating substance, which opposes electron flow and can store charge when supplied current from a source of voltage. A capacitor in an AC circuit allows for electron current flow even when the circuit is incomplete, because the constant reversal of electron flow in AC circuits allows for the capacitor plates to become alternately charged. In effect, the electron supply in the operating room can be physically isolated from the outside environment; as long as the electron movement *within the circuit* continues to alternate (AC current).

ELECTRICAL CIRCUIT SHOCK HAZARDS

An electrical shock can occur any time a person completes an electrical circuit by contacting the circuit at two points and having current, generated by a voltage source, pass through them. The damage an electrical current causes is twofold, with the disruption of electrical activity on a cellular level, such as in native pacemaker activity, and in the generation of heat through tissues. The severity of shock damage is determined by the amount of current and duration of flow through the body.

Macroshock refers to large amounts of current, usually between 1 mA and 6000 mA. Ventricular fibrillation can occur with macroshocks greater than 100 mA depending on the victim's skin resistance, which can vary widely. *Microshock* refers to currents in the range of 10 μA to 100 μA (0.01 mA to 0.1 mA), which can be devastating in a patient with a direct conductor to their heart, such as a central venous catheter or pacing wire. Microshock bypasses the normal skin resistance and subsequently can cause VF with very low amperage. This concept is similar to the usage of a neuraxial block instead of systemic opioids; since the shock is given very close to a sensitive structure, less energy is needed to have the same effect.

The two primary defenses against microshock are the vigilance of the anesthesia provider and an intact equipment ground wire. When caring for a patient at risk for microshock, the provider should never touch an electrical device and the pacing wire or central venous catheter at the same time, as this could complete an electrical circuit, sending current directly to the patient's myocardium. The ubiquitous disposable polyvinyl chloride gloves found in operating rooms provide both a barrier to infection and insulation from microshock to the anesthesia provider, and should always be worn for these reasons when touching the patient. Operating room electrical equipment ground wires provide three main functions: a low-resistance conduit for fault currents, which decreases the potential for macroshock; the dissipation of leak currents, which reduces risk of microshock; and feedback to the LIM (this is discussed more below).

GROUNDING

There are two ways in which the term *grounding* is used in understanding electrical circuits. Electrical power, supplied commercially to a home or business can be grounded or, in the case of operating rooms, ungrounded (recall that, as discussed above, current does not actually flow from the power station into the operating room). Electrical devices can also be grounded or ungrounded, depending on their usage and function. Grounded power is what is typically supplied to residences for several reasons, so that large voltages do not enter the home either from natural causes such as lightning or from equipment failure.

As anyone who has been in the operating room more than a few times can attest, it can get a little bit messy from time to time. With numerous machines, wires, cords, and fluids mixing together, the potential for electrical hazards surely exists. The main ways in which disaster is averted in this regard stems from the ungrounded power supply, in which the current is isolated from the ground potential. The current potential difference of the standard 120 volts exists only between two wires of the power system, therefore denying the possibility of a circuit between the power system and the ground. In order to provide an ungrounded power supply, an isolation transformer must be used, which when provided grounded current from a power source uses the previously described property of induction to generate a current in ungrounded wiring, thereby creating an ungrounded isolated power supply.

When a person comes into contact with one of side of an isolated ungrounded power system they will not receive a shock, as they are not completing a circuit. If faulty electrical equipment with a broken ground wire were to be plugged into an isolated power system, it would neither cause shock to the person using it nor trip the circuit breaker, but it would convert the ungrounded power supply to a grounded one. This scenario is termed a *first fault.* A second fault is required to create an electrical shock hazard.

Leakage current is generated by the capacitance inherent in all AC currents and the devices powered by them, which through their metal components allow a small current amount to the ground. This phenomenon undermines the isolation in the ungrounded power supply to the operating room, and thereby created a need for its detection via the LIM.

LINE ISOLATION MONITOR

The purpose of the LIM is to detect degradation of the isolated power supply, thereby decreasing the overall risk for shock to operating room staff and patients. Imagine a water delivery system such that, when a certain number of leaky hoses is connected to it, an alarm occurs (but does not shut off the water); the LIM is essentially the same thing for electricity in the OR. The LIM usually will alarm in two scenarios. If any faulty ungrounded piece of equipment is plugged into the OR, it creates a grounded system, this is known as a first fault. The LIM should alarm in the case of a first fault, as the potential for current flow greater than 5 mA (in recent LIMs) exists. The OR power supply now becomes grounded, and shock may occur in the case of a second fault. The second scenario in which LIMs commonly alarm is in the presence of excess leakage current from the numerous devices plugged into the power supply within an OR. Leakage current naturally occurs secondary to inductance in all AC circuits, and while there is no first fault in this instance, the LIM will still detect the potential for current flow. The system is still safe to use, and usually the amount detected is less than 5 mA.

Of note, the National Fire Protection Association code 99–1984 did not require hospitals to have isolated power supplies in areas where nonflammable anesthetics were used. A 1990 revision of this code had the caveat that "wet patient care areas be provided with special protection against electric shock." In this revision, an isolated power supply "shall be permitted as a protective means capable of limiting ground fault current without power interruption" (Figure 8.1). This is important primarily because an isolated power supply will still allow function of vital electronic machinery in the event of a first fault, while a ground fault circuit interrupter (GFCI) will stop a potentially hazardous current, and the machinery being supplied along with it. The GFCI outlets are commonly used in bathrooms or other potentially wet areas; they function by disconnecting the circuit (turning off) when excessive current flow is detected. The disadvantage of this system in contrast to the LIM is that if a fault occurs, the power supply is cut off (which could be problematic with life-sustaining equipment). The increasing use of GFCIs in ORs has been implemented in some hospitals instead of a LIM because of the lower cost associated with installation.

OPERATING ROOM FIRE SAFETY

Although the use of flammable anesthetic gas is no longer prevalent in the modern world, the risk of fire in the

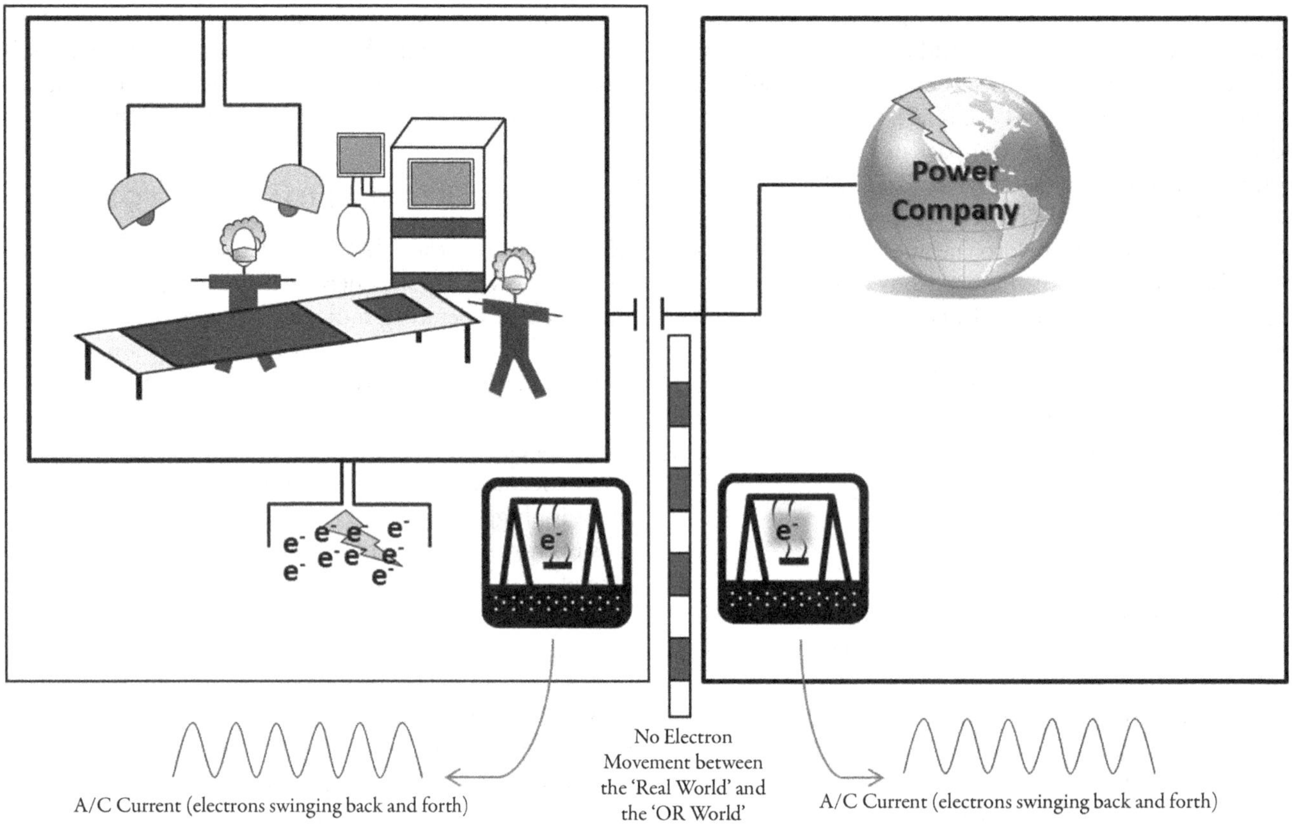

Figure 8.1 OR power supply when properly isolated. Image courtesy of George Williams, MD.

operating room still exists. In fact, with the use of electrosurgery units, lasers, drills, fiber-optic cables, and readily available fuel sources (drapes, towels, high oxygen content) fires still occur at a regular rate across the country. The classic fire triad consists of an *ignition source*, a *fuel*, and an *oxidizing agent*. Basic fire safety seeks to separate these three components from one another.

There are two main kinds of operating room fires. Most often seen are fires related directly to the patient, and of these the most notorious are head and neck surgeries under regional anesthesia (monitored anesthesia care technique). In these types of surgeries, the patient is being supplied oxygen, is underneath a fuel (drapes), and the surgeon may be using an ignition source (bovie). Although less common, fires not directly involving the patient can also occur, as in the classic example of desiccated CO_2 absorbent in the anesthesia machine. Operating room fires may seem theoretical in reading but, unfortunately, they are still commonly seen once a year or more in many larger institutions.

The National Fire Protection Association (NFPA) publishes the standards that govern safe practices across all professional areas, with NFPA standard 99 being specifically applicable to the practice of anesthesiology. These standards are included in a more than 200-page document available online (nfpa.org) and are updated every few years; as such, the full details of these requirements are not commonly read.

REFERENCES

1. Miller Ronald, Eriksson Larsed, Fleisher Lee A, et al. *Miller's Anesthesia*. 7th ed. Philadelphia, PA: Elsevier; 2010.
2. Morgan M, Edward G, Mikhail M, Murry M. *Clinical Anesthesiology*. 4th ed. Philadelphia, PA: McGraw-Hill; 2006.
3. Guideline 7: Automated External Defibrillation in Basic Life Support. New Zealand Resuscitation Council website. http://www.nzrc.org.nz/assets/Uploads/Guidelines/guideline-7-aug11.pdf. Published August 2011. Accessed March 26, 2015.

FURTHER READING

1. Barash P, Cullen B, Stoelting R, Cahalan M, Stock M. Clinical Anesthesia. 7th ed. Philadelphia, PA: Lippincott Williams & Wilkins, 2013.
2. How to Use an Automated External DefibrilatorDefibrillator. National Heart, Lung, and Blood Institute website. http://www.nhlbi.nih.gov/health/health-topics/topics/aed/howtouse. Published: December 2, 2011. Accessed March 26, 2015.

QUESTIONS

1. The fourth letter in the AICD code refers to:
   A. Antibradycardic pacing chamber

B. Tachycardia detection
C. Shock chamber
D. Programmability
E. Response to the event

2. A line isolation monitor will:
   A. fault if one side of the secondary circuit becomes ungrounded
   B. protect against microshock
   C. fault if one side of the secondary circuit becomes grounded
   D. isolate the main power source
   E. sound for electrical overload on a circuit

3. Which of the following is not a safety parameter on the modern anesthesia machine responsible for prevention of the attachment of the wrong gas cylinder to the yoke?
   A. minimum oxygen to nitrous ratio controller device
   B. low pressure oxygen alarm
   C. vaporizer interlock device
   D. pin index safety system
   E. oxygen flush mechanism

4. Which statement is FALSE regarding biphasic AEDs verses monophasic AEDs?
   A. Monophasic AEDs use less energy for defibrillation.
   B. Biphasic AEDs analyze cardiac rhythms more efficiently than monophasic AEDS.
   C. Biphasic AEDs are more successful in defibrillation attempts than monophasic AEDs.
   D. Biphasic AEDs are capable of compensating for impedance.
   E. When using monophasic AEDs, one should begin defibrillation at high energy levels.

5. Which of the following IS NOT considered a possible complication associated with radial artery cannulation?
   A. thrombosis
   B. necrosis or skin infection
   C. nerve damage
   D. embolism of air bubbles
   E. cardiac arrhythmias during guidewire insertion

6. When a patient presents with an AICD presents for a nonemergent surgery, the anesthesiologist should:
   A. Place a magnet over the device to convert it to asynchronous mode.
   B. Cancel the case because the patient has a condition that requires an AICD.
   C. Call the representative for the device to obtain additional key information about the device.
   D. Place a magnet near the device to turn off the antitachycardia capability.
   E. Insist that the surgeon use bipolar electrocautery.

7. Removing which of the following would have the LEAST effect on preventing an operating room fire?
   A. Reducing ambient temperature
   B. Decreasing oxygen concentration
   C. Spraying saline mist on the field during electrocautery
   D. Using nonflammable drapes

8. Which of the following BEST describes the line isolation monitor's primary function?
   A. Reduce electron flow when macroshock occurs
   B. Measure the amount electricity being used
   C. Alarm if OR electrical grounding possible
   D. Minimize the risk of OR fire

9. Which of the following BEST characterizes the type of current used to power OR devices?
   A. Direct flow of electrons from the power company
   B. Triphasic modulation
   C. Alternating current
   D. Induction current

ANSWERS

1. A. Antibradycardia pacing chambers. The ICDs are similar to pacemakers in that they have a four-place generic code to indicate lead placement and function. Newer ICDs have many programmable features, but essentially they measure each cardiac R-R interval and categorize the rate as normal, too fast (short R-R interval), or too slow (long R-R interval).

Table 8.1 **NASPE/BPEG (NORTH AMERICAN SOCIETY OF PACING AND ELECTROPHYSIOLOGY/BRITISH PACING AND ELECTROPHYSIOLOGY GROUP) GENERIC DEFIBRILLATOR CODE (NBD) "N" NASPE, "B" BRITISH "D" DEFIBRILLATOR.**

POSITION 1	POSITION 2	POSITION 3	POSITION 4
Shock chambers	Anti-tachycardia Pacing chambers	Tachycardia detection	Antibradycardia Pacing chambers
O = none	O = none	E = electro gram	O = none
A = atrium	A = atrium	H = hemo dynamic	A = atrium
V = ventricle	V = ventricle		V = ventricle
D = dual (A + V)	D = dual (A + V)		D = dual (A + V)

Be mindful that defibrillator coding is different from pacemaker coding.

Adapted from *Miller's Anesthesia*, p. 1402 Miller Ronald, Eriksson Larsed, Fleisher Lee A, et al. Miller's Anesthesia, 7th ed. Philadelphia, PA: Elsevier; 2010 (p.1402)

2. C. Line isolation monitors are used in operating rooms to monitor the isolation of the transformer. The LIM reads 0A (no leakage current) when the current is not able to make a complete loop. However, there are small leaks present all the time that slightly degrade the

isolation of the system. If the ungrounded side of the circuit becomes grounded due to a short, then touching the circuit allows the current to make a complete loop and could therefore shock the patient. Line isolation monitors are present to measure the potential for current flow from the isolated power source to the ground. It measures the degree of isolation between the ungrounded live wires and the ground. It also predicts the amount of current that could potentially flow if a second short circuit developed. The sounding of the isolation monitor alarm means that one side of the secondary circuit has been grounded.

3. D. Pin index safety system. The pin index safety system prevents the incorrect attachment of cylinders to the anesthesia machine and provides backup gas supply if pipeline supply is depleted. Minimum oxygen/nitrous oxide ratio controller device: prevents hypoxic gas mixture delivery to the patient. Oxygen flush mechanism allows the anesthesia provider to flush the breathing circuit. The vaporizer interlock device prevents the use of more than one inhalation anesthetic at a time; if a vaporizer is in use, then the others cannot be turned on. The low pressure oxygen alarm detects in adequate oxygen supply at the common gas outlet.
4. A. Monophasic AEDs do not use less energy. The biphasic defibrillator is able to compensate for impedance and is able to assess rhythms more accurately than the monophasic defibrillator. The biphasic defibrillator has proven to terminate VF more successfully than the traditional monophasic defibrillator, in the controlled setting of an electrophysiology laboratory. Biphasic defibrillation waveforms and impedance compensation together allow effective defibrillation at lower energies than with monophasic, non-impedance-compensated waveforms. Defibrillation success is defined as termination of VF into an organized rhythm or asystole 5 seconds after shock, regardless of the hemodynamic response.
5. E. Radial artery cannulation is often used to monitor the hemodynamics of patients with uncontrolled blood pressure, patients needing multiple blood gas analyses, and patients with other conditions necessitating tight blood pressure control. However, possible complications can arise such as thrombosis, hematoma, bleeding, vasospasm, embolization of air bubbles, necrosis of overlying skin, nerve damage, infection, and loss of digits. The occurrence of these complications can be decreased by taking the following steps: Limit your attempts, use appropriate size catheter depending on the size of the artery. Use heparinized saline (or normal saline) infusion through the catheter at a rate of 2–3 mL/h. Adequate perfusion can be monitored by placing a pulse oximeter on an ispilateral finger.
6. C. The manufacturer should be contacted. Most ICDs should have their antitachycardia therapy disabled before the use of any device that causes EMI (electromagnetic interference). In general, most ICDs will suspend antitachycardic features of the ICD, thereby disabling the device, when a magnet is appropriately placed to activate the magnet switch on an ICD. Some devices will be temporarily deactivated, while other devices will be permanently deactivated. In general, magnets will not affect an ICD's antibradycardia pacing mode or rate. Because of the vast number of devices and their different programmability programming, it is best to have the device interrogated and to call and communicate with the manufacturer to determine the device's response to a magnet.
7. A. The three factors that contribute to OR fires include: ignition, fuel source, and oxidizer. Reduced oxygen concentration would be effective and is commonly employed. Spraying saline mist during electrocautery has not been demonstrated as safe or effective in preventing fires, but conceptually could minimize the potential for spark (ignition) formation. Use of a nonflammable drape, though not commonly available, would remove the fuel source for a fire. Reduction in temperature alone does not address one of the three elements of fire and therefore is the *least* best answer.
8. C. The LIM is designed to alarm if there is more than 5 mA of current escaping from the devices in the room, at which point there is risk for current to pass from the dysfunctional device into a person that is grounded to the room (not to the rest of the world, as discussed). The LIM does not reduce electron flow. While the LIM is monitoring the amount of escaped current, it is not monitoring kilowatt hours or similar measures of electricity consumption. The LIM could lead to lack of grounding if the anesthesiologist is not vigilant, however, its function is not best described as reducing the risk of OR fires.
9. C. All power in the United States is provided in AC (alternating current) format. A power adapter (as is commonly used for wireless phones) is needed to convert this current from AC to DC power. AC power is not triphasic but appears as a sine wave (this was a distractor). Induction current is also a distractor, though energy could be transferred through an induction field, OR devices do not use this technology, though some portable devices do.

9.

STATISTICS AND COMPUTERS

Carlos A. Artime, Ariana Rojas, and George W. Williams

INTRODUCTION

Statistics is the branch of mathematics involved with the collection, analysis, and interpretation of data. There are two general types of data: *quantitative* and *qualitative.* Qualitative (or *categorical*) data consist of values that can be separated into different categories defined by a nonnumeric characteristic. Quantitative data, on the other hand, are numerical counts or measurements.

Qualitative data can be classified as *nominal* or *ordinal.* Nominal data is classified into names or categories in which no order or ranking can be imposed (e.g., color or marital status). Ordinal data is classified into categories that can be ordered or ranked, but precise differences between the ranks do not exist (e.g., ASA physical status or Mallampati classification).

Quantitative data can be *continuous,* covering a range of values without gaps or interruptions (e.g., weight or temperature); or *discrete,* meaning that the data can only have values equal to integers (e.g., number of prior surgeries).

SAMPLE AND POPULATION

In statistics, two key concepts of importance are those of *population* and *sample. Population* refers to a defined group or collection of entities that one is interested in analyzing or making inferences about. A population could be very specific (i.e., all of the CA-1 residents at an institution) or could be infinitely broad (i.e., stars in the universe). When gathering data about every member of a population is impractical, one may analyze a *sample,* or a subset, of the population in order to make inferences about the entire population.

There are two distinct statistical methodologies: (1) descriptive statistics, which summarizes the data from a sample, and (2) inferential statistics, in which the data from a sample are analyzed to make inferences or conclusions about the population that the sample was derived from.

DESCRIPTIVE STATISTICS

Measures that are commonly used in descriptive statistics include measures of central tendency and measures of dispersion (or variability).

MEASURES OF CENTRAL TENDENCY

- *Mean*: the mathematical average
- *Median*: the central data point if data are ordered from smallest to largest
  - If there are an even number of data points, the median is the mathematical average of the two central values.
- *Mode*: the most common value in a set of data

MEASURES OF DISPERSION

- *Standard deviation*: a measure of the spread of data around their mean
  - calculated by taking the square root of the sum of the squares of the differences of each data point from the mean divided by the number of data points minus 1.

$$s = \sqrt{\frac{\sum (x - \bar{x})^2}{n-1}}$$

  - where s = standard deviation, x = each value, $\bar{x}$ = mean, and n = number of values
- *Variance*: the square of the standard deviation
- *Standard error of the mean*: an estimate of how close the sample mean is likely to be to the population mean
  - calculated by dividing the standard deviation by the square root of the sample size

$$SE_{\bar{x}} = \frac{s}{\sqrt{n}}$$

- *Interquartile range*: the range of the values of a set of data between the 25th and 75th percentile

INFERENTIAL STATISTICS

Inferential statistics are based on *probability*, or the measure of the likelihood that an event will occur. As stated earlier, inferential statistics allow one to analyze the data from a sample in order to make inferences or conclusions about the population that the sample was derived from. This is accomplished by determining the probability that a characteristic in the sample is a characteristic if the population.

Hypothesis Testing

The most common inferential statistical method used in scientific studies is statistical hypothesis testing. Hypothesis testing involves proposing two mutually exclusive hypotheses about a population and then performing a statistical test of sample data to determine which hypothesis should be concluded. The *null hypothesis* (H_0) is the hypothesis that there is no difference between compared groups. The *alternative hypothesis* (H_A) is the hypothesis that there is, in fact, a difference. To perform hypothesis testing, an inferential statistic is calculated based on descriptive statistics of the sample data, and is then used to determine the probability that the degree of difference seen in the sample or a larger difference is due to chance (the p-value). Based on this probability, H_0 is either accepted or rejected. This is known as significance testing.

Significance testing, however, does not guarantee that the correct conclusion is reached. There are two types of errors that can be reached:

- *Type I error* (α) falsely rejects the null hypothesis, in other words, concluding there is a difference when there is not one (a false positive)
- *Type II error* (β) falsely accepts the null hypothesis, in other words, concluding there is no difference when there, in fact, is one (a false negative)

The *power* of a test is the strength of the ability of the test to detect when H_0 is false. It is calculated as $1 - \beta$. The smaller the type II error, the greater the power of the test and the more likely it is to detect an actual difference.

Which inferential statistic to calculate depends on four primary questions:

- How many groups of measurements are being compared?
- Are the measurements continuous or categorical?
- Are the measurements paired or independent?
- Is the data parametric or nonparametric?

Two measurements are paired when they come from the same subject (e.g., blood pressure before and after induction). This is determined by a study's design. It has to do with the way the measurements are obtained rather than the property of the measurements themselves.

Data is *parametric* if it follows a mathematical distribution, usually a normal (Gaussian) distribution, also known as a bell curve. *Nonparametric* data does not follow a mathematical distribution.

Table 9.1 shows which statistical test should be performed for which scenario.

Correlation and Regression

When the goal of a statistical analysis is to establish a relationship between two continuous variables, a *correlation coefficient* is calculated. This value, symbolized by *r*, measures the strength of a linear relationship, whereby an *r* value of 0 indicates no correlation, and an *r* value of +1 or −1 indicates a perfectly linear positive or negative correlation, respectively. It is important to note that though a strong correlation between two variables may imply a cause-and-effect relationship, this is NOT necessarily the case.

This same concept can be used to predict a relationship between two variables. A continuous dependent, or outcome, variable can be predicted from an independent variable using a *linear regression*. When a dependent variable

Table 9.1 STATISTICAL TESTS

	PARAMETRIC, CONTINUOUS DATA	NONPARAMETRIC, CONTINUOUS DATA	CATEGORICAL DATA
One group compared to a known mean	One-sample T-test	Wilcoxon Test	Chi-squared Test
Two independent groups	Student's T-test	Mann Whitney Test	Chi-squared Test (Fisher's Exact Test if sample sizes are small)
Two paired groups	Paired T-test	Wilcoxon Test	McNemar's Test
Three or more groups	ANOVA (Analysis of variance)	Kruskal-Wallace Test	Chi-squared Test

is predicted using multiple independent variables, this is termed a *multiple regression*. A *logistic regression* is a regression analysis that uses an independent variable or variables to predict a categorical dependent variable (usually a binary outcome).

Correlation coefficients have been used to compare two methods of making the same measurement; however, good correlation does not indicate good agreement. For this purpose, Bland and Altman proposed producing a graphical plot of the mean of two measurements against the difference between the two measurements. To identify outliers, the mean difference is plotted on the line along with the 95% limits of agreement, calculated as 1.96 times the standard deviation of the differences. It is analyzed visually and clinically, taking into account the size of the bias, the width of the limits of agreement, and any trends or variability in the differences.

Risk Ratios

In studies where the strength of the relationship between two nominal characteristics is to be explored, such as between an exposure and an outcome, two ratios can be calculated: the *odds ratio* and the *relative risk*. See Table 9.2.

The relative risk (RR) is the ratio of the incidence of disease in the exposed group to the incidence of disease in the unexposed group, and can be calculated as the experimental event rate (a/(a + b)) divided by the control event rate (c/(c + d)):

$$RR = \frac{a/(a+b)}{c/(c+d)}$$

The absolute risk reduction (ARR) assesses the reduction in risk compared with the baseline risk, and is the absolute value of the difference between the event rate and the control rate. The number needed to treat (NNT), or the reciprocal of the ARR, is the number of patients that need to be treated to prevent one occurrence of disease.

The odds ratio (OR) is another way to look at risk and is the odds that a person with the exposure develops disease (a/b) divided by the odds that a person without the exposure develops disease (c/d):

$$\mathrm{OR} = \frac{\mathrm{a/b}}{\mathrm{c/d}} = \frac{\mathrm{ad}}{\mathrm{bc}}$$

Table 9.2 CALCULATING A RISK RATIO

	DISEASE	NO DISEASE
Exposure	a	b
No exposure	c	d

The RR is used in cohort studies because prevalence is needed to calculate risk, while the OR is used in case-control studies because prevalence is not needed. When an outcome is rare, the OR approximates the RR.

Meta-Analysis

A meta-analysis is a type of study in which the data from a number of individual studies are combined so as to arrive at an overall conclusion. Meta-analyses are performed to increase statistical power by increasing the sample size and improve estimates of the size of an effect. The basis of the effect size is dependent on the type of outcome. If an outcome is numerical, the effect size is based on means, while nominal outcomes are based on odds ratios or proportions.

COMPUTERS

This component of the chapter seeks to roughly cover the different aspects of informatics as it relates to the medical field. Informatics can be defined as a pure and applied science responsible for the assembly, storage, recovery, and distribution of recorded knowledge. When this interdisciplinary science is applied in the service of patients and in the different specialized health areas such as nursing, dentistry, biology, and public health it is called medical informatics. Medical informatics embraces multiple fields but has scientific and applied components. The nonpractical aspects of information and management of the knowledge is part of the scientific component. On the other hand, how health providers are going to use that knowledge in function of patients is part of the applied component. There are different terms for this relatively new science, such as *health informatics* (Figure 9.1).

The objectives of medical informatics are optimization of diagnostic skills and intervention decisions owing to the quality improvement of clinical assessment processes, design and application of different structures to facilitate data collection, development of knowledge, and creation of tools with the purpose of using the theoretical information and putting it in the service of patients (Figure 9.2).

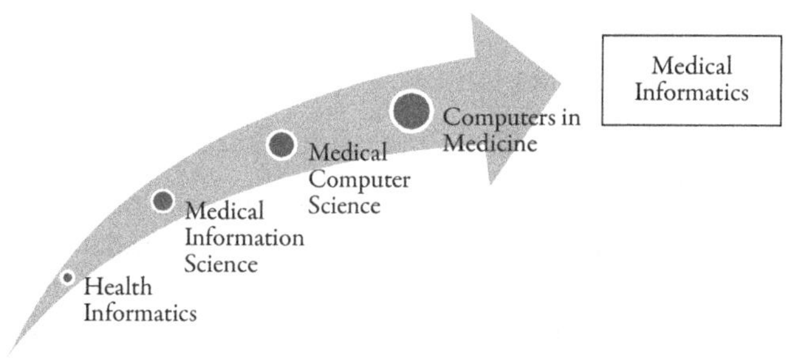

Figure 9.1 Previous terms for medical informatics.

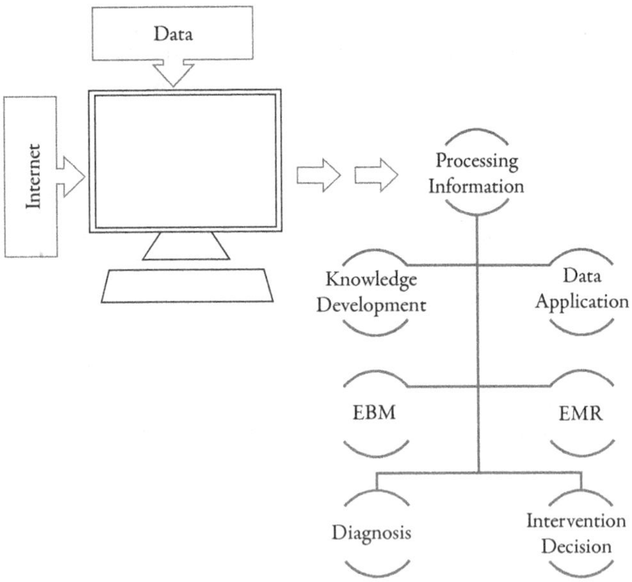

Figure 9.2 Medical informatics systematically organizes and processes the information in order to optimize knowledge development, data use, and management of electronic medical records (EMRs). It also facilitates evidence-based medicine (EBM), which increases the quality of the decision-making process.

BASIC COMPUTER KNOWLEDGE

The health system manages a dense amount of data records, thus healthcare professionals require some proficiency in medical informatics and at least a basic knowledge of computers and their physical components, systems, and programs.

Computers have been used in medicine since the 1970s, when the minicomputer was developed. This computer device was no longer orientated to a selective group, but was rather manufactured at the level of institutional departments. The era of personal computers started in the1980s, with the development of the microcomputer. From that time, the power of computing was reachable at an individual level and health professionals had access to it.

A computer is an electronic device composed of many parts that come together to gather, retrieve, and process data. All the physical parts of the computer are collectively called hardware. On the other hand, *software* refers to all the different programs running in the computer that give instructions to the hardware.

COMPUTER HARDWARE

Central Processing Unit

The central processing unit (CPU) is the center of all computer operations. It has two main incomes: data and instructions (from the software). The instructions have to be given with a specific language in order to understand the way that the data is going to be used. It is comparable with an operating room (OR) control office, which receives information from all the different departments and processes it systematically in order to organize a surgery schedule.

Without going into details, the CPU stands on the motherboard, which is the main circuit board of the computer and has spaces where not only the CPU but also the main memory and other components of the hardware of computer, such as graphic and sound cards, can be attached. The information is transported through the computer as bits on buses, like cars on a highway (Figure 9.3). It can also be seen this way: the motherboard is the skeleton where the nervous system sits, the nerves are the computer buses, and the data in the form of bits are the action potentials that travel through those nerves.

The speed at which information is transported and processed through the computer depends on several components within the CPU. The first is the internal clock, which determines the speed at which the instructions are executed. Caches can be defined as standby areas for data and instructions waiting to be used with the purpose to have them available. The CPU buses are effective information carriers. The internal clock speed is measured in megahertz (mHz), which describes the number of calculations that can be performed in a second. Modern processors are capable of performing millions of these calculations each minute. A fast internal clock is like a skilled anesthesia resident (after a nice cup of coffee) who can quickly execute any task needed. Cache memory property can be compared to having a drug kept in a fanny pack or pocket in order to have it immediately available, instead of needing to walk to the drug cart or hospital pharmacy to acquire it. The cache allows the data to be instantly accessible for the computer to use. Modern processors have primary and secondary memory caches, with the intention of estimating (or predicting) when information may be needed in order to make it readily accessible. Finally, computer buses must have sufficient capacity in order to facilitate a fast CPU; this is like having a broad aisle where many residents and patients can walk

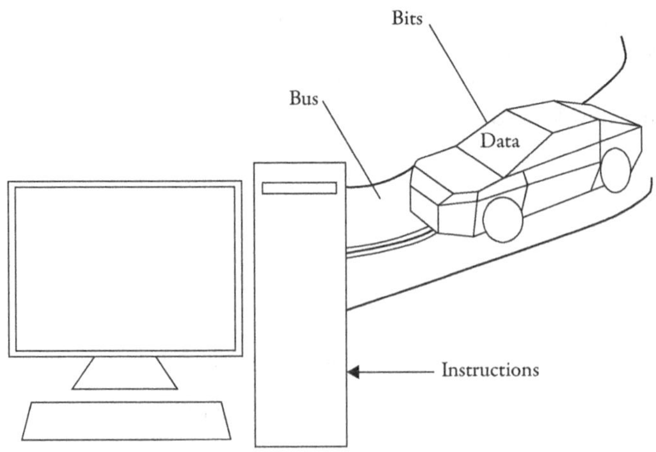

Figure 9.3 Computer data buses are like highways, and the bits are the form of data transportation. The instructions are given in order to determine how to use the data.

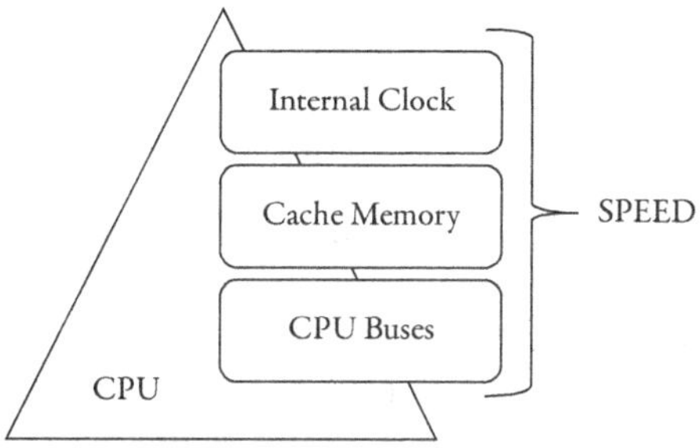

Figure 9.4 CPU speed. Determined by three components: Internal clock, cache memory, and CPU buses. Buses carry information in form of bits, older computers used to have 8 bits (not so wide) but nowadays computers generally have between 16 and 32 bits.

quickly through. If the aisle were narrow, not even skilled anesthesia residents (post coffee, with a fast internal clock) with the drugs needed in their pocket (data available for use in the cache memory) could perform rapidly to accomplish a task. These three factors determine the promptness and effectiveness of the processor (Figure 9.4).

The aforementioned CPU buses allow communication between the different parts of the computer; the system of buses is needed in order to achieve the coupling and the correct functioning of the keyboard, mouse, monitor, and memory stores. The capacity of the buses determines the ability to transport the data (bits) and it is proportional to the width of the bus, meaning that wider buses have more capacity and speed because more data can be transported. A main bus and several peripheral buses are attached to the motherboard. Examples of peripheral buses are the mouse, keyboard, removable disk drive, universal serial bus (USB), and others. The USB has a standardized plug and allows the attachment and removal of peripherals. One of the most important things about the USB is that it does not need a previous configuration, thus no software drive is needed to achieve communication between the new peripheral bus and the computer, because once the USB is plugged into one of the ports the operation system will identify it.

Memory

Information is stored in different modules of the computer. Random access memory (RAM) is a temporary storage used to execute some programs. The CPU cache memory uses static RAM (SRAM), a smaller memory module that reads and writes the data faster. In contrast, the storage memory uses dynamic RAM (DRAM) and requires periodical refreshment in order to retain information; it is larger but the time needed to refresh the data makes it slower. The storage memory can be fixed or removable, with fixed storage memory residing in the hard disk (where a huge amount of information can be store), and data is retained even when the computer is turned off. The hard disk is an important component of the hardware. Indeed, computers must have it in order to function properly. Compact disks (CDs) and "Flash" drives are examples of removable storage memory; the former uses a digital optical format to store the data, and the latter uses electronic rewritable storage called flash memory (Figure 9.5).

COMPUTER SOFTWARE

The hardware has all the necessary tools to process information, but in order to know how to manage the data it needs to receive instructions from the software, which is defined as all the computer programs. The collection of programs that coordinate and manage the activities within the computer is called the operating system (OS) and controls the CPU, memory storage, and other specific tasked programs. Moreover, the OS coordinates data movement between the different internal memories and determines where and when these memories are to be stored, and it also establishes the regulations to which all programs must adhere. Windows, Apple, and Linux are examples of OSs, and every mobile device and smartphone has its own OS. Without going into detail, the OS separates a given program assignment into handy pieces and organizes them in order to give them to the CPU systematically.

COMPUTER FAILURE

As patients, computers present a series of symptoms and signs when there is a problem in their system. First it is important to determine the etiology; it can be an analytical failure (software) or a physical failure (hardware). For example, a hard disk can be impaired by overheating, unexpected power failure, or any other mechanical or manufacture fault, which are physical problems, but it can also become damaged by OS corruption (virus), accidental deletion of

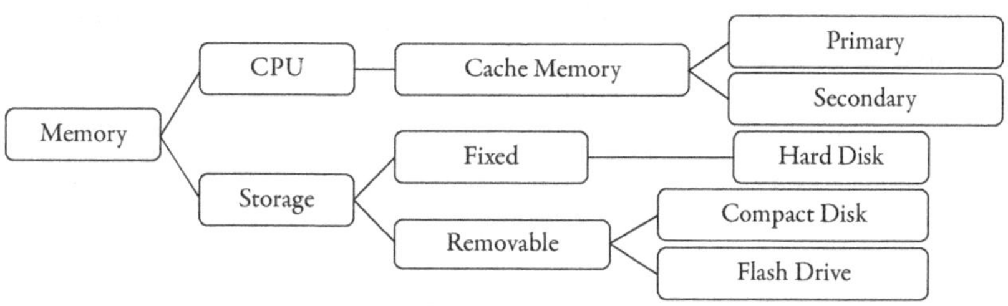

Figure 9.5 Memory stores the data and makes it accessible when needed.

main running programs, and other analytical problems. Computer viruses are intrusive small software programs that get into the system, interfering with its functions. A virus can use the e-mail program to spread itself from one computer to another (attached documents and instant messaging) or can be downloaded through the World Wide Web (The Web). In order to stay informed about current threats and avoid further infections, the computer must be updated with last antivirus tools.

COMPUTERIZED PATIENT RECORDS

Data is a broad term, used to describe facts or information, even though it could have different connotations depending on the discipline trying to define it; data can be numerical or descriptive or can exist as a media or other format. Medical records have data gathered from patients and stored for further analysis, review, and legal support documentation. Data should be handled properly in order to avoid issues in terms of acquisition, privacy, confidentiality, integrity, storage, and disposal. Data access and other components are protected and regulated by security guidelines.

The Health Insurance Portability and Accountability Act (HIPPA), established as law since August 1996, covers the privacy of protected health information (PHI) such as identity information (names, social security numbers, medical record numbers, and others), telephone numbers, ages, e-mail addresses, photographs, tattoos, or any other identifying aspect. Secure electronic communication is also ensured by HIPAA by promoting authentic, encrypted, and timed/dated messages and methods of research data collection, management, and analysis. Any healthcare provider using any electronic device to access or use patient information is covered by HIPAA.

There are three main elements that must be considered for maintaining protection and security of electronic PHI. The first is confidentiality, which indicates that only authorized users can access data, keeping the computer in a secure place, having individual passwords, and maintaining updated software are some options to achieve it. Second, ensuring the availability of the information is important. Environmental threats or technical failure may prevent access to the material; thus, backups and storage of these copies in different locations (off-site) could help to locate data if needed. The last element is data integrity, which guarantees the information has not been modified (whether by accident or transgression) after it was recorded; keeping track of the information used during the project may promote data integrity.

Research settings are also covered by HIPAA and many other laws and policies. Researchers must obtain authorization in order to collect and use data in a study, this consent could be given by an organizational committee, such as the Institutional Review Board, which may have some requirements for authorization, such as explanations of how the data is going to be collected, uses, shares, and protected. Actually, there are specific data collection, retention, and disposal methods that must be followed.

Electronic medical records (EMRs) are important in order to have a systematic and organized manner to process the dense amount of data managed by the health system. Furthermore, it is essential for clinicians and other healthcare providers to have some level of informatics expertise in order to ensure the proper introduction, modification, and management of data into the system. Nonetheless EMRs are meant to be transferred between clinicians and through different specialties; therefore, it is important to have a standard way to share knowledge and use common medical terminology to express it. On the other hand, computing records facilitate evidence-based medicine (EBM), which enhances clinical expertise, bringing higher healthcare quality.

CONCLUSION

This chapter presents just the tip of the iceberg. Informatics provides an unlimited world of tools that can be used to improve the quality and care of the health system. However, some level of proficiency in informatics is needed to be able to apply it properly.

REFERENCES

1. Pace NL. Experimental design and statistics. In: Barash PG, Cullen BF, Stoelting K, et al., eds. *Clinical Anesthesia*. 7th ed. Philadelphia, PA: Lippincott Williams & Wilkins; 2013:219–238.
2. Rosenbaum SH. Statistical methods in anesthesia. In: Miller RD, ed. *Miller's Anesthesia*. 7th ed. Philadelphia, PA: Churchill Livingstone/Elsevier; 2010:3075–3084.
3. Dawson B, Trapp RG. *Basic and Clinical Biostatistics*. 4th ed. New York, NY: McGraw-Hill; 2001.
4. Bland JM, Altman DG. Statistical methods for assessing agreement between two methods of clinical measurement. *Lancet*. 1986;327:307–310.

FURTHER READING

1. C. William Hanson. Medical Informatics. In: Miller RD, ed. *Miller's Anesthesia*. 7th ed. Philadelphia, PA: Churchill Livingstone/ Elsevier; 2010:69–80.
2. James Caldwell. Medical Informatics. In: Miller RD, Manuel C. Pardo Jr., ed. *Basics of Anesthesia*. 6th ed. Philadelphia, PA: Saunders/Elsevier; 2011: 26–32.
3. Collaborative Institutional Training Initiative at the University of Miami. CITI Program. https://www.citiprogram.org. Accessed November 9, 2014.

QUESTIONS

1. The speed at which information is transported and processed in the CPU depends on:

   A. Storage memory, internal clock, and CPU buses.

B. Operational system, storage memory, and CPU buses.
C. Cache memory, operational system, and internal clock.
D. CPU buses, operational system, and cache memory.
E. CPU buses, cache memory, and internal clock.

2. Which of the following statements is true regarding the hardware and software of the computer?
A. Both are computer programs.
B. The hardware receives instructions from the software in order to know what to do with the data.
C. The hardware of the computer controls and sends the instructions in order to process the information.
D. Both are memories within the CPU.
E. Both are physical components of the computer.

3. Which of the following statements is true regarding the operating system (OS)?
A. The OS is an element of the computer hardware.
B. The OS is a group of programs that coordinate the activities within the computer.
C. The OS determines the CPU speed.
D. The OS determines the storage capacity of the computer.
E. The OS is one of the programs of the computer.

4. According to HIPAA, what prerequisites are required in order to have a secure electronic communication?
A. Authentication, encryption, and clear time and date.
B. Time and date stamping and authentication.
C. Authentication and time stamping.
D. Authentication, different passwords, and encryption.
E. Authentication, encryption, and different passwords.

5. What are the three main elements of data protection?
A. Technology, storage, and privacy.
B. Confidentiality, backups, and disposal.
C. Availability, integrity, and storage.
D. Confidentiality, availability, and integrity.
E. Confidentiality, availability, and storage.

6. What statement is false regarding protected health information (PHI) in the Health Insurance Portability and Accountability Act (HIPAA)?
A. PHI refers to any information that can be paired to a patient.
B. PHI can be kept as oral, written, and electronic records.
C. Tattoos can serve as examples of PHI.
D. All the elements that identify the patient can be examples of PHI, except their names.
E. Authorization is required in order to be able to release elements of PHI.

7. Which of the following will increase the power of a statistical test?
A. Decrease the sample size
B. Raise the signifiance level from .05 to .1
C. Decrease the probablity of Type I error
D. Increase the probablity of Type II error
E. Increased variance in the sample data

8. Considering the data set below, which of the following statements is TRUE? 1,2,2,3,3,4,4,5,5,5
A. The mean is greater than the median
B. The data are normally distributed
C. The mode is 3.5
D. The distribution of the data is skewed to the right
E. None of the above

9. In which of the following scenarios would a chi-squared test be most appropriate? Assume the data are normally distributed.
A. Comparing time to intubation between patients with a Mallampati score of 1–2 and patients with a Mallampati score of 3–4.
B. Comparing time to intubation between patients with Mallampati scores of 1, 2, 3, and 4 (four groups).
C. Compairing systolic blood pressure before and after induction with propofol.
D. Comparing Modified Cormack-Lehane laryngeal view scores (I, IIA, IIB, III, IV) in thin and morbidly obese patients.
E. Comparing Modified Cormack-Lehane laryngeal view scores (I, IIA, IIB, III, IV) in morbidly obese patients before and after application of pressure on the thyroid cartilage.

10. Consider Table 9.3. What is the odds ratio for PONV in smokers vs. nonsmokers?

Table 9.3 PONV IN SMOKERS VERSUS NONSMOKERS

	PONV	NO PONV
Smoker	10	20
Nonsmoker	15	15

A. 0.5
B. 2
C. 0.33
D. 3
E. 0.66

11. Which of the following examples of different types of data is incorrect?
A. ASA physical status is an example of an ordinal variable.
B. Mallamapti classification is an example of a discrete variable.
C. Systolic blood pressure is an example of a continuous variable.
D. Gender is an example of a nominal variable.
E. Gender is an example of a categorical variable.

12. For a sample of 100 patients, the mean height is 66 inches and the standard deviation is 6 inches. What is the standard error of the mean (SEM)?

A. 11
B. 0.09
C. 0.6
D. 6.6
E. 60–72

ANSWERS

1. E. Post-coffee residents (fast internal clock) with the drugs needed in their pocket (cache memory) will perform rapidly through wide aisles (wide CPU buses) to accomplish a task. These three factors determine the promptness and effectiveness of the processor.
2. B. The hardware needs to receive the instructions from the software in order to know what to do with the information.
3. B. The OS is a group of programs that coordinate the activities within the computer; it is not a single program but forms part of the software of the computer and sets rules and regulations to the main programs and other specific task programs within the system.
4. A. HIPAA legislation of secure electronic communication covers three requirements: The authentication of the sender and recipient, encryption of the message (conversion of the data into a form that cannot be understood by an unauthorized user), and the specific time and date.
5. D. The three main elements of data protection are confidentiality (only authorized people can access the data), availability (data must be accessible and secure from physical or electrical damage), and integrity (the data have not been modified).
6. D. All the elements that identify patients can be examples of PHI, including their names, as that option, exclude names is the false statement. The rest of the options are true.
7. B. Power equals (1 – β), therefore anything that decreases the probability of Type II error (β), increases the power. Raising the significance level of the test (i.e., increasing α), decreases β and increases power (and vice versa). Decreasing the sample size increases β and decreases power. Increased variance and a smaller observed difference in the sample data both decrease the power.
8. E. The mean of the data set is 3.4 ([1 + 2 + 2 + 3 + 3 + 4 + 4 + 5 + 5 + 5]/10). The median is the average of 3 and 4, or 3.5. The mode is 5. The data do not have a normal distribution, as the data points are more concentrated on the higher values (Figure 9.6). A distribution is skewed to the side of the tail, therefore this distribution is skewed to the left (i.e., has a negative skew).

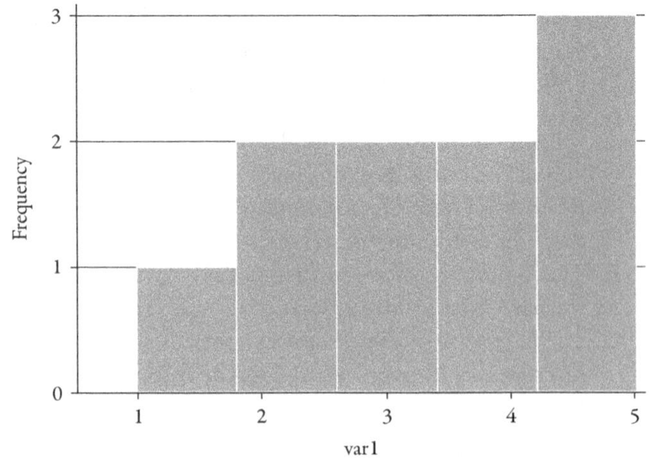

Figure 9.6 Data set.

9. D. The scenario in answer D compares categorical variables in two unpaired groups, therefore the chi-squared test is most appropriate. Answer A compares continuous variables in two independent groups, therefore a student's T-test is most appropriate. Answer B compares continous variabes in four indpendent groups, therefore ANOVA is the most appropriate test. Answer C compares continuous variables in two paired groups, therefore the paired T-test is most appropriate. Answer E compares categorical variables in two paired groups, therefore McNemar's test is most appropriate.
10. A. The odds ratio is the odds of PONV in smokers (10/20 = 0.5) divided by the odds of PONV in nonsmokers (15/15 = 1), or 0.5/1 = 0.5. The relative risk is the risk of PONV in smokers (10/30 = 0.33) divided by the risk of PONV in nonsmokers (15/30 = 0.5), or 0.33/0.5 = 0.66.
11. B. Nominal data is classified into names or categories in which no order or ranking can be imposed (e.g., gender). Ordinal data is classified into categories that can be ordered or ranked, but precise differences between the ranks do not exist (e.g., ASA physical status or Mallampati classification). Nominal and ordinal variables are both examples of categorical or qualitative variables. Quantitative (numerical) data can be *continuous*, covering a range of values without gaps, or interruptions (e.g., systolic blood pressure); or discrete, meaning that the data can only have values equal to integers (e.g., number of children). Although typically systolic blood pressure is expressed as an integer, such as 124, it is conceivable that it could be 124.3 if the measuring device were precise enough.
12. C. The standard error of the mean is the standard deviation divided by the square root of the sample size. $6/\sqrt{100} = 0.6$

SECTION III

PRINCIPLES OF PHARMACOLOGY

10.

GENERAL CONCEPTS IN PHARMACOLOGY

Karel Riha

INTRODUCTION

The study and practice of anesthesiology is dependent on the knowledge of drugs and the way they exert an effect on a patient's mind and body. Successful anesthesia involves the use of drugs to create analgesia, amnesia, sedation or hypnosis, and possibly paralysis with minimal untoward physiologic effect or with counteraction of an untoward effect with the use of adjunct drugs. To accomplish this, the practitioner must have a command of the science behind the use of drugs and the knowledge of how to observe their effects and manage administration based on those effects. This concept is the basis of the study of pharmacology, and it is one of the foundations of the study of anesthesiology. As such, it is likely to be covered extensively in the ABA Basic Examination and warrants thoughtful study and understanding of its basic tenets. This section serves as an introduction to those concepts and refers heavily to other texts and sources to explain the intricate mathematical derivations and details of the models described, which are likely beyond the scope of the examination and this discussion. Topics covered in this chapter include a general introduction to pharmacokinetics and pharmacodynamics, a more detailed look into pharmacokinetic principles such as volume of distribution, protein binding, partition coefficients, tissue uptake of drugs, ionization and pKa, and compartmental/exponential models of drug distribution and clearance. The chapter then discusses the pharmacokinetics specifically relevant to spinal and epidural administration of drugs and then the general concepts of tolerance and tachyphylaxis.

PHARMACOKINETICS AND PHARMACODYNAMICS

Pharmaco*kinetics* is the set of processes and conditions that describe how a drug is administered and spreads through the body and the models that predict what its concentration will be in different places in the body based on the time course after administration and the amount of drug that was given (*drug availability*). It may help to remember that *kinetics* deals with movement (physics, kinesiology, etc.), in this case movement of a drug through the body. A thorough understanding of pharmacokinetics will result in knowledge of how a drug is taken into the body, how it *spreads* through the body, how it *reaches* its target site, and how quickly and by what mechanism it is eliminated from the body. The general terms for these concepts are *absorption, distribution*, and *clearance.*

Administration of a drug can occur in a number of methods: intravenous (bypasses the need for absorption), oral, transcutaneous, intramuscular, subcutaneous, intranasal, inhalational, intrathecal, epidural, and perineural. All but intravenous administration require some type of absorption to occur for drug distribution and/or clearance and are just a sampling of the possible routes of administration available for a drug. Drug distribution then describes where a drug goes in the body after it is absorbed. One of the most important concepts here is the idea of volume of distribution of a drug, which refers to the apparent volume that a drug spreads into to achieve its final concentration in the plasma after administration and distribution to tissues. This is determined by the physical characteristics of the drug and not by the characteristics of the patient to whom it is administered. Also important in the discussion of distribution is the availability of the drug to spread throughout the body (including to its effect sites), which is partially dependent on protein binding and ionization.

Finally, the concept of clearance is important to determine the cessation of drug effect and its removal from the body. Because drugs are distributed to several places in the body and have variable propensity to stay in different tissues, the time course of clearance and the manner in which drugs are taken back into plasma and delivered to the organs that perform elimination are described by very complex mathematical models. Another layer of complexity is added when examining the physical methods of clearance, whether it involves renal filtration and elimination through the nephron or hepatic uptake and biliary elimination or enzymatic modification of the drug molecule and inactivation.

Pharmaco*dynamics* is the study of the *effect* of any given drug on the body, including the action of the drug on its effect site (usually binding to a receptor), the change in a receptor that occurs due to drug binding (or not binding), the biologic signal that results in a cell due to the action of the drug, and the physiologic or clinical effect of that biologic signal being activated or deactivated. It may help to recall that something that is *dynamic* results in change, or *effect*. Essentially, it is a study of the effect of a drug as a product of its dosage. There are four major classes of drug targets: g-protein coupled receptors, voltage-gated ion channels, ligand-gated ion channels, and enzymes. A simplistic way of looking at drug action is to consider the receptor in an equilibrium of active and inactive states, and the action of the drug is to disturb that natural equilibrium. It may do so by keeping the receptors more in the activated stated and functioning toward maximal capacity (agonists), keeping them in an activated state but unable to function at maximal capacity (partial agonists), competitively or noncompetitively preventing a receptor from being activated by its endogenous agonist or similar agent (antagonist), or forcing the receptor into the inactive state and reducing even its baseline activity at equilibrium (inverse agonist).

Additionally, drugs can be further classified based on potency, efficacy, and affinity to receptors. Potency refers to the relative concentration of a drug required to create a given effect. For example, any drug that creates an effect at a concentration of 1 mg/dL has a higher potency than one that creates the same effect at a concentration of 2 mg/dL. Efficacy refers to the ability of a drug to create an "amplitude" of effect; highly efficacious drugs create a near 100% possible effect on a receptor, while poorly efficacious drugs are unable to create a maximal effect even at complete receptor binding. Affinity is the ability of a drug to bind and stay bound to a receptor. Drugs with high affinity do not tend to dissociate from their receptors (possibly creating a termination of effect), while low affinity drugs easily dissociate and possibly have short-lived effect on a receptor. These three concepts are intrinsic to a particular drug and dependent on the molecular structure and not on the amount of drug administered or on the physiologic conditions encountered when administering a drug.

DOSE RESPONSE

The next concept in pharmacodynamics is that of the dose-response relationship. Typically, drugs produce a dose-response curve that is sigmoidal in shape (Figure 10.1), indicating that low doses of drugs produce little effect, increasing doses proportionally and almost linearly increase effect, and higher doses produce a ceiling effect that is not exceeded even with a large amount of additional drug. The principles of efficacy, potency, and affinity can be seen in the dose-response curve. The maximal effect indicates efficacy, comparing dose response curves for two drugs demonstrates potency, and drugs with higher affinity for their target receptors will bind more strongly to their receptors and create a higher slope of curve in the linear portion (more increase in effect for less additional drug given) (see Figure 10.1). Dose-response relationships are key in the study of pharmacology and are the typical way to describe the actions of any drug in a quantitative fashion. Additionally, they serve as one of the best methods to show variability in drug response among individuals in a population. Comparing the dose-response curves of multiple individuals to a given drug will show a great deal of variable response intrinsic to the individual. These differences cannot easily be determined to be either pharmacokinetic or pharmacodynamic in origin, but are easily observed, and several potential explanations exist for this, which are beyond the scope of this discussion.

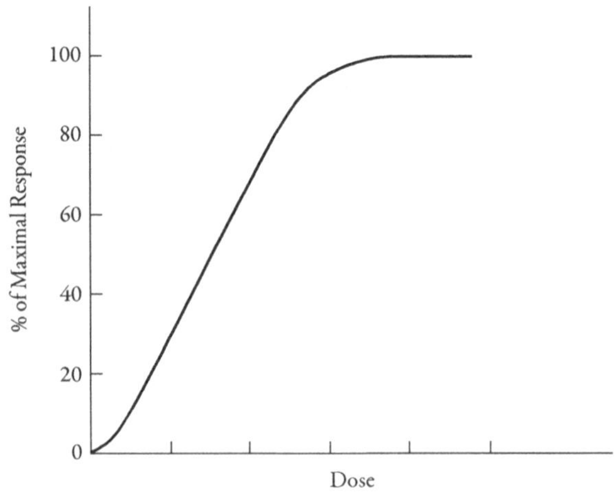

Figure 10.1 A dose response curve for an intravenously administered drug. Note the sigmoidal shape of the curve and the fact that it is nearly linear between 20% and 80% maximal effect of the drug. Diagram courtesy of Shruti Deshpande, MD.

DRUG INTERACTION

The final concept in pharmacodynamics is that of drug interaction. Drugs are rarely given individually in the practice of anesthesiology, so understanding the potential for a change in activity of one drug based on the presence of another is essential. Drug interaction can occur from drugs that act on the same receptor, where similar drugs are given and potentially interfere with each other's effects. For example, when an agonist and antagonist of a single receptor are administered, the net effect will be to shift the dose-response curve of the agonist to the right (higher dose of agonist is required to achieve the same effect), and possibly shift it out of the range of dosing where no effect is seen at all. Alternatively, noncompetitive antagonists generally have a separate binding site on the same receptor, so the effect will be to both shift the dose-response curve to the right and decrease the maximal effect of the agonist simultaneously. More important to the practice of anesthesiology are the drug interactions that take place between drugs that have different receptor sites of action. These interactions are not as well described, but they are measured by the effects of both drugs observed in a clinical scenario. For example, there is a well-described relationship between inhalational anesthetics and opioids in humans. In patients who are receiving intravenous opioids, the dose of inhalational anesthetic required to meet the same level of hypnosis is greatly reduced (up to 60%). This indicates a synergistic interaction on inhalational agents in the presence of opioids given the fact that the opioids themselves have little hypnotic effect. Clearly, the presence of and knowledge of the different types of interactions is crucial to the practice of anesthesiology.

PROTEIN BINDING

Protein binding is an important feature of many drugs that are transported in the blood. The primary plasma proteins that bind drugs in humans are albumin and α1-acid glycoprotein. Albumin binds many drugs that are weak acids and α1-acid glycoprotein binds drugs that are bases (such as local anesthetics). The important concept when considering protein binding of a drug is that the free (or unbound) drug molecules in plasma are the biologically active component of all the drugs carried in the bloodstream. As such, it is important to have an idea of the relative amount of protein binding involved for each drug and the amount of protein available in plasma to participate in binding. The former is an intrinsic characteristic of the drug itself and varies from different classes of drugs. The latter is a function of the patient's physiologic condition relative to the general patient population. Drugs that are highly protein bound will have a larger difference in the amount of free drug if there is a condition or disease state that affects the amount of protein available. This drug availability can relate to the patient's physiology in varying circumstances. For example, a drug with a free fraction (ratio of unbound drug/total drug in plasma) of 1 will still have a free fraction of 1 if all proteins are taken out of the plasma. Conversely, a drug with a free fraction on 0.1 in a normal patient (it is highly protein bound) will suddenly have a free fraction of 1 if all plasma proteins are removed, which is a very dramatic change. The only clinically relevant variable in protein binding in general anesthetic practice is the protein concentration available for drug binding. Disease states that alter protein concentration include renal disease, hepatic disease, heart failure, cancer, and pregnancy.

PARTITION COEFFICIENTS

Partition coefficients describe a drug's intrinsic characteristics of separation between two substances (or mediums) at equilibrium. They are important in a discussion of pharmacology in that each drug has specific partition coefficients that, in part, describe its availability to a receptor in the body to create an action. For example, blood/gas partition coefficients for volatile anesthetics define the ratio of anesthetic present in the blood or in gas form. Agents with low blood/gas partition coefficients typically have a faster onset of action because they have low solubility in the blood and have a faster rate of increase in alveolar concentration. Another example of this concept is the tissue/blood partition coefficient of local anesthetics. Drugs with a high tissue/blood coefficient are demonstrated to have an equilibrium that favors drug presence in the tissues over blood, indicating a higher degree of lipophilicity than another drug with a lower coefficient. Partition coefficients are an observation of how a particular drug distributes between phases; they do not describe why a drug separates in that way or describe a physical characteristic of the drug. They merely allow inferences of drug properties such as lipophilicity, solubility, or ionization.

IONIZATION AND PKA

Many drugs are acids or bases in chemical structure. Ionization of these drugs in plasma or tissues is dependent on two factors. The first is the acid-base environment of the solution or location of action. In anesthesiology we are primarily concerned with the pH of the plasma, which delivers drug to the tissues, and the pH at the effect site, where the drug binds to a receptor. The second concern is the intrinsic structure of the molecule and its propensity to either donate or accept hydrogen ions and exist either as an ionized or unionized molecule. This intrinsic nature of each molecule is defined as the *pKa*, or the pH at which the dissociation of hydrogen ions is equal both onto and off of the molecule. Stated differently, the pKa is the pH at which a molecule exists in 50% ionized and 50% unionized equilibrium. Bases typically have a pKa that is above neutral (7.0) and exist primarily in an ionized state in environments below their pKa. Acids have a pKa below 7 and exist in an ionized state in environments above their pKa. As an example, we examine two local anesthetics: mepivacaine and bupivacaine. Mepivacaine has a pKa (7.6) relatively close to physiologic pH (7.4), where bupivacaine's pH is more basic (8.1). The result is that mepivacaine has a much larger proportion of unionized molecules in plasma or in the tissues than bupivacaine.

More importantly and more clinically relevant is that the unionized drug much more easily crosses cell membranes and reached the effect site than does the ionized state. We can infer that drugs with a higher fraction of unionized molecules will therefore be more readily available to the effect site than those with a lower fraction. Looking back at the example of mepivacaine and bupivacaine, we see that the much more unionized mepivacaine also has a faster onset of action than does bupivacaine in clinical practice. This is at least in part due to the availability of unionized molecules to reach the effect site receptors.

TISSUE UPTAKE

When a drug is administered into the plasma, it is delivered throughout the body, but its presence in the plasma does not result in any discernible activity for most drugs. The drug must first exit the plasma and reach the site of its target receptor, and it relies on its physical characteristics as well as transport mechanisms to reach the effect site. Tissue uptake for almost all drugs in clinical use today is dependent on blood flow to the tissue, that is to say: (1) the uptake capacity of the tissue is far greater than the drug being made available and (2) a change in blood flow will result in a change in tissue uptake. Second, tissue uptake of drugs is usually dependent on a concentration gradient between the blood and tissue that creates an impetus for the drug to leave the circulation and enter the tissue. Once the concentration of drug is greater in the tissue, it will reenter plasma until an equilibrium is reached. Lipophilic drugs are often able to freely diffuse out of plasma and into tissues, but hydrophilic drugs that diffuse across membranes usually do so with the aid of a transmembrane channel, which are ubiquitous in capillaries except in the brain. In the brain, again, lipophilic drugs are able to cross membranes easily and quickly, but hydrophilic drugs typically require active transport across cell membranes. The same requirement for active transport often exists for drugs in their elimination organs as well. Thus, *tissue uptake* of a drug is dependent on the blood flow to the target tissue, the *availability* of unionized and unbound drug in the plasma, the presence of a *concentration gradient* to drive the molecules out of plasma, and the *physical characteristics* of the drug and its ability to cross cell membranes or the presence of *transmembrane proteins* to facilitate entry of the drug into the intended tissue.

COMPARTMENT AND EXPONENTIAL MODELS OF PHARMACOKINETICS

Considering the distribution of a drug in the body and how much drug is in the plasma at any time requires conceptualization of where the drug goes in the body. We have already established that the plasma is the initial location of the drug from which it is distributed to a target tissue. This implies that there are at least two compartments of distribution of a drug. We can consider the plasma as the central compartment from which a drug is distributed to peripheral compartments. First let us look at just the central compartment and treat the model as if there were only one compartment; the layers of complexity will be added with the same basic principles. Measurement of the plasma concentration of a drug at different times after administration into the plasma will show a decrement in concentration over time that follows a simple exponential decrement curve. This follows under the principles of first order kinetics, which is discussed in the section on drug clearance, but the concept is that the drug enters the body and is cleared from the same compartment at a rate proportional to the rate constant, k, for that drug.

What can be inferred as a result is that adding a compartment to the model involves a rate constant associated with that movement (recall that the drug moves into and from this next compartment). In fact, we can add an infinite number of compartments, each with a rate constant into and out of plasma and each of which corresponds to a separate tissue that is supplied by the blood. In order to keep the concept manageable, we conventionally reduce several compartments into one and finish with models that involve two or three compartments (Figure 10.2). The two peripheral compartments used correspond to those tissues that receive a large amount of blood flow and have rapid tissue uptake and equilibration of drug concentration (fast compartment) and those tissues that receive relatively less blood flow and equilibrate more slowly with the plasma concentration (slow compartment). The result of these complex interactions on the plasma concentration of a drug is depicted in the graph in Figure 10.3. There is a three-phase decrement in the plasma concentration: the first phase is of rapid distribution of the drug from the plasma to the tissues

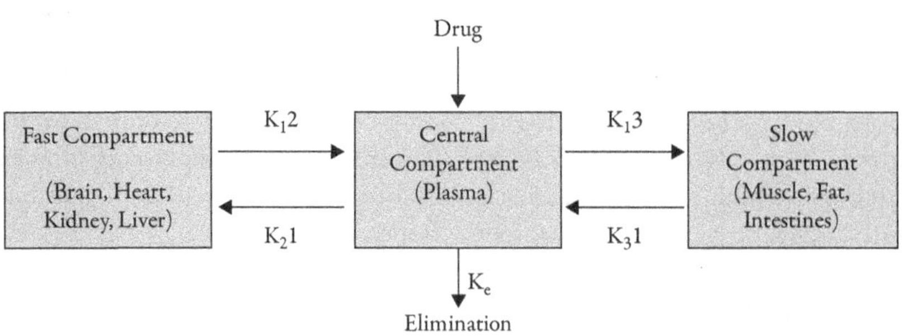

Figure 10.2 A schematic showing the possible distribution locations and complexity involved in the three-compartment pharmacokinetic model. Diagram courtesy of Shruti Deshpande, MD.

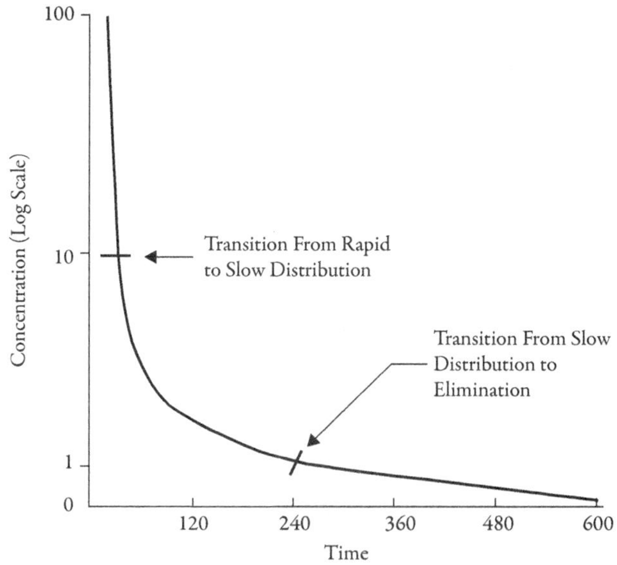

Figure 10.3 Exponential decay curve adjusted for the three compartment exponential model. Note the distinct three-phase morphology of the curve, corresponding to the various phases of drug distribution, redistribution (slow phase), and elimination. Diagram courtesy of Shruti Deshpande, MD.

that receive the most blood flow, the second is of continued movement of drug into the slow compartment tissues but also of return of drug from some of the fast compartment tissues in which the concentration has exceeded plasma concentration, and the third is of efflux from both peripheral compartments into the plasma but primarily of elimination of the drug from the plasma. In the third phase, both peripheral compartments have a drug concentration that is higher than in the plasma.

The mathematical basis behind these multicompartmental models of pharmacokinetics are referred to as exponential models. Miller's *Anesthesia* provides a very elegant and thorough derivation of the mathematical basis for the equation, but the description for the three-compartment model discussed is contained in the equation: $C(t) = Ae^{-\alpha t} + Be^{-\beta t} + Ce^{-\gamma t}$. A, B, and C are called coefficients, and α, β, and γ are called exponents, and each contributes to the model of drug movement between its corresponding compartment and the central compartment. With this in mind, it is important to note that this model only predicts the plasma concentration of a drug and not its pharmacodynamic effect. Some drugs' effects may closely mirror the plasma concentration, while others may show a significant lag time and prolonged effect after the start of clearance from the plasma.

PHARMACOKINETIC CONSIDERATIONS OF NEURAXIAL DRUG ADMINISTRATION

Neuraxial drug administration provides a different perspective of drug administration and delivery to target tissues and receptors. The presumption until now has been of drug injection into the plasma and circulation of the drug to target sites based on blood flow and distribution from the plasma. Administration of a drug into the neuraxial space (epidural or intrathecal) produces a different set of pharmacokinetic concerns that govern distribution of the drug to its receptors. The first difference, and common to both techniques, is the matter of drug dose. Generally speaking, drugs are administered at much lower doses in neuraxial injection than would be required to create an equivalent effect with intravenous dosing. The reason this is possible is that the drugs are already deposited very close to the effect sites and do not have to undergo transport across capillary membranes and into the tissue space to achieve their target. Epidural injection concerns vary based on the type of drug injected. If local anesthetics are used, the site of action is in the spinal nerve root and a high concentration of drug bathing the dura around the spinal nerves allows very rapid transfer to the neuronal ion channels where the drug acts. The same is true of other drugs, such as opioids, which cross the dura to reach the subarachnoid space and act in the spinal cord. The primary pharmacokinetic concern in epidural injection is of distribution of the drug away from the site of action by absorption into the plasma. High rates of plasma absorption may occur with drugs that easily cross the capillary membranes, such as lipid-soluble drugs. Additionally, lipid-soluble drugs may be stored in the epidural fat as depots until ultimately transferred into the plasma. Occasionally, vasocontricting agents are added to drug mixtures injected into the epidural space to limit blood flow and loss of drug to systemic circulation. Also, epidural injection is typically intended for a specific set of spinal levels, so the location of injection and spread of anesthetics should be toward the appropriate spinal nerve roots. In this regard, location of injection along with dose, volume, and concentration of injectate are the primary determinants in the speed of onset of action as well as the spread across spinal nerve root dermatomes.

Intrathecal injection bypasses many of the concerns associated with epidural injection, and as a result the doses used in these injections are even lower. The drug is now bathing the cerebrospinal fluid around the target site and only has to cross a minimal barrier to reach the intended receptors. The primary concern with administration of spinal anesthesia is the spread of drug throughout the cerebrospinal fluid and the possible unintended administration of drug to receptors in the brain and high spinal cord. This is especially apparent in the case of local anesthetics, which are used to create surgical anesthesia at very particular spinal levels and where blockade of neuronal function above those levels can be detrimental to a patient. Determinants of drug spread through the cerebrospinal fluid include the baricity of solution injected coupled with the patient's position (hyperbaric drugs will fall in the CSF with gravity and avoid spread in the cephalad direction), dose, and injection site. Volume and concentration of drug have little effect on the spread when the dose is held constant. Termination of action of intrathecal medications is through systemic absorption into the plasma and distribution of the drug away from the effect site. This may be done through diffusion of drug into the capillary or through turnover of CSF and loss of drug into the systemic circulation.

TOLERANCE AND TACHYPHYLAXIS

Tolerance is the requirement of increased dose of a drug to produce the same effect after repeated doses over time. It involves a right shift of the dose-response curve, or a decrease in efficacy of a given dose of drug. There are several different mechanisms for tolerance, but the most relevant to this discussion are pharmacokinetic and pharmacodynamic tolerance. *Pharmacokinetic* tolerance is the development of decreased ability to deliver a drug in adequate concentration to the effect site. This is most commonly due a significant increase in the clearance rate of the drug (which is often inducible in enzymatically cleared drugs), but is also possibly explained by changes in the distribution pattern of the drug within the body. *Pharmacodynamic* tolerance is a change in receptor function and response to a given concentration of drug present at the effect site. Reasons for this may be a change in the concentration of receptors on the cell membrane and reduction in cumulative effect or possibly a change in intracellular signaling secondary to receptor activation, also called desensitization. Opioids demonstrate a classic pharmacodynamic tolerance effect based on receptor down-regulation, desensitization, and physical modification of the receptor interfering with its function.

Tachyphylaxis is different from tolerance in that it is a much more acute loss of effect and requirement of increased dosage than seen in classical tolerance; this effect can be seen even after a single dose of a drug. Mechanisms for this vary from rapid receptor desensitization, depletion of signaling molecules acutely preventing transmission from the cell membrane to the site of cellular action, or a very rapid down-regulation of receptors. Examples of drugs that demonstrate tachyphylaxis are nitroglycerin (possibly due to saturation or impairment of nitric oxide production), ephedrine (through depletion of catecholamine stores), and beta agonists (through receptor down-regulation).

TERMINATION OF ACTION

Pharmacologic effect of drugs is dependent on the presence of an effective drug concentration at the site of drug action (biophase), which is in turn dependent on their plasma concentration. Once the effective drug concentration at the site of action falls below a certain threshold, the pharmacodynamic action of a drug is terminated. Redistribution is a classic mechanism by which pharmacodynamic effect is terminated (e.g., IV anesthetics). Systemic clearance permanently removes drugs from the body by eliminating the drug or its metabolite.

$$\text{CL (clearance)} = \frac{\text{Rate of elimination}}{\text{Plasma drug concentration}}$$

And similarly . . .

$$\text{Half time is a derived parameter} = \frac{0.693 \times V}{CL}$$

Context sensitive half time is a concept introduced in early 1990s as an attempt to better describe elimination half time (terminal half time) characteristics for IV drugs used in anesthesiology. It is defined as the time required for the plasma concentration to decrease by 50% for a drug administered as a long-term infusion. Propofol in ICU settings has been studied: unfortunately a 50% decrease in a plasmatic concentration does not always have a clinical correlation. Awakening times for prolonged infusion of propofol at a constant rate are similar after 24, 48, 72, and 96 hours of administration. Patients may need the plasma concentration to fall by ¾ or more before awakening—the time taken for this is known as decrement time.

BIOTRANSFORMATION

Drug metabolism occurs in different organs. The liver plays an important role for biotransformation of many drugs used in anesthesiology. Some drugs are partially or completely metabolized by other tissues: plasma (suxamethonium, cisatracurium, esmolol, remifentanil), intestinal mucosa, or lung parenchyma. Hepatic metabolism decreases the concentration of the active drug in plasma and thus promotes elimination of the drug from its site of action. This enzymatic process is a conversion of lipid-soluble, nonpolar drugs into more hydrophilic polar compounds, which can undergo glomerular filtration or can be secreted into bile. These enzymatic changes carried out by hepatocytes are divided into two types: phase 1 reactions and phase 2 reactions.

Phase 1 Reactions

Phase 1 reactions are nonsynthetic and occur in endoplasmic reticulum. Oxidation, reduction, and hydrolysis oxidation of drugs during phase I is mediated by the cytochrome P 450 (CYP) family. This enzymatic system is present in all tissues, with the highest concentration in the liver. It exhibits genetic polymorphism responsible for interindividual variations of drug responses. For example, CYP 3A4 metabolizes acetaminophen, fentanyl, alfentanyl, sufentanyl, and midazolam. Among drugs inhibiting CYP 3A4 are SSRIs, antifungals, protease inhibitors, and grapefruit juice. Drugs stimulating CYP 3A4 are barbiturates, steroids, rifampicin, and St. John's Wort. Propofol is metabolized mostly by CYB 2B6 and partly by CYP 3A4 intestinally.

Phase 2 Reactions

Phase 2 reactions are synthetic, involving conjugation of a drug or drug metabolite previously oxidized, reduced, or hydrolyzed. Conjugation with glucuronide is the most important mechanism (opioids). It occurs in the endoplasmic reticulum of hepatocytes. Sulfate conjugation may occur in the gut mucosa or cytoplasm of liver cell (heparin, norepinephrine, and acetaminophen). Drug acetylation, glycine conjugation, or methylation are other examples of phase 2 reactions. The final product of biotransformation is more hydrophilic and less polar and can be excreted from the body by the kidneys or bile.

DRUG EXCRETION

Many drugs are excreted through proximal tubular secretion (e.g., morphine, neostigmine, and lidocaine) or distal tubular secretion. Biliary secretion plays an important role in excretion of drugs with higher molecular weight over 500 Da. Ionized or partly ionized drugs and their metabolites are usually eliminated from hepatocytes by active transport to the biliary canaliculus (e.g., vecuronium, need for dose reduction in patients with biliary obstruction). Small amounts of most drugs are secreted unchanged in saliva and in milk. Breastfeeding is thus not advisable in patients being treated with opioids, hypnotics, and anxiolytics.

IMPACT OF LIVER DISEASE

Tests measuring proteosynthetic dysfunction in patients with end-stage liver disease (ESLD), such as prealbumin, albumin, and coagulation studies, warn us of potential pharmacokinetic alteration of drugs metabolized by hepatocytes. Hepatic dysfunction can affect pharmacokinetics of IV anesthetics due to (1) decreased synthesis of proteins by hepatocytes, (2) increase in the volume of distribution, and (3) reduction of hepatic metabolism. Pharmacodynamic effects of opioids, IV anesthetics, and benzodiazepines can be enhanced in patients with end-stage liver failure. Cisatracurium is a preferred nondepolarizing muscle relaxant in patients with ESLD, because it is eliminated by Hoffmann elimination and plasmatic ester hydrolysis. Hoffman elimination is spontaneous degradation of a drug in plasma and tissue at normal body pH and temperature; therefore, this type of metabolism requires no significant organ function to take place. Notably, the effect of succinylcholine may be prolonged in severe hepatic dysfunction due to decreased production of pseudocholinesterase by hepatocytes.

IMPACT OF RENAL DISEASE

Drugs depending on renal elimination should be used with caution or avoided (morphine, pancuronium, and meperidine). Elimination of vecuronium is primarily hepatic; only about 20% undergoes renal elimination. Similarly rocuronium undergoes primarily hepatic biotransformation and hepatobiliary excretion, but the duration of action seems to have greater variability. Cisatracurium is a preferred nondepolarizer by many anesthesiologists in patients with renal insufficiency, again resulting from metabolism by Hoffman elimination. Suxamethonium can be used safely in renal failure if potassium levels are under control. Synthetic opioids undergo hepatic elimination and usually do not represent a problem in renal insuffiency (e.g., fentanyl, etc.). Intravenous induction agents are used in reduced and titrated doses due to hemodynamic fragility, impaired volume status, and possible hypoproteinemia.

DRUG INTERACTIONS

Drug interaction is the modification of the effect of one drug by another drug. Many of these reactions are clinically unimportant, while other drug interactions are an integral part of medical and anesthetic practice. Drug interactions are often described in terms of following phenomena:

Summation: additive effect produced by two or more drugs with similar action given simultaneously (e.g., nitrous oxide and halogenated inhalational agent).

Antagonism: attenuation or prevention of pharmacological responses to agonists by other drugs (opioids and naloxone, neostigmine, and nondepolarizing muscle relaxants).

Potentiation: enhancement of the effects of one drug by another drug when both drugs have dissimilar pharmacological profiles (e.g., digoxin and thiazides).

Synergism: supra-additive effects of two or more drugs with similar pharmacological properties where the end effect is greater than anticipated from summation (concomitant administration of benzodiazepines and IV induction agents). Synergism is often interpreted by isoboles (graph showing equally effective combination of drugs) (Figure 10.4). Current evidence suggests that isoboles can be used to differentiate between additive and synergistic effects when the drugs concerned act at the same biophase (same receptor, same enzyme). The practical meaning of isoboles is to show coexistent effects of two drugs so that the lowest dose necessary to produce effect is found. Isoboles cannot be used for drugs that have different mechanisms of action.

Other types of drug interactions are possible. Pharmaceutical reactions are due to chemical or physical reactions that occur in vitro (e.g., concomitant infusion of sodium bicarbonate [$NaHCO_3$] and calcium salt forms precipitates and

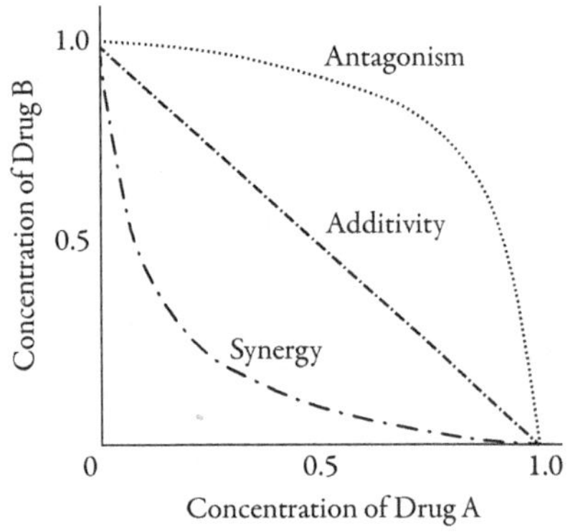

Figure 10.4 Isobole example. Diagram courtesy of Shruti Deshpande, MD.

is best avoided if only one drug is added to each unit of a crystalloid solution). No additives should be incorporated in infusions of colloids, blood, or lipids.

Pharmaco*kinetic* interactions also occur in the human body. For per os (PO) administered drugs they can occur during dissolution or absorption of PO given medication. A universal type of pharmacokinetic interaction is interaction during distribution. For example, uptake and elimination of inhalational anesthetic agents are influenced by minute ventilation and cardiac output; therefore, respiratory depressants (opioids) and negative inotropes will reduce speed of inhalational induction.

Pharmacokinetic metabolic reactions occur predominantly in the liver. The activity of P450 and other microsomal enzymes can be inductive or inhibitory (Figure 10.5). Pharmaco*dynamic* interaction (drug interactions) are used by anesthesiologists every day in clinical practice, for example, administration of a benzodiazepine prior to intravenous administration of anesthetics, as they lower the total dose of intravenous anesthetic needed to achieve unresponsiveness. Similarly, intravenously administered opioids will lower the MAC of inhalational anesthetic agents or dose requirements of continuous infusion of propofol. Drug interactions are described by sophisticated response surfaces—three-dimensional surfaces showing the expected effect of any combination of two drugs (Figure 10.6). Two agonists administered concomitantly can have either additive, supra-additive, or infra-additive effect.

Inductive	or	Inhibitory
Barbiturates		Imidazols (ketoconazole, omeprazole, cimetidine, etomidate) macrolide antibiotics, SSRI, HIV protease inhibitors, statins)
Antiepileptics Chronic Alcohol Grapefruit juice Hydrocarbons (smoked/grilled meats) Steroids St. John's Wort		

Figure 10.5 Pharmacokinetic metabolic reactions in the liver.

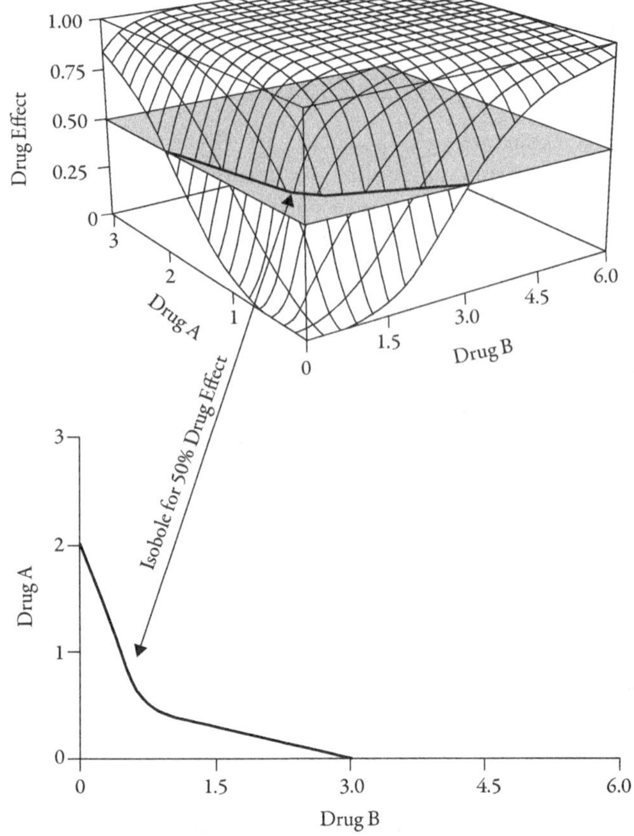

Figure 10.6 Response surface example. Diagram courtesy of Shilpa Dabhade, MD.

HERBAL SUPPLEMENTS

During the last 3 decades, there has been a noticeable increase in dietary supplements and natural remedies often used in conjunction with prescription medicines. The ASA recommends discontinuation of all herbal supplements 2 weeks before surgery. Some of these supplements can interfere with coagulation (garlic, ginger, ginkgo, ginseng, vitamin E, feverfew), hemodynamics (ephedra), or post-anesthetic recovery (valerian, kava kava). Well-controlled, randomized, and double-blinded studies are needed to strengthen current recommendations.

ADVERSE DRUG REACTIONS

Adverse drug reactions (ADRs) are responsible for 3%–5% of admissions and occur in more than 10% of inpatients.

Type A (Augmented)

Type A reactions are predictable, dose dependent, and related to primary pharmacological effect and make up 80% of all ADRs (overdose of opioids, muscle relaxants, insulin, etc).

ALLERGIC				NONIMMUNE	
Type I	Type II	Type III	Type IV	Anaphylactoid	Idiosyncratic
Intolerance	Cytotoxic	Immune	Delayed		
Anaphylactic		Complex			

Figure 10.7 Adverse drug reactions: Type B (Bizarre).

Type B (Bizarre)

Type B reactions are often unpredictable and dose independent (Figure 10.7). Allergic reaction is a hypersensitivity reaction and can be antibody- or cell mediated.

Anaphylaxis

Anaphylaxis is an acute reaction with a production of allergen-specific antibody (Ig E, IgG). This reaction leads to mast cell degranulation and subsequent release of mediators of anaphylactic reaction: histamine, tryptase, leukotriens, and prostaglandins. Reaction occurs within minutes, and is rarely delayed to hours. Generalized and/or systemic symptoms include hypotension, changes in heart rate, cutaneous flushing, itching, bronchospasm, an angioedema, and all may not occur in every anaphylactic reaction. When severe reactions are seen they are life threatening (anaphylactic shock). Treatment includes immediate discontinuation of the suspected allergen (prevents further recruitment of mast cells), airway maintenance, adequate oxygenation, rapid volume expansion, and epinephrine (e.g., 0.1 mg IV initially and titrated to effect). Secondary treatment includes administration of steroids, antihistamines, and calcium.

Incidence of anaphylactic reaction ranges from 1:10,000 to 1:20,000 anesthetics. The following laboratory tests can be used to biochemically assess for the presence of an allergic reaction: urine methylhistamine, serum tryptase, complement assays, and positive wheel and flare 30 minutes after intradermal injection of a specific allergen. Common causes of allergic reactions include antibiotics, radio-contrast media, latex, chlorhexidine, and dextran. Anaphylactic reactions to local anesthetics are rare, with esters more, and even less likely with amides. Muscle relaxants represent more than half of anaphylactic reactions resulting from anesthetic drugs; succinylcholine and rocuronium are the most common instigating agents.

Anaphylactoid

Anaphylactoid (nonallergic) reaction is a result of direct drug action on mast cells with a release of similar mediators as in true anaphylactic reaction. Allergen-specific antibody production does not occur. Large and rapidly administered doses of IV morphine or vancomycin are common examples of agents that result in an anaphylactoid response. Serum tryptase level may be used to differentiate between anaphylactic and anaphylactoid reaction. The treatment and supportive therapy for both types of reactions is the same.

Idiosyncratic Reaction

Idiosyncratic reactions are reactions that have a genetic predisposition. Examples include malignant hyperthermia, pseudocholinesterase deficiency (plasma cholinesterase variants), and cytochrome p450 variants.

REFERENCES (NON ANNOTATED)

Miller R, ed. *Miller's Anesthesia.* 7th ed. Philadelphia, PA: Churchill Livingstone; 2009.

Barash P, et al., eds. *Clinical Anesthesia.* 6th ed. Philadelphia, PA: Lippincott Williams & Wilkins; 2009.

Barash P, Cullen B, Stoelting R, Cahalan M, Stock M. *Clinical Anesthesia.* 7th ed. Philadelphia, PA: Lippincott Williams & Wilkins; 2013.

Butterworth JF, et al., eds. *Morgan and Mikhail's Clinical Anesthesiology.* 5th ed. New York, NY: McGraw Hill; 2013.

Cross M. *Physics, Pharmacology, and Physiology for Anaesthetists: Key Concepts for the FRCA.* 2nd ed. Cambridge, UK: Cambridge University Press; 2014.

Calvey N. *Principles and Practice of Pharmacology for Anaesthetists.* Malden, MA: Blackwell; 2008.

Miller R, Pardo M. *Basics of Anesthesia.* 6th ed. Philadelphia, PA: Elsevier; 2011.

Hemmings H, Egan T. *Pharmacology and Physiology for Anesthesia.* Philadelphia, PA: Saunders; 2013.

FURTHER READING

Barash P, Cullen B, Stoelting R, Cahalan M, Stock M. *Clinical Anesthesia.* 7th ed. Philadelphia, PA: Lippincott Williams & Wilkins, 2013.

QUESTIONS

1. Which of the following local anesthetic drugs will have the most rapid onset of action after administration into the epidural space?

   A. Drug A—pKa 8.1
   B. Drug B—pKa 7.9
   C. Drug C—pKa 7.6
   D. Drug D—pKa 8.5

2. A researcher is studying the effects of ketamine on the function of the NMDA receptor in a lab. She discovers that in the presence of ketamine, she needs to increase the concentration of glutamate available to preserve receptor function. Additionally, even at extremely high doses of glutamate, the response by the receptor cannot reach its highest level. The correct term for this relationship of ketamine to the NMDA receptor is:

A. Inverse agonism
B. Noncompetitive antagonism
C. Partial agonism
D. Competitive antagonism

3. You are asked by a pharmaceutical company to study a drug that will create the ideal spinal anesthetic. Which of the following factors is the most important in determining the potential spread of the drug in the intrathecal space?

A. Dissolving the drug in a hyperbaric solution
B. Decreasing the dose of the drug to avoid cephalad spread
C. Increasing the concentration so the drug can be in a smaller volume
D. Adding a vasoconstrictor to prevent systemic absorption of the drug

4. Which of the following BEST describes anaphylaxis during the intraoperative period?

A. 1:100,000 case incidence
B. Opioids are the most common cause
C. Type A drug reaction
D. Neuromuscular blocking agents are the most common cause
E. IgA mediated

5. Herbal medicines should be discontinued

A. 1 week before surgery
B. 2 weeks before surgery
C. 24 hours before surgery
D. Do not need to be discontinued

ANSWERS

1. C. With the information given, drug C is the logical choice for having the most rapid onset of action. The local anesthetic with the lowest pKa will have the highest fraction of nonionized drug available for transport across cell membranes and should subsequently have the most rapid onset of action. Other factors can also affect onset of action, including overall drug dose, drug concentration, lipid solubility, and protein binding. For example, a drug with a lower nonionized fraction may have a faster onset of action if it is more lipid soluble and has a higher concentration gradient in order to reach the effect site. However, without that information, pKa is the only available measure to predict the onset of action of a drug.

FURTHER READING

Barash P, et al., eds. *Clinical Anesthesia*. 6th ed. Philadelphia, PA: Lippincott Williams & Wilkins; 2009:536–537.

2. B. The fact that there was a right shift of the dose-response curve (increasing dose of glutamate for same effect) and an inability to reach maximal effect indicates that ketamine is a noncompetitive antagonist at the NMDA receptor. Noncompetitive antagonism involves a separate binding site on the same receptor for the antagonist such that the agonist is no longer able to create the same conformational change or effect in the receptor necessary for normal response. Competitive antagonism shifts the dose response curve to the right but does not reduce the maximal efficacy because the binding site can be overcome and cleared of antagonist by high concentrations of agonist. Inverse agonsim refers to a drug binding a receptor and preventing its change into the active form (thereby reducing any baseline receptor function that existed previously). Partial agonism is seen when a drug activates a receptor, but is unable to do so to its maximal effect.

FURTHER READING

Miller R, ed. *Miller's Anesthesia*. 7th ed. Philadelphia, PA: Churchill Livingstone; 2009:496–498.

3. A. Baricity and patient position have uniformly been shown to have the greatest effect on spread of anesthetic in the intrathecal space. Drug dose has a lesser effect, and site of injection can also have a clinically relevant effect on the spread of spinal anesthetic. Concentration and volume of drug have very little effect on the spread of anesthetic in the intrathecal space.

FURTHER READING

Barash P, et al., eds. *Clinical Anesthesia*. 6th ed. Philadelphia, PA: Lippincott Williams & Wilkins; 2009:936–940.

4. D. Recall that the incidence of intraoperative anaphylaxis ranges from 1:10,000 to 1:20,000 anesthetics, so they are much more common than mentioned in answer A. Opioids are not the most common cause, but neuromuscular blockers are. A type A drug reaction is a reaction expected from the dosing range given (i.e., overdose), and therefore is not anaphylaxis based on the mechanism. IgA not associated with anaphylactic reactions. IgE is the classically taught pathway for anaphylactic reactions, and IgG has additionally been demonstrated to initiate anaphylaxis.
5. B. Recall that herbal medicines have clinical efficacy by a variety of mechanisms, and many inhibit coagulation, affect anesthetic requirement, or have hemodynamic consequences. As such, the ASA recommends discontinuation of all herbal medications 2 weeks prior to surgery.

11.

ANESTHETICS

GASES AND VAPORS

Mehernoor F. Watcha and Catherine P. Seipel

PHYSICAL PROPERTIES AND COMPARATIVE PHARMACODYNAMICS

The force of attraction between the molecules of a substance determines whether it exists in solid, liquid, or gaseous phases. Solids have fixed volumes and three-dimensional shapes, with reduced energy and higher attraction between molecules. Fluids such as liquids and gases have no fixed shape and occupy the entire volume of the container to conform to its shape and exert pressure on the container walls. Liquids, unlike gases, have a fixed volume and are difficult to compress because of the greater attraction between their molecules. Gases have no fixed shape or volume but can be compressed into smaller volumes. The pressure, volume, and temperature relationships of gases follow the laws of physics.

A substance can change from one phase to another depending on the temperature and pressure. The temperature at which a substance changes from solid to liquid at ambient pressures is called its melting point. The temperature at which a liquid changes to gas at atmospheric pressure is called the boiling point. A substance, such as oxygen or nitrogen, that is normally in the gaseous phase at room temperature and atmospheric pressure is termed a permanent gas. Changes in ambient pressure cause changes in the boiling and melting temperatures. Gases can be liquefied by increasing the pressure or by cooling (e.g., nitrous oxide). However, there is a critical temperature above which a gas cannot be liquefied by increasing the pressure. When the amount of liquid in a closed container is smaller than the container, there is a surface between it and the air above. The liquid turns into a gas at the surface by evaporation and exerts pressure on the wall of the container. This is termed a vapor, as the substance is normally a liquid at room temperature and atmospheric pressure. Evaporation continues until there is equilibrium between the vapor and the liquid and there is no further increase in the vapor concentration at the saturated vapor pressure for that temperature. As long as there is some liquid in the container, the vapor pressure is independent of the volume of the liquid. However, increasing the temperature will increase the saturated vapor pressure until it reaches atmospheric pressure at the boiling point.

An ideal inhalation agent will be potent in low concentrations, be pleasant to inhale, have a rapid onset and offset of action, undergo minimal metabolism, and have minimal side effects, while also being inexpensive, nonexplosive, nonflammable, nontoxic, and safe to administer with a carbon dioxide absorbent. The physical characteristics of potent inhalation agents govern their clinical effects and the practicality of administration. The potent inhalation agents used in current clinical practice (isoflurane, desflurane, sevoflurane, and halothane) have a vapor pressure below atmospheric pressure at room temperatures of 20°C and are liquid under normal circumstances. The relationship between vapor pressure and the boiling point is listed in Table 11.1, which shows that the higher the vapor pressure, the lower is the boiling point of the agent. Desflurane has a boiling point of 23.5°C. It is therefore packaged in a specialized bottle to prevent boiling in open containers at room temperature and to allow transfer to a vaporizer without exposure to atmosphere. These volatile anesthetic drugs can be evaporated in vaporizers before being added to the breathing circuits for administration to the patient. Desflurane has a vapor pressure of 700 mmHg at 20°C at sea level, and so a variable bypass vaporizer can deliver an unpredictable concentration. Specially designed vaporizers are required, where desflurane is heated and a 2-atmosphere pressure maintained in the vaporizer for accurate metered delivery. Fresh gas from the anesthesia machine mixes with the gas from the vaporizer so that the inspired gas concentration will differ from the dialed-in concentration on the vaporizer depending on the fresh gas flow rate, the breathing system volume, and the amount absorbed in the circuit.

Table 11.1 PHYSICAL CHARACTERISTICS OF POTENT INHALATIONAL ANESTHETICS

PROPERTY	HALOTHANE	ENFLURANE	ISOFLURANE	SEVOFLURANE	DESFLURANE	NITROUS OXIDE
Vapor Pressure (mmHg)	243	172	238	157	669	38770
Boiling point (°C)	50	57	49	59	24	−88
Blood/gas partition coefficient	2.5	1.9	1.46	0.65	0.42	0.46
Oil/gas partition coefficient	220	98	97	53	18.7	1.4
Minimum Alveolar Concentration to prevent movement response to incision in 50% (MAC) (30–60 yr)	0.75	1.63	1.17	1.8	6.6	104
Metabolism (%)	20	2.4	0.2	2-5	0.02	–

With high flow rates the inspired gas concentration (FI) will be closer to the fresh gas concentration.

The aim of anesthesia is to establish and maintain a constant anesthetic level at the effector site in the brain during the procedure and rapid elimination during the recovery phase. When a patient receives a potent inhaled anesthetic, it is delivered to the lungs, taken up in the blood stream, and then moved to the site of action in the brain. Equilibrium is established between the concentrations of anesthetics in the alveoli, blood, and brain. In clinical practice it is not possible to measure the concentration of anesthetics in the brain and difficult to measure the concentration in blood. Therefore, the alveolar concentration is used clinically as an indicator of the administered dose of anesthetic. In a mixture of gases in a container each gas exerts a pressure proportional to its fractional mass at a given volume and temperature. This partial pressure is the pressure it would have if it alone occupied the volume. The inspired concentration (FI) is usually used (fractional volume of inhaled anesthetic) rather than partial pressures and is equal to the partial pressure divided by ambient (atmospheric) pressure.

It is important for the anesthesiologist to know the factors that control the relationship between the delivered concentration from the anesthesia machine and the concentrations achieved in various tissues at different times. The movement of inhaled anesthetic from the machine to the alveoli is dependent on the inspired partial pressure (PI), the alveolar ventilation, and the characteristics of the breathing system. During induction, higher inspired concentrations offset the uptake in the blood. With time, the inspired concentration should be reduced or the continuous increase in anesthetic concentrations at the effector site may result in toxicity. Increased alveolar ventilation increases the rise in alveolar partial pressures (PA) and induction of anesthesia. Controlled ventilation increases the rise in PA during induction and the risk of overdosage if the higher inspired concentrations continue to be maintained. The breathing system volume may buffer this rise but can be countered by high gas inflow from the anesthetic machine.

When anesthetics are delivered to the subject, there is uptake from the lungs into the bloodstream for delivery to the effector sites in the brain. The uptake of anesthetics is dependent on the product of three factors: solubility (l), cardiac output (Q), and alveolar to venous partial pressure difference (PA–PV). The blood/gas partition coefficient describes how that anesthetic partitions itself between the two phases when equilibrium has been achieved. A larger blood/gas partition coefficient produces a greater uptake and hence a lower ratio of the fraction of alveolar to inspired gas concentrations (FA/FI) in the lungs. Because the anesthetic partial pressure in the alveoli is transmitted to the arterial blood and thence to all tissues (especially the brain), the development of an adequate brain anesthetic partial pressure may be delayed in the case of highly blood-soluble agents, such as ether and methoxyflurane, with a consequent delay in induction of anesthesia. For this reason these drugs are no longer used in current clinical practice. Induction with drugs having a low blood/gas partition coefficient such as sevoflurane is rapid. Induction with the moderately soluble agents (enflurane, isoflurane, or halothane) is slower and compensated by delivering a higher concentration than the planned alveolar concentration ("overpressure"). There is a minimal clinically relevant difference in induction of anesthesia with 5% halothane and 8% sevoflurane, despite a nearly fourfold greater solubility of halothane.

The initial high inspired concentration is required to offset the uptake of anesthetic from the alveoli and is termed the concentration effect. When a mixture of anesthetic gases is used, there is an independent second gas effect, where high volume uptake of the less soluble gas (usually nitrous oxide) accelerates the increase in alveolar concentrations of the concurrently administered second gas. The converse effect is seen during recovery, when the faster elimination of nitrous oxide results in diffusion hypoxia unless supplemental oxygen is administered. Nitrous oxide can also diffuse into air-filled cavities in the body. As nitrous oxide is 35 times more soluble in blood compared with nitrogen, it will diffuse more rapidly into air-filled spaces than nitrogen can diffuse out. If the space is elastic (e.g., intestinal loops, venous air embolism) the walls will expand, and if the air-filled space has rigid walls (e.g., pleura, middle ear, etc.) the pressure inside will increase. Nitrous oxide is contraindicated in these conditions.

The effect of increased cardiac output on uptake is explained by the fact that a greater passage of blood through the lungs removes more anesthetic and thereby lowers the alveolar anesthetic concentration. The effect of a change in cardiac output is analogous to the effect of a change in solubility. As already noted, doubling solubility doubles the capacity of the same volume of blood to hold anesthetic. Doubling cardiac output also would similarly double the volume of blood exposed to anesthetic and slow induction. Conversely, in shock the reduced cardiac output is associated with a more rapid induction and a greater risk for cardiovascular toxicity. The presence of a left-to-right intracardiac shunt has a minimal effect on uptake if cardiac output is normal. However, a right-to-left shunt is associated with a slower uptake, as some blood does not get exposed to the anesthetic in the alveoli and the amount of anesthetic delivered to the brain may be lower.

The alveolar to venous anesthetic partial pressure difference results from tissue uptake of anesthetic. The presumption that alveolar and arterial anesthetic partial pressures are equal is reasonable in normal patients who have no barrier to diffusion of anesthetic from alveoli to pulmonary capillary blood and who do not have ventilation/perfusion ratio abnormalities.

The factors that determine the fraction of anesthetic removed from blood traversing a given tissue are analogous to the factors affecting FA/FI. These are tissue solubility, tissue blood flow, and arterial to tissue anesthetic partial pressure difference. Again, uptake is the product of these three factors. If any one factor approaches zero, uptake by that tissue becomes negligible. While blood/gas partition coefficients range from 0.45 for desflurane to 15 for methoxyflurane, tissue/blood partition coefficients (i.e., tissue solubility) range from 1 for lean tissues to 3.4 for other tissues. The lower flow of blood to lean tissues maintains the arterial to tissue anesthetic partial pressure difference for a longer time compared with the brain. With its high perfusion per gram, the brain equilibrates rapidly with the anesthetic partial pressure brought to it in arterial blood. Uptake of anesthetic by muscle continues long after uptake by the brain has ceased.

Fat has a tissue/blood coefficient ranging from 2.3 (nitrous oxide) to 51 (halothane) to 61 (methoxyflurane). That is, each milliliter of fat tissue contains 2.3 times more nitrous oxide than, or 51 times as much halothane as, a milliliter of blood having the same nitrous oxide or halothane partial pressure. This enormous capacity of fat for anesthetic means that most of the anesthetic contained in the blood is transferred to the fat. However, the anesthetic partial pressure in that tissue rises very slowly because of the large capacity of fat and the low perfusion. Thus, fat is a depot for anesthetic and uptake from other tissues continues even after administration of the anesthetic has stopped. During recovery from anesthesia, tissue concentrations of anesthetics continue to maintain PA levels even when the inspired concentrations have been turned to zero at the end of the procedure. Recovery is prolonged when soluble anesthetics have been used compared with the insoluble ones.

During recovery from anesthesia the reverse of the phenomenon seen during induction occurs. The rate of decrease of PA at the end of anesthesia can be affected by metabolism of the anesthetics. Modern anesthetics undergo minimal metabolism, and recovery is dependent on the rate of elimination. As inspired concentrations cannot be reduced below zero, there is no opposite phenomenon to the concentration effect. However, elimination can be increased with higher minute ventilation, but the lower carbon dioxide tensions may result in apnea, delaying tracheal extubation readiness. Elimination is also dependent on the solubility of the agent in blood and tissues and the duration of administration (context-sensitive elimination). Prolonged administration can result in a reservoir of anesthetics in tissue and recovery of swallowing, breathing, and chemical ventilatory drive may be prolonged compared with awakening, which is dependent on the brain concentration of anesthetics.

The physical characteristics of potent inhaled anesthetics have a major influence on their actions and must be understood by clinicians who administer these agents clinically (Table 11.1).

MECHANISM OF ACTION OF ANESTHETICS

General anesthesia is a composite state with independent but overlapping components of amnesia, sedation, loss of consciousness, immobility and reduced autonomic responses to noxious stimuli, and analgesia with or without muscle relaxation. A wide variety of substances with different chemical structures possess the ability to induce the anesthetic state, and their mechanism of action is still not completely understood at the molecular and cellular level. Inhalation anesthetics hyperpolarize neurons and reduce excitability in the postsynaptic neuron. They also inhibit excitatory synapses and enhance inhibitory synapses. The reduction in presynaptic action potential reduces presynaptic calcium influx, which amplifies the reduction in neurotransmitter release. There is no single specific anatomic site of action of anesthetics, and these drugs inhibit electrical activity at the peripheral sensory neurons, spinal cord, brain stem, and cerebral cortex. The immobility in response to surgical incision is the result of action on the spinal cord, while unconsciousness is the effect on the cerebral cortex, perhaps by its effect on gamma amino-butyric acid type A ($GABA_A$) receptors in the ventrolateral preoptic and tuberomamillary nuclei. The thalamic area metabolism is reduced under anesthesia, and this may reduce ascending stimuli to the cortex. Depression of hippocampal neurotransmission may be responsible for the amnestic effects of anesthetics. This is discussed in more detail in the section on the effect of volatile anesthetics on the central nervous system.

Meyer and Overton established the strong relationship between the solubility of a gas in the hydrophobic solvent olive oil and potency as a general anesthetic. They put forward a unitary theory of anesthesia suggesting that all anesthetic target sites must have a nonpolar character, and this theory led to investigations of the lipid membranes and the hydrophobic sites on the interior of proteins as a possible site of action. This theory stated that accumulation of anesthetic molecules in the hydrophobic (or lipophilic) regions of the bipolar neuronal lipid membrane caused distortion and expansion (thickening) due to volume displacement. Proponents of the unitary theory of anesthetics suggested that accumulation of critical amounts of anesthetic results in sufficient membrane thickening to reversibly alter membrane ion channel function and induce the state of general anesthesia. However, changes in membrane density seen with anesthetics can be duplicated by changes in temperature without inducing anesthesia. There are also deviations from the Myer-Overton rule, where some compounds are less potent than predicted by the oil/gas partition coefficient and some are ineffective in producing immobility to stimuli and actually cause convulsions despite their marked solubility in olive oil. In addition enantiomers with identical chemical composition and olive oil solubility have different anesthetic potencies. These findings led to the abandonment of the unitary lipid theory of anesthetic action, and current investigations have focused on the identification of specific protein-binding sites for anesthetic effects.

The strongest evidence for a direct action of anesthetics is present for the $GABA_A$ receptor, the N-methyl-D-aspartate (NMDA) receptors, and the two-pore potassium channels. The $GABA_A$ receptor is a ligand-gated chloride ion channel that may mediate the inhibition of response to noxious stimuli by propofol and etomidate. Other drugs such as ketamine, xenon, and nitrous oxide inhibit the ligand-gated calcium ion channels in NMDA receptors. Halogenated agents may also act on the two-pore potassium channels.

In summary, there is no single mechanism for the anesthetic state, and each component of general anesthesia may be the result of action at a different site. The search for mechanisms of anesthesia has moved to finding the site of action for each anesthetic for each component of anesthesia. The $GABA_A$ receptor is the probable site of action for loss of consciousness with propofol and etomidate. A better understanding of each component of anesthesia is necessary for a systematic search for new anesthetics.

EFFECTS ON THE CENTRAL NERVOUS SYSTEM

Anesthetic drugs act at different sites in the central nervous system (CNS) to produce the effects of immobility in response to surgical stimuli, unconsciousness (hypnosis), amnesia, and sedation, with different doses being required for each effect. Volatile anesthetic doses are usually expressed in fractions of the minimum alveolar concentration that will prevent a movement response to surgical incision in 50% of subjects (MAC). The MAC is additive, meaning that 0.5 MAC of isoflurane plus 0.5 MAC of N_2O is approximately equal to 1 MAC. The failure to show a relationship between electroencephalography (EEG) and immobility in response to surgical stimuli has led to the hypothesis that movement response to surgical stimuli is not a result of cerebral cortical activity but an effect at the spinal level. This has been confirmed by experiments that have shown removal of the forebrain does not alter MAC values (Table 11.2). Selective administration of antagonists of various receptors suggests the NMDA type glutamate receptors contribute to this effect, but not the nicotinic acetylcholine or the $GABA_A$ receptors. An integrated theory for the mechanism of anesthetic-induced immobility during surgical stimulation is still not established.

Hypnosis or alteration of the level of consciousness is another poorly understood effect of volatile anesthetics and is seen at doses of less than 0.5 MAC (Table 11.3). Earlier

Table 11.2 FACTORS THAT INCREASE AND DECREASE MAC

FACTORS THAT INCREASE MAC	FACTORS THAT DECREASE MAC
Medications—MAO Inhibitors, Ephedrine, Levodopa	Increasing age (↓ 6% per decade)
Drugs—Acute amphetamine administration, Cocaine	Metabolic acidosis
Hyperthermia	Hypoxia
Chronic ethanol use	Hypothermia
Hypernatremia	Hyponatremia
	Lithium
	Pregnancy
	Acute ethanol use
	Alpha 2 agonists
	Ketamine
	Opioids
	Lidocaine
	Barbiturates
	Anemia
	Benzodiazepenes
	Neuromuscular blockers

Table 11.3 MINIMUM ALVEOLAR CONCENTRATION (MAC) VALUES FOR VARIOUS END-POINTS

DESCRIPTION	MAC VALUE
Surgical MAC—consistently stops movement to surgical stimulus	1.2–1.3 MAC
MAC awake	0.15–0.5 MAC
Loss of awareness and recall	0.4–0.5 MAC

theories of an anatomic structure that controls consciousness have been replaced by the concept that consciousness requires coherent synchronicity and functional connectivity of various cortical structures. Functional imaging of the human brain has shown suppression of thalamic activity by some but not all anesthetics and has led to the theory that the mechanism of unconsciousness is related to deafferentation of the thalamic neurons. Activity in the gamma band (40–90 Hz) of the EEG is observed during natural sleep and after administration of anesthetics. However, hypnosis occurs at lower doses of volatile anesthetics than those required to show thalamic suppression.

Amnesia is a desired effect of anesthetics and is achieved at lower doses (<0.25 MAC) than required for hypnosis. Explicit memory is impaired at lower anesthetic concentrations than implicit memory. There is evidence that theta rhythms (4–12 Hz) of the EEG in the hippocampal area are suppressed by anesthetics and benzodiazepines. As with other CNS actions of anesthetics, the cellular mechanisms remain unclear.

In summary, the exact mechanisms of action of various anesthetics on the CNS are not clearly known but are probably at different sites for different end points. A clearer understanding of the actions of anesthetic agents at the cellular and molecular level may lead to the development of newer drugs that will have selective effects of only one of the components of general anesthesia (amnesia, sedation, immobility, or unconsciousness).

Inhalation anesthetics also have an effect on the CNS by alterations in the cerebral blood flow (CBF) and intracranial pressure. The inhaled anesthetics in current clinical use have reasonably similar effects in clinical practice on the cerebral metabolic rate (CMR), EEG, and CBF, but can have different effects on intracranial pressure, CSF production, and CBF autoregulation. All potent agents depress cerebral metabolism and spontaneous cortical neural activity until an isoelectric EEG is obtained. Further increases in the dose of inhaled anesthetics do not alter the CMR. The exception is halothane.

There is a dose-dependent increased cerebral blood flow with all inhaled anesthetics despite the decreased CMR. Autoregulation of brain blood flow is diminished at different MAC levels with different inhalation agents, with better preservation with sevoflurane compared with isoflurane and desflurane. The changes in CBF can be attenuated by hypocapnia and IV adjuvants. Intracranial pressures will increase or decrease proportionate to CBF changes. Greater increases are seen with halothane and possibly with desflurane from airway irritation.

In recent years there has been increasing concern about the effect of anesthetics on the developing brain. Animal studies have clearly established an apoptotic effect in many different species. There are epidemiological studies suggesting delayed development in children exposed to anesthetics at a young age, but it is unclear whether this is an effect of the anesthetic or of the condition that led to the need for anesthesia. Many studies are under way to answer this most important question.

EFFECTS ON THE CARDIOVASCULAR SYSTEM

Volatile anesthetics produce a dose-related decrease in arterial blood pressure. The magnitude of this reduction is similar at equianesthetic concentrations of various potent inhalation agents, but the mechanism varies. Halothane decreases blood pressure by a direct reduction in cardiac output from reduced myocardial contractility, while the newer agents isoflurane, desflurane, and sevoflurane maintain cardiac output and reduce blood pressure by decreased systemic vascular resistance. Desflurane has an effect of increasing sympathetic outflow in humans (but not animals), especially when concentrations above 5%–6% are administered. This is associated with hypertension, tachycardia, and release of epinephrine, norepinephrine, and plasma antidiuretic hormone and may precipitate ischemia in patients with vascular disorders. This effect is attenuated by the concomitant administration of opioids, clonidine, or beta blockers. These effects of desflurane are thought to be triggered by the airway receptors and are not seen with sevoflurane.

Negative inotropic effects of anesthetics are seen in isolated cardiac muscle strips by decreased maximal velocity of shortening, peak developed force, and rate of force development. Simultaneous changes in autonomic nervous system activity and systemic and pulmonary hemodynamics complicate left ventricular systolic function assessment in the intact animal. In a normal heart, volatile anesthetics produce a dose-dependent depression of left ventricular (LV), right ventricular (LV), and left atrial (LA) myocardial contractility. The volatile anesthetics also affect LV diastolic function and LV–arterial coupling. In the usual doses used clinically, the echocardiographic indices of myocardial function in intact animals are not affected by isoflurane, sevoflurane, and desflurane, but are with halothane. However, in animals where the neural control of the heart has been eliminated, there is a mild and similar dose-dependent depression of myocardial contractility with these agents.

Heart failure is not just a result of impaired contractility but also of altered LV diastolic function. Volatile anesthetic administration is associated with a dose-related prolongation of LV isovolumic relaxation, and this may contribute to impaired coronary blood flow during early diastole. The vasodilation effects of anesthetics may compensate for declines in contractility at lower doses, but the mechanical matching between LV and arterial vasculature degenerate at higher concentrations and contribute to reduced cardiac function in vivo when volatile anesthetics are administered. In the failing myocardium the dependence of LV relaxation on afterload is enhanced and any beneficial effect of volatile anesthetics on LV afterload are limited. The LV end diastolic pressure and chamber dimensions are reduced by these drugs in the failing heart. Cardiac output decreases may be profound in the presence of LV dysfunction.

The effects of volatile anesthetics on the heart rate depend on baroreceptor reflex activity, although these agents depress sinoatrial node activity. Halothane attenuates the baroreceptor response and so does not change the heart rate markedly. Isoflurane and desflurane cause dose-related increases in heart rate as the preserved baroreceptor activity increases in response to afterload decreases. This response may be decreased at extremes of age (neonatal and geriatric) and by administration of opioids and increased by surgical stimulation. Volatile anesthetics increase resting afferent activity and enhance baroreceptor sensitivity by a calcium ion dependent mechanism to reduce overall sympathetic activity and responses to decreased blood pressure. These actions of volatile anesthetics on baroreceptor control of circulation may be profound in elderly patients with autonomic dysfunction and other subjects with essential hypertension, diabetes, or heart failure.

Volatile anesthetics slow sinoatrial node discharge, shorten the cardiac action potential, and prolong atrioventricular conduction time and the QTc interval. This may result in bradycardia and atrioventricular conduction abnormalities and a potential for polymorphic ventricular tachycardia (torsades de pointes) in patients with congenital long QT intervals. The myocardium can be sensitized to the arrhythmogenic effects of epinephrine by volatile anesthetics (in particular halothane). Much higher doses of epinephrine are required to produce ventricular arrhythmias when desflurane or sevoflurane are used compared with halothane.

Volatile anesthetics cause relatively weak direct coronary artery vasodilation, but reductions in heart rate, preload, afterload, and inotropic states will determine the net effect on coronary vasculature. Coronary vasodilation may cause redistribution away from ischemic myocardium, and treatment of hypotension with phenylephrine will restore subendocardial blood flow. Coronary steal did not occur in a canine model of coronary artery disease with the administration of isoflurane, halothane, desflurane, or sevoflurane. Most studies suggest that myocardial oxygen supply and demand rather than the anesthetic are of greater importance in outcome in patients with coronary artery disease.

There is now substantial evidence that volatile anesthetics provide protective effects during myocardial ischemia and reperfusion injury when given before (preconditioning) or immediately after (postconditioning) ischemia, and the effect lasts beyond the time for elimination of the anesthetic drug. Anesthetic preconditioning in experimental ischemia is dose related. In elderly patients undergoing coronary artery bypass surgery, desflurane and sevoflurane (but not propofol) maintained contractile function and were associated with decreased release of troponin I, a marker of myocardial damage. Sevoflurane preconditioning reduced the postoperative release of biochemical markers of LV (brain natriuretic peptide) and renal (cystatin C) dysfunction. There are a number of potential sites of action for the cardioprotective effects of volatile anesthetics during reperfusion including G-protein coupled ligands, nitric oxide, protein kinases, and mitochondrial and sarcolemmal potassium adenosine triphosphate (ATP) channels. The clinical implication is that sevoflurane and desflurane reduce myocardial injury and improve outcomes during surgery in patients with ischemic cardiac disease.

Alterations in the intracellular calcium homeostasis are thought to be the basis for the effects of volatile anesthetics on the myocardium. The structure and function of voltage-dependent calcium channels are directly altered by volatile anesthetics with inhibition of calcium influx via the sarcoplasmic reticulum. These drugs also depress sodium–calcium exchange independent of the voltage-dependent calcium channel effect, and this may be the cause of increased negative inotropic effects of volatile anesthetics on the neonatal myocardium.

Nitrous oxide is commonly administered along with volatile anesthetics, and when this is done the systemic vascular resistance and blood pressure are higher because of the effect of increased sympathetic nervous system activity induced by nitrous oxide. In isolated heart preparations, nitrous oxide produces mild direct negative inotropic effect. It does not substantially alter LV function or have a direct effect on coronary vasculature in vitro. The cardiovascular effects of nitrous oxide are difficult to evaluate in patients, as they will also be receiving volatile anesthetics, opioids, or other adjuvants. Modest increases in pulmonary and systemic vascular resistance are probably related to the effects of sympathetic stimulation.

Xenon is an odorless, tasteless, inert anesthetic gas with a low blood/gas partition coefficient, does not undergo biotransformation, and has analgesic properties not mediated by opioid or alpha adrenergic receptors. It causes minimal systemic and pulmonary hemodynamic effects, maintains myocardial contractility, reduces epinephrine and cortisol responses to surgical stimulation, and protects the myocardium during ischemia. However, the MAC of xenon is high (71%). Despite the other characteristics that make it an ideal anesthetic, xenon has not been used in routine clinical practice, as it is very expensive and difficult to manufacture.

EFFECTS ON THE RESPIRATORY SYSTEM

Inhaled anesthetics affect different respiratory functions including the control of ventilation, pulmonary blood flow, airway smooth muscle tone, mucus secretion, surface tension in the alveoli, and pulmonary inflammatory responses. The ventilatory control system consists of a sensory limb, with peripheral and central mechanical airway and chemoreceptors, and a control center in the brain stem to integrate these inputs and produce an output to the motor system through phrenic and spinal nerves to the respiratory muscles including the diaphragm and abdominal and intercostal muscles. All volatile anesthetics with the exception of xenon have a dose-dependent effect of decreased tidal volume and increased respiratory rate, which partially offsets decreased minute ventilation at higher MAC equivalent levels. Xenon increases tidal breathing while decreasing the respiratory rate in contrast to other potent inhalation agents. There is a relative increase in dead-space ventilation with an increased arterial partial pressure of carbon dioxide ($PaCO_2$) in anesthetized patients. At equipotent MAC concentrations, this increase in $PaCO_2$ is greater with desflurane and isoflurane compared with sevoflurane. The addition of nitrous oxide at an equivalent MAC level and respiratory response to surgical stimulation attenuates the effects of volatile anesthetics on the $PaCO_2$. Acidemia from the accumulation of carbon dioxide may cause organ dysfunction of the heart (arrhythmias), lung (pulmonary hypertension), and brain (increased intracranial pressures), with a potential for serious complications in those with underlying diseases.

Arterial carbon dioxide tension is the most important stimulus to ventilation. The apneic threshold is the highest $PaCO_2$ level at which a patient stays apneic and this is 4–5 mmHg below resting $PaCO_2$. Volatile anesthetics depress ventilation and apneic thresholds to a similar degree. Assisted ventilation to lower CO_2 tensions during anesthesia will eventually decrease it below the apneic threshold, at which point controlled ventilation is required. The duration of apnea before an anesthetized subject starts breathing spontaneously will depend on the depth of anesthesia. Intentional hyperventilation to eliminate volatile anesthetics, rebreathing carbon dioxide, and maintenance of relative hypercapnia are steps used to shorten emergence time at the end of an anesthetic.

Volatile anesthetics also attenuate the ventilatory response to hypoxia by an effect on peripheral chemoreceptors in the carotid sinus and elsewhere. The magnitude of this depressant effect varies among different agents and the order of sensitivity from high to low is halothane, isoflurane, sevoflurane, and desflurane. The profound depression of ventilatory response to hypoxemia has clinical importance, suggesting a risk for postoperative hypoxemia occurs for some time after discontinuation of anesthetic agents. This may be most important in patients who are dependent on the hypoxic drive for ventilation (e.g., chronic lung failure).

The effect of clinically relevant concentrations of inhaled anesthetics on pulmonary vasculature is minimal compared with its effect on systemic vascular resistance. The pulmonary vasodilator effects are offset by reduced cardiac output with little or no change in pulmonary blood flow and arterial pressures. However, volatile anesthetics have a potential to attenuate hypoxic pulmonary vasoconstriction, a process by which the body reduces blood flow to underventilated areas of the lung and increases flow to the ventilated areas to improve ventilation perfusion matching. In human patients undergoing one-lung ventilation, arterial oxygenation is similar when isoflurane, desflurane, sevoflurane, or propofol is administered.

Volatile anesthetics have clinically important bronchodilator relaxant effects on the airway smooth muscle tone by both direct depression of smooth muscle contractility and by indirect actions via the inhibitory effect of increased $PaCO_2$ tensions on reflex neural pathways. The direct effects involve inhibition of cell membrane voltage-dependent calcium channels resulting in decreased intracellular calcium. The bronchodilator effects of volatile anesthetics can be attenuated by injury to the bronchial epithelium, by the reduction in functional residual capacity (FRC) with induction of anesthesia, and by intraoperative hypothermia. The bronchodilator effect of volatile anesthetics on the distal airways can be countered by airway constriction from the irritant effects on the laryngeal and tracheal receptors in the upper airway, particularly if desflurane is used. The bronchoconstriction responses are enhanced in chronic smokers, airway stimulation in lightly anesthetized patients, and use of anesthetic adjuvants that release histamine. Volatile anesthetics are an effective method of treating status asthmaticus when conventional therapy has failed. While halothane has been used successfully for this condition, the drug is not readily available any more in the United States. In view of the airway irritant effects of desflurane and isoflurane, sevoflurane has been used for managing status asthmaticus unresponsive to beta 2 adrenoreceptor therapy. Sevoflurane has the advantage of a quicker onset, lack of pungency, and a lower risk of cardiovascular depression and cardiac arrhythmias compared with halothane.

Mucus from ciliated respiratory epithelium captures inhaled particles and transports them out of the airway by ciliary motion. Volatile anesthetics reduce this motion and alter the characteristics of the mucus particularly in the mechanically ventilated patient even if the inspired gases are warmed and humidified. Pulmonary surfactant plays a role in removing foreign particles from the airway in addition to enhancing the bactericidal actions of alveolar macrophages. Its major effect is to decrease the work of breathing by reducing surface tension in the alveolus. Prolonged administration of inhaled anesthetics may lead to postoperative respiratory complications from reduced mucus clearance and impaired surfactant production. These effects may be more pronounced in patients with lung injury (smokers, chronic bronchitis, cystic fibrosis, asthma, etc.). The effects of volatile anesthetics on acute lung injury have been described as both proinflammatory and protective, depending on the study conditions and the cell type examined.

EFFECTS ON NEUROMUSCULAR FUNCTION

All volatile anesthetics have a dose-related relaxant effect on skeletal muscle tone with enhancement of neuromuscular blockade. Recovery from neuromuscular blockade is faster with the elimination of volatile anesthetics. Desflurane has a greater enhancement effect of rocuronium compared with sevoflurane or isoflurane at equipotent MAC equivalent concentrations, and recovery from vecuronium is faster when desflurane is reduced to a 0.25 MAC concentration compared with an equipotent reduction of isoflurane. The mechanism of action may be a result of action on the postsynaptic nicotinic acetylcholine receptor.

Malignant hyperthermia is an acute uncontrolled increase in skeletal muscle metabolism triggered by exposure to volatile anesthetics in genetically susceptible subjects. This condition is inherited as an autosomal dominant disorder with a variable penetration and involves the ryanodine receptor genes typically located on the long arm of chromosome 19. The ryanodine receptor mediates the release of calcium ions from the sarcoplasmic reticulum, and subjects with mutations in the RYR1 gene can develop an uncontrolled hypermetabolic state called malignant hyperthermia when exposed to triggering agents such as potent inhalation anesthetics. The clinical symptoms include increased oxygen consumption, lactate formation, rapid rises in body temperature, acidosis, and rhabdomyolysis with hyperkalemia. Early diagnosis and treatment with dantrolene is essential for a good outcome.

EFFECTS ON RENAL FUNCTION

In the early 1980s methoxyflurane was used for anesthesia, and metabolism of this volatile anesthetic resulted in fluoride production, which was associated with high-output renal failure after prolonged exposure to methoxyflurane anesthesia. In 2006, generic formulations of sevoflurane were introduced with different water contents. In the original patented preparation of sevoflurane, water was added to inhibit the degradation of sevoflurane to hydrogen fluoride when exposed to the metal halides and oxides in the vaporizers. The generic versions have low water content, and it is unclear whether this will cause renal dysfunction.

Sevoflurane is catalyzed by carbon dioxide absorbents to form compound A (fluoromethyl-2,2-difluoro-1-[tri fluoromethyl] vinyl ether), which has been shown to be nephrotoxic in rats. The production of compound A is increased in low-flow breathing systems, by warm or dry CO_2 absorbents, and by barium hydroxide lime. Dry barium hydroxide has also been associated with fires and is not used in the US and European markets. Renal toxicity from compound A varies by species. Compound A is metabolized to cysteine derivatives, which are handled in one of two ways. In some species, including humans, the cysteine conjugates are acetylated to mercapturic acid, which is not toxic. In other species, including the rat, the cysteine conjugates are converted by beta-lyase enzymes in the kidneys to a toxic intermediary that is responsible for renal cell necrosis of the cortical medullary tubules in the proximal tubule. This can result in elevated serum creatinine, blood urea nitrogen, proteinuria, and other markers of renal damage. However, in humans the acetylation pathway is dominant. Patients with existing renal disease who received sevoflurane did not show greater signs of renal failure compared with those receiving desflurane. This study was designed to increase compound A exposure by using low-flow states (<1 L/min) for more than 2 hours with barium hydroxide absorbents and minimal use of adjuvants. The widespread use of sevoflurane in millions of patients for more than 15 years all over the world without a well-documented case of renal injury suggests that compound A–induced nephrotoxicity in humans is not a major problem.

EFFECTS ON HEPATIC FUNCTION

Several hundred cases of hepatotoxicity have been attributed to halothane, while hepatic injury attributable to isoflurane and desflurane is rare. Current volatile anesthetics, specifically halothane, can affect hepatic function in two ways. The first mechanism is by direct hepatocyte toxicity and occurs in approximately 20% of adults. This mechanism is often mild, associated with a small increase in alanine aminotransferase (ALT) and aspartate aminotransferase (AST) and low morbidity. Injury by direct hepatocyte toxicity does not require previous anesthetic exposure.[2]

The second mechanism, halothane hepatitis, is less common but significantly more severe. Patients with halothane hepatitis will demonstrate markedly elevated levels of ALT, AST, and alkaline phosphatase; hepatic necrosis; fulminant hepatic failure; and a mortality of 50%–75%.[2] Clinical investigation suggests that halothane hepatitis may have an allergic or hypersensitivity mechanism. With repeated exposure, individuals may develop an immune reaction to anesthetic metabolites, which can manifest as fever, rash, arthralgia, or eosinophilia. In susceptible individuals, T-cells and B-cells are sensitized to trifluoro-acetate (TFA)-protein adducts created in the biotransformation of halothane.[2]

The incidence of hepatic injury is related to the degree of metabolism of the anesthetic. From greatest to least, the incidence of injury is halothane > enflurane > isoflurane > desflurane. Because all of these anesthetics are biotransformed in a manner similar to halothane, one can conclude that they may all cause hepatitis in the same manner, though with a lesser incidence.

In addition to these mechanisms, hypoxic injury to hepatocytes can cause postoperative hepatic dysfunction. The liver relies on two sources of blood for oxygen delivery. The first is the well-oxygenated hepatic artery, the second the poorly oxygenated portal vein. Fortunately, volatile anesthetics increase oxygen-rich hepatic artery blood flow with little effect on oxygen-poor portal vein flow.

Other factors that contribute to hepatic injury include retraction or compression from local surgery (abdominal procedures, cholecystectomy), preexisting hepatic dysfunction (cirrhosis, hepatic resection for hepatocellular carcinoma), and genetic polymorphisms in enzymatic function. Lastly, hepatic enzyme induction from medications can increase the oxygen demand of hepatocytes.

EFFECTS ON HEMATOLOGIC AND IMMUNE SYSTEMS

The effects of volatile anesthetics on hematologic and immune systems have been widely examined in both in vivo and in vitro animal models. These studies have shown in animal models that volatile anesthetics affect interferon stimulation of natural killer (NK) cell cytotoxicity.[3] While human studies are more difficult to interpret due to a wide range of patient factors and drugs administered, a single retrospective study examining patients with primary melanoma found that survival was decreased in patients who received general anesthesia for resection, instead of local anesthesia. In this study, this decrease in survival was attributed to the use of general anesthesia.[4]

BIOTRANSFORMATION AND TOXICITY

Biotransformation of volatile anesthetics largely occurs in the liver, due to its large size, dual blood supply, and abundance of drug-metabolizing enzymes. The major enzymatic reactions that occur are oxidation, hydrolysis, and conjugation. These drug reactions are further divided into two categories: phase 1 and phase 2 reactions. Phase 1 reactions create a polar functional group by oxidation (hydroxyl group) or hydrolysis (amino group). Phase 2 reactions, through conjugation (of glucuronic acid, sulfate, or glycine) to a drug or drug metabolite, create an even more polar group. The end result of these two reactions is a compound that is easily excreted by the kidneys or gastrointestinal or biliary tract. Glucuronidation is the most important phase 2, conjugation reaction.[2]

The most notable phase 1 enzymes are the cytochrome P450 enzymes (CYPs). Most of these enzymes metabolize multiple drugs. Frequently, more than one enzyme may be used in the metabolism of a drug. In humans, CYP3A4 and CYP3A5 make up greater than half of the total CYP; and CYP2E1 is responsible for the phase 1, oxidative metabolism of halogenated anesthetics.[2]

METABOLISM OF INDIVIDUAL ANESTHETICS

Nitrous oxide is not metabolized in human tissue. However, when combined with vitamin B_{12}, nitrous oxide can be metabolized to N_2 by human intestinal flora. Nitrous oxide oxidizes vitamin B_{12} and inhibits its coenzyme function. An example of this coenzyme inhibition is the ability of nitrous oxide to decrease methionine synthase activity, which is necessary for DNA synthesis and methylations. Fortunately, in clinically relevant doses of nitrous oxide, this effect is unlikely.

One-quarter of halothane is metabolized into three compounds: trifluoroacetic acid (TFA, major metabolite), chloride, and bromide. The TFA-chloride metabolite can react with tissue proteins to form TFA-proteins that are implicated in halothane immune-mediated hepatotoxicity. Isoflurane and desflurane are metabolized to a lesser degree than halothane. However, metabolism of these anesthetics can also create TFA-proteins as they are structurally very similar to halothane. Approximately 5% of sevoflurane is biotransformed. Metabolism of sevoflurane does not produce TFA-protein adducts.

Elimination of volatile anesthetics occurs mainly through exhalation, though insignificant amounts are also eliminated through skin and viscera.

The rate of emergence from an anesthetic depends on alveolar ventilation, tissue solubility, duration of anesthetic, and cardiac output. More soluble anesthetics will distribute throughout the alveoli, vessel-rich group organs, muscle, and fat, creating a "reservoir" of volatile anesthetic. A longer duration of anesthetic will also contribute to rate of emergence, as more anesthetic may be deposited into the "reservoir." Elimination of highly soluble volatile anesthetics, such as halothane and isoflurane, is particularly affected by the duration of anesthetic. The insoluble anesthetics, sevoflurane, desflurane, and nitrous oxide, in contrast, are minimally affected by the duration of anesthesia.

TOXICITY

Sevoflurane and sodium hydroxide– or potassium hydroxide–based carbon dioxide absorbents interact to form byproducts; the most notable byproduct is compound A (fluoromethyl-2-2-difluoror-1-(trifluoromethyl) vinyl ether). Of the CO_2 absorbers, Baralyme is associated with higher compound A production than soda lime. Newer calcium hydroxide–based absorbents do not degrade anesthetics to carbon monoxide or compound A.

The clinical significance of compound A toxicity has been highly debated since early studies demonstrated that high levels of compound A lead to renal failure and death in animal models. However, two decades of intense research of sevoflurane and nephrotoxicity have shown that compound A does not lead to clinically significant renal toxicity in humans.[2] Despite this statement, sevoflurane should be used judiciously in patients with preexisting renal disease and in accordance with approved package guidelines.

REFERENCES

1. Miller RD, Pardo MC Jr. *Basics of Anesthesia*. 6th ed. Philadelphia, PA: Elsevier Saunders; 2011.
2. Butterworth JF, McKey DC, Wasnick J, Priebe H-J, Maged M, eds. *Morgan and Mikhail Clinical Anesthesiology*. 5th ed. New York, NY: Lange Medical Books, McGraw-Hill Education; 2013.
3. Evers AE, Maze M, Karash ED. *Anesthetic Pharmacology*. 2nd ed. Cambridge, UK: Cambridge University Press; 2011.
4. Barash PG, Cullen BF, Stoelting RK, Cahalan MK, Stock M, Ortega R. *Clinical Anesthesia*. 7th ed. Philadelphia, PA: Lippincott Williams & Wilkins, 2013.

FURTHER READING

Martin J. Inhaled anesthetics: metabolism and toxicity. In: Miller R, Eriksson L, Fleisher L, Wiener-Kronish J, Young W, eds. *Miller's Anesthesia*. 7th ed. Philadelphia, PA: Churchill Livingstone; 2010:633–666.

Schlagenhauff B; Ellwanger U; Breuninger H; Stroebel W; Rassner G; Garbe C. Prognostic impact of the type of anaesthesia used during the excision of primary cutaneous melanoma. *Melanoma Res*. 2000;10(2):165–169.

Snyder G, Greenberg S. Effect of anaesthetic technique and other perioperative factors on cancer recurrence. *BJA*. 2010;105(2):106–115.

QUESTIONS

1. A compound is being considered as a new potent anesthetic agent. Which of the following properties will ***NOT*** increase the speed of induction with the new agent compared with currently available drugs?
   A. New agent increases minute ventilation compared with current drugs.
   B. New agent has lower blood/gas partition coefficient compared with current drugs.
   C. New agent maintains or slightly increases cardiac output compared with current drugs.
   D. New agent is metabolized at a much faster rate compared with current drugs.

2. The order in which the following effects occur with increasing concentrations of anesthetics (from low to high) is:
   A. Amnesia, loss of consciousness, immobility with surgical stimulation, isoelectric EEG
   B. Loss of consciousness, isoelectric EEG, amnesia, immobility with surgical stimulation
   C. Amnesia, immobility with surgical stimulation, loss of consciousness, isoelectric EEG
   D. Loss of consciousness, immobility with surgical stimulation, isoelectric EEG, amnesia

3. Identify the ***FALSE*** statement below:
   A. Desflurane stimulates airway receptors to cause bronchoconstriction.
   B. Autoregulation of cerebral blood flow is better preserved with sevoflurane compared with isoflurane.
   C. Cardiac output is maintained with clinical doses of desflurane and sevoflurane, but blood pressure decreases because of reduced myocardial contractility.
   D. Xenon administration is associated with a greater reduction in tidal volumes compared with other agents.

4. Identify the ***TRUE*** statement:
   A. A rapid rise in sevoflurane concentration is associated with greater bronchoconstriction compared with desflurane.
   B. Desflurane causes increased sympathetic outflow when inspired concentrations are rapidly increased.
   C. Xenon is an inert, odorless, tasteless gas that is associated with quick induction and undergoes extensive biotransformation resulting in a rapid emergence.
   D. Volatile anesthetics are contraindicated in patients undergoing coronary arterial bypass, because they increase myocardial damage.

5. All of the following factors increase minimum alveolar concentration (MAC) except:
   A. Hyperthermia
   B. Hypernatremia
   C. Methamphetamines
   D. Hyponatremia
   E. Ephedrine

6. Which of the following statements about halothane hepatitis is least likely to be true?

A. Previous exposure to halothane is necessary to develop halothane hepatitis.
B. Halothane hepatitis carries a mortality of greater than 50%.
C. Sevoflurane causes hepatitis in a similar autoimmune manner.
D. Hepatitis results from immune sensitization to trifluoroacetic acid–tissue compounds.
E. Halothane causes more cases of autoimmune hepatitis than any other volatile anesthetic.

7. Which of the following anesthetics has the smallest blood/gas partition coefficient?

A. Isoflurane
B. Sevoflurane
C. Desflurane
D. Nitrous oxide
E. Halothane

8. According to the NIOSH, the recommended maximum exposure for health care workers to volatile anesthetics when used in combination with N_2O is:

A. 2 ppm
B. 2.5 ppm
C. 25 ppm
D. 0.5 ppm
E. 5 ppm

ANSWERS

1. C. The speed of induction of anesthesia is dependent on the rate of rise of anesthetic gas concentrations in the brain. The uptake of anesthetics from the lungs into the bloodstream for delivery to the effector sites in the brain is dependent on the product of gas solubility, cardiac output, and alveolar to venous partial pressure difference. Increased ventilation, higher inspired gas concentrations, low solubility, and decreased cardiac output along with the presence of a second gas will speed induction, while higher cardiac output and increased metabolism will reduce alveolar concentrations.
2. A. Amnesia occurs at about 0.25 MAC, while loss of consciousness occurs at approximately 0.5 MAC. Immobility with surgical stimulation requires 1 MAC, while isoelectric EEG requires higher concentrations.
3. D. Xenon has minimal or no effects on respiration. The other statements are true and are discussed in the section "Effects on the Respiratory System."
4. B. Sevoflurane causes bronchodilation and is used in uncontrolled status asthmaticus. A rapid rise in desflurane increases heart rate and sympathetic outflow. Xenon does not undergo biotransformation. Volatile anesthetics provide myocardial protection from ischemia. Hence, the correct answer is B.
5. D. Hyponatremia decreases minimum alveolar concentration. Hyperthermia, hypernatremia, amphetamines, and ephedrine are all factors that increase minimum alveolar concentration.
6. C. There is a single case report of hepatitis after sevoflurane in a pediatric patient after appendectomy. This patient also suffered from iatrogenic acetaminophen toxicity, and the hepatitis may also have been attributed to that factor.
7. C. Desflurane has the smallest blood/gas partition coefficient, with a value of 0.42. The next smallest is nitrous oxide, 0.46.
8. D. The recommended limits for health care workers' exposure to volatile anesthetics when used in combination with N_2O is 0.5 ppm.

12.

OPIOIDS

Priscilla J. Garcia

The term *opiate* specifically describes drugs derived from opium, which includes morphine, its semisynthetic derivatives, and codeine. The term *opioid* refers to all exogenous substances, both synthetic and natural, that bind to opioid receptors and produce an agonist effect. Opioids are classified as naturally occurring, semisynthetic, or synthetic. Naturally occurring opioids include morphine, codeine, papaverine, and thebaine. Semisynthetic opioids are derived from morphine, but with modifications made to the molecule, and include heroin and buprenorphine. The most common synthetic opioids include fentanyl, sufentanil, remifentanil, alfentanil, meperidine, methadone, and butorphanol.[1] *Opioids* can further be classified as agonists (morphine, fentanyl), partial agonists (buprenorphine), and mixed agonist-antagonists (nalbuphine, butorphanol), depending on their interaction with opioid receptors.[2]

MECHANISM OF ACTION

Opioids bind to stereospecific opioid receptors both centrally in the CNS and peripherally outside the CNS. Opioid receptors are found in the periaqueductal gray matter, the ventromedial medulla, the dorsal horn of the spinal cord, and peripheral sensory neurons.[3] The levorotatory form of opioid has the agonist activity. Binding to the opioid receptor results in the activation of pain-modulating (antinociceptive) systems, similar to the action of endogenous endorphins such as endorphin, dynorphin, and enkephalin. Opioids in the ionized state bind the anionic opioid receptor site. The opioid receptor activation results in a decrease in neurotransmission mostly from presynaptic inhibition of neurotransmitter release.[4] Opioid receptor activation increases potassium conductance, leading to hyperpolarization of cellular membranes.

Opioid receptors belong to the guanine (G) protein-coupled receptor family and are classified as μ, δ, σ, or κ receptors. Activation of the G protein-coupled receptor results in both the inhibition of adenyl cyclase and in ion movement across calcium and potassium channels. This results in decreased neuronal activity.[1] Mu receptors are primarily responsible for spinal and supraspinal analgesia. Activation of the μ_1 subtype (supraspinal, spinal) is thought to produce analgesia, while the μ_2 subtype (spinal) is thought to produce hypoventilation and physical dependence.

PHARMACOKINETICS AND PHARMACODYNAMICS

Pharmacokinetics is the study of drug movement through the body. It refers to the relationship between a drug dose and its concentration at the effect site(s) versus time through the processes of absorption, redistribution, biotransformation, and elimination. It is how the body affects a drug. Pharmacodynamics examines the effects of the drug on the body, including both therapeutic and toxic responses. These effects determine a drug's efficacy, potency, and therapeutic ratio.[5]

IV

The intersubject variability in response to opioids is due to pharmacokinetic and pharmacodynamic parameters. Opioids are weak bases that dissociate into protonated and free-base fractions in solution, in which the proportion depends on the pH and pKa. The free-base fraction is more lipid soluble than the protonated fraction. Highly lipid-soluble opioids have a faster onset of action.[1] However, the ionized state is necessary for strong binding at the anionic opioid receptor site.[6] Opioids can also be bound to plasma proteins, which include albumin and α_1-acid glycoprotein. Only the unbound, unionized fraction is diffusible. Therefore, the speed of onset of opioid effect is influenced by both the lipid solubility and its protein binding.[1] Plasma concentration levels peak within minutes of

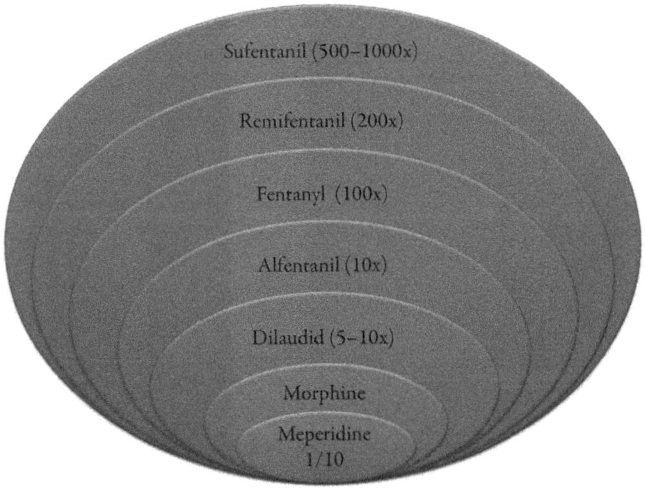

Figure 12.1 Relative potency of opioids displayed graphically. Image courtesy of the University of Texas Health Science Center at Houston Medical School. Image courtesy of George Williams, MD.

opioid administered through intravenous bolus or after a brief infusion. Redistribution terminates the action of smaller doses of opioids, but larger doses require biotransformation to lower plasma levels. In general, most opioids depend on the liver for biotransformation. The main pharmacodynamic difference between the different opioids is the potency and rate of equilibration between plasma and the site of drug effect (Figure 12.1).

MORPHINE

PHARMACOKINETICS

Morphine is the "gold standard" by which other opioids are compared. It can be given via oral, intravenous, rectal, intramuscular, subcutaneous, epidural, or intrathecal routes. It undergoes extensive first-pass metabolism in the liver and requires a higher dose than when given parenterally. It is usually administered intravenously in the immediate perioperative period. Its peak effect is delayed as compared with other narcotics such as fentanyl, taking 15 to 30 minutes to reach its peak effect when administered intravenously.[6] Its duration of action is approximately 4 hours.[4]

METABOLISM AND EXCRETION

Morphine undergoes conjugation in the liver with glucuronic acid to form morphine-3-glucuronide (M3G) and morphine-6-glucuronide (M6G). Morphine-3-glucuronide has neuroexcitatory activity and produces myoclonus, delirium, and seizures. Morphine-6-glucuronide produces analgesia and ventilatory depression via its action on μ receptors.[4] It has an even greater opioid agonist activity and a longer half-life than morphine itself. Both M3G and M6G are excreted by the kidney and will accumulate in patients with renal problems.[3] Infants and newborns preferentially metabolize morphine to M3G compared with adults and have longer clearance times for morphine metabolites.

EFFECT ON CIRCULATION

Morphine induces a histamine release and should be used with caution in patients with reactive airway disease or hypovolemia.[3] Morphine can also be associated with bradycardia. In general, opioids do not significantly impair cardiovascular function or contractility. However, hypotension may occur due to bradycardia, venodilation, and decreased sympathetic reflexes.[5]

EFFECT ON RESPIRATION

All opioids produce a dose-dependent ventilatory depression through their interactions with μ_2 receptors. The depressant effect on the brain stem ventilatory centers decreases the responsiveness to carbon dioxide, which can be seen as an increase in the resting $PaCO_2$, and shifts the carbon dioxide response curve to the right.[6] Opioids increase the apneic threshold (the highest $PaCO_2$ at which a patient stays apneic) and decrease hypoxic drive.[5] Of note, the triad of myosis, hypoventilation, and coma suggest opioid overdose.[6]

EFFECT ON OTHER ORGANS

Skeletal muscle rigidity can be seen when large doses of opioids are given quickly intravenously. Opioids can also cause spasm of the smooth muscle of the gastrointestinal system leading to constipation, biliary colic, and delayed gastric emptying. Spasm of the sphincter of Oddi can be relieved with naloxone or glucagon. Patients can also have nausea and vomiting due to the direct stimulation of the chemoreceptor trigger zone in the floor of the fourth ventricle.[6] Morphine and its related opioids (i.e., codeine) depress the cough reflex.

Opioids decrease the minimum alveolar concentration (MAC) of volatile anesthetics in a dose-dependent manner, but reach a ceiling effect of a 50% decrease in MAC. However, even in large doses they do not by themselves reliably produce unconsciousness. Opioids act as cerebral vasoconstrictors and can decrease cerebral blood flow and intracranial pressure in the absence of hypoventilation.[4]

FENTANYL

PHARMACOKINETICS

Fentanyl is a synthetic opioid agonist that is 75 to 125 times more potent than morphine.[4] It has a faster onset and shorter duration of action than morphine. However, when multiple doses of fentanyl are given, or when there is a continuous infusion of fentanyl, there is progressive saturation of inactive tissue sites, which results in a prolonged plasma concentration of fentanyl. The analgesia duration and ventilatory depression will be prolonged as well.[6] Context-sensitive half-time is the time required for the plasma drug concentration to decrease by 50% after termination of an infusion. If the continuous infusion of fentanyl lasts longer than 2 hours, the context-sensitive half-time greatly increases and is higher than that of sufentanil.[6]

METABOLISM AND EXCRETION

Fentanyl's short duration of action is due to rapid redistribution. It is metabolized by hepatic cytochrome P450 enzymes (CYP3A) into inactive compounds. Norfentanyl, the principal metabolite, is structurally similar to normeperidine.

EFFECT ON CIRCULATION

Fentanyl generally has a favorable effect on hemodynamics due to a lack of histamine release and absence of direct myocardial depression, and it helps suppress the stress response to surgery.[6] However, bradycardia can be seen.

INDICATIONS AND CONTRAINDICATIONS

Fentanyl is often used to blunt the circulatory response to endotracheal intubation as well as for analgesia.

REMIFENTANIL

PHARMACOKINETICS

Remifentanil's analgesic properties are similar to fentanyl. It has a unique ester linkage that allows it to be hydrolyzed to inactive metabolites by nonspecific plasma and tissue esterases. Therefore, remifentanil has a brief action, is rapidly titratable (due to rapid clearance and small volume of distribution), has rapid onset and offset, and is noncumulative.[6] Its peak effect is within 1.1 minutes.

METABOLISM AND EXCRETION

Remifentanil is unique among the opioids by undergoing metabolism to inactive metabolites by nonspecific plasma and tissue esterases. It has a predictable drug effect due to little variability between individuals.

SIDE EFFECTS AND TOXICITY

Remifentanil has a short recovery time. It does pass through the placenta but without neonatal effects. It may be associated with acute opioid tolerance.

SUFENTANIL

PHARMACOKINETICS

Sufentanil is an analog of fentanyl and has an analgesic potency that is 5 to 10 times that of fentanyl. Its effect time is similar to fentanyl. The context-sensitive half-time for sufentanil is less than that for fentanyl and alfentanil. Small doses have a rapid redistribution to inactive tissues, but large or repeated doses can lead to a cumulative effect.

SIDE EFFECTS AND TOXICITY

Sufentanil can have a more profound depression of ventilation and bradycardia than fentanyl. Use of a large dose may lead to skeletal muscle rigidity, making ventilation difficult.

ALFENTANIL

PHARMACOKINETICS

Alfentanil is an analog of fentanyl that is less potent (one-fifth to one-tenth) and has one-third the duration of action of fentanyl.[6] It has a rapid onset of action due to low pKa, which results in almost 90% of the drug existing in the nonionized form. The nonionized form crosses the blood-brain barrier. Its quick onset is useful to blunt the response to a single, brief stimulus.

METABOLISM AND EXCRETION

There is a tenfold interindividual variation in systemic clearance, most likely from differences in the CYP3A4 enzyme activity.[6]

SIDE EFFECTS AND TOXICITY

Alfentanil can have a more profound depression of ventilation and bradycardia than fentanyl. Use of a large dose may lead to skeletal muscle rigidity, making ventilation difficult.

HYDROMORPHONE

Hydromorphone is a derivative of morphine. It is approximately 5 to 8 times more potent than morphine. Intravenous hydromorphone causes less pruritus and nausea than morphine.[3]

MEPERIDINE

PHARMACOKINETICS

Meperidine is a synthetic opioid and is structurally similar to atropine. Is it approximately one-tenth as potent as morphine.

METABOLISM AND EXCRETION

Meperidine has extensive hepatic metabolism with 90% of the drug initially undergoing demethylation to normeperidine. Normeperidine is half as active an analgesic as meperidine, but stimulates the CNS, causing myoclonus and seizures.[6] Normeperidine is renally excreted.

SIDE EFFECTS AND TOXICITY

The side effects resemble those of morphine, except that meperidine tends to cause an increase in heart rate (not bradycardia) due to its structural similarity to atropine. Large doses can cause a decrease in myocardial contractility, which is unique among the opioids. Its normeperidine metabolite can cause delirium and seizures when it accumulates. Orthostatic hypotension occurs more frequently and with a greater degree than morphine. Meperidine impairs ventilation and crosses the placenta.[6] It can also lead to serotoninin syndrome if given to patients on antidepressant drugs.

INDICATIONS AND CONTRAINDICATIONS

Meperidine is used for analgesia as well as for suppressing postoperative shivering. It is not an effective antitussive.

OPIOID ANTAGONISTS—NALOXONE

Opioid antagonists are structurally similar to the agonists except with minor changes. The antagonists bind the μ opioid receptors and displace the opioid agonist. The binding of the pure antagonist to the mu receptor does not activate the mu receptor. Naloxone quickly reverses opioid-induced analgesia and ventilatory depression.[4] However, it has a short duration of action (30 to 45 minutes) and may need to be redosed to avoid renarcotization. The abrupt reversal of analgesia from naloxone may lead to sympathetic stimulation, resulting in tachycardia, hypertension, pulmonary edema, and cardiac dysrhythmias including ventricular fibrillation.

EPIDURAL AND INTRATHECAL

Neuraxial opioids primarily target μ receptors present in the substantia gelatinosa of the spinal cord. Analgesia is dose related and is specific for visceral rather than somatic pain.[6] Analgesia results from the diffusion of the drug across the dura to the μ receptors of the spinal cord as well as the systemic absorption of the drug, producing effects similar to those from intravenous administration of opioid. Lipid solubility is a primary determinant of how well a drug will penetrate the dura. Fentanyl and sufentanil are 800 and 1600 times, respectively, more lipid soluble than morphine. After epidural administration, fentanyl will peak in the CSF in 20 minutes, and sufentanil in 6 minutes, versus morphine in 1 to 4 hours.[6] Epinephrine decreases systemic absorption of the opioid but does not influence diffusion across the dura into the CSF.[6] Lipid solubility is also important in opioid cephalad spread. The more lipid-soluble drugs (i.e., fentanyl) will have limited cephalad movement because they have greater uptake into the spinal cord; less lipid-soluble drugs (i.e., morphine) will have more cephalad spread because they remain in the CSF longer. Morphine will ascend due to the bulk flow of CSF. Coughing or straining can affect the spread, but body position cannot (which is different when compared with local anesthetics).[6]

SIDE EFFECTS

The most frequent side effects of neuraxially administered opioids are pruritus, nausea and vomiting, urinary retention, and depression of ventilation. Pruritus is the most common and is due not to histamine release but rather to the cephalad migration of the opioid in the CSF and its interaction with opioid receptors in the trigeminal nucleus. Opioid antagonists like naloxone are effective in relieving opioid-induced pruritus. Antihistamines may also be indirectly effective, but this is likely due to their sedating properties. Urinary retention occurs more often with neuraxial opioids than with intravenous or intramuscular administration. This is thought to be due to opioid receptors in the sacral spinal cord, which inhibit sacral parasympathetic nervous system outflow, causing detrusor muscle relaxation, increased maximum bladder capacity, and urinary retention.[6] Depression of ventilation may occur within minutes or can be delayed for hours. Early depression occurs within 2 hours and is usually associated with systemic absorption of the lipid-soluble opioids such as fentanyl or sufentanil. Delayed respiratory depression occurring after 2 hours is usually associated with cephalad spread of the opioid in the CSF and its interaction with receptors in the ventral medulla. It most often occurs 6 to 12 hours after intrathecal or epidural administration of morphine. Factors that increase the risk of delayed depression of ventilation include concomitant use of parenteral opioids or other sedatives, high opioid dose, low opioid lipid solubility, lack of opioid tolerance, advanced age, increased intrathoracic pressure, and possibly patient position.[6]

REFERENCES

1. Fukuda K. Intravenous opioid anesthetics. In: Miller RD, ed. *Miller's Anesthesia*. 6th ed. Philadelphia, PA: Elsevier Churchill Livingstone; 2005:379–437.
2. Coda B. Opioids. In: Barash PG, Cullen BF, Stoelting RK, Cahalan MK, Stock MC, eds. *Clinical Anesthesia*. 6th ed. Philadelphia, PA: Lippincott Williams & Wilkins; 2009:465–497.
3. Power R. Analgesics I: opioids. In: Estrada C, Stayer S, Mann D, Carling N, Patel N, Hopkins P, eds. *Condensed Review of Pediatric Anesthesiology*. Electronic book; 2013:22–29.
4. Stoelting R. Opioids. In: Stoelting RK, Miller RD, eds. *Basics of Anesthesia*. 5th ed. Philadelphia, PA: Churchill Livingstone Elsevier; 2007:112–122.

5. Morgan G, Mikhail M, Murray M. Nonvolatile anesthetic agents. In: *Clinical Anesthesiology*. 4th ed. New York, NY: McGraw-Hill; 2006:179–204.
6. Stoelting R, Hillier S. Opioid agonists and antagonists. In: *Handbook of Pharmacology and Physiology in Anesthetic Practice*. 2nd ed. Philadelphia, PA: Lippincott Williams & Wilkins; 2006:81–117.

FURTHER READING

Stoelting R, Hillier S. *Pharmacology and Physiology in Anesthetic Practice*. 4th ed. Philadelphia, PA: Lippincott Williams & Wilkins; 2005.

QUESTIONS

1. Which of the following characteristics regarding opioids is FALSE?
   A. Opioids are weak bases.
   B. Speed of onset of opioid effect is influenced by both lipid solubility and protein binding.
   C. μ_1 subtype (supraspinal, spinal) is thought to produce hypoventilation and physical dependence.
   D. Most opioids depend on liver for biotransformation.

2. Opioid agonists produce the following:
   A. Amnesia
   B. Nausea and vomiting due to action on the GI tract
   C. Dilated pupils
   D. Unconsciousness at high doses
   E. Minimal pruritus

3. Opioid-induced nausea is best minimized when the opioid is given through which of the following routes?
   A. Intravenous
   B. Intramuscularly
   C. Oral
   D. Intrathecal
   E. None of the above

4. Fentanyl has a long elimination half-life, but a short duration of action due to:
   A. Rapid redistribution
   B. Rapid renal excretion
   C. Small percent nonionized at pH 7.4
   D. Large percent protein bound
   E. High hepatic extraction ratio

5. Remifentanil has brief clinical duration of action compared with the other opioids due to its:
   A. Large volume of distribution
   B. High protein-bound fraction
   C. Lower pKa
   D. Metabolism by nonspecific plasma and tissue esterases
   E. Rapid redistribution

6. Which of the following regarding alfentanil is FALSE?
   A. Has a rapid onset due to its low pKa
   B. Is one-fifth to one-tenth less potent than fentanyl
   C. Has less associated depression of ventilation and bradycardia than fentanyl
   D. Lowers the MAC of volatile agents
   E. Has a smaller volume of distribution than fentanyl

7. Drugs with effects that are not significantly altered in patients with renal failure include all the following EXCEPT:
   A. Fentanyl
   B. Remifentanil
   C. Sufentanil
   D. Morphine
   E. Alfentanil

8. Meperidine differs from other opioids in all the following EXCEPT for:
   A. Produces tachycardia
   B. Decreases myocardial contractility
   C. Is associated with serotonin syndrome
   D. Less respiratory depression
   E. Higher degree of orthostatic hypotension

9. Naloxone administered to reverse opioid-induced analgesia and depression of ventilation is associated with all the following except:
   A. Pulmonary edema
   B. Bradycardia
   C. Cardiac dysrhythmias
   D. Hypertension
   E. Sudden pain

10. Compared with opioids administered intravenously, opioids given neuraxially are associated with all the following EXCEPT:
   A. Less pruritus
   B. Urinary retention
   C. Delayed respiratory depression
   D. Analgesia for visceral pain
   E. Equivalent serum concentrations

ANSWERS

1. C. Activation of the μ_1 subtype (supraspinal, spinal) is thought to produce analgesia, while the μ_2 subtype (spinal) is thought to produce hypoventilation and physical dependence. Opioids are weak bases that dissociate into protonated and free-base fractions in solution, in which the proportion depends on the pH and pKa. The free-base fraction is more lipid soluble than the protonated fraction. Highly lipid-soluble opioids have a faster onset of action.[1] However, the ionized

state is necessary for strong binding at the anionic opioid receptor site.[6] Opioids can also be bound to plasma proteins, which include albumin and α_1-acid glycoprotein. Only the unbound, unionized fraction is diffusible. Therefore, the speed of onset of opioid effect is influenced by both the lipid solubility and its protein binding.[1] Redistribution terminates the action of smaller doses of opioids, but larger doses require biotransformation to lower plasma levels. In general, most opioids depend on the liver for biotransformation.

2. D. Opioid agonists can produce unconsciousness at high doses but do not produce reliable amnesia. Nausea is mediated through the chemoreceptor trigger zone in the floor of the fourth ventricle.[6] Pupils are constricted with opioid agonism.
3. E. Patients have nausea and vomiting due to the direct stimulation of the chemoreceptor trigger zone in the floor of the fourth ventricle.[6] No specific route of administration has been shown to decrease the incidence of opioid-induced nausea.
4. A. Fentanyl's short duration of action is due to rapid redistribution.[4] It is metabolized by hepatic cytochrome P450 enzymes (CYP3A) into inactive compounds.
5. D. Remifentanil is unique among the opioids in its lack of accumulation with repeated dosing or prolonged infusions due to its metabolism by blood and tissue esterases.[6]
6. C. Alfentanil is an analog of fentanyl that is less potent (one-fifth to one-tenth) and has one-third the duration of action of fentanyl.[6] It has a rapid onset of action due to low pKa, which results in almost 90% of the drug existing in the nonionized form. The nonionized form crosses the blood-brain barrier. Its quick onset is useful to blunt the response to a single, brief stimulus. There is a 10-fold interindividual variation in systemic clearance, most likely from differences in the CYP3A4 enzyme activity.[6] It can have a more profound depression of ventilation and bradycardia than fentanyl. Use of a large dose may lead to skeletal muscle rigidity, making ventilation difficult. It has a smaller volume of distribution than fentanyl.
7. D. Morphine undergoes conjugation in the liver with glucuronic acid to form morphine-3-glucuronide (M3G) and morphine-6-glucuronide (M6G). Morphine-3-glucuronide has neuroexcitatory activity and produces myoclonus, delirium, and seizures. Morphine-6-glucuronide produces analgesia and ventilatory depression via its action on μ receptors.[4] It has an even greater opioid agonist activity and a longer half-life than morphine itself. Both M3G and M6G are excreted by the kidney and will accumulate in patients with renal problems.[3] Also, meperidine's metabolite normeperidine is half as active an analgesic as meperidine, but stimulates the CNS, causing myoclonus and seizures when it accumulates.[6] It is renally excreted. Generally, the effects of drugs in the fentanyl series are not significantly altered by renal failure.
8. D. The side effects resemble those of morphine except that it tends to cause an increase in heart rate (not bradycardia) due to its structural similarity to atropine. Large doses can cause a decrease in myocardial contractility, which is unique among the opioids. Its normeperidine metabolite can cause delirium and seizures when it accumulates. Orthostatic hypotension occurs more frequently and with a greater degree than morphine. Meperidine impairs ventilation and crosses the placenta.[6] It can also lead to serotonin syndrome if given to patients on antidepressant drugs.
9. B. Opioid antagonists are structurally similar to the agonists except with minor changes. The antagonists bind the μ opioid receptors and displace the opioid agonist. The binding of the pure antagonist to the μ receptor does not activate the μ receptor. Naloxone quickly reverses opioid-induced analgesia and ventilatory depression.[4] However, it has a short duration of action (30 to 45 minutes) and may need to be redosed to avoid renarcotization. The abrupt reversal of analgesia from naloxone may lead to sympathetic stimulation resulting in tachycardia, hypertension, pulmonary edema, and cardiac dysrhythmias including ventricular fibrillation.
10. A. The most frequent side effects of neuraxially administered opioids are pruritus, nausea and vomiting, urinary retention, and depression of ventilation. Pruritus is the most common and is due not to histamine release but rather to the cephalad migration of the opioid in the CSF and its interaction with opioid receptors in the trigeminal nucleus. Urinary retention occurs more often with neuraxial opioids than with intravenous or intramuscular administration. This is thought to be due to opioid receptors in the sacral spinal cord, which inhibit sacral parasympathetic nervous system outflow, causing detrusor muscle relaxation, increased maximum bladder capacity, and urinary retention.[6] Depression of ventilation may occur within minutes or can be delayed for hours. Early depression occurs within 2 hours and is usually associated with systemic absorption of the lipid-soluble opioids such as fentanyl or sufentanil. Delayed depression occurring after 2 hours is usually associated with cephalad spread of the opioid in the CSF and its interaction with receptors in the ventral medulla. It most often occurs 6 to 12 hours after

intrathecal or epidural administration of morphine. Factors that increase the risk of delayed depression of ventilation include concomitant use of parenteral opioids or other sedatives, high opioid dose, low opioid lipid solubility, lack of opioid tolerance, advanced age, increased intrathoracic pressure, and possibly patient position.[6] Epidural administration of morphine, fentanyl, and sufentanil produce opioid blood concentrations similar to those produced by intramuscular injections of an equivalent dose.[4]

13.

INTRAVENOUS ANESTHETICS

Alina Bodas, Vera Borzova, and Ricardo Riveros

ETOMIDATE

MECHANISM OF ACTION

Etomidate is a short-acting intravenous anesthetic introduced for clinical use in 1972.[1] Etomidate interacts with a stereoselectivity on gamma amino-butyric acid type A (GABAA). Etomidate is composed by two isomers: the R(+), which is responsible for the anesthetic effect, and the S(-) with minimal effect inducing transmission on GABAA receptor[2] (Figure 13.1). The effect of etomidate on GABA receptors contrasts with the absence of effect on other ion channels.

PHARMACOKINETICS AND PHARMACODYNAMICS

Plasma protein binding of etomidate is high (75%), but less than propofol (98%) and barbiturates (85%). Because of its high solubility in fat, etomidate has a large central and peripheral volume of distribution, 4.5 L/kg and 74.9 L/kg respectively. After an induction dose of etomidate (0.2–0.6 mg/kg), plasma concentration follows a pharmacokinetic profile of the three-compartment model. Etomidate has a rapid onset and short duration of activity. The redistribution of etomidate out of the central nervous system (CNS) into peripheral tissues (mainly muscle) is responsible for the short duration of action (4–8 min) after an induction dose.

METABOLISM AND EXCRETION

Etomidate is metabolized in the liver by hepatic esterases to inactive metabolites including carboxylic acid and an ethanol-leaving group. Elimination is mostly renal (78%) and to a lesser extent biliary (22%) for the carboxylate metabolite. Etomidate plasma clearance is 15–20 mL/min/kg with a terminal metabolic half-life of 2–5 hours. Because etomidate has a context-sensitive half-life shorter than propofol (Figure 13.2), the use of etomidate infusion for sedation and anesthesia was advocated during the first decade of clinical availability.[3,4] However, the demonstration of secondary effects (adrenal toxicity) precludes the use of etomidate for infusion.

EFFECT ON CIRCULATION

Of the intravenous anesthetics, etomidate provides the least cardiovascular depression, including minimal changes in blood pressure and heart rate. Therefore, etomidate is commonly used for induction of general anesthesia in patients with poor cardiac function such as those with ischemic heart or valvular disease.[5] On the other hand, etomidate does not inhibit sympathetic tone during laryngoscopy, and opioids frequently are given to blunt these responses.

Etomidate offers a favorable profile as an induction agent in the setting of intravascular volume depletion. In a pig model of moderate hemorrhage, the pharmacokinetic and pharmacodynamic of etomidate were minimally affected.[6] Therefore etomidate has been used as a hypnotic agent for rapid sequence induction in the setting of hemorrhagic shock.

EFFECT ON RESPIRATION

Compared with barbiturates and propofol, etomidate produces less apnea, rarely induces allergic reactions, and induces no histamine release. Etomidate does not inhibit sympathetic response to direct laryngoscopy.

EFFECT ON OTHER ORGANS

Etomidate is capable of causing reduced cerebral metabolic rate and reduced cerebral blood flow and intracranial pressure while maintaining cerebral perfusion pressure.[5] Electroencephalographic changes associated with use of etomidate are similar to those observed with barbiturates.[7]

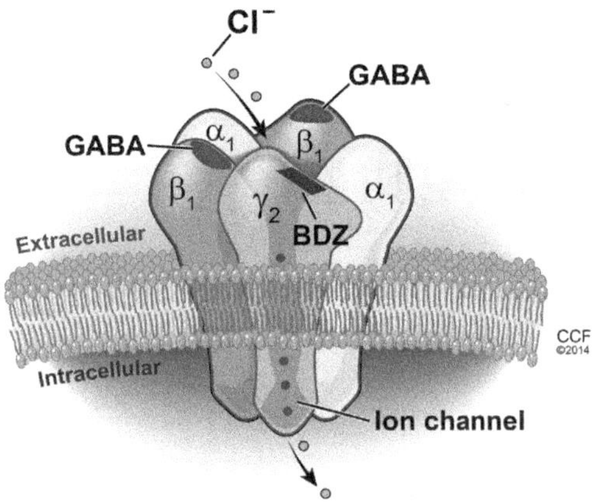

Figure 13.1 GABAA receptor.

Different effects associated with using etomidate are seen on evoked potentials. On auditory evoked potentials, etomidate decreases amplitude and increases latency[8]; Somatosensory evoked potential amplitudes are increased,[9] while motor evoked potential amplitudes are decreased; the latter effect is minimal when compared with propofol and barbiturates.[10] Etomidate produces minimal hepatic metabolic inhibition of cytochrome P450 without having an effect on the metabolism of other anesthetic or analgesic drugs.[11]

SIDE EFFECTS AND TOXICITY

After a single dose for induction of anesthesia, etomidate can cause pain on injection and myoclonic movements. The type of solvent used for etomidate preparation is responsible for pain on injection as follows: aqueous solutions > propylene glycol > medium chain length or cyclodextrines. Myoclonic movements are not associated with electroencephalographic changes and can be attenuated using premedication opioids such as benzodiazepines or dexmedetomidine or by splitting the induction dose.[12]

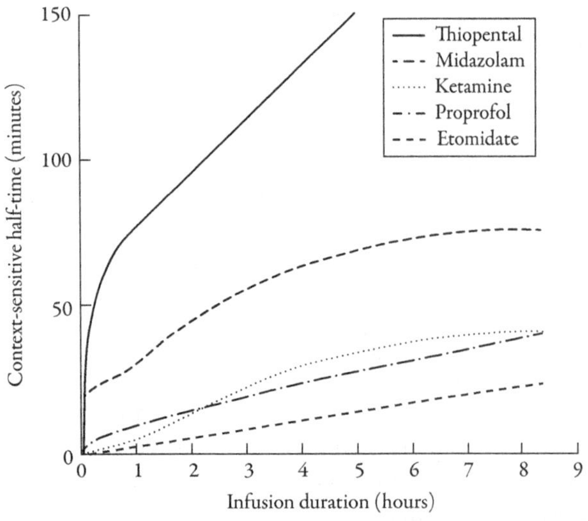

Figure 13.2 Context-sensitive half-life of the intravenous anesthetics.

Postoperative nausea and vomiting (PONV) has been considered as an adverse effect of etomidate. Early studies reported similar incidences of PONV compared with barbiturates.[13,14] Comparing etomidate in lipid emulsion with propofol for induction of anesthesia, the incidence of nausea is similar between both medications, while the incidence of vomiting is higher with etomidate.[15,16]

Adrenal cortical inhibition is a well-recognized adverse effect of etomidate. Etomidate's effect on the adrenal axis is through blockade of 11β-hydroxylase, an important enzyme in the synthesis of cortisol. Adrenal suppression lasts 6–8 hours after a single induction dose and more than 24 hours after infusion of etomidate.

INDICATIONS AND CONTRAINDICATIONS

Currently the use of etomidate is approved as an anesthetic induction agent and for anesthetic maintenance in short surgical procedures. Given the risk for adrenal toxicity, etomidate is not indicated for use for prolonged infusion. A controversy exists about the use of a single dose of etomidate in critically ill patients. Effects of a single dose of etomidate in patients with septic shock include adrenal suppression, an increase in 28-day mortality, and nonbenefit of steroid replacement therapy.[17] However, other studies have failed to demonstrate such effect on mortality.[18–20] Therefore further larger studies to define the role of a single induction dose of etomidate on clinical outcomes in critically ill patients are needed.

PROPOFOL

MECHANISM OF ACTION

Propofol is the most common parenteral anesthetic used in the United States. Propofol is a lipid formulation composed as 1% emulsion in 10% soybean oil, 2.25% glycerol, and 1.2% egg phosphatide. In order to inhibit bacterial growth, disodium EDTA (0.05 mg/mL) or sodium metabisulfite (0.25 mg/mL) is added. However, it is recommended to discard any unused propofol after 4 hours of removal of its sterile packaging. Because the lipid emulsion of propofol is associated with hyperlipidemia and pain on injection, a new aqueous solution, fospropofol, offers an alternative as an induction agent without the adverse effects. Fospropofol, which is a prodrug of propofol, is hydrolyzed by the endothelium to propofol, phosphate, and formaldehyde, which is converted to formic acid then transformed to CO_2 and water by tetrahydrofolate dehydrogenase.[21]

Propofol inhibits the response to noxious stimuli, which is mediated by its action on $GABA_A$ receptors by specific activity on B3 subunits, whereas the sedative effects are mediated by the B2 subunit in the same receptor. The agonistic action of propofol on $GABA_A$ receptors increases the activity of glycine-gated chloride channels resulting in a hyperpolarization of neurons secondary to an increase in chloride conduction, which is responsible for the inhibitory neurotransmission in the spinal cord and brain stem.

PHARMACOKINETICS AND PHARMACODYNAMICS

Propofol is highly bound to plasma proteins (98%), including albumin and red blood cells. After an induction dose of 1.5 to 2.5 mg/kg, the pharmacokinetics of propofol follows a three-compartment model, with central compartment and the slow and fast distribution compartments of 9.3 L, 44.2 L, and 266 L, respectively. The elimination half-life B is 1.8 hours. The clearance of propofol is faster than barbiturates, facilitating shorter recovery and discharge after a surgical procedure.[22] After infusion, propofol has a context-sensitive half-life shorter than 25 minutes for an infusion lasting up to 3 hours, and 40 minutes for infusions lasting up to 8 hours. Propofol used for infusion for more than 3 days increases the risk of hypertriglyceridemia, and monitoring of triglyceride in plasma is recommended.[23]

The pharmacokinetic profile of propofol changes with patient's age. Neonates have a reduced clearance, having risk for delayed emergence after anesthesia or sedation with propofol. The induction and maintenance doses of propofol are higher in children due to a higher volume of distribution and clearance of the medication. In geriatric patients, the elimination of propofol is slower and clearance decreases in patients older than 60 years of age. Since the volume of the central compartment in patients older than 65 years is reduced, an increase in the rate of propofol infusion can represent a significant rise in plasma concentration. Therefore, the induction and maintenance doses of propofol administered to geriatric patients need to be reduced between 30% and 75%.[24]

The induction dose of propofol in obese patients should be adjusted to the ideal body mass. Propofol does not exhibit an accumulation pattern in obese patients. It is recommended to adjust the maintenance doses based on the maintenance lean body mass, because higher concentrations during emergence and hemodynamic instability can be observed when the dose is calculated based on total body weight.

METABOLISM AND EXCRETION

Propofol is metabolized in the liver. The initial step is an oxidation to 1,4-di-isopropylquinol, followed by coupling with glucuronic acid and production of glucuronides; all of these metabolites are renally excreted. Extrahepatic metabolism of propofol has been described in organs such as the kidneys, small intestine, brain, and lungs.[25] Since propofol has a high hepatic extraction ratio, there is a relationship between its elimination, cardiac output, and hepatic blood flow.[26]

Since propofol is highly bound to protein and has a high extraction ratio in pathological states such hypoalbuminemia or anemia, a higher free fraction is not compensated by higher clearance or elimination; therefore, intensified effects of propofol are expected in patients with these disease processes.

EFFECT ON CIRCULATION

Propofol induces a dose-dependent decrease in arterial blood pressure after induction of anesthesia. This effect can be explained by a decrease in peripheral vascular resistance *and* myocardial contractility.[27] Propofol should be used with caution in patients with hypovolemia, cardiac failure, and hypertension, because they are prone to develop greater decreases in arterial blood pressure after an induction dose. After induction of propofol no significant changes are seen in heart rate.

EFFECT ON RESPIRATION

Propofol produces a respiratory depression with decrease in tidal volume, increase in respiratory frequency, and reduction in the inspiratory time followed by apnea that can last at least 30 seconds. The effect of propofol on tidal volume is more significant than the decrease on respiratory rate. Compared with tiopenthal, an induction dose of propofol causes slightly more pronounced respiratory depression.[28]

A propofol maintenance infusion dose (50–120 mcg/kg/min) decreases the ventilatory response to CO_2 and to hypoxia. Propofol does not induce bronchospasm and may be used as induction agent in patients with asthma or chronic obstructive pulmonary disease. Propofol decreases vagal (muscarinic receptors) and metacholine-induced bronchoconstriction. The use of metabisulfite as a preservative ablates the bronchodilator effect of propofol.[29]

EFFECT ON OTHER ORGANS

Propofol decreases cerebral blood flow, cerebral metabolic rate, and intracranial pressure. Propofol can produce dose-dependent EEG burst suppression. Despite the beneficial neurological effects, no outcome studies of propofol as a neuroprotective agent have been performed. After an induction dose, propofol can induce transient choreiform movements and opisthotonus. These movements are not associated with seizure activity, are transient, and infrequently occur. Propofol does not trigger malignant hyperthermia and may be a good choice for patients at risk to develop this condition. At subhypnotic doses such as a 10–20 mg bolus followed by 10 mcg/kg/min, propofol has antiemetic activity. Propofol does not affect renal, hepatic, or hematologic functions.

SIDE EFFECTS AND TOXICITY

A propofol induction dose can cause pain on injection and in some cases thrombophlebitis in the vein used to infuse propofol. The incidence of pain on injection is similar to that with etomidate. Strategies to decrease the incidence of pain on injection include avoiding small veins, avoiding use of those on the dorsum of the hand, and adding lidocaine to the propofol solution. Other side effects previously discussed include myoclonic movements that are transient, apnea after induction dose that can last more than 30 seconds, and decrease of systemic blood pressure associated with low vascular resistance and decreased myocardial contractility.

Propofol is considered a safe anesthetic in general; however, propofol infusion syndrome (PRIS) is a serious and lethal adverse effect associated with high doses (>4 mg/kg for single dose or >67 mcg/kg/min for infusion) for a prolonged period (48 hours) of propofol. Propofol infusion syndrome is clinically characterized by severe metabolic acidosis, hyperkalemia, rhabdomyolysis, lipemia, hepatomegaly, renal failure, and myopathy. The pathophysiology of PRIS remains unclear. Factors that have been implicated as potential causes include a failure in the mitochondrial respiratory chain as well as genetic factors related with inborn error in the fatty acid oxidation.

INDICATIONS AND CONTRAINDICATIONS

Propofol is the most common parenteral intravenous anesthetic used in clinical practice. Indications for the administration of propofol include induction and maintenance of anesthesia, and sedation for procedures in or outside of the operating room. Based on the physiological patient condition, an induction dose can be between 1.0 and 2.5 mg/kg. After an induction with propofol, a maintenance dose is recommended between 100 and 200 mcg/kg/min. Adjustments are made based on physiological patient status, surgical needs, and use of other intravenous anesthetics. The use of propofol and an opioid for total intravenous anesthesia has demonstrated reduction in the incidence of postoperative nausea and vomiting.[30]

Propofol provides a reliable level of sedation that is easy to titrate and a rapid recovery after infusion. Therefore, propofol is suitable for use in sedation in the intensive care unit (ICU) and during short surgical procedures and as a supplement for patients receiving regional anesthesia.

Propofol should be used with caution in patients with limited cardiac reserve such those with cardiac failure, those undergoing cardiac surgery, and those with hypovolemia or hypertension, as they are prone to develop greater decreases in arterial blood pressure after an induction dose.

Anaphylactoid reactions with the current propofol formulation are uncommon, and have been reported in patients with multiple other allergies. Therefore, in patients with history of multiple allergies, propofol should be used with caution. Patients with known allergies to egg and soy products may have an allergic response to propofol; as such, cautious use should be considered in these patients.[31]

BENZODIAZEPINES

MECHANISM OF ACTION

Benzodiazepines bind to specific benzodiazepine receptors. This binding modulates and increases the efficiency of the inhibitory GABA neurotransmitter system through the coupling of the GABA receptor with the chloride ion channel. This results in the hyperpolarization of the postsynaptic cell membrane and renders postsynaptic neurons resistant to the effects of the excitatory neurotransmitters. Clinically it produces anxiolysis, sedation, and hypnosis.

PHARMACOKINETICS AND PHARMACODYNAMICS

The three benzodiazepine receptor agonists available in clinical practice are short-acting midazolam (Versed), intermediate-acting diazepam (Valium), and long-acting lorazepam (Ativan). All three are highly lipophilic and produce a rapid CNS response. The high lipophilicity also leads to the large volume of distribution of benzodiazepines. Redistribution from the highly perfused central compartment to the less perfused peripheral compartment is responsible for the termination of the clinical effect of the benzodiazepines after the initial doses.

METABOLISM AND EXCRETION

All benzodiazepines are metabolized in the liver by oxidation and glucuronide conjugation. Water-soluble glucuronide conjugates are excreted by the kidney. Unlike lorazepam, which has no active metabolites, diazepam produces two active metabolites that can prolong its drug effect. Prolonged infusion of midazolam can result in accumulation of active metabolites especially in the presence of renal impairment.

EFFECT ON CIRCULATION

Benzodiazepines decrease systemic vascular resistance and lead to a small reduction in the arterial blood pressure. Their ability to preserve homeostatic reflex mechanisms results in overall stable hemodymanics even in the presence of ischemic and valvular heart disease. Midazolam can increase cardiac output and decrease filling pressure in patients with elevated left ventricular pressures. When given in combination with opioids, benzodiazepines can decrease systemic blood pressure via the synergistic reduction in sympathetic tone.

EFFECT ON RESPIRATION

Benzodiazepines produce dose-dependent respiratory depression, modestly attenuate upper airway reactivity, and depress the swallowing reflex. All of the benzodiazepines can cause apnea if used in sufficient doses. Apnea is more likely in the presence of opioids. Benzodiazepines and opioids produce synergistic (supra-additive) respiratory depression.

EFFECT ON OTHER ORGANS

All benzodiazepines reduce the cerebral metabolic oxygen consumption and cerebral blood flow. The ratio of cerebral blood flow to cerebral metabolic oxygen consumption remains relatively normal. Importantly, cerebral vasomotor response to carbon dioxide is preserved during midazolam administration. Midazolam has little effect on intracranial pressure. All benzodiazepines increase the seizure threshold, including a seizure caused by local anesthetics, and all can be used to treat status epilepticus. Lorazepam is the most efficacious of all the benzodiazepines in treating status epilepticus.

SIDE EFFECTS AND TOXICITY

The most significant side effect of midazolam is respiratory depression, which can be reversed with flumazenil. Flumazenil is a competitive benzodiazepine receptor antagonist. Flumazenil is cleared rapidly and may require repeated boluses or a continuous infusion to prevent resedation. Reversal of the sedation and respiratory depression with flumazenil does not produce adverse cardiovascular effects even in the presence of ischemic heart disease. It can, however, precipitate withdrawal in individuals physically dependent on benzodiazepines. Lorazepam and diazepam can cause venous irritation and thrombophlebitis.

INDICATIONS AND CONTRAINDICATIONS

Midazolam, lorazepam, and diazepam have amnestic, sedative, anxiolytic, hypnotic, anticonvulsant, and centrally mediated muscle-relaxing properties. Clinically, benzodiazepines are used to provide anxiolysis and anterograde amnesia prior to surgery and during moderate and deep sedation. Midazolam is the most frequently used drug due to the rapid onset and short duration of action. Long-term administration of benzodiazepines leads to a decrease of efficacy (tolerance) most likely related to the down-regulation of the benzodiazepine–GABA receptor complexes.

Midazolam appears to have a role in prevention of postoperative nausea and vomiting. In several studies intravenous midazolam was shown to reduce postoperative nausea and vomiting similar to intravenous ondansetron and dexamethasone.

Small intravenous doses of midazolam can be administered safely to the mother during a cesarean section without significant unwanted effects on the newborn baby, though the risk of anterograde amnesia remains for the mother.

KETAMINE

MECHANISM OF ACTION

Ketamine is a unique intravenous anesthetic with significant analgesic effect. It is structurally related to phencyclidine (PCP). Ketamine antagonizes the effect of glutamate on the N-methyl-D-aspartate (NMDA) receptor, thus inhibiting the excitatory response and producing a dissociative state of hypnosis and analgesia. It also binds to nicotinic, muscarinic, and opioid receptors. Ketamine has two stereoisomers, S(+) and R(-), with S(+) being more potent. Ketamine is water soluble and exists in an aqueous solution.

METABOLISM AND EXCRETION

Ketamine is metabolized by hepatic microsomal cytochrome P450 enzymes to form active metabolites norketamine and hydroxynorketamine that are excreted by the kidney. The elimination half-life of ketamine is 2–3 hours. Ketamine can be given intravenously, intramuscularly, intranasally, orally, and rectally. Bioavailability of oral ketamine is 20%–30% due to first-pass metabolism.

EFFECT ON RESPIRATION

Ketamine produces minimal respiratory depression when used alone. Ketamine preserves autonomic reflexes better than other intravenous agents. Despite that, aspiration can occur in the presence of full stomach and airway reflexes should not be assumed to be protective. Ketamine is a potent bronchodilator and can be used for intravenous induction in the presence of bronchospasm. Ketamine is known to increase salivation and lacrimation and can lead to laryngospasm, especially in the lightly anesthetized child.

EFFECT ON CIRCULATION

Ketamine has a significant effect on the cardiovascular system and produces an elevation in blood pressure, heart rate, and cardiac output that can lead to an increase in myocardial oxygen consumption. Coronary blood flow might be limited in the presence of a stenotic coronary lesion, and myocardial ischemia can ensue. Ketamine-induced tachycardia and systemic hypertension can be attenuated by prior administration of a benzodiazepine. Despite the central cardiovascular stimulation, ketamine can cause myocardial depression in the seriously ill patient with depleted catecholamine reserves. Ketamine is well tolerated in children with congenital heart diseases. It does not change either the direction or magnitude of the shunt, and it helps to maintain systemic oxygenation. Caution should be used in patients with pulmonary hypertension, because ketamine causes more pronounced elevation in pulmonary than systemic vascular resistance. This effect is less pronounced in children, and ketamine has been used safely in pediatric pulmonary hypertension.

EFFECT ON OTHER ORGANS

The dissociative anesthesia caused by ketamine is characterized by profound analgesia, variable amnesia in a patient who might appear conscious with open eyes, and relatively well preserved reflexes. Ketamine dilates pupils, causes horizontal and vertical nystagmus, and increases salivation and lacrimation.

Ketamine increases cerebral metabolic rate, cerebral blood flow, and intracranial pressure. Hyperventilation would attenuate this increase. Ketamine also elevates intraocular pressure through elevation of the systemic blood pressure and increase in intracranial pressure.

SIDE EFFECTS AND TOXICITY

Ketamine anesthesia can produce hallucinations, vivid dreaming, and illusions that can cause fear, confusion, and euphoria. These adverse effects can be attenuated by the use of benzodiazepine premedication. Ketamine was shown to accentuate neonatal brain cell apoptosis in animal models. There is not enough evidence to support the restriction of the use of ketamine in human neonates at the present time.

INDICATIONS AND CONTRAINDICATIONS

Ketamine is useful for patients with reactive airway disease; patients with septic shock; healthy trauma victims; patients with hypovolemia, cardiomyopathy, cardiac tamponade, and restrictive pericarditis; and patients with congenital heart disease with right-to-left shunt. Intramuscular injection of ketamine can be used in the emergency situation in the absence of intravascular access and in combative and uncooperative patients without intravenous lines. Subanesthetic doses of ketamine can provide postoperative analgesia and have opioid-sparing effects. Ketamine is a good choice for procedural sedation for painful procedures, especially in children.

In patients with elevated intracranial and intraocular pressure, pulmonary hypertension, ischemic heart disease, vascular aneurysms, and psychiatric disorders, ketamine should be used cautiously if at all. Nonetheless, there is emerging evidence that ketamine does not cause elevation of intracranial pressure in traumatic brain injury, though further studies are warranted.

BARBITURATES

INTRODUCTION

Barbiturates were the earliest nonopioid intravenous anesthetics that were used in clinical practice. Although synthesized in the 1860s, it was not until 1920 that IV barbiturates became available for widespread use. Thiopental was introduced into clinical practice in the mid-1930s and became the most commonly used IV barbiturate in anesthetic practice. The principal barbiturate in clinical use today is phenobarbital for the treatment of intractable status epilepticus. Even though barbiturates are infrequently used in modern anesthetic practice (as of 2011, thiopental is no longer manufactured), understanding their metabolism and pharmacology offers further insight into the understanding of anesthetic medications.

METABOLISM

With the exception of phenobarbital, barbiturates are hepatically metabolized. The metabolites are inactive and excreted in the urine. Barbiturates are known to induce the action of hepatic enzymes. For this reason they are to be avoided in patients with acute intermittent porphyria. Barbiturates can stimulate the hepatic enzyme (aminolevulinic acid synthetase) responsible for producing porphyrins that are intermediaries in heme synthesis.

Phenobarbital is renally cleared. Alkalinizing the urine enhances its excretion.

PHARMACOKINETICS

Rapid redistribution explains the termination of action of a single dose of barbiturate. When a continuous infusion of barbiturate is used, the recovery time increases, as termination of action becomes dependent on uptake into adipose tissue (a slower process, as blood flow to adipose tissue is proportionally lower) and hepatic metabolism.

Thiopental

First-order kinetics (a constant fraction of the drug is cleared from the body per unit time) are observed in standard induction doses (3–5 mg/kg). At higher doses, as receptors are saturated, zero-order kinetics (a constant amount of the drug is cleared per unit of time) are observed (see the Pharmacology chapter for more details). Thiopental can readily accumulate in tissue because it is a lipophilic drug that has a relatively high volume of distribution and a low rate of hepatic clearance. Obese patients are thus at greater risk for prolonged clearance of thiopental.

MECHANISM OF ACTION

Barbiturates enhance the activity of the inhibitory neurotransmitter GABA. By binding to the $GABA_A$ receptor, barbiturates enhance the action of GABA, causing increased influx of chloride and hyperpolarization of the cell membrane. This increases the excitability threshold of the postsynaptic neuron. Furthermore, barbiturates inhibit the synaptic transmission of excitatory neurotransmitters such as glutamate and acetylcholine.

PHARMACODYNAMICS

Barbiturates act to depress consciousness and produce some degree of amnesia. They are not known to have analgesic properties; in fact, at low blood concentrations, they can decrease the pain threshold.

ONSET OF ACTION

There are four key factors that determine the speed with which a drug enters the CNS: the lipid solubility, ionization (pKa), level of protein binding, and plasma drug concentration. Thiopental, for instance, is very lipid soluble and has a pKa of 7.6, meaning that at close to physiologic pH about half the drug is in its nonionized and therefore lipophilic form, able to cross readily into the CNS. The implications of this pKa are such that when the patient is acidotic, more of the drug is in the nonionized form, so less drug is needed to induce the desired clinical effect. The converse is also true, so that in an alkalotic patient more drug may be needed. Protein binding also affects the onset of action, as only free unbound drug can cross the blood-brain barrier. Barbiturates are highly bound to albumin, and pH and disease states that affect the amount of protein in the body affect barbiturate protein binding. While hepatic or liver disease may decrease total body protein, this usually bears little clinical significance. Finally the plasma concentration of the drug determines how quickly it crosses the blood-brain barrier based on its concentration gradient. Plasma concentration is determined by the dose of the drug and the speed with which it is given.

TERMINATION OF ACTION

The most important factor governing termination of action is plasma disappearance of the drug. As drug is cleared from the plasma more drug that is in the CSF can travel down its concentration gradient out of the CSF and to the liver to be metabolized. Lipid solubility, the degree of ionization, and CSF concentration gradients all play an important role. Two main mechanisms account for the decrease of barbiturates in the plasma: (1) redistribution to peripheral tissue (muscle then fat) and (2) metabolism and clearance by the liver.

EFFECT ON CEREBRAL METABOLIC RATE

Barbiturates decrease the $CMRO_2$, causing progressive slowing of the EEG and decreased ATP consumption. At an isoelectric EEG no further decrease in $CMRO_2$ is noted. Cerebral blood flow and, therefore, intracranial pressure are also reduced by barbiturates.

SIDE EFFECTS AND CONTRAINDICATIONS

Cardiovascular

Barbiturates depress the cardiovascular system by causing peripheral vasodilation, leading to venous pooling. They also have negative inotropic effects (decreased calcium influx into cells), decreased ventricular filling from venous pooling of blood, and decreased sympathetic output from the autonomic nervous system. Caution must be given if using a barbiturate in hypovolemic patients, as a significant decrease in cardiac output and hemodynamic instability may occur.

Respiratory

Barbiturates cause central respiratory depression and transient apnea after administration. Recovery of respiratory function after a one-time dose is fairly quick, with respiratory parameters returning to normal about 15 minutes after a single induction dose of thiopental.

Contraindications to barbiturate use include the following:

1. Respiratory compromise
2. Hemodynamic instability
3. Status asthmaticus
4. Acute intermittent porphyria

DEXMEDETOMIDINE

Dexmedetomidine is a highly selective alpha-2 agonist that has shown to have a broad set of uses. Alpha-2 adrenergic receptor agonists have several effects: sedation, anxiolysis, hypnosis, analgesia, and sympatholysis.

METABOLISM

Dexmedetomidine is metabolized extensively by the liver and excreted in the urine. More than 90% is protein bound.

PHARMACOKINETICS

The elimination half-life of dexmedetomidine is 2–3 hours. The context-sensitive half-life is from about 4 minutes after a 10-minute infusion to about 250 minutes after an 8-hour infusion.

EFFECTS ON THE CENTRAL NERVOUS SYSTEM

Dexmedetomidine produces sedative and hypnotic effects by affecting alpha-2 agonists in the locus ceruleus and spinal cord. Sedation and anxiolysis are mediated primarily via the locus ceruleus, and analgesia is mediated primarily via the spinal cord. Although the effects of dexmedetomidine alone on cerebral blood flow and intracranial pressure are not well characterized, some studies support a decrease in cerebral blood flow in healthy volunteers. Dexmedetomidine is known to decrease the minimum alveolar concentration of inhalational anesthetics, and in higher concentrations it can affect memory and recall.

RESPIRATORY EFFECTS

While dexmedetomidine does reduce minute ventilation, it retains the ventilatory response to increasing CO_2 levels. Dexmedetomidine appears to decrease tidal volume without affecting respiratory rate. The combination of dexmedetomidine with an opioid enhances analgesia but does not appear to potentiate further respiratory depression.

CARDIOVASCULAR EFFECTS

The overall effects of dexmedetomidine on the cardiovascular system include a decrease in heart rate, decreased systemic vascular resistance, and decreased cardiac output, myocardial contractility, and blood pressure. A bolus dose of dexmedetomidine causes a biphasic response, with an initial increase in blood pressure and decrease in heart rate. This initial increase in blood pressure is likely due to its effects on peripheral alpha-2 receptors.

DOSAGE AND USES

Dexmedetomidine is not indicated for the induction or maintenance of anesthesia. Rather, it functions as a postoperative sedative and as an adjunct medication to reduce hypnotic and opioid requirements. Generally, it is administered as a bolus dose followed by an infusion. The usual loading dose is 1 mcg/kg over 10 minutes; however, ranges between 0.5 and 2.5 mcg/kg have been described. Infusing over 10 minutes decreases the hypertension seen with a rapid bolus. The typical infusion rate is anywhere from 0.2 to 1 mcg/kg/h. There is a growing body of evidence that another possible role for dexmedetomidine is the attenuation of emergence delirium that is observed in some pediatric patients. Research into the optimal dosage for this indication is ongoing.

REFERENCES

1. Bergen J, Smith D. A review of etomidate for rapid sequence intubation in the emergency department. *J Emerg Med.* 1997;15:221–230.
2. Tomlin S, Jenkins A, Lieb W, Frank N. Stereoselective effects of etomidate optical isomers on gamma-aminobutyric acid type A receptors and animals. *Anesthesiology.* 1998;88:708–717.
3. Kay B. Total intravenous anesthesia with etomidate: I. A trial in children. *Acta Anaesthesiol Belg.* 1977;28:107–113.
4. Bird T, Edbrooke D, Newby D, Hebron B. Intravenous sedation for the intubated and spontaneously breathing patient in the intensive care unit. *Acta Anaesthesiol Scand.* 1984;28:640–643.
5. Batjer H. Cerebral protective effects of etomidate: experimental and clinical aspects. *Cerebrovasc Brain Metab Rev.* 1993;5:17–32.
6. Johnson K, Egan T, Layman J, Kern S, White L, McJames S. The influence of hemorrhagic shock on etomidate: a pharmacokinetic and pharmacodynamic analysis. *Anesth Analg.* 2003;96:1360–1368.
7. Ghoneim M, Yamada T. Etomidate: a clinical and electroencephalographic comparison with thiopental. *Anesth Analg.* 1977;56:479–485.
8. Thornton C, Heneghan C, Navaratnarajah M, Bateman P, Jones J. Effect of etomidate on the auditory evoked response in man. *Br J Anaesth.* 1985;57:554–561.
9. Sloan T, Ronai A, Toleikis J, Koht A. Improvement of intraoperative somatosensory evoked potentials by etomidate. *Anesth Analg.* 1988;67:582–585.
10. Taniguchi M, Nadstawek J, Langenbach U, Bremer F, Schramm J. Effects of four intravenous anesthetic agents on motor evoked potentials elicited by magnetic transcranial stimulation. *Neurosurgery.* 1993;33:407–415, discussion 415.
11. Atiba J, Horai Y, White P, Trevor A, Blaschke T, Sung M. Effect of etomidate on hepatic drug metabolism in humans. *Anesthesiology.* 1988;68:920–924.
12. Forman S. Clinical and molecular pharmacology of etomidate. *Anesthesiology.* 2011;114:695–707.
13. Giese J, Stanley T. Etomidate: a new intravenous anesthetic induction agent. *Pharmacotherapy.* 1983;3:251–258.
14. Zacharias M, Clarke RS, Dundee JW, Johnston S. Evaluation of three preparations of etomidate. *Br J Anaesth.* 1978;50:925–929.
15. Mayer M, Doenicke A, Nebauer A, Hepting L. [Propofol and etomidate-Lipuro for induction of general anesthesia: Hemodynamics, vascular compatibility, subjective findings and postoperative nausea]. *Anaesthesist.* 1996;45:1082–1084.
16. St Pierre M, Dunkel M, Rutherford A, Hering W. Does etomidate increase postoperative nausea? A double-blind controlled comparison of etomidate in lipid emulsion with propofol for balanced anaesthesia. *Eur J Anaesthesiol.* 2000;17:634–641.
17. Sprung C, Annane D, Keh D, et al. Hydrocortisone therapy for patients with septic shock. *N Engl J Med.* 2008;358:111–124.
18. Tekwani KL, Watts HF, Rzechula KH, Sweis R, Kulstad E. A prospective observational study of the effect of etomidate on septic patient mortality and length of stay. *Acad Emerg Med.* 2009;16:11–14.
19. Ray D, McKeown D. Effect of induction agent on vasopressor and steroid use, and outcome in patients with septic shock. *Crit Care.* 2007;11:R56.
20. Jabre P, Combes X, Lapostolle F, et al. Etomidate versus ketamine for rapid sequence intubation in acutely ill patients: a multicentre randomised controlled trial. *Lancet.* 2009;374:293–300.
21. Brunton L, Chabner B, Knollman B. *Goodman and Gilman's The Pharmacological Basis of Therapeutics.* 12th ed. New York, NY: McGraw-Hill Medical; 2011.
22. Schuttler J, Ihmsen H. Population pharmacokinetics of propofol: a multicenter study. *Anesthesiology.* 2000;92:727–738.
23. McKeage K, Perry C. Propofol: a review of its use in intensive care sedation of adults. *CNS Drugs.* 2003;17:235–272.
24. Bienert A, Wiczling P, Grzeskowiak E, Cywiński J, Kusza K. Potential pitfalls of propofol target controlled infusion delivery related to its pharmacokinetics and pharmacodynamics. *Pharmacol Rep.* 2012;64:782–795.
25. Takata K, Kurita T, Morishima Y, Morita K, Uraoka M, Sato S. Do the kidneys contribute to propofol elimination? *Br J Anaesth.* 2008;101:648–652.
26. Upton R, Ludbrook G, Grant C, Martinez A. Cardiac output is a determinant of the initial concentrations of propofol after short-infusion administration. *Anesth Analg.* 1999;89:545–552.

27. Kirkpatrick T, Cockshott I, Douglas E, Nimmo W. Pharmacokinetics of propofol (diprivan) in elderly patients. *Br J Anaesth.* 1988;60:146–150.
28. Goodman N, Black A, Carter J. Some ventilatory effects of propofol as sole anaesthetic agent. *Br J Anaesth.* 1987;59:1497–1503.
29. Miller R, Fleisher L, Johns R, et al., eds. *Miller's Anesthesia.* 6th ed. Philadelphia, PA: Elsevier Churchill Livingstone; 2005.
30. Visser K, Hassink E, Bonsel G, Moen J, Kalkman C. Randomized controlled trial of total intravenous anesthesia with propofol versus inhalation anesthesia with isoflurane-nitrous oxide: postoperative nausea with vomiting and economic analysis. *Anesthesiology.* 2001;95:616–626.
31. Murphy A, Campbell E, Baines D, Mehr S. Allergic reactions to propofol in egg-allergic children. *Anesth Analg.* 2011;113(1):140–144. Epub April 5, 2011.

FURTHER READING

Barash P, Cullen B, Stoelting R, Cahalan M, Stock M. *Clinical Anesthesia.* 7th ed. Philadelphia, PA: Lippincott Williams & Wilkins; 2013:479–500.
Cote C, Lerman J, Anderson B. Pharmacokinetics and pharmacology of drugs used in children. In: Cote C, Lerman J, Anderson B. *A Practice of Anesthesia for Infants and Children.* 4th ed. Philadelphia, PA: Elsevier Saunders; 2013:1053.
Miller R, ed. *Miller's Anesthesia.* 6th ed. Philadelphia, PA: Elsevier; 2006:326–334, 355–359.
Miller R, ed. *Miller's Anesthesia.* 7th ed. Philadelphia, PA: Elsevier; 2010:719–768.
Stoelting R, Hillier S. *Pharmacology and Physiology in Anesthetic Practice.* 4th ed. Philadelphia, PA: Lippincott Williams & Wilkins; 2005.
Talke P, Caldwell J, Kirkegaard-Nielsen H, Stafford M. The effects of dexmedetomidine on neuromuscular blockade in human volunteers. *Anesth Analg.* 1999;88:633–639.

QUESTIONS

1. All of the following anesthetics have effects on GABA receptors **EXCEPT**:
   A. Nitrous oxide
   B. Etomidate
   C. Isoflurane
   D. Fospropofol

2. Adrenal insufficiency associated with etomidate:
   A. May last for >96 hours after a single dose
   B. Is only associated with etomidate infusion administration
   C. Does not improve with steroid replacement therapy
   D. Is an uncommon effect in patients in septic shock

3. Ketamine induction is appropriate in all patients EXCEPT:
   A. 28-year-old male with splenic laceration and hepatic contusion after motor-vehicle accident.
   B. 12-year-old with acute lymphoblastic leukemia in septic shock for central line placement.
   C. 20-year-old with systemic lupus erythematosus for pericardiocentesis of cardiac tamponade.
   D. 78-year-old male with intermittent chest pain for exploratory laparotomy for small bowel obstruction.
   E. 2-month-old with tetralogy of Fallot with hypercyanotic spell for complete repair.

4. All of the following are indications for dexmedetomidine administration, EXCEPT:
   A. Postoperative sedation in the intensive care unit of a 35-year-old female who underwent a temporal lobe tumor resection and is being weaned from the ventilator
   B. As an adjuvant to maintenance of anesthesia in a 75-year-old male with a history of diabetes and hypertension so as to decrease the minimum alveolar concentration of hypnotic agents
   C. As an adjuvant to neuromuscular blockade in a 20-year-old female with myasthenia gravis
   D. As an adjuvant to treating postoperative pain in a 45-year-old male with a history of heroin addiction who is now in the ICU after suffering rib fractures from a fall.

ANSWERS

1. A. Nitrous oxide. The only general anesthetics that do not have significant effects on $GABA_A$ or glycine receptors are ketamine, nitrous oxide, cyclopropane, and xenon. These agents inhibit a different type of ligand-gated ion channel, the N-methyl-D-aspartate (NMDA) receptor. Xenon is particularly rare, expensive, and currently impractical for clinical use.

FURTHER READING

Patel PM, Patel HH, Roth DM. General anesthetics and therapeutic gases. In: Brunton LL, Chabner BA, Knollmann BC, eds. *Goodman and Gilman's The Pharmacological Basis of Therapeutics.* 12th ed. New York, NY: McGraw-Hill; 2011.

2. C. Does not improve with steroid replacement therapy. Adrenal suppression lasts 6–8 hours after a single induction dose and more than 24 hours after infusion of etomidate. Effects of a single dose of etomidate in patients with septic shock include adrenal suppression, an increase in 28-day mortality, and nonbenefit of steroid replacement therapy.

FURTHER READING

Ray DC, McKeown DW. Effect of induction agent on vasopressor and steroid use, and outcome in patients with septic shock. *Crit Care.* 2007;11:R56.
Sprung CL, Annane D, Keh D, et al. Hydrocortisone therapy for patients with septic shock. *N Engl J Med.* 2008;358:111–124.

Tekwani KL, Watts HF, Rzechula KH, et al. A prospective observational study of the effect of etomidate on septic patient mortality and length of stay. *Acad Emerg Med.* 2009;16:11–14.

3. D. Intermittent chest pain in 78-year-old male is a symptom of coronary artery disease until proven otherwise. The emergent nature of the planned surgery might not allow for sufficient time for full investigation. Tachycardia and hypertension caused by sympathetic effects of ketamine will increase myocardial oxygen consumption and can lead to acute coronary ischemia. All other patients are appropriate candidates for ketamine infusion.

FURTHER READING

Miller R, ed. *Miller's Anesthesia.* 7th ed. Philadelphia, PA: Elsevier; 2010:746

4. C. There is no evidence that dexmedetomidine decreases the dose requirement for neuromuscular blocking drugs. While the added hypnotic and analgesic benefits may help attenuate muscle movement while under anesthesia, dexmedetomidine has not been demonstrated to have effects on the peripheral actions of neuromuscular blocking medications.

14.

LOCAL ANESTHETICS

Chris D. Glover and Kim-Phuong Nguyen

MECHANISM OF ACTION

Local anesthetics prevent the transmission of the action potential by reversibly binding to voltage-gated Na+ channels located on nerve fibers. This action prevents the influx of Na+ ions, thereby decreasing the rate of depolarization in response to a nerve stimulus and preventing the achievement of the threshold potential. Local anesthetics also block other ion channels (K+, Ca2+, G protein coupled receptors); but the significance of these actions is still unclear.

The structure of local anesthetics consists of a lipophilic group (typically an aromatic benzene ring), an intermediate chain, and a hydrophilic group (typically a tertiary amine) (Figure 14.1). The tertiary amine on the hydrocarbon backbone of local anesthetics is a weak base (unconjugated neutral or nonionized form), which can accept a hydrogen ion to form a conjugated acid (positively charged or ionized form). At physiologic pH, local anesthetics exist in these two forms. The ratio of the two forms depends on the pKa (the dissociation constant of the local anesthetic) and the surrounding pH. In other words, the pKa is the pH at which the ratio of ionized and nonionized drug is equal.

The target site of local anesthetics is located inside the Na channel pore, and therefore local anesthetics must cross the nerve lipid bilayer membrane into the cell interior to reach its site. As a consequence, the potency of each local anesthetic is closely related to its lipid solubility. The lipid solubility of a local anesthetic is determined by the degree of alkyl group substitution on the amide group and the benzene ring.[1] Unlike inhaled anesthetic agents, there is no measurement of local anesthetic potency that is analogous to the minimum alveolar concentration. The neutral lipophilic form crosses the lipid membrane much faster than the cationic form. The percentage of local anesthetic found in the neutral form at normal tissue pH of 7.4 is inversely proportional to the pKa, and thus, local anesthetics with lower pKa will have a faster onset of blockade. Upon entry of the local anesthetic inside the cell, the lower pH shifts the equilibrium toward the positively charged form, which antagonizes the Na+ channels more potently than the neutral form. Lipid solubility usually parallels intrinsic local anesthetic potency. Thus, highly lipid soluble local anesthetics are more potent and usually have a longer duration of action than less lipid soluble ones.[2] In addition to lipid solubility, the minimum concentration of local anesthetic that will block nerve conduction depends on other factors such as the nerve fibers, temperature, tissue vascularity, and tissue pH.

The onset of action also depends on the route of administration and the dose or concentration of the drug. Local anesthetics injected in the subarachnoid space where the nerves lack a sheath achieve a quicker onset of nerve block in comparison with peripheral nerves. The amount of drug needed for desheathed fibers is a hundredfold lower than for encased fibers. For peripheral nerves, the amount of drug that reaches the nerves depends on the proximity of injection and the diffusion of the drug. While chloroprocaine may theoretically have a slower onset than lidocaine because its pKa of 9.1 favors the positively charged form, higher concentration of 3% solution (typical clinical concentration) will result in a faster onset because of a greater diffusion gradient.

Protein binding largely determines the duration of action of the local anesthetic. Increased protein binding is associated with increased duration of action, because the local anesthetics more slowly diffuse from a lipid-rich environment to the bloodstream. Agents that have a high affinity for protein remain bound to the nerve membrane and Na+ channel longer. The rate of vascular uptake from the injection site also plays a role in the duration of action by removing the agent from the area of effect. Injection of local anesthetic at areas of high vascularity such as the intercostal site will result in higher plasma concentration. Adding a vasoconstrictor such as epinephrine slows the vascular absorption and, therefore, prolongs the block, with the most prominent effect in drugs with intermediate duration rather than long-acting agents.

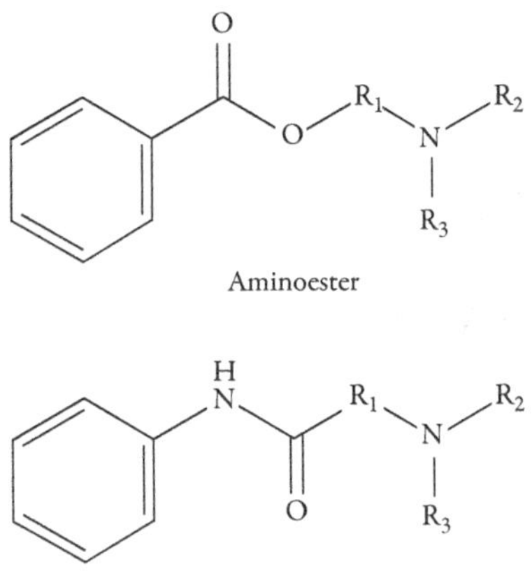

Figure 14.1 The structure of local anesthetics. Image courtesy of George Williams, MD.

Local anesthetics produce a differential blockade with an ordered progression starting at temperature, followed by proprioception, motor function, sharp pain, and then light touch.[1] Historically, this was felt to be related to the size of the fibers; however, experimental findings show that small myelinated fibers (Aγ motor and Aδ) are the most susceptible, followed by larger myelinated (Aα and Aβ) over small nonmyelinated C fibers, which mediate dull pain.[2] The potency of the local anesthetic as well as the concentration and volume determines the quality of the nerve blockade.

PHARMACOKINETICS

The concentration of local anesthetics in plasma is determined by the amount of drug injected, the amount of intravascular absorption, the rate of tissue distribution, the rate of biotransformation, and the excretion of the drug. The blood concentration of local anesthetics is also influenced by patient-related factors including age, cardiovascular status, and renal and hepatic function.

UPTAKE

In general, the plasma concentration of a local anesthetic is directly proportional to the dose injection (in a nearly linear fashion) regardless of the speed of injection or the concentration. The rate of systemic absorption of a local anesthetic depends a number of factors including site of injection, total dose, physiochemical properties of the drugs (Table 14.1), and presence of vasoconstrictive or other adjuvants. For instance, injection of a drug in more vascular tissue results in higher plasma concentration of local anesthetic in a shorter time. The order of increasing rate of absorption by injection site is subcutaneous < sciatic < femoral < brachial plexus < epidural < caudal < intercostal < intravenous. In addition, more lipid-soluble agents are absorbed more quickly in neural and nonneural tissue than less lipid-soluble ones, resulting in lower systemic absorption. Vasoconstrictive drugs such as epinephrine reduce the rate of systemic absorption.

Table 14.1 PHYSIOCHEMICAL PROPERTIES OF LOCAL ANESTHETICS

LOCAL ANESTHETIC	PKA	RELATIVE LIPID SOLUBILITY	% PROTEIN BINDING	ONSET	DURATION OF ACTION (H)	SINGLE MAX DOSE (MG)/ + EPINEPHRINE
Amides						
Lidocaine	7.9	1	64	Fast	0.5–3	300/500
Mepivacaine	7.6	0.3	77	Fast	1–4	400/500
Prilocaine	7.9	0.4	55	Fast	0.5–3	600
Bupivacaine	8.1	8	95			
				Slow (peripheral)	4–12	175/225
				Mod (epidural)	2–5	175/225
				Fast (spinal)	1–4	20
Ropivacaine	8.1	2.5	94			
				Slow (peripheral)	5–8	250
				Mod (epidural)	2–6	200
Esters						
Cocaine	8.6	NA	67	Fast	0.5–1	150
Tetracaine	8.5	12	94	Fast	2–6	20
Procaine	8.9	0.3	6	Fast	0.5–1	1000
Chloroprocaine	8.7	2.3	N/A	Fast	0.5–1	800/1000

Evers A. *Anesthetic Pharmacology, Physiologic Principles, and Clinical Practice.* Philadelphia, PA: Churchill Livingstone Elsevier; 2004:507–535.

DISTRIBUTION

The rate of distribution of a local anesthetic is described by a two-compartment model: the rapid phase involving uptake in highly perfused tissues that reach rapid equilibration, and the slow phase depending on less perfused tissues and specific properties of the individual local anesthetic. Therefore, more highly perfused organs show higher concentrations of local anesthetic drug than less well perfused organs do. Pulmonary tissue rapidly extracts local anesthetics.

BIOTRANSFORMATION AND EXCRETION

Despite being placed near nerves, only a small fraction (1%–2%) actually reaches the nerve membrane. Amide and ester type local anesthetics differ in their metabolism. Ester local anesthetics are metabolized by plasma cholinesterases and red cell esterases except for cocaine, which is metabolized by carboxylesterases in the liver. Para-aminobenzoic acid (PABA), a metabolite of ester local anesthetics, may cause allergic reactions in susceptible individuals. Amides are mainly degraded by liver enzymes via aromatic hydroxylation, N-dealkylation, and amide hydrolysis. The rate of degradation is dependent on the individual amide local anesthetic, and its metabolites are excreted by the kidneys. Only small amounts of local anesthetics are excreted unchanged in urine.

Patients with decreased hepatic or renal function should have appropriate dose adjustment of amide local anesthetics because of the increased risk for systemic toxicity. Liver disease has a minimal effect on ester local anesthetics. Drugs that increase liver enzymes (barbiturates) increase the systemic clearance of amide local anesthetics. Pregnancy may cause decrease clearance of the local anesthetic. There is some evidence that young infants and elder patients may have decreased clearance and increase absorption, and therefore, may be at increased risk for systemic toxicity.

COMPARISON OF DRUGS AND CHEMICAL GROUPS

Local anesthetics are classified as amino amides or amino esters based on the type of chemical bond linking the lipophilic phenyl ring with the hydrophobic tertiary amine. Because local anesthetics are weak bases, they are poorly water soluble and dispensed as hydrochloride salts resulting in acidic (pH 4–7) solutions. Ester local anesthetics are relatively unstable in solution as compared with amides.

AMIDE LOCAL ANESTHETICS

Lidocaine

Lidocaine has a number of clinical applications, which include wound infiltration, peripheral nerve block, bier block, epidural block, topical skin ointment or jelly, and nebulization to the upper airway. Due to concerns about neurotoxicity and transient neurologic symptoms, its use for spinal anesthesia has fallen out of favor. Intravenous infusions of lidocaine to achieve low plasma levels (<5 mcg/mL) may result in systemic analgesia and can be used to treat chronic neuropathic pain. Lidocaine causes peripheral vasodilation, so the addition of epinephrine can prolong the duration of action by decreasing the systemic absorption of lidocaine. In addition, lidocaine possesses anti-inflammatory effects by inhibiting the release of pro-inflammatory cytokines and preventing leukocyte adhesion.[3] These effects may be effective in the treatment of predominantly inflammatory conditions such as irritable bowel disease.

Prilocaine

Prilocaine has a similar profile and clinical application as lidocaine. The addition of epinephrine confers minimal advantage because prilocaine causes less vasodilation than lidocaine. While it may be useful for intravenous regional anesthesia due to its low risk for systemic toxicity, at doses greater than 500 mg, it causes methemoglobinemia from its metabolite o-toluidine, thereby limiting its use.

Mepivacaine

The profile for mepivacaine is also similar to lidocaine, but it has a slightly longer duration of action. Metabolism of mepivacaine is prolonged in the fetus and newborn, thus, it is not generally recommended for obstetric anesthesia. The addition of epinephrine may significantly prolong the duration of action even though mepivacaine has mild vasodilatory effects.

Bupivacaine

Standard formulations of bupivacaine consist of a racemic mixture of both the R and S enantiomers. Because of its ability to produce prolonged and intense sensory analgesia relative to motor blockade, bupivacaine is commonly used in local tissue infiltration, peripheral, spinal, and epidural blocks. If inadvertently injected intravenously during a nerve block, its high affinity for cardiac Na+ channels and high lipid solubility can result in refractory cardiac arrest. Unlike lidocaine, which enters and leaves the Na+ channel quickly, recovery from bupivacaine blockade during diastole is prolonged.

Levobupivacaine

Levobupivacaine is the preparation of the S-enantiomer of bupivacaine. While similar in the clinical profile and potency to bupivacaine, it has reduced CNS and cardiovascular toxicity, allowing for a larger dose to be given. However, it is currently unavailable in the United States.

Ropivacaine

Ropivacaine was developed as an alternative single enantiomer to racemic bupivacaine because of concerns about bupivacaine's cardiotoxicity. Like levobupivacaine, larger doses of ropivacaine can be administered. Its more favorable interaction at the cardiac Na+ channel and greater vasoconstriction ability contributes to its reduced cardiotoxicity. Ropivacaine may preferentially block C fibers, resulting in less motor blockade. However, the difference between bupivacaine and ropivacaine on cardiotoxicity becomes less clear when equipotent concentrations and dosages are compared.

ESTER LOCAL ANESTHETICS

Procaine

Procaine has low potency and short duration of action with a slow onset due to its high pKa, which limits its use.

Chloroprocaine

High concentrations of chloroprocaine can be used because of its relatively low potency and low toxicity. Plasma cholinesterases rapidly metabolize chloroprocaine, resulting in a very short plasma half-life. Among all local anesthetics, it is believed to have the lowest CNS and cardiovascular toxicity, with almost no maternal transmission to the fetus. These properties make it advantageous in obstetrical epidural analgesia. Despite lower levels of plasma esterases in the neonate, infusion of chloroprocaine has not been shown to cause increase plasma local anesthetic levels and may be used safely in epidurals for infants. Administration of epidural chloroprocaine can interfere with subsequent administration of epidural amide local anesthetics or opioids.

Tetracaine

Tetracaine has an intermediate to long duration of action, which can be further increased if a vasoconstrictor is added. It is mainly used as a spinal anesthetic, but repeated dosing may lead to cauda equina syndrome in animal studies.

Cocaine

Cocaine causes intense vasoconstriction and is used mostly as a topical agent to anesthetize the nasal airway before endotracheal intubation. Because cocaine inhibits the reuptake of catecholamines, it can cause hypertension, tachycardia, dysrhythmias, and other cardiac effects.

Benzocaine

Benzocaine has a slow onset with a short duration of action, and it is used mostly for topical anesthesia to anesthetize the oral and nasal mucous membranes in preparation for fiber-optic intubation. Large doses may cause methemoglobinemia.

MIXED TOPICAL ANESTHETICS

Eutectic mixture of local anesthetics (EMLA) cream is a mixture of lidocaine and prilocaine at a concentration of 2.5%. It is applied to intact skin surfaces under an occlusive dressing to provide dermal analgesia for minimal painful procedures such as intravenous catheter insertion. Neonates have decreased methemoglobin reductase activity, and therefore EMLA should be used with caution.

PROLONGATION OF ACTION

The duration of peripheral or neuraxial nerve blocks may be increased by adding various adjuncts to the local anesthetic. A number of agents including tramadol, neostigmine, and midazolam have been investigated but are generally not in routine clinical use.

EPINEPHRINE

Epinephrine prolongs the duration of blockade by decreasing the systemic absorption of the local anesthetic and allowing more local anesthetic to reach the nerve membrane. It may also bind to alpha 2 receptors directly in the brain and spinal cord. The alpha 2 adrenergic receptors in the spinal cord are known to activate endogenous analgesic mechanisms.[2] Maximum recommended doses should not exceed 0.2 mg, with typical concentrations between 1:200 k to 1:600 k. Epinephrine added to shorter-duration agents such as lidocaine appears to significantly extend their duration, with only modest prolongation when added to bupivacaine.

ALKALINIZATION

Adding sodium bicarbonate to the local anesthetic solution raises the pH and shifts the equilibrium in favor of the neutral base form, which speeds the movement of local anesthetic into the cellular interior. The unconjugated neutral form penetrates into the neural cytoplasm, and the protonated form actually binds to the Na+ channel. The pKa of clinical preparations of local anesthetics ranges from 7.6 to 8.9. Adding sodium bicarbonate to the solution to raise the pKa will increase the amount of neutral form and hasten the penetration of the local anesthetic into the neural tissue, thereby the onset of the block. However, alkalinization has only shown a modest improvement of less than 5 minutes in the onset of the block, and in fact may decrease the duration of action in lidocaine solutions.

ALPHA 2 ADRENERGIC AGONISTS

Clonidine produces analgesia via supraspinal and spinal adrenergic receptors[4] as well as direct inhibitory effects on peripheral nerve conduction of A and C fibers. Clonidine improves the duration of the block by 2 hours in both intermediate- and long-acting agents. In general, studies have shown that clonidine enhances the local anesthetics in intrathecal, epidural, and peripheral nerve applications.[5,6] Dexmedetomidine is being studied, but is currently not FDA approved for clinical use as an additive to local anesthetics.

OPIOIDS

The administration of opioids with local anesthetics in the central neuraxial sites results in synergistic analgesia, except for chloroprocaine. The mechanism of decreased opioid effectiveness with chloroprocaine is unclear, but it does appear to be caused by direct antagonism of opioid receptors. While there exist peripheral opioid receptors, studies have not shown an increase in efficacy of peripheral nerve blockade with the addition of opioids. Lastly, evidence does not support the use of intra-articular injection of local anesthetic with opioids for postoperative analgesia.

STEROIDS

In animal studies, addition of dexamethasone prolongs the conduction block in peripheral nerves. Perineural administration of dexamethasone has increased the duration of brachial plexus blocks with some reported cases of a 50% increase in the duration of analgesia.[7,8]

EXTENDED DURATION FORMULATIONS

Research and trials are ongoing using liposomal encapsulation of local anesthetics, and the duration of action is based on the properties of the liposome. Local anesthetics may also be incorporated into biodegradation polymer microspheres for sustained release.[9] The indications, efficacy, and safety of these formulations are yet to be determined.

SIDE EFFECTS AND TOXICITY OF LOCAL ANESTHETICS

Complications and side effects from local anesthetics have been known since the time Dr. Bier first injected cocaine into the subarachnoid space. In fact, the side-effect profile associated with cocaine prompted a search for agents with less toxic profiles. While local anesthetics remain essential to the practice of anesthesia with a broad range of applications, a deep understanding of their toxic effects must be attained to safely administer these drugs.

Toxicity to local anesthetics results when high concentrations of these agents are observed in the plasma via inadvertent intravenous or intrathecal injection. Patient conditions that increase risk of developing of toxicity include systemic acidosis, hypercapnia, hypercarbia, and decreased protein binding. Toxicity from local anesthetics covers a range of signs and symptoms. Low dose exposures lead to mild disturbances in the nervous system, whereby patients report circumoral numbness, dizziness, and tinnitus. As dose exposure increases, this excitability is replaced by CNS depression with seizure activity and coma. Cardiovascular system signs associated with increased drug exposure include hypotension, prolongation of the PR and QRS complex, and ultimately cardiovascular collapse.

Lipid solubility as a direct measure of potency influences absorption of these agents. Agents that are more lipid soluble are absorbed more slowly, leading to higher potential levels of accumulated drug, precipitating increased risk when these agents are used. Toxicity is proportional to the dose injected, site of injection, and use of a vasoconstrictor. Sites with highest rates of absorption and concentration are: IV >> intercostal >> caudal >> epidural >> brachial plexus >> femoral >> sciatic >> subcutaneous injections.[10,11]

Metabolism of the vast majority of esters occurs via hydrolysis with pseudocholinesterase, with cocaine being the lone exception. Toxicity with ester local anesthetics is inversely related to the hydrolysis by cholinesterase that occurs with these agents. The metabolites are largely inactive, but one worth mentioning is PABA, which is thought to promote an immune response in susceptible individuals.[12] This makes up the vast majority of reported allergy to local anesthetics.[13] Signs associated with this rare complication include dermatitis, bronchospasm, and anaphylaxis. Confirmation can be made via tryptase testing or intradermal testing in patients where the true etiology of such a clinical scenario remains unclear.

Where local anesthetics are deposited also plays a critical role, as there is minimal cholinesterase in the cerebrospinal fluid when compared with the plasma.[14] Parturients and those with pseudocholinesterase deficiency will have a higher likelihood of developing high levels of local anesthetics, resulting in systemic toxicity.[15] Among the esters, chloroprocaine undergoes such rapid hydrolysis that it is an unlikely candidate in causing systemic toxicity. Tetracaine, given its slower metabolism, is a far more likely candidate among ester local anesthetics.

Toxicity from amide local anesthetics occurs at a much higher frequency, given their complex metabolism. These agents undergo biotransformation by hepatic microsomes and then excretion by the kidneys. This is a much slower process when compared with ester hydrolysis, and results in sustained increases in the plasma for this class of local anesthetics.[16]

Some formulations of amides contain methylparaben and metabisulfite, which are used as preservatives in multidose vials. These preservatives are similar to PABA and can cause allergic reactions, although this occurs at a far lower incidence when compared with esters.[17] This rate has been further decreased by introduction of preservative-free local anesthetic solutions. Less than 1% of adverse events associated with local anesthetics are allergic in nature.[18]

The majority of the signs and symptoms attributable to local anesthetic allergy are more likely manifestations of toxicity from high plasma levels of local anesthetics.

The following section emphasizes potential pitfalls with local anesthetic use in everyday practice. Signs of toxicity, additives, and methemoglobinemia are also discussed. The two classes of local anesthetics, given their molecular structure and metabolism, lends to the potential reactions seen. Toxicity associated with local anesthetics can be broken down into three broad categories: myotoxicity, neurotoxicity, and cardiac toxicity.

MYOTOXICITY

Local anesthetic injection into muscle can result in histopathologic changes signifying injury in skeletal muscle. Presenting complaints from patients include muscle pain and muscle dysfunction. Potency of agents seems to correlate with the amount of injury seen. The mechanism of injury seems related to mitochondrial dysfunction and calcium homeostasis.[19] This effect however is reversible, with muscle regeneration occurring within 2 weeks of injury.[20,21]

NEUROTOXICITY

Central nervous system toxicity results from local anesthetics crossing the blood-brain barrier. Not surprisingly, toxicity correlates with the potency of local anesthetics in that agents that are highly lipid soluble can predispose to CNS symptoms in dose ranges that are small compared with less lipid-soluble agents. Central nervous system symptoms are initially excitatory at low doses, with sedation and coma noted at higher doses. At low doses, sensory signs include tinnitus, facial tingling, restlessness, circumoral numbness, and vertigo, with progression to seizures, CNS depression, coma, and cardiac arrest as dose accumulation occurs. Associated hypoxia and metabolic acidosis potentiates possible CNS injury. An important point to mention is that use of neuromuscular drugs does nothing to underlying seizure activity. A benzodiazepine should be administered to stop seizure activity in patients with signs of local anesthetic toxicity. A further breakdown of the signs and symptoms associated with local anesthetic toxicity is noted in Figure 14.2.

Direct neurotoxicity of local anesthetics can result from injection of local anesthetics near the nerve fascicle, which results in histopathologic changes consistent with neuronal injury. The degree of injury seems related to intraneural placement, concentration, and length of exposure to the local anesthetic, although the exact mechanism of injury remains unclear.[22,23] This phenomenon is quite rare, with an incidence of radiculopathy and paraplegia at 0.03% and 0.0008% respectively.[24] While direct neurotoxicity is rare, two conditions associated with local anesthetic deposition neuraxially should be discussed.

Transient neurologic symptoms (TNS) are a transient hyperalgesia noted along the back and lower extremities following an uneventful spinal anesthetic. Incidence has been reported to be as high as 40% of cases. The injury pattern is largely short-lived, with a majority of patients reporting complete resolution by the second postoperative day. The agent most implicated with this condition is lidocaine. Lithotomy positioning, as well as obesity and early ambulation are thought to play a role in development of TNS. Another risk factor is ambulatory surgery. The dose of local anesthetic and baricity are not considered risk factors in the development of TNS.[25] Treatment is largely supportive, with administration of nonsteroidals and trigger point injections.

Cauda equina syndrome is a persistent paralysis in the lower extremities with associated sensory loss in the perineum and varying levels of urinary and fecal incontinence. The mechanism of this injury is thought to be associated with injury to the sacral nerve roots from trauma, ischemia, infection, or neurotoxicity.[26]

This prolonged neural toxicity was initially reported following spinal anesthesia in the 1990s with the use of

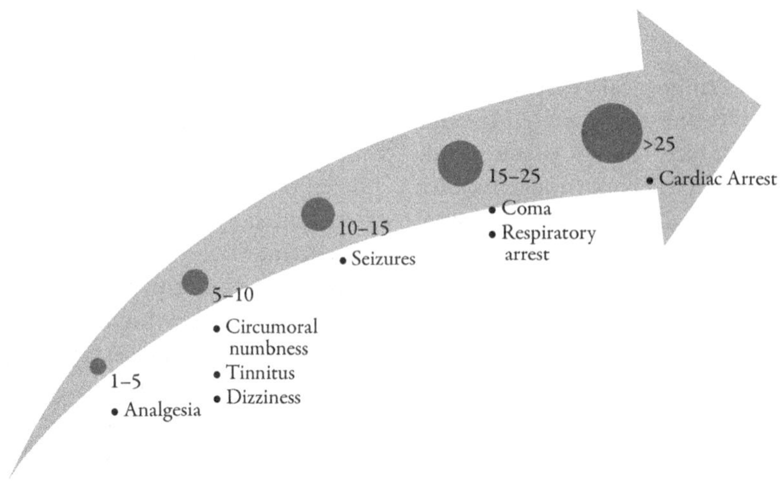

Figure 14.2 Lidocaine plasma concentrations (mcg/mL) with associated presentations.

microcatheters, which allowed for the accumulation of high concentrations of hyperbaric lidocaine or chloroprocaine near nerve roots.[27,28] Another reported instance postulated an injury pattern resulted from direct neurotoxic effects of an intrathecal dose of lidocaine that was to be used for epidural administration.[29]

CARDIAC: DIRECT AND INDIRECT EFFECTS

Cardiac toxicity of local anesthetics is the most dreaded complication associated with overdose, given the poor recovery profile of patients receiving bupivacaine infusions. The more potent agents such as bupivacaine, ropivacaine, and levobupivacaine predispose patients to develop cardiac collapse and complete heart block.

The mechanism of injury is not completely understood, but in this section we discuss the physiologic changes noted. Toxicity from local anesthetics results in disruption in the baroreflex, leading to an inability of the heart to respond to changes in blood pressure.[30] This is further exacerbated by direct local anesthetic action on the smooth muscle surrounding blood vessels. At low doses, one sees vasoconstriction, while vasodilation occurs with higher doses. In the pulmonary vasculature, hypertension occurs with increasing local anesthetic concentrations.[31]

Electrical conductance and contractility are adversely impacted with increasing concentrations of local anesthetics. The primary ion channel affected in myocytes is a heart-specific voltage-gated sodium channel, but other cations such as calcium and potassium are also antagonized with toxicity.[32] Clinically, one sees hypotension and prolongation of the PR and QRS complex. Specific mention should be given to bupivacaine regarding cardiac toxicity, as it binds avidly to sodium channels when compared with other local anesthetics. The term "fast in slow out" is used to describe the slow dissociation that occurs during diastole for this agent. The end result is propagation or perpetuation of the conduction defect seen in patients exposed to toxic doses of bupivacaine.[32,33]

Treatment is supportive, with the understanding that prolonged resuscitation may be needed in those with bupivacaine cardiotoxicity. A distress call should be sent out to obtain available help and a critical events checklist should be used to facilitate the treatment algorithm. The airway should be secured and seizure suppression via benzodiazepines should be initiated. Hemodynamic support with epinephrine should be used to treat hypotension. Intralipid administration has been shown to improve resuscitation in cases of refractory local anesthetic toxicity. The proposed mechanism for its benefit lies in its ability to reverse local anesthetic-induced inhibition of fatty acid metabolism and its ability to serve as a lipid sink in sequestering local anesthetics.[34,35] Dose should start at 1.5 mg/kg over 1 minute followed by an infusion at 0.25 mL/kg/min. The maximum dose of intralipid should not exceed 10 mL/kg over the first 30 minutes. Propofol should not be used as an alternative to intralipid, as the intralipid dose needed would further compound the hypotension seen. Box 14.1 covers the algorithm discussed.

Methemoglobinemia

Methemoglobinemia (MetHb) occurs when an oxidizing reaction within erythrocytes converts iron in hemoglobin from a ferrous state to a ferric one. This life-threatening condition results from the inability of the oxidized version of hemoglobin to bind and unload oxygen and carbon dioxide, leading to shortness of breath, cyanosis, and mental status changes.[36] A leftward shift in the oxyhemoglobin disassociation curve is also noted. Methemoglobin is usually maintained at less than 1% of total Hb.[37]

The most common etiology in the development of methemoglobinemia is medication administration. The list is extensive, so emphasis here is placed on common local anesthetics known to cause methemoglobinemia. This

Box 14.1 THE ABCS OF LOCAL ANESTHETIC TOXICITY (LAST)

Assistance (Call for help)

AIRWAY

- 100% oxygen
- Intubate if needed

BRAIN

- Benzodiazepines for seizure suppression

CARDIAC

- Epinephrine <1 mcg/kg
- ACLS/PALS
- AVOID vasopressin
  - Beta blockers
  - Calcium channel blockers
  - Local anesthetics

SAVE

- Lipid Emulsion Therapy (20%)
  - Bolus 1.5 mL/kg IV over 1 minute
  - Repeat bolus *2 for persistent cardiac instability
  - Continuous infusion 0.25 mL/kg/min
  - Max 10 mg/kg over 30 min for initial dosing

includes prilocaine, benzocaine, and lidocaine.[38] Neonates and those less than 3 months of age are at particular risk for developing methemoglobinemia, given lower amounts of NADH-cytochrome b5 reductase in this patient population. This enzyme is responsible for reducing methemoglobin into hemoglobin. Another contributing factor in neonates is fetal hemoglobin's propensity to be more easily oxidized than adult hemoglobin.

Signs and symptoms of methemoglobinemia are dependent on the level of methemoglobin present systemically (Table 14.2). Signs and symptoms include mental status changes, shortness of breath, and cyanosis, with a characteristic chocolate appearance on blood sampling. The sine qua non for this condition is a lack of improvement in cyanosis with 100% oxygen administration.[39] Patients often present with dysrhythmias, seizures, coma, and death when methemoglobin exceeds 50%.

Arterial sampling of blood usually reveals a characteristic chocolate brown color. Diagnosis is made using multiwave co-oximetry. Standard pulse oximetry lacks the specificity to delineate methemoglobin and carboxyhemoglobin. As methemoglobin absorbs light equally between the two wavelengths on a pulse oximeter, the oxygen saturation is a constant 85% even as the concentration of methemoglobin rises.

Treatment should be initiated if the patient exhibits signs of methemoglobinemia or if the methemoglobin concentration is greater than 30%. Methylene blue 1–2 mg/kg over 5 minutes with a max dose of 7 mL/kg will serve as a cofactor in reducing methemoglobin to hemoglobin. Doses beyond this can result in toxicity, which can worsen hemolysis and methemoglobinemia. Methylene blue should be avoided in those with glucose 6-phosphate dehydrogenase deficiency, as methylene blue would cause further oxidation. Exchange transfusions should be considered in those with glucose 6-phosphate dehydrogenase deficiency or refractory methemoglobinemia.[40]

Table 14.3 contains a brief list of additives that are commonly combined with local anesthetics.

Table 14.2 METHEMOGLOBINEMIA SERUM LEVELS AND ASSOCIATED SYMPTOMS

METHEMOGLOBIN %	SYMPTOMS
<10%	None
10–20%	Cyanosis
20–30%	Headache, tachycardia, dizziness
30–50%	Fatigue, respiratory distress, tachycardia
50–70%	Acidosis, seizures, coma, dysrhythmias
>70%	Death

Table 14.3 ADDITIVES TO LOCAL ANESTHETICS AND THEIR ASSOCIATED MECHANISM OF ACTION

ADDITIVES	MECHANISM OF ACTION
Epinephrine	Local vasoconstriction Alpha 2 adrenergic agonism
Clonidine Dexmedetomidine	Alpha 2 adrenergic agonism
Opioids	Opioid receptor agonism
Ketamine	NMDA receptor antagonism
Dexamethasone	Unknown
Sodium bicarbonate	Alkalinization

Epinephrine is added to local anesthetics to facilitate detection of intravascular injection in the epidural space and prolongation of peripheral nerve blockade. In the epidural space, activation of alpha-adrenergic receptors enhances analgesia seen when these agents are used. The prolongation noted with peripheral blockade is primarily mediated via local vasoconstriction, which then results in decreased vascular reuptake via epinephrine's alpha 1 receptor agonism effect.[41,42] This effect occurs more frequently in short- and intermediate-acting agents and is not noted to be of significance in long-acting local anesthetics (ropivacaine, bupivacaine, levobupivaine).

Clonidine and alpha-adrenergic-receptor-specific agonists such as dexmedetomidine mediate analgesic effects at supraspinal and spinal adrenergic receptors. Clonidine prolongs block duration while decreasing local anesthetic requirements.[43] Systematic reviews have consistently shown an analgesic benefit when clonidine is added to local anesthetics.[44] Dexmedetomidine has alpha-2-receptor specificity on a scale of 1600:1 and has increased duration of analgesia and improved onset with significantly lower pain scores for the first 24 hours.[45]

Sodium bicarbonate potentiates local anesthetic action via two pathways: (1) It increases the extracellular pH, resulting in alkalinization with an increase in the amount of unionized local anesthetic available, resulting in shorter block onset. (2) It causes local anesthetics to go from an unionized to ionized form intracellularly.[46]

Opioids can be used in the epidural and subarachnoid space given the presence of mu receptors along the lamina of the cortex and the substantia gelatinosa in the spinal cord.[47] Lipophilicity and molecular weight are thought to play roles in onset of analgesia and duration of analgesia. Lipophilicity also accounts for the ability of opioids to migrate in the epidural space. Agents such as fentanyl and sufentanil owe their rapid onset of action to their high lipophilicity, which facilitates rapid systemic absorption. Hydrophilic agents are not as well absorbed, and this leads to agents such as morphine having prolonged duration, cephalad migration, and slower onset when given neuraxially. Side effects for opioids are dose dependent. The four most common side effects seen include pruritis, urinary retention, ventilator depression, and nausea/vomiting. Of note, one must pay particular attention to the bimodal respiratory depression associated with epidural administration of morphine.[48] Although opioid receptors are present in the peripheral axons of sensory afferents, there seems to be no clinical benefit of adding opioids to local anesthetics for peripheral nerve blocks.[49]

SUMMARY

General practice guidelines for the safe administration of local anesthetics include avoidance of local anesthetics containing preservatives and avoiding the use of lidocaine in spinal anesthesia. There remains no local anesthetic whose toxicity profile relegates its use as the preferred agent in the field of anesthesia. Intralipid and resuscitation equipment should be readily available in any area where local anesthetic administration occurs. Vigilance through administration and proper patient selection remain keys in preventing or mitigating potential toxicity.

REFERENCES

1. Barash P. *Clinical Anesthesia*. 6th ed. Philadelphia, PA: Lippincott Williams & Wilkins; 2013:561–579.
2. Miller R, ed. *Miller's Anesthesia*. 7th ed. Philadelphia, PA: Churchill Livingston Elsevier; 2010:913–939.
3. Giddon D, Lindhe J. In vivo quantitation of local anesthetic suppression of leukocyte adherence. *Am J Pathol.* 1972;68:327–338.
4. Eisenach J, De Kock M, Klimscha W. Alpha 2 adrenergic agonists for regional anesthesia: a clinical review of clonidine (1984–1995). *Anesthesiology*. 1996;85:655.
5. Popping D. Clonidine as an adjuvant to local anesthetics for peripheral nerve and plexus blocks. *Anesthesiology*. 2009;111:406.
6. Colin J. Should we add clonidine to local anesthetic for peripheral nerve blockade? A qualitative systematic review of the literature. *Region Anesth Pain M*. 207;32:330.
7. Parrington S. Dexamethasone added to mepivacaine prolongs the duration of analgesia after supraclavicular brachial plexus blockade. *Reg Anesth Pain Med*. 2010;35:422.
8. Cummings K. Effect of dexamethasone on the duration of interscalene nerve blocks with ropivacaine or bupivacaine. *Br J Anesthesia*. 2011;107:446.
9. Curley J. Injectable biodegradable bupivacaine/polyester microspheres. *Anesthesiology*. 2006;104:110–121.
10. Evers A. *Anesthetic Pharmacology, Physiologic Principles, and Clinical Practice*. Philadelphia, PA: Churchill Livingstone Elsevier; 2004:507–535.
11. Wildsmith J, Tucker T, Cooper S, Scott D, Covino B. Plasma concentrations of local anaesthetics after interscalene brachial plexus block. *Br J Anaesth*. 1977;49(5):461–466.
12. Eggleston S, Lush L. Understanding allergic reactions to local anesthetics. *Ann Pharmacother*. 1996;30(7–8):851–857.
13. Sidhu S, Shaw S, Wilkinson J. A 10-year retrospective study on benzocaine allergy in the United Kingdom. *Am J Contact Dermat*. 1999;10(2):57–61.
14. Kambam J, Horton B, Parris W, Hyman S, Berman M, Sastry B. Pseudocholinesterase activity in human cerebrospinal fluid. *Anesth Analg*. 1989;68(4):486–488.
15. Oropollo A. Abnormal pseudocholinesterase levels in surgical population. *Anesthesiology*. 1978;48(4):284–286.
16. Miller R, Pardo M, Stoelting R. *Basics of Anesthesia*. 6th ed. Philadelphia, PA: Elsevier/Saunders; 2011:xii, 817.
17. Larson CE. Methylparaben: an overlooked cause of local anesthetic hypersensitivity. *Anesth Prog*. 1977;24(3):72–74.
18. Stoelting R, Miller R. *Basics of Anesthesia*. 5th ed. Philadelphia, PA: Churchill Livingstone; 2007:xii, 697.
19. Nouette-Gaulain K, Sirvent P, Canal-Raffin M, et al. Effects of intermittent femoral nerve injections of bupivacaine, levobupivacaine, and ropivacaine on mitochondrial energy metabolism and intracellular calcium homeostasis in rat psoas muscle. *Anesthesiology*. 2007;106(5):1026–1034.
20. Benoit P, Belt W. Destruction and regeneration of skeletal muscle after treatment with a local anaesthetic, bupivacaine (Marcaine). *J Anat*. 1970;107(Pt 3):547–556.
21. Benoit P. Reversible skeletal muscle damage after administration of local anesthetics with and without epinephrine. *J Oral Surg*. 1978;36(3):198–201.
22. Miller R, ed. *Miller's Anesthesia*. 7th ed. Philadelphia, PA: Elsevier; 2010.
23. Barash P, Cullen B, Stoelting R, Cahalan M, Stock M. *Clinical Anesthesia*. 7th ed. Philadelphia, PA: Lippincott Williams & Wilkins, 2013:xviii, 1640.
24. Brull R, McCartney C, Chan V, El-Beheiry H. Neurological complications after regional anesthesia: contemporary estimates of risk. *Anesth Analg*. 2007;104(4):965–974.
25. Zaric D, Pace N. Transient neurologic symptoms (TNS) following spinal anaesthesia with lidocaine versus other local anaesthetics. *Cochrane Database Syst Rev*. 2009;2:CD003006.
26. Kane R. Neurologic deficits following epidural or spinal anesthesia. *Anesth Analg*. 1981;60(3):150–161.
27. Rigler M, Drasner K, Krejcie T. Cauda equina syndrome after continuous spinal anesthesia. *Anesth Analg*. 1991;72(3):275–281.
28. Lambert D, Hurley R. Cauda equina syndrome and continuous spinal anesthesia. *Anesth Analg*. 1991;72(6):817–819.
29. Drasner K, Rigler M, Sessler D, Stoller M. Cauda equina syndrome following intended epidural anesthesia. *Anesthesiology*. 1992;77(3):582–585.
30. Pickering A, Waki H, Headley P, Paton J. Investigation of systemic bupivacaine toxicity using the in situ perfused working heart-brainstem preparation of the rat. *Anesthesiology*. 2002;97(6):1550–1556.
31. Liu P, Feldman H, Covino B, Giasi R, Covino B. Acute cardiovascular toxicity of intravenous amide local anesthetics in anesthetized ventilated dogs. *Anesth Analg*. 1982;61(4):317–322.
32. Guo X, Castle N, Chernoff D, Strichartz G. Comparative inhibition of voltage-gated cation channels by local anesthetics. *Ann N Y Acad Sci*. 1991;625:181–199.
33. Clarkson C, Hondeghem L. Mechanism for bupivacaine depression of cardiac conduction: fast block of sodium channels during the action potential with slow recovery from block during diastole. *Anesthesiology*. 1985;62(4):396–405.
34. Weinberg G, VadeBoncouer T, Ramaraju G, Garcia-Amaro M, Cwik M. Pretreatment or resuscitation with a lipid infusion shifts the dose-response to bupivacaine-induced asystole in rats. *Anesthesiology*. 1998;88(4):1071–1075.
35. Weinberg G, Ripper R, Murphy P. Lipid infusion accelerates removal of bupivacaine and recovery from bupivacaine toxicity in the isolated rat heart. *Reg Anesth Pain Med*. 2006;31(4):296–303.

36. Cortazzo J, Lichtman A. Methemoglobinemia: a review and recommendations for management. *J Cardiothorac Vasc Anesth.* 2013.
37. Anderson S, Hajduczek J, Barker S. Benzocaine-induced methemoglobinemia in an adult: accuracy of pulse oximetry with methemoglobinemia. *Anesth Analg.* 1988;67(11):1099–1101.
38. Nguyen S, Cabrales R, Bashour C. Benzocaine-induced methemoglobinemia. *Anesth Analg.* 2000;90(2):369–371.
39. Curry S. Methemoglobinemia. *Ann Emerg Med.* 1982;11(4):214–221.
40. Coleman M, Coleman N. Drug-induced methaemoglobinaemia: treatment issues. *Drug Saf.* 1996;14(6):394–405.
41. Kroin JS, et al. Clonidine prolongation of lidocaine analgesia after sciatic nerve block in rats is mediated via the hyperpolarization-activated cation current, not by alpha-adrenoreceptors. *Anesthesiology.* 2004;101(2):488–494.
42. Sinnott C, Strichartz G. Levobupivacaine versus ropivacaine for sciatic nerve block in the rat. *Reg Anesth Pain Med.* 2003;28(4):294–303.
43. Gabriel J, Gordin V. Alpha 2 agonists in regional anesthesia and analgesia. *Curr Opin Anaesthesiol.* 2001;14(6):751–753.
44. Brummett C, Williams B. Additives to local anesthetics for peripheral nerve blockade. *Int Anesthesiol Clin.* 2011;49(4):104–116.
45. Brummett C, Norat M, Palmisano J, Lydic R. Perineural administration of dexmedetomidine in combination with bupivacaine enhances sensory and motor blockade in sciatic nerve block without inducing neurotoxicity in rat. *Anesthesiology.* 2008;109(3):502–511.
46. Ibusuki S, Katsuki H, Takasaki M. The effects of extracellular pH with and without bicarbonate on intracellular procaine concentrations and anesthetic effects in crayfish giant axons. *Anesthesiology.* 1998;88(6):1549–1557.
47. Cousins M, Mather L. Intrathecal and epidural administration of opioids. *Anesthesiology.* 1984;61(3):276–310.
48. Karaman S, Kocabas S, Uyar M, Hayzaran S, Firat V. The effects of sufentanil or morphine added to hyperbaric bupivacaine in spinal anaesthesia for caesarean section. *Eur J Anaesthesiol.* 2006;23(4):285–291.
49. Murphy D, McCartney C, Chan V. Novel analgesic adjuncts for brachial plexus block: a systematic review. *Anesth Analg.* 2000;90(5):1122–1128.
50. Neal J, Mulroy M, Weinberg G. American Society of Regional Anesthesia and Pain Medicine checklist for managing local anesthetic systemic toxicity: 2012 version. *Reg Anesth Pain Med.* 2012;37(1):16–18.

SUGGESTED READING

Miller R, Pardo M. *Basics of Anesthesia.* 6th ed. Philadelphia, PA: Elsevier; 2011.

QUESTIONS

1. Which of the following injection sites would result in the higher systemic plasma concentration after injection of a local anesthetic with the same concentration and dose?
    A. Intercostal
    B. Epidural
    C. Brachial plexus
    D. Sciatic nerve
    E. Subcutaneous

2. The addition of epinephrine to which of the following local anesthetics results in the least effect in the duration of action?
    A. Lidocaine
    B. Mepivacaine
    C. Bupivacaine
    D. Procaine
    E. Chloroprocaine

3. An emergency cesarean section is posted for a 25-year-old G1P0 at 39 weeks with fetal distress who has a functional laboring epidural. Which of the following properties accounts for the more rapid onset of epidural block with 3% 2-chloroprocaine versus 2% lidocaine?
    A. Ester versus amide local anesthetic
    B. pKa
    C. Protein binding
    D. Concentration
    E. Lipid solubility

4. Which agent is least indicated in the treatment of local anesthetic toxicity?
    A. Epinephrine
    B. Amiodarone
    C. Esmolol
    D. Midazolam
    E. Propofol

5. All of the following are conditions that predispose patients to local anesthetic toxicity EXCEPT:
    A. Acidosis
    B. Increased protein binding
    C. Hypercapnia
    D. Decreased clearance of local anesthetics
    E. Hypercarbia

6. You are scheduled to anesthetize a 90-kg male for cholecystectomy whose past history is significant for G6PD deficiency. Micrognathia leads you to pursue an awake fiber-optic intubation. Versed is administered, and Hurricane spray © is used to topicalize the airway. Multiple attempts are needed to intubate this patient, with cyanosis noted on securing the breathing tube. Breath sounds are bilateral and equal on exam, but oxygen saturations remain at 85% on 100% oxygen with ventilation. What is the most appropriate initial step in managing this patient?
    A. Pull back ETT tube
    B. Methylene blue infusion
    C. Ascorbic acid
    D. Dextrose administration
    E. Exchange transfusion

7. All of the following are considered risk factors in the development of transient neurologic symptoms EXCEPT:
    A. Lidocaine use
    B. Obesity
    C. Early ambulation
    D. Hyperbaric of local anesthetic
    E. Lithotomy

ANSWERS

1. A. The plasma concentration of local anesthetic is directly proportional to the dose injection, regardless of the speed of injection or the concentration. Injection of local anesthetic in more vascular tissue results in greater systemic absorption. The order of increasing rate of absorption by injection site is subcutaneous < sciatic < femoral < brachial plexus < epidural < caudal < intercostal < intravenous.
2. C. Epinephrine is frequently added to local anesthetic solutions to produce vasoconstriction, which decreases the systemic absorption of the local anesthetic, thereby prolonging the duration of action. The extent to which epinephrine prolongs the duration depends on the specific local anesthetic. Epinephrine appears to extend the blockade of shorter-duration local anesthetics such as lidocaine, with only modest effects with bupivacaine.[2]
3. D. While local anesthetics cross the lipid membrane much faster in their neutral lipophilic form than their cationic form, and alkalinization of the local anesthetic shifts the equilibrium in favor of the neutral base, which increases onset, the most important determinant of onset of blockade is the local anesthetic dose or concentration. Protein binding affects the duration of action. Despite a pKa of 8.9, 3% 2-chloroprocaine demonstrates a more rapid onset of action due to its higher concentration and a greater diffusion gradient. In humans, 1.5% lidocaine produces a more rapid onset of epidural anesthesia than 1.5% chloroprocaine, however, 3% chloroprocaine results in more rapid onset than 2% lidocaine.[2]
4. C. Calcium channel blockers and beta blockers worsen myocardial function and should be avoided in local anesthetic toxicity. Propofol should not be used, as it is emulsified in 10% lipid solution and the subsequent volume needed to deliver enough lipid would result in significant cardiovascular compromise. However, it would stand to reason that propofol may be useful in small doses for seizure suppression if benzodiazepines are unavailable. Benzodiazepines remain the preferred agent in abolishing seizures. Epinephrine/amiodarone are first-line agents for arrhythmias encountered and have a role in those with local anesthetic toxicity.50
5. B. All the conditions listed except for choice B result in more unbound local anesthetics in plasma, allowing for a lower threshold for central nervous system toxicity.
6. C. This is a case of methemoglobinemia complicated by a patient history of glucose 6 phosphate dehydrogenase deficiency. This enzyme is responsible for generating NADPH, which is the substrate used to reduce methemoglobinemia to hemoglobin. Methylene blue administration is the primary treatment for methemoglobinemia. In those with G6PD deficiency, methylene blue can cause further hemolysis in this subgroup. Pulling the tube back is not warranted given the physical exam findings. Dextrose should be administered to those with methemoglobinemia, as it is necessary to form NADPH. Ascorbic acid, riboflavin, and cimetidine have been used with varying success and are considered second-line agents in treatment of methemoglobinemia. Exchange transfusion can be used in patients with severe methemoglobinemia or in those where methylene blue therapy has failed. No pharmacologic therapy exists for hereditary methemoglobinemia.
7. D. Baricity and dose of local anesthetic have no association with the development of transient neurologic symptoms.

15.

MUSCLE RELAXANTS

Mark Harbott and Kaylani Govindan

INTRODUCTION

Neuromuscular blocking agents are used during general anesthesia for providing muscle relaxation to facilitate tracheal intubation and immobility during surgery. The two major classes of muscle relaxants are depolarizing and nondepolarizing agents.

The cell membrane of the neuron and muscle fiber at the neuromuscular junction are separated by a narrow gap called the synaptic cleft. Acetylcholine (Ach) molecules are stored in tiny vesicles at the terminal neuron, and these vesicles fuse with the terminal membrane to release Ach into the synaptic cleft during an action potential. These Ach molecules diffuse across the synaptic cleft to bind to the nicotinic cholinergic receptors on the motor end plate. Activation of these receptors is required for muscle contraction. The Ach receptor consists of five glycoprotein subunits, two identical alpha and single beta, delta, and epsilon subunits. The Ach molecules bind only to the two alpha subunits, and this causes the miniature end plate potential whereby cations (sodium and calcium in, potassium out) flow through the open Ach receptor channel. The action potential propagates along the muscle membrane and T-tubule, releasing calcium from the sarcoplasmic reticulum, which allows the contractile proteins actin and myosin to interact to cause muscle contraction. The Ach is rapidly hydrolyzed by the enzyme acetylcholinesterase into acetate and choline. The sodium channels in the muscle membrane close when the generation of action potential ceases, causing muscle relaxation.[1]

MECHANISM OF ACTION

The neuromuscular blockers are structural analogs of Ach, and they act as either agonists (depolarizing) or antagonists (nondepolarizing) at the receptors on the end plate of the neuromuscular junction.[2]

MECHANISM OF ACTION OF DEPOLARIZING AGENTS

Succinylcholine is the only depolarizing agent in use in the United States. Structurally it consists of two Ach molecules. It readily binds to the two alpha subunits of the Ach receptor, generating a muscle action potential, but unlike Ach, it is not metabolized by acetylcholinesterase and it persists at high concentration, providing a continuous stimulation of the receptor. This depolarization causes opening of the sodium channel, resulting in depolarization of the receptor (Phase I block). Continued binding of the agent renders the receptor incapable of transmitting further impulses. Prolonged end plate depolarization causes ionic changes in the receptor resembling that of nondepolarizing agents. This results in a Phase II block.[2]

Immediately after injection of succinylcholine, fasciculations are observed due to agonist effect of succinylcholine. This is followed by paralysis due to the desensitization of the motor end plate.

MECHANISM OF ACTION OF NONDEPOLARIZING AGENTS

Nondepolarizing agents are competitive antagonists at the nicotinic Ach receptors. They bind to the Ach receptor, but are unable to induce ion channel opening. An end plate potential does not develop, as Ach is blocked from binding to the receptors. Neuromuscular blockade is produced with the blockade of only one alpha subunit.

Chemically these are benzylisoquinolones or steroidal compounds. Their action can be overcome by increasing the concentration of Ach in the synaptic cleft. This blockade can be antagonized with anticholinesterase agents like neostigmine.

PHARMACOKINETICS AND PHARMACODYNAMICS

PHARMACOKINETICS AND PHARMACODYNAMICS OF SUCCINYLCHOLINE

The dose of succinylcholine required for tracheal intubation in adults is 1–1.5 mg/kg, and this dose produces profound block within 60 seconds. Smaller doses (0.5 mg/kg) may also produce adequate intubating conditions.

Succinylcholine has a rapid onset of action and an extremely short duration of action (<10 min). The rapid onset of action is due to its low lipid solubility. As it enters the circulation, most of it is metabolized by pseudocholinesterase, and only a fraction of the injected dose reaches the neuromuscular junction. As the serum levels fall, the drug diffuses away from the neuromuscular junction, limiting the duration of action.

Abnormal Responses to Succinylcholine

The duration of action is prolonged by high dosage or abnormal metabolism. Hypothermia decreases the rate of hydrolysis, and low levels of pseudocholinesterases are seen in pregnancy, liver disease, renal failure, and certain drug therapies. Low levels produce only modest prolongation of action, and this usually goes unnoticed clinically.

Rarely, there are patients who are unable to effectively metabolize succinylcholine (or mivacurium) secondary to a congenital abnormality in butyrylcholinesterase (pseudocholinesterase). Normal butyrylcholinesterase is inhibited by the compound dibucaine. Abnormal butyrylcholinesterase is not inhibited to the same degree. The genes that code for production of the abnormal butyrylcholinesterase may be homozygous or heterozygous. Dibucaine inhibits normal butyrylcholinesterase 80%, atypical heterozygous butyrylcholinesterase shows 50%–60% inhibition, and atypical homozygous butyrylcholinesterase shows 20%–30% inhibition. The *dibucaine number* is proportional to pseudocholinesterase function and independent of the amount of enzyme. The dibucaine number provides a qualitative estimate the adequacy of pseudocholinesterase.

The duration of action of succinylcholine will be prolonged by as much as 4–8 hours in patients who have a homozygous deficiency, whereas those who are heterozygous for the deficiency will see a more modest prolongation of the order of 50%–100% (see Table 15.1).[3] Prolonged paralysis from atypical pseudocholinesterase should be treated with mechanical ventilation until recovery of muscle function.

PHARMACOKINETICS AND PHARMACODYNAMICS OF NONDEPOLARIZING AGENTS

All neuromuscular blocking agents are injected intravenously as their uptake via oral absorption is minimal, which is due to the presence of quaternary amines in their bulky ring structure. They penetrate membranes poorly and do not enter cells or cross the blood-brain barrier. The nondepolarizing agents are categorized into short-, intermediate-, and long-acting drugs, based on their elimination half-lives (Table 15.2). The volume of distribution of these agents is equal to the extracellular fluid (ECF) volume.

Onset time is determined by the time required to reach a critical level at the site of action, which corresponds to 100% blockade and reflects the time required for drug transfer from the plasma to the neuromuscular junction. The factors that modify the access of the drug to and from the neuromuscular junction are cardiac output, distance of the muscle from the heart, and muscle blood flow. The blockade usually occurs sooner at well-perfused central muscles like vocal cords and diaphragm than at the peripheral muscles of the hand and foot.

The onset of nondepolarizers can be quickened by using a larger dose, which may prolong the duration of blockade, or by using a priming dose. Giving 10%–15% of the intubating dose a few minutes prior to induction will occupy enough receptors so that paralysis will occur quickly when the rest of the dose is given. Precurarization involves giving a small dose of nondepolarizer prior to administering succinylcholine to prevent fasciculations.

Potent drugs have a slower onset because a large proportion of the receptors must be occupied. If more drug molecules are available (low potency) blockade of the receptors will be faster, resulting in rapid onset. Duration of action is determined by the time required for the drug concentration to fall below a certain level. Drugs with rapidly decreasing plasma concentrations have a shorter duration of action, while slowly eliminated drugs have a long duration of action.[1]

Table 15.1 DURATION OF ACTION OF SUCCINYLCHOLINE

TYPE OF BUTYRYLCHOLINESTERASE	INCIDENCE	DIBUCAINE NUMBER	RECOVERY FROM SUCCINYLCHOLINE OR MIVACURIUM
Homozygous typical	Normal	70–80	Normal
Heterozygous atypical	1/480	50–60	Increased by 50%–100%
Homozygous atypical	1/3200	20–30	Prolonged to 4-8 hours

Table 15.2 CLASSIFICATION OF NONDEPOLARIZING AGENTS

SHORT DURATION AGENTS	ELIMINATION HALF-LIFE (MINUTES)
Mivacurium	20
Intermediate-duration agents	
Atracurium	20
Cisatracurium	23
Rocuronium	90
Vecuronium	70
Long-duration drugs	
Doxacurium	95
D-tubocurarine	90
Pancuronium	140

INDIVIDUAL AGENTS

Mivacurium

Structure

Benzylisoquinolone derivative. It is a mixture of 3 isomers cis-trans, trans-trans and the cis-cis isomer, out of which the first two are pharmacologically active.

Metabolism and Excretion

Mivacurium, like succinylcholine, is metabolized by pseudocholinesterase, thereby prolonging the action in patients with pseudocholinesterase deficiency. In contrast to succinylcholine, mivacurium blockade can be reversed with anticholinesterases. The duration of action can be prolonged in pregnancy and in patients with renal or hepatic failure because of decreased plasma cholinesterase levels.

Atracurium

Structure

Atracurium is a bisquartenary ammonium benzylisoquinolone.

Dose

Intermediate-duration drug with an onset of action of 2-3 minutes and an elimination half-life of 20 minutes. The duration of action does not depend on age, kidney function, or hepatic function. Onset can be shortened and duration prolonged by increasing the dose, but it is not recommended to exceed 0.5 mg/kg because of histamine release and possible hypotension. The duration of action can be prolonged by hypothermia and acidosis.

Metabolism and Excretion

Atracurium is degraded via two pathways: Ester hydrolysis catalyzed by nonspecific esterases and a spontaneous nonenzymatic, pH-dependent degradation called Hofmann elimination. The nonspecific esterases are also involved in the elimination of esmolol and remifentanil. The end products of degradation are laudanosine and acetate fragments. Laudanosine has been known to induce seizures at extremely high doses, and is metabolized by the liver and excreted by the kidneys.

Cisatracurium

Structure

Cisatracurium is a stereoisomer of atracurium that is four times more potent.

Dose

The onset time is longer (3–5 min) due to the potency of drug, and the elimination half-life is 22–25 min. At a dose of 0.1–0.15 mg/kg, onset is faster (2 min) and the duration of action is prolonged to 45–60 minutes.

Metabolism and Excretion

Cisatracurium undergoes degradation by organ-independent Hoffman elimination (compare with atracurium). The metabolites have no residual neuromuscular blocking effects. Metabolism and elimination are not affected by kidney or liver failure.

Rocuronium

Structure

It is a monoquartenary steroid that is structurally similar to vecuronium.

Dose

It has a rapid onset of action and an intermediate duration of action (30–40 min). A dose of 1mg/kg produces intubating conditions similar to that of succinylcholine, making it suitable for rapid sequence induction, but the duration is prolonged to 60 minutes.

Metabolism and Excretion

Rocuronium undergoes no metabolism and is eliminated primarily by the liver and minimally by the kidneys and has no active metabolites. Its duration of action is prolonged in severe hepatic failure but is not significantly affected by renal disease.

Vecuronium

Structure

It is a monoquartenary aminosteroid produced by demethylation of the pancuronium molecule. The absence of a methyl group beneficially alters the side effects (cardiovascular stability) without affecting the potency.

Dose

An intubating dose of 0.8–0.12 mg/kg produces intubating conditions in 3 minutes, lasting up to 90 minutes. Women are more sensitive to vecuronium (greater degree of blockade and longer duration of action), which may be due to the larger volume of distribution, increased fat, and muscle mass in men.

Metabolism and Excretion

Vecuronium is primarily excreted in the bile and secondarily by the kidneys (25%). Vecuronium undergoes spontaneous deacetylation to produce 3-OH, 17-OH, and 3,17-(OH)2 metabolites, of which 3-OH is the most potent and has 60% of the activity of vecuronium. It is excreted by the kidneys and may be responsible for prolonged paralysis seen in ICU patients. Renal failure, sepsis, and high-dose corticosteroid therapy all increase the risk for this prolonged paralysis.

Pancuronium

Structure

It is a bisquartenary aminosteroid, consisting of a steroid ring with two molecules of Ach.

Metabolism and Excretion

It has a slow onset of action and a long duration (1.5–2 h after a dose of 0.15 mg/kg). It is metabolized by the liver and excreted by the kidneys. The 3-OH metabolite has some neuromuscular blocking activity. Clearance is decreased in renal disease, thereby prolonging the duration of action. Patients with liver disease may require a higher initial dose due to increased volume of distribution but lower maintenance dose secondary to decreased plasma clearance.

Doxacurium

Structure

It is a benzylisoquinolone compound closely related to mivacurium and atracurium.

Dose

A dose of 0.05 mg/kg produces adequate intubating condition in 5 minutes, and has a long duration of action lasting up to 150 minutes.

Metabolism and Excretion

The primary route of elimination is renal excretion, and there is a minor degree of slow hydrolysis by plasma cholinesterase. The duration of action is prolonged in patients with renal disease.

ABNORMAL RESPONSES TO NONDEPOLARIZING AGENTS

Neonates: Neonates are sensitive to muscle relaxants because of the immaturity of neuromuscular junction, but their increased ECF volume provides a larger volume of distribution.

Hypothermia: Hypothermia prolongs blockade by decreasing metabolism and decreasing excretion.

Respiratory Acidosis: Respiratory acidosis potentiates the blockade of most nondepolarizers and antagonizes the reversal, which is of clinical relevance in a postoperative hypoventilating patient.

Myasthenia Gravis: Myasthenic patients are resistant to succinylcholine, requiring larger doses to produce blockade, and sensitive to the nondepolarizing neuromuscular blocking drugs. Also, these patients are already on anticholinesterase therapy with pyridostigmine, making reversal inadequate. Generally, neuromuscular agents are avoided in these patients to decrease the need for postoperative mechanical ventilation.

Myasthenic Syndrome: These patients are *very* sensitive to both depolarizing and nondepolarizing neuromuscular blocking agents.

Myotonia: Myotonic patients have a sustained dose-related contracture response to succinylcholine, making mechanical ventilation difficult. Hyperkalemia may result from increased muscle membrane fragility. The response to nondepolarizers is normal, while reversal with neostigmine may result in a myotonic contracture. It is better to avoid succinylcholine in these patients and use short- or intermediate-duration nondepolarizer with neuromuscular monitoring. Mechanical ventilation should be continued until the effects of muscle relaxants have worn off, thereby avoiding the need to use reversal agents. Myotonic patients have been reversed successfully with sugammadex.

Muscular Dystrophy: Administration of succinylcholine in children with muscular dystrophy results in hyperkalemia and rhabdomyolysis. There have been several reports of fatal cardiac arrests in previously undiagnosed latent muscular dystrophy. The response to nondepolarizers and anticholinesterases are usually normal. Succinylcholine should be avoided if the onset of symptoms occurred in childhood or adolescence. The probability of latent muscular dystrophy in young boys (<10 years) is a good reason to avoid succinylcholine in this age group. Nondepolarizers should be carefully titrated and anticholinesterases are not contraindicated and sugammadex may be a good choice.

Amyotrophic Lateral Sclerosis and Multiple Sclerosis: Contractures may occur in response to succinylcholine, and resistance to nondepolarizers may be appreciated.

PROLONGATION OF ACTION/ SYNERGISM

A mixture of two nondepolarizing muscle relaxants is considered to be either additive or synergistic. Additive interactions are observed after two chemically related agents such as atracurium and mivacurium are administered or after the coadministration of steroidal neuromuscular blockers. Combinations of structurally dissimilar blockers (steroid with a benzylisoquinolinium) produces a synergistic response. The advantages of combining two neuromuscular blockers include rapid onset and short duration of action (mivacurium-rocuronium combination) and also a possible reduction in cardiovascular side effects. Pharmacodynamic response to the use of two nondepolarizers depends on the specific drugs used and the sequence of their administration. Approximately three half-lives are required for the clinical changeover and for the block to take on the characteristics of the second drug. The prolongation of action of the first maintenance dose of mivacurium administered after atracurium is thought to be additive. This is attributed to relative concentrations of these drugs at the receptors, which still remain occupied by the first administered drug. With further incremental doses of the second drug, more receptors are occupied by that drug and taking on its clinical profile.

The interaction between succinylcholine and nondepolarizers depends on the doses used and the order of administration. Small doses of nondepolarizer are administered before succinylcholine to prevent fasciculation. This has an antagonistic effect on the depolarizing block by succinylcholine, necessitating a higher dose.

SIDE EFFECTS AND TOXICITY

Muscle relaxants are not benign drugs. There are a wide variety of both minor and major side effects. A thorough understanding of the nature of these effects is critical for the anesthesiologist's day-to-day practice.

SIDE EFFECTS AND TOXICITY OF SUCCINYLCHOLINE

Succinylcholine is the muscle relaxant often assumed to have the most serious side effects, but all muscle relaxants may have life-threatening side effects.

Cardiovascular

Succinylcholine is able to act at all cholinergic receptors in the body, including the muscarinic receptors in the heart, which explains the relatively high incidence of cardiovascular side effects. Sinus tachycardia is fairly common, due to the ability of the drug to release catecholamines.[1] Sinus bradycardia may occur with some frequency, particularly in children. A variety of cardiac dysrhythmias may occur as well, including both junctional and ventricular dysrhythmias.

Hyperkalemia

Succinylcholine will increase serum K by about 0.5 meq/L secondary to potassium leak from cells during the depolarization process in healthy patients. Patients with preexisting hyperkalemia (e.g., renal failure) will not exhibit any greater increase in potassium levels.

Extrajunctional Proliferation and Hyperkalemia

Each Ach receptor at the neuromuscular junction is composed of five subunits. The combination of these subunits determines whether a receptor is classified as a *mature* versus immature (*extrajunctional*) receptor. Normal Ach receptors are composed of two alpha, one beta, one delta, and one epsilon subunit, whereas extrajunctional receptors have a gamma subunit substituted for the epsilon subunit (see Figure 15.1).

In healthy muscle cells, almost all of the receptors are junctional in nature. During certain disease processes (burns, denervation injuries, immobilization, severe sepsis), proliferation of extrajunctional receptors may occur. When Ach binds to extrajunctional receptors, the response is different because the receptor has altered morphology. In particular, when an agonist binds to an extrajunctional receptor, the ion channels remain open for longer, which results in increased potassium leak from the cell. In addition, it is thought that agonists have higher affinity for the extrajunctional receptor. When succinylcholine is given in patients with proliferation of these abnormal receptors, life-threatening hyperkalemia with consequent arrhythmias may occur.

The *enhanced* affinity of agonists like Ach and succinylcholine to these receptors is in in contrast to the *decreased* affinity of antagonists for these receptors, which explains the resistance of patients with burns and denervation injuries to nondepolarizing agents.

The proliferation of these abnormal receptors may occur within hours of the initial injury, burn, or immobility, and it is generally thought that succinylcholine should be avoided if the injury has taken place more than 24 hours prior.

Increase in Intragastric Pressure

Succinylcholine routinely causes an elevation in intragastric pressure in addition to an elevation in the tone of the lower esophageal sphincter, and therefore does not contribute to an increased risk of aspiration.[1]

Increase in Intraocular Pressure

The underlying mechanism has not been clearly elucidated, although it has been established that succinylcholine causes an average increase in intraocular pressure of about 5 to 15 mmHg. The use of succinylcholine in open globe procedures remains somewhat controversial, although pretreatment with nondepolarizers may limit the increase in pressure and therefore allow for more liberal use of the drug during a rapid-sequence induction for open globe procedures. Of

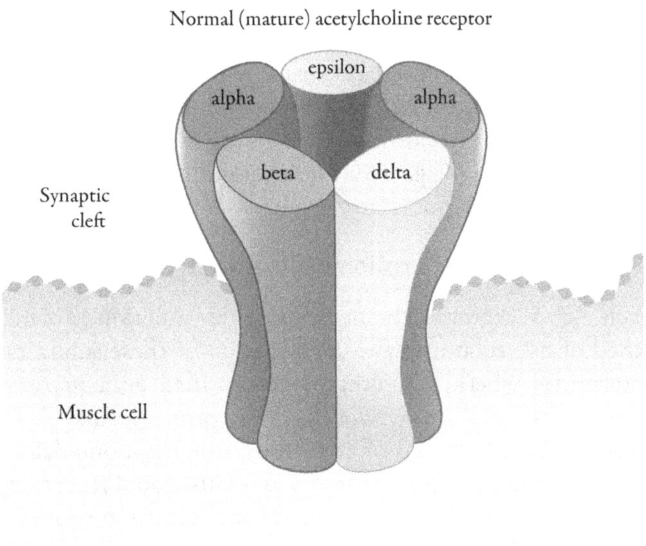

Figure 15.1 Normal acetylcholine receptor showing the five subunits around a central ion channel. Adapted from Miller R, ed. *Miller's Anesthesia*. 7th ed. Philadelphia, PA: Elsevier; 2010.

greater importance is selection of a technique that avoids hypoxia, hypercarbia, or "bucking" on the endotracheal tube.

Increase in Intracranial Pressure

This effect may be reliably offset by pretreatment with a nondepolarizer. In emergency situations, the transient rise in intracranial pressure must be weighed against the risk of inadequate anaesthesia during intubation if succinylcholine is not used, which could result in far greater increases in intracranial pressure.

Postoperative Myalgias

This is commonly seen a day or two after administration of the drug. The intensity of the myalgias does not appear to be related to the degree of fasciculations witnessed. Pretreatment with small doses of nondepolarizers may decrease the severity of the myalgias.

Malignant Hyperthermia

Succinylcholine is likely to be a potent triggering agent for the development of malignant hyperthermia in susceptible patients when used concomitantly with a volatile anesthetic.[4]

Phase II Block

With large doses of succinylcholine or an infusion, the characteristic of the block may change to mimic the clinical conditions associated with a nondepolarizing agent.

SIDE EFFECTS AND TOXICITY OF NONDEPOLARIZING DRUGS

Although nondepolarizing drugs are widely considered to be safer than depolarizing drugs, there are many important and potentially serious side effects to consider.

Cardiovascular

Hypotension and tachycardia may be seen with atracurium and mivacurium, secondary to the histamine-releasing effect of these benzylisoquinoliniums. This effect is not seen with cisatracurium. Pancuronium may cause an increase in heart rate. Although both vecuronium and atracurium were once thought to cause bradycardia, this response occurs only when opioids are administered as well, so the bradycardia is likely to be secondary to the opioid effect.

Respiratory

Benzylisoquinoliniums that release histamine (atracurium and mivacurium) may result in bronchospasm, particularly in patients with preexisting reactive airways disease.

Critical Illness Polyneuromyopathy

Nondepolarizing muscle relaxants (NDMRs) used in the critical care environment for extended periods of time may be a risk factor for the development of the syndrome called critical illness polyneuromyopathy, where patients exhibit signs of muscle weakness and difficulty in weaning from the ventilator. It is important to note that the use of muscle relaxants is only one of the many risk factors believed to contribute to the problem. Other risk factors include female sex, multiorgan failure, hyperglycemia, hepatic failure, electrolyte abnormalities, TPN (Total parenteral nutrition), corticosteroid use, and sedatives.[5] Most of the evidence shows that the use of NDMRs in critically ill patients is a co-risk factor and not an independent one.[6]

SIDE EFFECTS AND TOXICITY COMMON TO DEPOLARIZING AND NONDEPOLARIZING DRUGS

Hypersensitivity Reactions

Both depolarizing and nondepolarizing agents are often cited as the leading cause of hypersensitivity reactions during anesthesia, with latex and antibiotics as the second and third most common causes respectively.[7] All NDMRs can cause nonspecific histamine release from mast cells,[8] and the effect is significantly more potent with the benzylisoquinoliniums than the aminosteroids. Most of these reactions are likely to go unnoticed clinically, unless there is massive histamine release, which would result in major effects on the hemodynamic and respiratory systems. Most of the allergic reactions to neuromuscular blockers are thought to be mediated by interaction of the quaternary ammonium ion in NDMRs with IgE on mast cells. The estimated incidence of these reactions is approximately 100 per one million procedures,[9] and can be life threatening.

INDICATIONS AND CONTRAINDICATIONS

SUCCINYLCHOLINE

This remains the agent of choice for rapid-sequence intubations, where the concern for aspiration of gastric contents outweighs the potential risks and side effects of using the drug. There is no other muscle relaxant that can provide the same depth of muscle paralysis as quickly as succinylcholine can.

Succinylcholine is contraindicated in patients with denervation or burn injuries after the first 24 hours of injury. There is controversy about when succinylcholine can be safely used again in burn patients. Patients who are immobile for extended periods may also experience extrajunctional receptor proliferation, and succinylcholine should also be avoided in these patients (see Figure 15.1).

The use of succinylcholine in pediatrics has declined steadily over the years because of the fear of using the agent in a patient with an undiagnosed muscle myopathy and consequent hyperkalemia. In otherwise healthy children who are ambulating normally, the use of succinylcholine is unlikely to cause major complications.

There is some controversy regarding the use of succinylcholine in patients with open globe injuries. There has been a long-cited theoretical risk of extrusion of ocular contents if the drug is used. In situations where a patient with an open globe injury requires a rapid-sequence induction, it is up the individual physician to decide whether or not the risks of using succinylcholine are greater than the risk of using rocuronium in a rapid-sequence dose, particularly if the airway exam is nonreassuring and the potential exists for a failed intubation and consequent need for mask ventilation (with possible aspiration in a full stomach situation). In this scenario, the risk of ensuing hypoxia and hypercarbia are likely to be far more deleterious to intraocular pressure than the transient moderate rise caused by succinylcholine (which may be prevented in the first place by pretreatment with a small dose of a nondepolarizing agent).

NONDEPOLARIZING AGENTS

The use of these drugs in clinical anesthesia practice is to facilitate intubation and to provide surgical relaxation where appropriate (e.g., intra-abdominal surgery, where relaxation of the abdominal muscles is essential for the operation). Most anesthesiologists will use muscle relaxants in the adult population for intubation, although many choose to forego using a muscle relaxant for intubation in young children. Many studies have however demonstrated that significantly better intubating conditions can be expected with the use of a NDMR than without.[10–12]

When used for tracheal intubation, nondepolarizers have different onset times to maximal effect, and this should be taken into account when preparing to intubate. Cisatracurium has been shown to have the slowest onset time, whereas rocuronium has the fastest when the ED95 dose is used.[13]

Residual paralysis at the conclusion of surgery needs to be avoided. It is imperative to use only as much relaxant during a procedure as is required to assist the surgical technique or prevent undesirable movement in precarious situations (such as a patient who is in headpins for neurosurgical or orthopedic procedures). As an example, assuming there is sufficient anesthetic depth, it is usually appropriate to maintain the train-of-four count at 2–3 twitches for abdominal muscle relaxation during abdominal surgery. Use of a twitch monitor is essential to monitor the level of muscle relaxation, as predicting duration of action of these agents based purely on their pharmacological properties can be unreliable.[14]

In circumstances where the physician deems that succinylcholine is contraindicated but the patient still requires a rapid-sequence induction, larger doses of nondepolarizers may be utilized as an alternative. Rocuronium, when administered with a dose of 1.2 mg/kg will shorten onset time to around 30–60 seconds. This dose is four times the ed95 and results in significant prolongation of the drug's duration of action, anywhere from 60 to 80 minutes compared with 20–35 minutes when the drug is given at a standard intubating dose of 0.6 mg/kg.

In the 1980s NDMRs were commonly used for most patients on mechanical ventilation in intensive care units, but their use has steadily decreased over the years for concerns primarily related to risk for development of polyneuromyopathy, possible awareness, and other hazards such as risk for deep vein thrombosis, corneal abrasions, and anaphylaxis.[15]

ANTAGONISM

A thorough appreciation of the conditions under which antagonism of muscle relaxants may take place is critical for the clinician to appropriately adjust drug dosing under these circumstances.

MECHANISM OF ANTAGONISM

Only NDMRs can be effectively antagonized by pharmacological agents. Succinylcholine is metabolized by pseudocholinesterase (butyrylcholinesterase), which occurs naturally.

In order to completely mitigate the effects of NDMRs on muscle cells, the drug needs to be completely eliminated from the body. There are a variety of pathways of elimination for the various nondepolarizers, including hepatic metabolism, hepatic excretion via the bile, renal excretion, and enzymatic metabolism and nonspecific Hoffman degradation in the plasma. However, in most clinical scenarios, complete elimination takes significantly more time to occur that would be clinically useful.

The NDMRs are competitive antagonists at the neuromuscular junction. When using a nondepolarizing agent, these drugs act in a noncompetitive fashion by binding to the nicotinic receptor at the neuromuscular junction, but they compete with Ach for binding sites. If the ratio of Ach to neuromuscular blocker is high, Ach will occupy a sufficient number of receptors to result in depolarization of the muscle cell. Acetylcholinesterase is a naturally occurring enzyme produced within the muscle cell at the neuromuscular junction. It rapidly breaks down Ach as it is released, resulting in a very small amount of Ach reaching the nicotinic receptor during normal action potentials. Inhibition of acetylcholinesterase results in less breakdown of Ach, which competes more effectively with nondepolarizing agents resulting in antagonism of neuromuscular block.

Drugs that inhibit acetylcholinesterase allow clinicians to effectively antagonize the actions of NDMRs. There are a number of acetylcholinesterase inhibitors in clinical use, including neostigmine, pyridostigmine, physostigmine, and edrophonium.

CLINICAL ANTAGONISM

Neuromuscular blockade should only be reversed when clinical monitoring dictates it—usually at least one twitch should be seen at the time of reversal. It takes up to 10 minutes for the full reversal effect of neostigmine. There is evidence suggesting that residual neuromuscular blockade after seemingly adequate reversal results in significant morbidity in patients recovering from general anesthesia. In particular, the incidence of hypoxemia, upper airway obstruction, subjective complaints of weakness, longer Post Anesthesia Care Unit stays, and delayed extubation are all factors thought to be related to inadequate reversal. This resulted in the recommendation that the train-of-four ratio should be at least 0.9 for full reversal, which is in contrast to the more traditional thinking that 0.7 is sufficient.[16]

Incomplete antagonism may also impair the body's ventilatory response to hypoxia, which may increase postoperative pulmonary complications in patients recovering from general anesthesia. Although residual block is a real concern with significant comorbidities, the incidence of this is relatively low. The efficacy of antagonism of NDMR blockade may be potentiated by hypothermia, volatile anesthetics, severe dehydration, calcium channel blockers, and so forth. Although many anesthesiologists believe that it is unnecessary to reverse a nondepolarizing agent if a few hours have passed since the last dose, there is some evidence that there is still a degree of neuromuscular block even hours after the last dose.[17,18] When consideration of elimination half-life is applied, this point is further emphasized. For example, a NDMB that has a 60-minute elimination half-life would require 5 hours to clear to 3% active circulating drug; this would only be lengthened in patients with hepatic or renal disease. In patients with marginal pulmonary function or metabolic reserve the consequences could be substantial.

SIDE EFFECTS

Acetylcholinesterase inhibitors not only act at the neuromuscular junction but also have widespread cholinergic effects at all nicotinic and muscarinic receptors. Because these agents can act at muscarinic receptors of the parasympathetic nervous system as well as on the autonomic ganglia of the cardiovascular, respiratory, and gastrointestinal systems, many unwanted side effects may occur. These include bronchospasm, tachycardia, and increased bowel motility. In an attempt to mitigate these effects, the anticholinergic agents that bind to cholinergic receptors are used in addition to acetylcholinesterase agents and include atropine and glycopyrrolate. These drugs themselves have important side effects, such as tachycardia, nausea, decreased bowel motility, and decreased salivation leading to a dry mouth. Atropine is able to cross the blood-brain barrier and cause confusion, which can be difficult to differentiate from emergence delirium in the recovery room. Glycopyrrolate is a quaternary amine and is unable to cross the blood-brain barrier. It does not cause confusion and may be the agent of choice in the operating room for use with acetylcholinesterase inhibitors. When a tertiary amine anticholingeric is administered with resulting central nervous system effects, it may be necessary to antagonize with an anticholinesterase that can cross the blood-brain barrier. As a result of this clinical pattern, the types of drugs administered are matched for both their duration of action and their physiologic effects.

For example, atropine has a faster onset than glycopyrrolate and a shorter duration of action. It is better suited for use with edrophonium, because the pharmacokinetics of the two drugs are better matched, as is the combination between neostigmine and glycopyrolate, which is commonly the combination used in clinical practice.

The clearance of acetylcholinesterase inhibitors is prolonged in patients with renal failure; however, so is the clearance of the NDMRs prolonged, which presumably prevents recurarization.

Reversal of clinical neuromuscular block will only be seen if there is a threshold concentration of neuromuscular blocker. Two molecules of acetylcholine need to bind to the nicotinic receptor in order for depolarization to occur. Only one molecule of NDMR is needed to block depolarization, so there needs to be a very high concentration of Ach to effectively antagonize the effect of the NDMR. Additionally, the use of acetylcholinesterase inhibitors have a ceiling effect at which additional doses do not result in any more Ach being available in the neuromuscular junction. If a sufficiently high concentration of NDMR is present in the junction, no amount of acetylcholinesterase inhibitor will be able to reverse the block, at least not until the agent undergoes its natural metabolism. This observation reiterates the importance of having an adequate return of TOF twitches prior to administering reversal.

Finally, it is important to keep in mind that acetylcholinesterase inhibitors also inhibit plasma cholinesterase to a degree, although it is probably still better to reverse mivacurium than not to.[14]

DRUG INTERACTIONS

Neuromuscular blocking drugs interact with multiple receptors in the body, and share their site of action with many other drugs. Many drugs can interact directly with the Ach receptor, while others cause changes to the structure of the receptor itself, which in turn modifies the response of the receptor when a neuromuscular agent is bound to it.

ANTIBIOTICS

Many antibiotics have effects on neuromuscular transmission, and the various classes of antibiotics may exert their effects through different mechanisms. The aminoglycoside antibiotics, for example, are able to inhibit the prejunctional release of acetylcholine, as well as decrease the sensitivity of the acetylcholine receptor to acetylcholine. Neomycin and streptomycin are the most likely drugs in the polymyxin class to cause clinically relevant potentiation of neuromuscular blockade, which occurs both pre- and postjunctionally. Of the lincosamides, clindamycin and lincomycin exert effects both pre- and postjunctionally, but clinical affects are not readily apparent.[1] On the other hand, tetracyclines exert their effect only at the postjunctional level. There is no convincing evidence to support the potentiation of neuromuscular block by the penicillins, cephalosporins, or metronidazole (see Figure 15.2).

ANTIEPILEPTICS

Antiepileptics may affect the response to neuromuscular blockers via both a direct effect at the neuromuscular junction as well as by affecting the metabolism of the paralytic agents. Chronic administration of antiepileptics can lead to either induction or inhibition of the cytochrome P450 system in the liver. Some medications may even induce one isoform of the P450 system while inhibiting another (see Table 15.3). It takes approximately 1–3 weeks for the induction effects to take place after a patient starts treatment with an antiepileptic medication. The older-generation medications (carbamazepine, phenytoin, and phenobarbital) are likely to increase the metabolism and elimination of the aminosteroid nondepolarizing agents because this class of neuromuscular blockers undergoes liver metabolism and elimination. There is no convincing evidence to

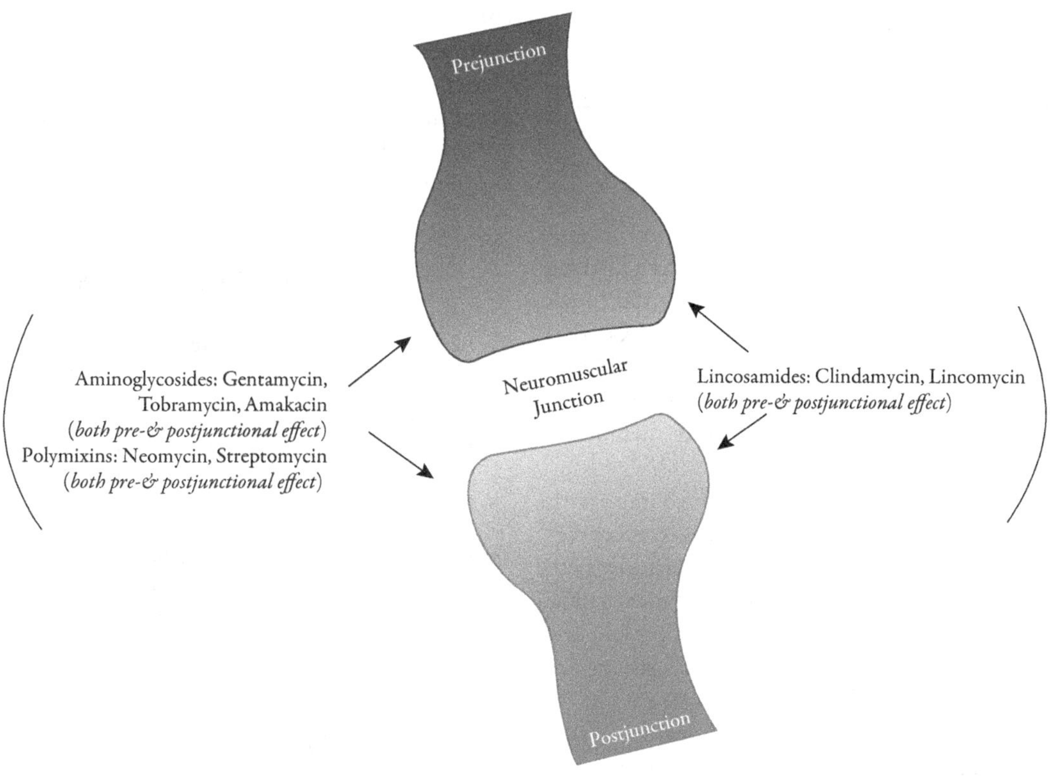

Figure 15.2 Antibiotic potentiation of neuromuscular blockade in the neuromuscular junction.

Table 15.3 ANTIEPILEPTICS INDUCTION OR INHIBITION OF THE CYTOCHROME P450 SYSTEM IN THE LIVER

DRUG	INDUCTION OF LIVER ENZYMES	INHIBITION OF LIVER ENZYMES
Phenytoin	✓	✓
Carbamazepine	✓	
Phenobarbital	✓	
Valproic acid		✓
Felbamate	✓	✓
Lamotrigine	✓	
Topiramate	✓	✓
Gabapentin	No effect	No effect
Ethosuximide	No effect	No effect
Vigabatrin	No effect	No effect

Modified with permission from Soriano SG, Martyn JA. Antiepileptic-induced resistance to neuromuscular blockers: mechanisms and clinical significance. *Clin Pharmacokinet*. 2004;43:71–81.

support that there is an increased requirement for atracurium or mivacurium in patients on anticonvulsants, most likely because these drugs are not dependent on processes in the liver for their elimination.

The protein α_1 acid glycoprotein is produced by the liver and binds and transports all nondepolarizing blockers when they enter the plasma. Chronic use of phenytoin, carbamazepine, and phenobarbital all induce the production of α_1 acid glycoprotein in the liver.[19] This results in increased binding of NDMRs, causing a decrease in the free fraction of the drug available at the nicotinic receptor at the neuromuscular junction and attenuation of the clinical response to the drug.

There are also direct effects of antiepileptics on the neuromuscular junction. When phenytoin is given as a loading dose, it can produce a mild degree of neuromuscular block and therefore also potentiates the block of NDMRs. This is believed to be secondary to the membrane-stabilizing effects of phenytoin. Carbamazepine may also induce neuromuscular block on its own as well as via its metabolite carbamazepine-10, 11-epoxide.[20]

It has also been postulated that long-term therapy with anticonvulsants may induce proliferation of Ach receptors at the neuromuscular junction as a response to chronic neuromuscular block, which could increase resistance to the effects of neuromuscular blockers. This might explain the enhanced sensitivity to succinylcholine in these patients, as well as a potential concern for hyperkalemia.

Although not originally thought to, recent evidence suggests that valproic acid may increase rocuronium requirements.[21] Other anticonvulsants (gabapentin, ethosuximide, vigabatrin, levetiracetam) do not appear to have significant effects on a patient's response to neuromuscular blockers.

Lithium

Lithium is used to treat bipolar disorder. It is able to potentiate the effects of NDMRs at the neuromuscular junction at both a pre- and postsynaptic level. A prolonged duration of action has been seen with both depolarizing and nondepolarizing agents.

Magnesium

Magnesium is able to potentiate the neuromuscular block produced by NDMRs. In clinical anesthesia practice, this is most relevant in the obstetric population where patients with preeclampsia may be treated with magnesium. It is postulated that magnesium has both a pre- and a postjunctional effect. Magnesium is able to inhibit calcium channels presynaptically and therefore limit the release of Ach into the synaptic cleft. Magnesium also has the ability to inhibit postjunctional membranes of many cells, including skeletal muscle cells. Careful titration of neuromuscular blockers is mandatory in patients receiving magnesium therapy in order to ensure adequate recovery after reversal.

Inhaled Anesthetics

Inhaled anesthetics have long been known to enhance neuromuscular block from NDMRs. Potentiation of neuromuscular block differs among the inhaled anesthetics and the order of degree of enhancement from most to least of commonly used anesthetic agents is: desflurane > sevoflurane > isoflurane > halothane > nitrous oxide = barbiturates = opioid = propofol anesthesia. The mechanism of the potentiation is believed to be multifactorial and includes enhanced affinity of the NDMR to the Ach receptor as well as a central effect on neurotransmission.[3]

REFERENCES

1. Barash P, Cullen B, Stoelting R, Cahalan M, Stock M. *Clinical Anesthesia*. 6th ed. Philadelphia, PA: Lippincott Williams & Wilkins; 2009.
2. Clark M. Lippincott's illustrated reviews. In: *Pharmacology*. 5th ed. Baltimore, MD: Wolters Kluwer Health/Lippincott Williams & Wilkins; 2012.
3. Miller RD, ed. *Miller's Anesthesia*. 7th ed. Philadelphia, PA: Churchill Livingstone/Elsevier; 2010.
4. Hopkins PM. Malignant hyperthermia: pharmacology of triggering. *Br J Anaesth*. 2011;107:48–56.
5. Confer J, Wolcott J, Hayes R. Critical illness polyneuromyopathy. *Am J Health Syst Pharm*. 2012;69:1199–1205.
6. Hermans G, De Jonghe B, Bruyninckx F, Van den Berghe G. Interventions for preventing critical illness polyneuropathy and critical illness myopathy. *Cochrane Database Syst Rev*. 2014;1:CD006832.
7. Mertes P, Alla F, Tréchot P, Auroy Y, Jougla E, Groupe d'Etudes des Réactions Anaphylactoïdes Peranesthésiques. Anaphylaxis

during anesthesia in France: an 8-year national survey. *J Allergy Clin Immunol.* 2011;128:366–373.
8. Claudius C, Garvey L, Viby-Mogensen J. The undesirable effects of neuromuscular blocking drugs. *Anaesthesia.* 2009;64(Suppl 1):10–21.
9. Mertes P, Demoly P, Malinovsky J. Hypersensitivity reactions in the anesthesia setting/allergic reactions to anesthetics. *Curr Opin Allergy Clin Immunol.* 2012;12:361–368.
10. Lieutaud T, Billard V, Khalaf H, Debaene B. Muscle relaxation and increasing doses of propofol improve intubating conditions. *Can J Anaesth.* 2003;50:121–126.
11. Combes X, Andriamifidy L, Dufresne E, et al. Comparison of two induction regimens using or not using muscle relaxant: impact on postoperative upper airway discomfort. *Br J Anaesth.* 2007;99:276–281.
12. Schlaich N, Mertzlufft F, Soltesz S, Fuchs-Buder T. Remifentanil and propofol without muscle relaxants or with different doses of rocuronium for tracheal intubation in outpatient anaesthesia. *Acta Anaesthesiol Scand.* 2000;44:720–726.
13. Bowman W, Rodger I, Houston J, Marshall R, McIndewar I. Structure: action relationships among some desacetoxy analogues of pancuronium and vecuronium in the anesthetized cat. *Anesthesiology.* 1988;69:57–62.
14. Fink H, Hollmann M. Myths and facts in neuromuscular pharmacology: new developments in reversing neuromuscular blockade. *Minerva Anestesiol.* 2012;78:473–482.
15. Greenberg S, Vender J. The use of neuromuscular blocking agents in the ICU: where are we now? *Crit Care Med.* 2013;41:1332–1344.
16. Murphy G, Brull S. Residual neuromuscular block: lessons unlearned. Part I: definitions, incidence, and adverse physiologic effects of residual neuromuscular block. *Anesth Analg.* 2010;111:120–128.
17. Caldwell J. Reversal of residual neuromuscular block with neostigmine at one to four hours after a single intubating dose of vecuronium. *Anesth Analg.* 1995;80:1168–1174.
18. Debaene B, Plaud B, Dilly M, Donati F. Residual paralysis in the PACU after a single intubating dose of nondepolarizing muscle relaxant with an intermediate duration of action. *Anesthesiology.* 2003;98:1042–1048.
19. Soriano S, Martyn J. Antiepileptic-induced resistance to neuromuscular blockers: mechanisms and clinical significance. *Clin Pharmacokinet.* 2004;43:71–81.
20. Nguyen A, Ramzan I. Acute in vitro neuromuscular effects of carbamazepine and carbamazepine-10,11-epoxide. *Anesth Analg.* 1997;84:886–890.
21. Kim M, Hwang J, Jeon Y, Do S. Effects of valproic acid and magnesium sulphate on rocuronium requirement in patients undergoing craniotomy for cerebrovascular surgery. *Br J Anaesth.* 2012;109:407–412.

FURTHER READING

Stoelting R, Hillier S. *Pharmacology and Physiology in Anesthetic Practice.* 4th ed. Philadelphia, PA: Lippincott Williams & Wilkins; 2005.

QUESTIONS

1. Which of the following is true about patients with pseudocholinesterase deficiency?
   A. Patients with heterozygous atypical pseudocholinesterase genes will have a prolonged block of up to 8 hours after succinylcholine administration.
   B. Patients with homozygous pseudocholinesterase genes will have a dibucaine number of 40–60.
   C. The adequacy of pseudocholinesterase can be determined quantitatively by the dibucaine number.
   D. Patients with homozygous atypical genes will have a prolonged block for up to 8 hours requiring mechanical ventilation after succinylcholine administration.

2. Which of the following correctly describes the response of neuromuscular blockers in patients with musculoskeletal disorders?
   A. Patients with myasthenia gravis are sensitive to both depolarizers and nondepolarizers.
   B. Patients with muscular dystrophy will have an exaggerated hyperkalemic response and rhabdomyolysis after succinylcholine administration.
   C. Myotonic patients will have an exaggerated contacture response after the administration of nondepolarizers.
   D. Patients with myasthenic syndrome are resistant to the effect of nondepolarizers.

3. A 42-year-old male with chronic renal insufficiency was admitted 3 days ago after sustaining a spinal cord injury from a fall, which resulted in paraplegia. The patient is scheduled for thoracic decompression and fusion. Which of the following statements is correct regarding the use of muscle relaxants during the procedure?
   A. The patient is likely have to increased sensitivity to rocuronium.
   B. Succinylcholine will bind with increased affinity to an Ach receptor consisting of five subunits: two alpha, one beta, one delta, and one gamma.
   C. If a rapid-sequence induction is chosen, administration of succinylcholine is the agent of choice to secure the airway.
   D. The patient will have a decreased response to standard doses of reversal agents.
   E. The patient will have an exaggerated release of potassium during succinylcholine administration because of his renal disease.

4. A patient who recently ate a full meal is brought emergently to the operating room after sustaining a gunshot wound to his abdomen. He satisfies criteria for shock. The anesthesiologist elects to proceed with a rapid-sequence intubation. Choose the correct statement:
   A. Rocuronium at a dose of 0.6 mg/kg will provide intubating conditions similar to succinylcholine at 1 mg/kg.
   B. Recovery from a dose of rocuronium of 1.2 mg/kg will take about 30 minutes on average.
   C. The use of succinylcholine in this patient may result in increased intragastric pressure and is therefore contraindicated.
   D. Maintenance of general anesthesia after induction should include ensuring that the patient has no twitches while the surgeon is working in the abdomen.
   E. Succinylcholine is not contraindicated in shock states.

5. Regarding reversal of nondepolarizing neuromuscular blockers:
   A. Neostigmine may inhibit butyrylcholinesterase and prolong the duration of subsequent doses of succinylcholine.
   B. The maximum effect of neostigmine is achieved 5 minutes after administration.
   C. When glycopyrrolate is used as part of neuromuscular reversal, it may contribute to symptoms of confusion in the postanesthesia care unit in certain patients.
   D. Higher doses of neostigmine may effectively antagonize the action of nondepolarizers when no twitches are evident, but this is avoided because of the higher incidence of unwanted anticholinergic effects.
   E. Neostigmine is a competitive agonist for the Ach receptor at the neuromuscular junction.

6. Which of the following statements regarding drug interactions with neuromuscular blockers is true?
   A. A patient with preeclampsia receiving magnesium will have a decreased response to nondepolarizing blockers during a general anesthetic.
   B. Chronic use of phenytoin may induce production of alpha-1 acid glycoprotein that can induce resistance to nondepolarizing agents.
   C. Chronic intake of carbamazepine causes resistance to succinylcholine.
   D. Lithium decreases the effect of nondepolarizing agents at the neuromuscular junction.
   E. Desflurane is less likely to enhance nondepolarizing block than propofol.

ANSWERS

1. D. Atypical pseudocholinesterase may be heterozygous or homozygous. Patients with heterozygous genes have a slightly prolonged block (20–30 min) whereas those with homozygous atypical genes will have a long blockade lasting up to 8 hours after administration of succinylcholine. This prolonged paralysis from atypical pseudocholinesterase should be treated with mechanical ventilation until the recovery of the muscle function. The abnormal pseudocholinesterase genes include dibucaine-resistant (1/100 of normal affinity for pseudocholinesterase and most common), fluoride resistant, and silent genes (no activity). The percentage of inhibition of pseudocholinesterase by dibucaine, a local anesthetic, is termed the dibucaine number. Normal pseudocholinesterase is inhibited by 80%, whereas only 20% of atypical pseudocholinesterase is inhibited and atypical heterozygous shows 40%–60% inhibition. The dibucaine number is proportional to pseudocholinesterase function and independent of the amount of enzyme. The dibucaine number provides a qualitative estimate of the adequacy of pseudocholinesterase.
2. B. Administration of succinylcholine in children with muscular dystrophy results in hyperkalemia and rhabdomyolysis. There have been several reports of fatal cardiac arrests in previously undiagnosed latent muscular dystrophy. Myasthenic patients are resistant to succinylcholine, requiring larger doses to produce blockade, and sensitive to the nondepolarizing neuromuscular blocking drugs. Myotonic patients have a sustained dose-related contracture response to succinylcholine, making mechanical ventilation difficult, while the response to nondepolarizers is normal. Patients with myasthenic syndrome are very sensitive to both depolarizing and nondepolarizing neuromuscular blocking agents.
3. B. This patient will have proliferation of abnormal extrajunctional receptors secondary to a denervation injury that is more than 24 hours old. These abnormal receptors have a different structure to normal Ach receptors in that they have five units composed of two alpha, one beta, one delta, and one gamma subunit, whereas normal receptors have an epsilon subunit substituted for a gamma. Acetylcholine and succinylcholine have enhanced binding to these abnormal receptors. Succinylcholine is contraindicated in these patients, because the proliferation of these receptors as well as the enhanced affinity will result in massive release of potassium. Nondepolarizers however have a decreased affinity for the abnormal Ach receptors, and this patient will likely exhibit resistance to nondepolarizers. Patients with preexisting kidney disease do not exhibit an exaggerated increase in potassium compared with normal patients.

FURTHER READING

Miller RD, ed. *Miller's Anesthesia*. 7th ed. Philadelphia, PA: Churchill Livingstone/Elsevier; 2010:865.

4. E. In order for rocuronium to mimic the onset and depth of neuromuscular blockade that succinylcholine can achieve, it needs to be administered in a dose that is four times the ED95, which is approximately 1.2 mg/kg. When a high initial dose like this is used, the duration of action will be significantly prolonged, often in excess of an hour. Although succinylcholine does cause an increase in intragastric pressure, it also increases tone in the lower esophageal sphincter, which prevents the raised intragastric pressure from causing movement of gastric contents into the esophagus. There is no need to maintain muscle relaxation to the extent that there is no response to a train-of-four stimulation from the twitch monitor. Adequate relaxation of abdominal skeletal muscle is seen at 2–3 twitches. Although succinylcholine does have cardiovascular side effects, it is not contraindicated in shock states.

5. A. The administration of succinylcholine after reversal with an anticholinesterase inhibitor (e.g., if the patient has laryngospasm post extubation requiring succinylcholine) can result in significant increased duration of action of succinylcholine, because its metabolism is dependent on the activity of butyrylcholinesterase, which is also inhibited in the plasma by the acetylcholinesterase inhibitors. Neostigmine takes at least 10 minutes to reach maximal effect, so this needs to be take into account when timing the administration of reversal agents. Glycopyrrolate is a quarternary amine and does not cross the blood-brain barrier. It should not enter the differential for confusion in the PACU. Although higher doses of anticholinesterase inhibitors might lead to increased anticholinergic effects, this is not the reason for avoiding a higher dose. The ceiling dose exists because there is a maximal effect of inhibitor in causing an increase in Ach in the synaptic cleft and increasing the dose will not lead to an increased concentration of Ach. Neostigmine inhibits the enzyme acetylcholinesterase at the neuromuscular junction and does not compete for binding to the Ach receptor.
6. B. Magnesium causes potentiation of the action of nondepolarizing agents via its pre- and postjunctional effects at the neuromuscular junction. Patients receiving magnesium therapy require decreased doses of nondepolarizing agents. Classic anticonvulsants such as phenytoin, carbamazepine, and phenobarbital can induce the liver to increase the production of alpha-1 acid glycoprotein, which is the transport protein for nondepolarizing agents which effectively decreases the clinically active free fraction of the muscle relaxant, resulting in resistance to its effects. There is no evidence to suggest that anticonvulsants cause succinylcholine resistance. Lithium has been shown to potentiate the action of neuromuscular blockers at the neuromuscular junction. Inhaled anesthetics have the ability to enhance nondepolarizing block to a far greater extent than propofol. The reasons for this are multifactorial and include enhanced affinity of the NDMR to the Ach receptor as well as a central effect on neurotransmission.

SECTION IV

CLINICAL SCIENCES

16.

ANESTHESIA PROCEDURES, METHODS, AND TECHNIQUES

Young Su, Salma El Marjiya-Villarreal, and George W. Williams

PREOPERATIVE EVALUATION

Preoperative evaluation of a patient is a basic element of the anesthesiologist's provision of care. There are several components of the preoperative evaluation that must be addressed when interviewing a patient. The goals of the preoperative assessment are ultimately to improve safety and outcome for the patient by identifying potential anesthetic difficulties with existing, as well as undiagnosed, medical conditions. The preoperative meeting also allows the anesthesiologist an opportunity to establish a relationship with the patient in order to appropriately inform about and discuss the anticipated risks and, hopefully, alleviate anxiety.[1] The preoperative assessment can be challenging in that it must be performed efficiently and thoroughly within a limited time frame, either due to emergency conditions, patient condition limitations, or scheduling plans. Unfortunately, there is very little literature to support a standard anesthetic workup, but some consensus has been provided by the American Society of Anesthesiologists as recommendations on the preoperative evaluation.[2]

TIMING OF EVALUATION

Preoperative assessment, ideally, should not be a rushed or time-constrained activity. In general, the preoperative evaluation timing should be based on the degree of surgical invasiveness. It is recommended that with escalating surgical invasiveness, the preoperative assessment should be performed before the day of surgery. Similar recommendations pertain to patients with high severity of disease. Patients with low surgical interventions or low severity of disease can be interviewed on the day of surgery.

PATIENT HISTORY

The patient interview is essential for the anesthesiologist to establish a relationship with the patient and also to obtain the majority of information required for a preoperative evaluation. This is an opportunity for the anesthesiologist to understand their patient's current health status and to determine anesthetic risk. The history should begin with the planned surgical condition and treatments related to the condition. Previous and current medical conditions of the nervous, respiratory, cardiac, hepatic, renal, gastrointestinal, and endocrine systems should be reviewed. It is not adequate to simply state the disease; it is also important to establish the severity of the disease and understand past and current treatments. Past surgeries and anesthetic type, as well as any related complications, should be investigated. This should include familial difficulties with anesthesia to identify possible malignant hyperthermia-prone patients. Medications, prescribed or over-the-counter, should be recorded, as should any allergies to drugs or substances. Additionally, tobacco, alcohol, or illicit drug use should be documented. While this review process seems extensive, it can be quickened by a screening questionnaire that covers most of these areas.

PHYSICAL EXAMINATION

Many studies have shown the high yield value of a history and physical exam in determining a diagnosis. One study found that 56% of correct diagnoses were made on history taking alone, and this increased to 73% with the physical exam in a general medicine clinic.[3] It is essential for the anesthesiologist to use these tools to gain the most information possible about the patient before proceeding to diagnostics. The physical exam should begin with vital signs, including the patient's body mass index (BMI), which is calculated from height and weight. A BMI of 40 or greater defines morbid obesity, while a BMI of 30–39.9 is obese; a BMI of 25–29.9 is overweight. Physical evaluation of the heart, lungs, and extremities (edema, pulses, rashes) is necessary, as well as a basic neurological exam to document any deficiencies. Of utmost importance is a thorough airway examination to determine any potential difficulties (this is reviewed more extensively later).

PREOPERATIVE LABORATORY TESTING

A routine test is defined as a test ordered in the absence of a specific clinical indication or a test that is set as customary. An indicated test is one that is ordered for a specific purpose. The ASA Practice Advisory for preanesthetic evaluation does not encourage routine preoperative testing, but instead recommends ordering labs tailored to the patient's medical condition(s) in order to gain information about the disease. The information is then used to guide management or to optimize the patient's medical condition.[2] Generally, exams performed within 6 months of surgery are acceptable if there has not been any significant change in the patient's medical history.[2] The ASA Task Force on Preanesthetic Evaluation has the following recommendations for laboratory testing:

1. Electrocardiogram (ECG): may be indicated for patients with known cardiac disease or related risk factors but not simply required due to advanced age.
2. Other cardiac evaluation such as consultations, noninvasive screening exams, or invasive functional exams should be considered after assessing the risks versus benefits and with patients with higher cardiovascular and surgical factors (there is more extensive discussion on this later).
3. Chest radiograph may be considered for patients with COPD, patients with recent upper respiratory infection, smokers, and patients with cardiac disease, but should not be unequivocally ordered for these patients.
4. Pulmonary evaluations other than chest x-ray include consultations, noninvasive screening tests (pulmonary function tests, pulse oximetry), and invasive exams (arterial blood gas): patients to consider for these exams should be carefully evaluated as to the risk versus benefit of these exams; however, these tests but may be beneficial in patients with asthma, COPD, and scoliosis with restrictive function. Also, surgical type and invasiveness should be considered. Predisposing risk factors for major perioperative pulmonary complications include cough, dyspnea, smoking, history of lung disease, obesity, and abdominal or thoracic surgery, with the most significant being site of surgery.[4]
5. Hemoglobin or hematocrit should not routinely be performed, but should be considered in patients with liver disease, extremes of age, history of anemia, bleeding or other hematological disorders, and highly invasive surgical procedures.
6. Coagulation studies should be considered in patients with history of bleeding disorders, renal dysfunction, liver dysfunction, use of anticoagulants, and highly invasive procedures.
7. Serum chemistries may be indicated in patients with endocrine disorders, renal dysfunction, liver dysfunction, and use of certain medications that might alter electrolytes.
8. Urinalysis is not generally indicated unless surgical hardware implantation may occur or when symptoms are present.
9. Pregnancy testing may be offered to all females of childbearing age. Generally, group practice or hospital policy will indicate guidelines for urine pregnancy testing prior to surgery.

ASA PHYSICAL STATUS CLASSIFICATION

In 1941, Dr. Meyer Saklad introduced a classification system for a patient to be able to withstand surgery. The term "physical state" was intended to correlate to the patient's preoperative condition and also be used for statistical purposes. This classification system has been expanded to six categories and is used today in an attempt to stratify a patient's health status. The classification has no relation to the operative procedure.[5] The six degrees of physical status are as follows:

ASA Physical Status 1: A normal healthy individual

ASA Physical Status 2: A patient with mild systemic disease.

Examples included mild diabetes, NYHA capacity I or IIa.

ASA Physical Status 3: A patient with severe systemic disease.

Examples include complicated or severe diabetes, NYHA capacity IIb.

ASA Physical Status 4: A patient with severe systemic disease that is a constant threat to life.

This class is for patients that are in an extremely poor physical state.

ASA Physical Status 5: A moribund patient who is not expected to survive without the operation.

ASA Physical Status 6: A declared brain-dead patient whose organs are being removed for donor purposes.

Any emergency operation is noted by placing an "E" after the classification.

Since the introduction of the classification, multiple studies have demonstrated a strong correlation between ASA classification and perioperative mortality. As ASA classification increases, so does postoperative mortality, as shown in several research studies.[6] It is important to note that the assigned ASA classification should reflect the patient's physical status, not perceived operative risk. As such, the ASA classification should arbitrarily be escalated by the anesthesiologist simply because the patient is not expected to do well clinically.

CARDIAC EVALUATION

The purpose of the cardiac evaluation is not to give "clearance" to the patient for the surgery from a cardiac standpoint, but rather to establish the patient's cardiac status and determine the best management of the patient during the perioperative period. The cardiac evaluation is intended to provide the patient, anesthesiologist, and surgeon information to determine the best treatment and the optimal care with that information. The American College of Cardiology and American Heart Association have published guidelines for the perioperative evaluation for noncardiac surgery, which are reviewed annually and revised as needed. The most recently updated guidelines were published in 2007.[7]

1. Recommendation for echocardiogram is reasonable for patients with dyspnea of unknown origin or in patients with known heart failure who have had a clinical change in status within the previous 12 months. There is also evidence that echocardiography is useful in asymptomatic patients with diastolic murmurs, continuous murmurs, late systolic murmurs, murmurs associated with ejection clicks, or grade 3 or louder systolic murmurs.
2. Recommendation for resting 12-lead ECG is reasonable in patients with at least one clinical risk factor undergoing a vascular surgery. It is also recommended for patients with known coronary heart disease, peripheral arterial disease, or cerebrovascular disease who are scheduled for any intermediate-risk surgery.
3. Noninvasive stress tests should be performed in patients with active cardiac conditions and in patients with three or more clinical risk factors (see Box 16.1) with poor functional capacity undergoing vascular surgery. Noninvasive stress tests may be performed in patients with one or two clinical risk factors with poor functional capacity requiring an intermediate-risk or vascular surgery if the test will change management. It is important to understand that these exams should be only performed when there will be a change in management.
4. Coronary revascularization, either coronary artery bypass graft or percutaneous coronary intervention, should be considered in patients with significant left main coronary artery stenosis and in patients with three-vessel disease with stable angina. Coronary revascularization has been shown to be useful in patients who have two-vessel disease with significant proximal LAD stenosis and either an ejection fraction less than 0.50 or identified ischemia on noninvasive testing. Patients with unstable angina, non-ST segment elevation myocardial infarction (MI) or acute ST-elevation MI will benefit from coronary revascularization.

Box 16.1 CLINICAL CARDIAC RISK FACTORS

1. High-Risk Surgery (intraperitoneal, intrathoracic, or vascular procedures)
2. History of Ischemic Heart Disease
3. History of Compensated or Prior Heart Failure
4. History of Cerebrovascular Disease
5. Diabetes Mellitus (on Insulin)
6. Renal Insufficiency (Creatinine > 2.9 mg/dL)

Adapted from Fleisher LA, Beckman JA, Brown KA, et al. ACC/AHA 2007 guidelines on perioperative cardiovascular evaluation and care for noncardiac surgery: executive summary: a report of the American College of Cardiology/American Heart Association Task Force on Practice Guidelines. *Circulation*. 2007;116:1971–1996; Fleisher LA. Cardiac risk stratification for noncardiac surgery: update from the American College of Cardiology/American Heart Association 2007 guidelines. *Cleve Clin J Med*. 2009;76:S10–S115.

Serious Cardiac Conditions

The ACC/AHA guidelines have identified four active cardiac conditions in which the patient should undergo evaluation and treatment before any noncardiac surgery. These conditions include unstable coronary syndromes, decompensated heart failure, significant arrhythmias, and severe valvular disease.[7]

1. Unstable coronary syndromes are classified as either unstable angina or recent MI. "Recent" is defined as an MI within the previous 30 days. Patients with severe angina or with stable angina who are sedentary may be included in this group. The rate of perioperative MI or death in this group is estimated to be as high as 28% due to the hypercoagulability of the disease state compounded with surgery.[8]
2. Decompensated heart failure is defined as New York Heart Association (NYHA) functional class IV, patients with worsening symptomatic heart failure or new-onset heart failure. The NYHA functional classification is

Table 16.1 NYHA CLASSIFICATION

Class I	No limitation on physical activity; ordinary activity does not produce fatigue, palpitations, or syncope
Class II	Mild limitation of physical activity; ordinary activity results in fatigue, palpitations, or syncope
Class III	Marked limitation on physical activity; less than ordinary activity results in fatigue, palpitations, or syncope; comfortable at rest
Class IV	Unable to perform any physical activity without discomfort; symptoms at rest

Adapted from Khosla A, Cattano D. Airway assessment. In: Hagberg CA, Artime CA, Daily WH, eds. *The Difficult Airway: A Practical Guide*. New York, NY: Oxford University Press; 2013:1–8.

used to assess the severity of functional limitations and correlates fairly well with prognosis (see Table 16.1).

3. Significant arrhythmias are classified as high-grade or Mobitz type II AV block, third-degree AV block, symptomatic ventricular arrhythmias, supraventricular arrhythmias with uncontrolled ventricular rate, and symptomatic bradycardia.
4. Severe valvular disease is defined as severe aortic stenosis or symptomatic mitral stenosis. Severe aortic stenosis is classified as mean pressure gradient greater than 40 mmHg, aortic valve area less than 1.0 cm^2, or symptomatic stenosis. Symptomatic mitral stenosis is manifested as progressive dyspnea on exertion, exertional presyncope, or heart failure.

Stepwise Approach to Perioperative Cardiac Assessment

The ACC/AHA Guidelines provide a step-by-step approach to decision-making for the cardiac patient in their need for cardiac testing. The algorithm is an excellent tool for all clinicians to follow for the recommended workup, and is based on evidence collected by the Task Force.[7]

1. Step 1: Deciding the level of urgency of the case. Emergency surgery does not allow for adequate workup but should proceed with perioperative surveillance if indicated (intraoperative cardiac monitoring and postoperative serial ECGs and troponins)
2. Step 2: Determining whether the patient has any of the four active cardiac conditions discussed above. If present, the recommendation is to evaluate and treat the condition as per the ACC/AHA guidelines before proceeding to the operating room.
3. Step 3: Determining the risk stratification of the surgery. Patients undergoing low-risk surgery would rarely benefit from a cardiac intervention or change in medical management prior to surgery and can proceed with the surgery without it. Table 16.2 lists the level of risk related to specific surgeries.

Table 16.2 CARDIAC RISK STRATIFICATION FOR NONCARDIAC PROCEDURES

RISK STRATIFICATION	EXAMPLES
High: Vascular (cardiac risk > 5%)	Aortic and other major vascular surgery Peripheral vascular surgery
Intermediate (cardiac risk 1%–5%)	Intraperitoneal, Intrathoracic surgery Carotid endarterectomy Head and neck surgery Orthopedic surgery Prostate surgery
Low (cardiac risk generally < 1%)	Endoscopic procedures Superficial procedures Cataract surgery Breast surgery Ambulatory surgery

Adapted from Fleisher LA, Beckman JA, Brown KA, et al. ACC/AHA 2007 guidelines on perioperative cardiovascular evaluation and care for noncardiac surgery: executive summary: a report of the American College of Cardiology/American Heart Association Task Force on Practice Guidelines. *Circulation*. 2007;116:1971–1996.

4. Step 4: Determining the patient's exercise ability without producing any cardiac symptoms. Functional capacity is expressed by metabolic equivalents (1 MET is defined as 3.5 mL O_2 uptake/kg per min, which is the resting oxygen uptake in a sitting position). Patients with a functional capacity of greater than or equal to 4 METs without cardiac symptoms will rarely require any intervention and can proceed with the operation. Table 16.3 gives the estimated MET requirements associated with specific activities.

Table 16.3 ESTIMATED METABOLIC EQUIVALENTS OF OXYGEN CONSUMPTION

1 MET	Eat, Dress, Use the Toilet
2–3 METs	Walk Indoors, Walk a block at 2-3 mph
4 METs	Light housework (washing dishes)
4–7 METs	Climb a flight of stairs, Walk at 4 mph, Run a short distance, Do heavy house work like scrubbing floors or lifting furniture
7–10 METs	Participate in moderate physical activities such as golf, bowling, dancing, doubles tennis
>10 METs	Participate in strenuous physical activities such as swimming, singles tennis, football, basketball, or skiing

Adapted from King MS. Preoperative evaluation. *Am Fam Physician*. 2000;62:387–396; Fleisher LA, Beckman JA, Brown KA, et al. ACC/AHA 2007 guidelines on perioperative cardiovascular evaluation and care for noncardiac surgery: executive summary: a report of the American College of Cardiology/American Heart Association Task Force on Practice Guidelines. *Circulation*. 2007;116:1971–1996.

5. Step 5: Determining further workup when the patient has a poor or unknown exercise tolerance. When this situation arises, proper cardiac evaluation is based on the patient's clinical risk factors and type of surgery. Patients with three or more clinical risk factors undergoing vascular surgery should be considered for cardiac evaluation and testing if it will change the medical management. For those patients undergoing intermediate-risk surgery, noninvasive testing should only be done if it will change medical management, otherwise, they can proceed with the surgery with heart rate control. Patients with one or two clinical risk factors should only be considered for noninvasive testing if it will change medical management regardless. Patients without any clinical risk factors can proceed with surgery without further testing.

Cardiac Risk Prediction

In 1977, Dr. Lee Goldman identified nine risk factors from the preoperative evaluation that have a statistically significant correlation with a perioperative life-threatening or fatal cardiac event. He weighted each factor according to its risk. The four-group risk index gives a predicted percentage possibility for life-threatening cardiac complications. Table 16.4 lists the criteria for the risk factors with the allotted points and the predicted percentage of complications.[9,10]

Table 16.4 GOLDMAN'S CARDIAC RISK INDEX

1. History:	
a. Age > 70 years old	**5 points**
b. Myocardial Infarction within 6 months	**10 points**
2. Cardiac Exam	
a. Signs of CHF, ventricular gallop, or JVD	**11 points**
b. Significant aortic stenosis	**3 points**
3. ECG	
a. Rhythm other than sinus or PACs	**7 points**
b. 5 or more PVCs per minute	**7 points**
4. General medical condition	
PO_2 < 60 or PCO_2 > 50 mmHg; K< 3 mEq/L; HCO_3 < 20 mEq/L; BUN > 50; Creatinine > 3 g/dL; abnormal SGOT, chronic liver disease	**3 points**
5. Operation	
a. Emergency	**4 points**
b. Intraperitoneal, intrathoracic, or aortic	**3 points**
Risk Index:	**% Complications**
0–5 Points	**Class I: 1%**
6–12 Points	**Class II: 7%**
13–25 Points	**Class III: 14%**
26–53 Points	**Class IV: 78%**

Adapted from Cardiac Risk Index in Noncardiac Surgery (Goldman, et.al.) website. http://medcalc3000.com/CardiacRisk_G.htm. Published 1998–2013. Accessed June 6, 2014; Goldman L, Caldera DL, Nussbaum SR, et al. Multifactorial index of cardiac risk in noncardiac surgical procedures. *N Engl J Med.* 1977;297:845–850.

AIRWAY EVALUATION

Performing an airway assessment entails taking a full medical history, including history of previous intubations, and performing an airway-oriented physical exam.

Central to the difficult airway (DA) algorithm is the necessity of preoperatively evaluating each patient for a possible DA (Figures 16.1 and 16.2). A difficult airway is defined as the clinical situation in which a conventionally trained anesthesiologist experiences difficulty with face mask ventilation, difficulty with tracheal intubation, or both.[11] The most recent ASA Practice Guidelines for the Management of the Difficult Airway begins with assessing the patient for possible difficult bag mask ventilation, supraglottic airway placement, direct laryngoscopy, intubation, or surgical airway access. Boxes 16.2–16.5 list characteristics that predict difficulties in those areas. If there is a good possibility that any one of these techniques could be difficult, the airway should be secured while the patient is still awake.

OTHER SPECIAL CONSIDERATIONS FOR PREOPERATIVE EVALUATIONS

Upper Respiratory Infection

For the adult patient with upper respiratory infection (URI) symptoms, a detailed history to elicit severity of

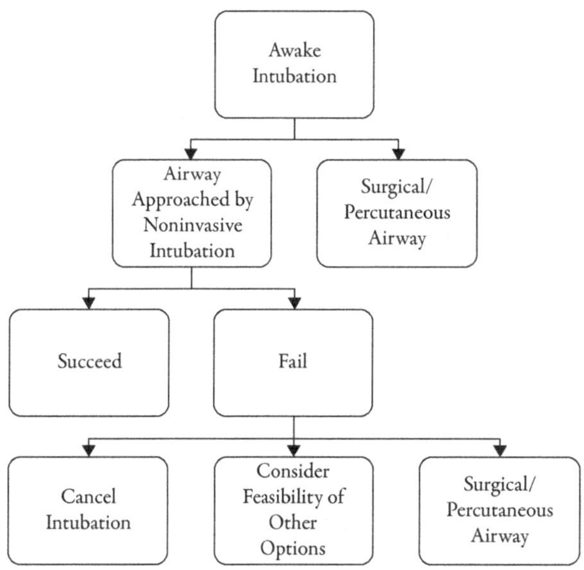

Figure 16.1 ASA difficult airway algorithm for awake intubation. Adapted from Zakaria, et al. Neurocritical Care Review, Procedural Skills and Monitoring (Williams, G). Page 409–410. Demos Medical Publishing: New York, NY. 2014.

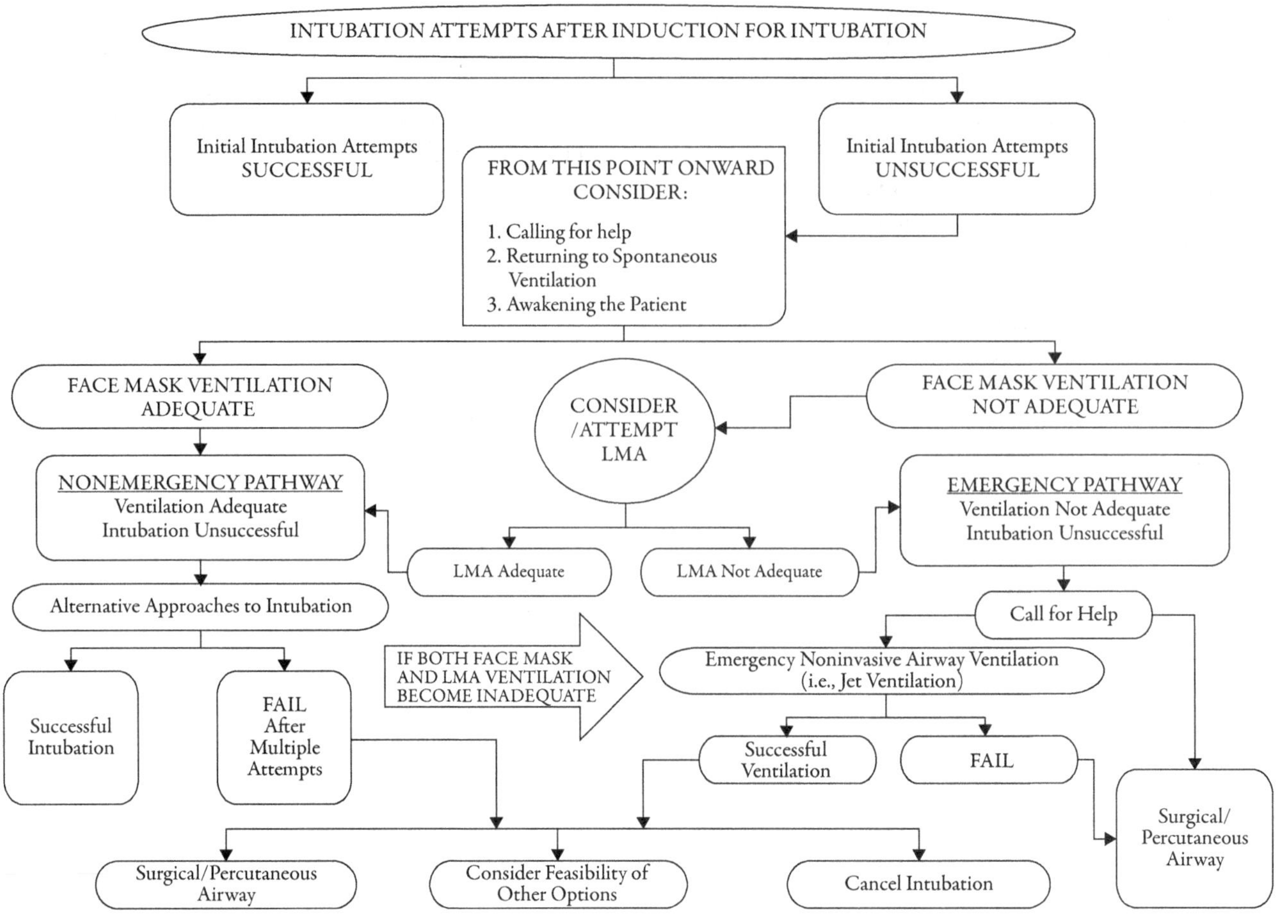

Figure 16.2 ASA difficult airway algorithm for intubation. Adapted from Zakaria, et al. Neurocritical Care Review, Procedural Skills and Monitoring (Williams, G). Page 409–410. Demos Medical Publishing: New York, NY. 2014.

the infection is important. It is prudent to cancel elective surgery for patients with severe symptoms, which include purulent secretions, productive cough, temperature higher than 38°C, or signs of pulmonary involvement. The surgery should be delayed for about 4 weeks, the time needed for airway hyperreactivity to resolve. There is very limited value for chest radiography, because positive findings usually lag behind clinical symptoms. Patients experiencing mild to moderate symptoms should be safe to proceed with surgery, but considerations for avoidance of ETT, additional postoperative pulse oximetry monitoring, and appropriate hydration to help avoid thick secretions should be instituted if possible. For pediatric patients, the Taid and Malviya algorithm for children with URI symptoms is a great tool for decision-making.[3]

Box 16.2 PREDICTORS OF DIFFICULT BAG-MASK VENTILATION

Age > 55 years

BMI > 26 kg/m^2

Lack of teeth

Presence of beard or mustache

History of snoring or diagnosis of OSA

+2 risk factors indicate difficult BMV

Adapted from Khosla A, Cattano D. Airway assessment. In: Hagberg CA, Artime CA, Daily WH, eds. *The Difficult Airway: A Practical Guide.* New York, NY: Oxford University Press; 2013:1–8.

Box 16.3 PREDICTORS OF DIFFICULT INTUBATION

Previous history of difficult intubation

Long upper incisors

Overbite

Limited TMJ movement

Limited mouth opening (<3cm)

Reduced neck extension

Short thyromental distance (<2 finger breadths)

Mallampati II or IV classification

Short, thick neck

Adapted from Henderson J. Airway assessment. In: Miller RD, ed. *Miller's Anesthesia*. Philadelphia, PA: Churchill Livingstone Elsevier; 2010:1573–1607.

Box 16.4 PREDICTORS OF DIFFICULT SUPRAGLOTTIC AIRWAY (SGA) PLACEMENT

Limited airway opening

Large incisors

Intraoral or pharyngeal tumor/pathology

Reduced atlantoaxial movement

Adapted from Campo SL, Denman WT. The LMA: it's role in the difficult airway. *Int Anesthesiol Clin*. 2000;38:29–45.

Obstructive Sleep Apnea

Obstructive sleep apnea (OSA) is a syndrome characterized by periodic, partial or complete obstruction of the upper airway during sleep, which results in arousal to restore airway patency. Preoperative evaluation of a patient with suspected OSA should occur prior to the day of surgery with enough time to initiate proper workup and treatment before the surgery. The preoperative evaluation of a patient with suspected OSA should begin with a comprehensive review of the medical records including airway difficulty, BMI (>35 kg/m^2), cardiovascular problems, and other medical conditions. If a sleep study is available, it is important to review the study to determine the patient's classification of OSA: mild, moderate, or severe. If a sleep study is not available, a patient and family interview to identify presence of OSA should be performed by inquiring about loud snoring with frequent pauses or arousals from sleep. Other important symptoms include daytime somnolence and easily falling asleep despite adequate sleep. Finally, a focused physical exam on neck circumference (>17 inches in men or >16 inches in women), midline or touching tonsils, craniofacial abnormalities of the airway, and large tongue size can reveal factors predisposing a patient to OSA. If a diagnosis of OSA is suspected, the anesthesiologist and surgeon should consider obtaining a sleep study and initiate OSA treatment within advanced timing of the surgery.

The extensive preparation and evaluation of a patient with OSA is focused on improving outcomes on these patients who will receive sedation and analgesics. It is highly recommended that patients with severe OSA undergo a period of CPAP (or NIPPV) treatments prior to the surgery. A specific postoperative management plan should be considered preoperatively and be in place in order to avoid the potential for respiratory depression, more commonly present in patients with OSA receiving sedation or narcotics due to airway collapse and sleep deprivation.[12]

Box 16.5 PREDICTORS OF DIFFICULT SURGICAL AIRWAY

Neck anatomy that is distorted due to trauma or pathology

Fixed or limited neck extension

Previous radiation to neck area

Large, thick neck

Adapted from Vissers RJ, Bair AE. Surgical airway management. In: Wall RM, Murphy MF, eds. *Manual of Emergency Airway Management*. Philadelphia, PA: Lippincott Williams & Wilkins; 2012:193–218.

Do-Not-Resuscitate Orders

It is important to review with the patient or designated caregiver any do-not-resuscitate (DNR) orders prior to proceeding with anesthesia. The nature of administering anesthesia involves interventions that can be viewed as "resuscitation." During the preoperative evaluation, a conversation needs to involve the patient's desires regarding interventions or treatments. There are three options for the patient in regard to their DNR order: full suspension of directives, limited resuscitation with regard to specific interventions, or limited resuscitation with regard to the patient's values. Full attempt at resuscitation removes the preexisting DNR orders during the surgery and in the immediate postoperative period. Limiting resuscitation with regard to specific procedures allows the patient to refuse specific interventions such as chest compressions. Limiting resuscitation with regard to the patient's values means the patient wishes the anesthesiologist to use their best clinical judgment to align with the patient's goals. This generally means that the anesthesiologist can use the necessary interventions to manage an event if it can be resolved without long-term sequelae. All of these items should be documented in the patient's medical record. Even if an institution has a policy of suspending DNRs for the operating room, it is still prudent to understand the desires and values of the patient.[13]

ALLERGIES

Allergies are classically defined as an immune response to an antigen. These hypersensitivity responses can be classified into four basic types. Type I reactions are anaphylactic or immediate hypersensitivity reactions. Active mediators are released from mast cells and basophils after binding to IgE. Examples include anaphylaxis, extrinsic asthma, or allergic rhinitis. Type II reactions are antibody-dependent cell-mediated cytotoxic reactions, which are IgG or IgM mediated; these cause either direct cell lysis, increased phagocytosis by macrophages, or increased killer T-lymphocytes. Examples include ABO-incompatible transfusion reactions, drug-induced immune hemolytic anemia, or heparin-induced thrombocytopenia. Type III reactions are immune complex reactions due to soluble antigens and antibodies depositing in the microvasculature. Examples include classic serum sickness from snake antivenom or antithymocyte globulin or immune complex injury. Type IV reactions are delayed hypersensitivity reactions and where sensitized lymphocytes react with specific antigens. These typically manifest in 18 to 24 hours, peak in 40 to 80 hours, and resolve in 72 to 90 hours. Examples include tissue transplant rejection, graft-versus host reactions, or contact dermatitis.

Intraoperative allergic reactions occur in 1 in 5,000 to 25,000 anesthetics, with a mortality rate of 3.4%. More than 90% of reactions occur within 5 minutes, with the most common life-threatening complication being circulatory arrest, which may only be manifested by refractory hypotension. Allergic drug reactions account for 6%–10% of all adverse reactions. Common antigenic agents administered during anesthesia include muscle relaxants, latex, antibiotics, blood products, and colloid volume expanders.

Patients often refer to adverse drug effects as allergies. Predictable adverse drug reactions occur in 80% of the adverse drug effects. Evaluation of a patient with an allergic reaction often starts with an initial history and physical. There are several tests for potential allergens, which include the leukocyte histamine release test, the radioallergosorbent test (RAST) through the detection of specific IgE toward particular allergens, the enzyme-linked immunosorbant assay (ELISA) through antigen-specific antibodies, and the intradermal test (skin test). Unfortunately, these tests do not exist for most anesthetic drugs.

Management of an allergic reaction can be divided into two stages. The initial therapy involves discontinuation of the antigen, maintenance of the airway, administration of oxygen, discontinuation of anesthetic agents, volume expansion (~2–4 liters), and epinephrine (5- to 10-microgram boluses as needed). After the initial treatment, antihistamines (0.5–1 mg/kg diphenhydramine), possible catecholamine infusions such as epinephrine and norepinephrine, bronchodilators (i.e., albuterol), corticosteroids (hydrocortisone or methylprednisolone), and vasopressin for refractory shock are commonly administered. An airway evaluation should also take place.

NPO GUIDELINES

For elective surgery, the ASA recommendations for NPO Guidelines are 2 hours for clear liquids, 4 hours for breast milk, 6 hours for solids and formula (for infants), 6 hours for a light meal, and 8 hours for a heavy meal that includes fried or fatty foods (see Figure 16.3). This may be modified for long-standing diabetes (reduced gastric motility) and other factors that increase risk for aspiration. However, ingestion of clear liquids 2–3 hours prior to surgery reduces irritability, thirst, and hunger. Additionally some studies suggest this may decrease the gastric volume and increase gastric pH.

"FULL STOMACH"

Patients who have not followed the NPO guidelines are considered to have a full stomach. Additionally, patients with incompetent gastroesophageal sphincters are at risk for pulmonary aspiration. Those at risk include pregnant women, diabetics; others with gastroparesis, hemorrhage, or obstruction; those requiring emergency surgery; those with gastroesophageal reflux disease; or those who have recently eaten or are experiencing nausea. Especially at risk are patients presenting with acute trauma.

Anesthetic Management Implications

Patients with a full stomach are at risk for aspiration under general anesthesia and as such require either rapid-sequence intubation with cricoid pressure in patients without serious airway deformity, or awake intubation with sedation and topical anesthesia, or avoidance of a general anesthetic altogether. In rapid-sequence intubation, the intravenous induction agent is given immediately followed by a rapidly acting neuromuscular blocking drug. Laryngoscopy and intubation are performed as soon as possible. Cricoid pressure (Sellick maneuver) is performed at the start of induction until confirmation of correct endotracheal tube placement. The pressure is downward displacement of the cricoid cartilage against the vertebral bodies. It is contraindicated in active vomiting (risk of esophageal rupture), cervical spine fracture, and laryngeal fracture. If intubation is difficult and desaturation occurs, gentle positive pressure ventilation can be used.

Prior to induction, gastric emptying can be increased with a prokinetic agent such as metaclopromide, gastric volume reduced through suctioning a nasogastric tube, and acidity reduced through a nonparticulate antacid such as sodium citrate (Bicitra), H2 receptor antagonist such as famotidine, and proton pump inhibitor such as lansoprazole. Induction is rapid sequence with cricoid pressure. Either a cuffed endotracheal tube, a combitube, or a proSeal laryngeal mask airway (LMA) (or its equivalent, such as an LMA supreme) is placed.

Gastric Emptying

Gastric emptying time is most rapid for clear liquids, slower for milk than clear liquids, and for human break

2 hours	4 hours	6 hours	8 hours
Clear liquids	Breast Milk (only choice in this category)	Formula, Light Meal	Heavy meal, Fried foods

Figure 16.3 NPO guidelines.

milk, faster than cow milk. Pregnancy and diabetes reduce the rate of gastric emptying. In diabetes this corresponds well with the onset of autonomic neuropathy, which can increase gastric emptying time by as much as 30 minutes to 2 hours.

COMMON CHRONIC MEDICATIONS

Patients often present with chronic medications, which often have anesthetic side effects. Often patients require such medications for their chronic medical conditions, and their interruption or continuation may have implications for their disease control.

ANTIHYPERTENSIVES

The angiotensin-converting enzyme (ACE) inhibitors block conversion of ACE and the renin-angiotensin-aldosterone system. Both ACE inhibitors and angiotensin receptor blockers (ARBs) have been known to cause refractory hypotension under general anesthesia requiring vasopressin.

ANTIANGINAL MEDICATIONS

Major classes of antianginal agents are nitrates, beta blockers, calcium channel blockers, and aspirin. The side effects of these medications are typically mild hypotension under general anesthesia, though not as profound as that seen with ACE inhibitiors. Nitrate administration after sidenifil is contraindicated due to an increased risk of hypotension.

ANTIHYPERGLYCEMIC MEDICATIONS

Treatment of diabetes usually consists of diet, oral hypoglycemic drugs, exercise, and exogenous insulin. Insulin is prepared in either pork, beef, human, or recombinant sources and can be either short acting, intermediate acting, or long acting. Perioperative glucose management depends on glucose monitoring. There are different protocols for insulin management. Miller recommends discontinuation of long-acting insulin and oral hypoglycemics 1–2 days preoperatively. On the day of surgery, a glucose-containing solution (2 mg/kg/min) is started at the normal time a meal would be eaten, then an insulin infusion at 0.5–1.25 units/h started for those on insulin. Glucose is to be checked every hour and infusion titrated. For patients who have diet-controlled diabetes and a short procedure, glucose is checked perioperatively and then every 3 hours until oral intake is resumed.

ANTIDEPRESSANTS

MAO is an enzyme that important in degradation of catecholamines. An MAO inhibitor (MAOI) binds irreversibly with the enzyme and increases the amine concentration at the presynaptic terminal.

Chronic MAOI use causes antihypertensive, antidepressive, and antinarcoleptic effects. The antihypertensive effect is by blocking breakdown of tyramine, which is then converted in the periphery to octopamine, which has a weaker effect than norepinephrine. The MAOIs are primarily used in psychiatry as antidepressants on the theory that depression is caused by decreased amine levels in the CNS. There are two forms of MAOIs, A—which acts on the 5-HT—epinephrine, norepinephrine, tyramine, dopamine; and B—tyramine and dopamine. Drug and food reactions are the great concern for patients taking MAOIs. Tyramine-containing foods such as red wine and aged cheese can lead to hypertensive crisis, while the sedative effects with alcohol, sedatives, and general anesthesia are cumulative. Meperidine can lead to hyperpyrexic coma and death. Interactions with tricyclic antidepressants can be disastrous. Recommendation is at least 2 weeks of discontinuation before elective procedures, although there is a controversy if there is no other effective medication available. In addition, tricyclic antidepressants have antihistaminic, anticholinergic, and sedative properties and slow cardiac conduction. Centrally acting anticholingerics combined with tricyclics can increase postoperative delirium. Lithium prolongs the action of neuromuscular blocking drugs and of benzodiazepines and barbiturates (in high doses).

ANTIPLATELET AGENTS

Patients with ischemic cardiac disease, especially after stent placement, are placed on platelet inhibitors (adenosine diphosphate [ADP] receptor inhibitors and glycoprotein IIb/IIIa receptor inhibitors). There is controversy over their application in the surgical population secondary to the increased risk of bleeding. Clopidigrel, in multiple studies, has been associated with increased risk for bleeding; however, in one small study, increased bleeding did occur in association with clopidigrel administration. A long-acting GP inhibitor, abixicimab, has been shown to increase bleeding, but shorter acting ones in the PURSUIT study did not.

PROPHYLACTIC ANTIBIOTICS

Surgical site infections (SSIs) are the second most common hospital-acquired infections. The anesthesiologist has the ability to control factors that are involved in SSIs, including timing and administration of antibiotics. The anesthesiologist must administer the antibiotic so that the blood and tissue concentrations of the antibiotic exceed the minimum inhibitory concentrations (MIC) of the bacteria likely to cause infection.

As a general concept, antibiotic prophylaxis should cover the organisms contained within the layers of tissue that are expected to be surgically incised (see Figure 16.4). For

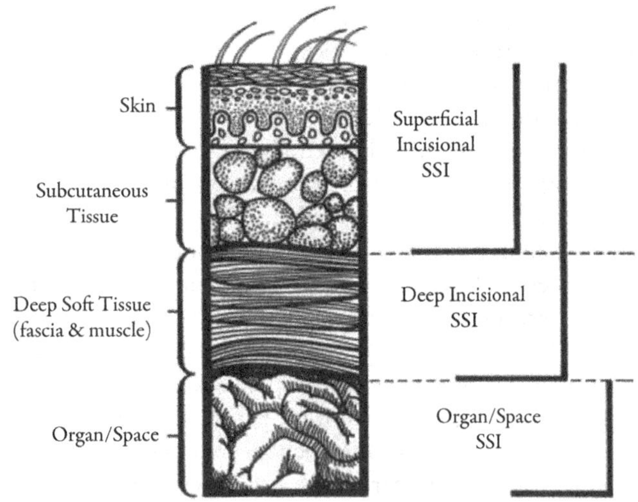

Figure 16.4 Cross-section of abdominal wall depicting CDC classifications of surgical site infection. Source: Healthcare Infection Control Practices Advisory Committee (HICPAC). Centers for Disease Control and Prevention website. http://www.cdc.gov/hicpac/SSI/figure-SSI.html. Accessed March 26, 2015.

example, in "clean" procedures, cefazolin is the antibiotic of choice because common skin microbes are killed by this antibiotic, thus reducing the likelihood of an SSI. Conversely, surgeries involving the intestines will require Gram-negative coverage and anaerobic coverage with antibiotics such as cefoxitin or cefotetan. Methicillin resistant staphylococcus aureus (MRSA) colonization should have vancomycin for prophylaxis. Cefazolin should be given 1 hour prior to surgical incision. Vancomycin should be given over 120 minutes to prevent "red man syndrome," and all antibiotics should be discontinued after 24 hours. If a tourniquet is to be used, antibiotics should be given prior to tourniquet inflation. Patients with allergies to beta-lactams should be given clindamycin or vancomycin in clean procedures. The National Surgical Infection Prevention Project—which included the Centers for Disease Control, Medicare, and surgical (American College of Surgeons) and anesthesia (American Society of Anesthesiologists) societies—recommends antibiotics for different surgical procedures.

Prophylactic Cardiac Risk Reduction

Administration of beta-adrenergic agents may reduce the risk of perioperative myocardial ischemia. The POISE trial, a landmark study evaluating the perioperative administration of beta-adrenergic blockers, demonstrated a 27% reduction in the MI rate, but an increased rate of 30-day all-cause mortality and stroke. This shows the administration of beta-adrenergic agents to be potentially both beneficial and dangerous. Current AHA guidelines recommend perioperative beta blockade as a Class I indication for patients previously receiving beta blockers, for those undergoing vascular surgery, for those who are at high cardiac risk, or for patients with a finding of cardiac ischemia on testing. In addition to beta blockers, other medications have been found to be helpful in prophylactic cardiac risk reduction, such as alpha-2 agonists (clonidine), statins, and calcium channel blockers. Nitroglycerin is not indicated as prophylaxis.

Risks of Administration

Vancomycin can cause "Red Man's Syndrome," characterized by a rash and hypotension, when given over 15 minutes and rarely occurring when given over 1–2 hours. It is important to note that a history of Red Man's Syndrome with vancomycin administration should not be considered a true allergy. Rapid and high dose infusion of gentamicin can cause hearing loss.

Drug Interactions

All antibiotics, with the exception of cephalosporins and erythromycin, can prolong the effects of neuromuscular blockers. Erythromycin (macrolide antibiotics) can inhibit the cytochrome P450 system and cause a prolonged effect from benzodiazepines.

PREOEPRATIVE ASSESSMENT

Comprehensive preoperative evaluation and management improves patient satisfaction and reduces perioperative mortality and morbidity. A preanesthesia visit should include a thorough anamnesis that reviews medications, allergies, comorbid conditions, and previous operations; a complete physical examination; an assignment of ASA score; necessary diagnostic exams; and discussion of the planned anesthesia.

VARIABILITY IN DRUG RESPONSE

There is a wide variability in the response of different patients to identical doses of the same drug. Drugs do not always produce the same effect in all subjects and may not even produce identical responses when given to the same patient on different occasions. The principal causes of variability in drug responses are physiological and pathological conditions (i.e., age, tobacco use, liver or renal disease).

DRUG INTERACTIONS

Drug interactions in anesthetic practice may occur between preexisting drug therapy and general (intravenous and inhalational) or local anesthetic agents, analgesics, muscle relaxants, and drugs used for premedication. Interactions may also occur between anesthetic agents and their adjuvant.

In vivo interactions with general anesthetics may occur and involve:

- Drugs with respiratory depressant properties (i.e., nitrous oxide, see Table 16.5): Influence the inhalational

Table 16.5 DRUGS WITH RESPIRATORY DEPRESSANT PROPERTIES

DRUG	CLINICAL USE	PROPERTIES	ADVERSE EFFECT	INTERACTION WITH ANESTHETIC DRUG
Nitrous Oxide (NO)	Potent analgesic Inhalational anesthestic	High diffusing capacity High solubility in blood Rapid induction and recovery	↓ myocardial contractility ↑ cerebral blood flow→↑ICP ↑POVN ↑PVR in patients with preexisting pulmonary hypertension ↑size air-filled spaces (high solubility in blood)→diffusion hypoxia Inhibits methionine synthetase→megaloblatic bone marrow changes with prolonged use. Peripheral neuropathy with prolonged use Possible teratogenic effect. Supports combustion→↑risk fires	↑uptake and ↓MAC of other inhalational agents

anesthetic metabolism, uptake, distribution, and elimination. The minimum alveolar concentration (MAC) value of many fluorinated agents, which reflects their potency in steady-state conditions, is reduced with the concomitant use of diazepam, opioid analgesics, hypnotics, tranquilizers, antidepressants, and certain antihypertensive agents.

- Antiarrhythmic and antianginal agents (Table 16.6): should always be continued until the immediate preoperative period to avoid the rebound phenomena (worsening of angina or reonset of arrhythmias), as the latter's risks far outweigh those of the drug interactions during anesthesia.
- Sympathomimetic amines (Table 16.7):
  Interactions with anesthetic drugs are mainly when administered during surgery. Arrhythmias induced by sympathomimetic amines during inhalational anaesthesia can usually be controlled by beta blockers.

ANTIHYPERTENSIVE AGENTS

Many anesthetic drugs cause hypotension. Perioperative hypotension risk is higher in treated hypertensive patients than in normotensive subjects. However, such adverse effects can be prevented by adjusting the drug dosage and closely monitoring the circulating volume and blood pressure (e.g., an intravenous infusion should be considered for all patients who are receiving ACE inhibitors prior to induction of anesthesia). In treating hypertensive patients, inhalational agents (which have negative inotropic and peripheral resistance effects) may lead to exaggerated falls in systemic blood pressure (e.g., sevoflurane lowers blood pressure and may interact with alpha or beta blockers or with other drugs that can produce vasodilation. In addition, induction agents in such patients can induce severe hypotension during general anesthesia or postural hypotension on recovery.

There are several drugs that modify electrolyte balance, see Table 16.8 to review these agents.

Muscle Relaxants

Volatile anesthetic agents increase the neuromuscular block induced by nondepolarizing muscle relaxants and induce dual block when patients are concomitantly receiving repeated doses of succinylcholine.

Cytochrome P450

Cytochrome P450 is responsible for metabolizing many of the anesthetic and other drugs that undergo liver metabolism. Many drugs influence cytochrome P450 by inducing *or* inhibiting its activity. The inducing drugs lead to acceleration of liver metabolism of many drugs, making it necessary to increase the dose of affected drugs in order to obtain the same therapeutic effect. The inhibitors inhibit liver metabolism of many drugs, leading to their dose increase in the blood and making it necessary to decrease the dose given to avoid toxicity. Barbiturates, phenytoin, carbamazepine, rifampicin, griseofulvin, alcohol (chronic consumption), and polycyclic hydrocarbons (tobacco smoke, grilled meat) all induce cytochrome P450. Imidazoles (cimetidine, etomidate, ketoconazole, omeprazole), amiodarone, macrolide antibiotics (erythromycin, clarithromycin), antidepressants, HIV protease inhibitors, ciclosporin, gestodene, and grapefruit juice all inhibit cytochrome P450.

NEPHROTOXIC AGENTS

There are many anesthetic (e.g., sevoflurane) and other drugs (e.g., aminoglycoside) with nephrotoxic effects. Their concomitant use can lead to kidney damage (including the formation of compound A, which is nephrotoxic, hepatotoxic, and cardiotoxic). See Table 16.9 for preoperative considerations with regard to outpatient cardiovascular drugs,

Table 16.6 ANTIARRHYTHMIC AND ANTIANGINAL AGENTS

DRUG	CLINICAL USE	MECHANISM OF ACTION AND CHARACTERISTICS	ADVERSE EFFECT	INTERACTION WITH ANESTHETIC DRUGS
Nitrates	Angina CHF MI	Venous dilation at normal therapeutic doses. Arteriosus and venous dilation at higher doses.	Systemic hypotension Reflex tachycardia	
β-adrenoceptor antagonists	Angina Antihypertensive Antiarrhythmic	Bind to β-adrenoceptors→ inhibit epinephrine & norepinephrine such adrenoreceptors→inhibit sympathetic effect	Bradycardia: Severe bradyarrhythmia → ↓BP	Inhalational agents and propranolol→ ↓liver blood flow.
Calcium channel blockers	Angina Antihypertensive Antiarrhythmic	Disrupt movement of Ca+2 through Ca+2 channels Inhibit Ca2+ entry into excitable cells Two types: Dihydropyridine and non-dihydropyridine CCB.	Headache, constipation, rash, nausea, flushing, edema (fluid accumulation in tissues), drowsiness, low blood pressure, and dizziness	*Verapamil and diltiazem,→heart block, which may be enhanced by inhalational anesthesia * Many volatile anesthetic agents have significant calcium channel-blocking activity or interfere with the mobilization of intracellular Ca2+→ additive and synergistic effects may occur leading to intraoperative hypotension
Amiodarone	Antiarrhythmic III class.	Inhibits adrenergic stimulation ↓A-V conduction and sinus node function ↑PR, QRS, and QT intervals α & β adrenergic blockade. Long elimination half-life	Bradyarrhythmias Complete AV block Pacemaker dependence in cardiosurgery patients who receive various anesthetic regimes Ventricular arrhythmias Liver and thyroid function test abnormalities Hepatitis/cirrhosis Pulmonary fibrosis (with prolonged use)	Anesthetic drugs and Amiodarone→ additive effects due its long t/2. Inhibits cytochrome P450→ increases serum levels of digoxin, oral anticoagulants, diltiazem, quinidine, procainamide, and phenytoin

Table 16.7 SYMPATHOMIMETIC AMINES

DRUGS	CLINICAL USE	MECHANISM OF ACTION AND PROPERTIES	ADVERSE EFFECT	INTERACTION WITH ANESTHETIC DRUGS
Cocaine	Promote mucosal surface anesthesia and vasoconstriction in ENT surgery	Inhibits the reuptake of noradrenaline Sympathomimetic amines with β-adrenergic activity	Dependence, irritability, paranoia, restlessness, anxiety	May precipitate dangerous or fatal tachyarrhythmias during inhalational anesthesia
Ephedrine	Hypotension, Nasal congestion Bronchospasm.	α- and β-adrenergic stimulation→norepinephrine release at sympathetic nerve endings (indirect).	Hypertension, dysrhythmias, myocardial ischemia, CNS stimulation, decrease in uterine activity.	Greater propensity to induce arrhythmogenic effects than directly acting catecholamines
Ketamine	Sedation Hypnotic	Blocks polysynaptic reflexes in the spinal cord, inhibiting excitatory neurotransmitter effects Dissociates thalamus from limbic cortex→ dissociative anesthesia Central sympathomimetic stimulation→↑ catecholamine levels	↑salivation Emergency Delirium ↑ICP Myoclonic movements Eyes: glaucoma, nystagmus, diplopia.	Nondepolarizing muscle relaxants are potentiated by ketamine
Theophylline	Asthma Bronchospasm Infantile apneic spells	Inhibits phosphodiesterase→bronch odilation and positive inotropic and chronotropic effects CNS stimulant Increase anesthetic requirements and MAC values	Nausea & vomiting Anorexia Dizziness Headaches Agitation, Tachyarrhythmias Ventric arrhythmias Palpitations Convulsions ↓BP & ↑RR	The use of ketamine, concomitantly with Theophylline→ Tachyarrhythmias and seizures
Levodopa	Parkinson Hypertension (in pregnancy)	Its decarboxylation produces dopamine (responsible for adverse effects)	Tachyarrhythmias Vasoconstriction	Cardiovascular dose-related effects.

Table 16.8 DRUGS THAT MODIFY ELECTROLYTE BALANCE

DRUGS	CLINICAL USE	MECHANISM OF ACTION AND PROPERTIES	ADVERSE EFFECT	INTERACTION WITH ANESTHETIC DRUGS
Digitalis	CHF Ventricular heart rate control in atrial fib/flutter PSVT.	**Positive inotropic**: inhibition of the Na/K ATPase pump→↑intracellular Na-Ca exchange→↑ intracellular calcium→↑contractility); **Neg. chronotropic**: direct suppression of AV node conduction→↑effective refractory period and ↓conduction velocity).	Mental depression, confusion, headaches, drowsiness, anorexia, nausea, vomiting, weakness, visual disturbances, delirium, EKG abnormalities (arrhythmias) and seizures.	Interacts with drugs that lower K^+ (most diuretics, corticosteroids, insulin), inducing supraventricular or ventricular ectopic beats during inhalational anesthesia
Potassium-sparing diuretics (spironolactone)	CHF Hypertension Hypokalemia Acne Vulgaris	Competitive binding of receptors at aldosterone-dependent Na-K exchange site in distal tubules→↑excretion of Na+, Cl-, and H2O and retention of K+ and H+	skin rash, headache, dizziness, and GI symptoms of nausea, vomiting, gas, and stomach pain	Risk of potentially fatal hyperkalemia in severe CHF patients
calcitonin	Osteoporosis (especially in bisphosphonate intolerance) Hypercalcemia	Lower calcium by: *Inhibits Ca^{2+} absorption by the intestines *Inhibits osteoclast activity in bones *Stimulates osteoblastic activity in bones. *Inhibits renal tubular cell reabsorption of Ca^{2+} allowing it to be excreted in the urine	Runny nose. Nasal discomfort, sores, or redness. Nosebleeds.	Depress cardiac contractility→ cardiac arrhythmias

Table 16.9 PREOPERATIVE CONSIDERATIONS

DRUG CLASS	CLINICAL CONSIDERATIONS	SURGERY WITH BRIEF NPO STATE	SURGERY WITH PROLONGED NPO STATE
Beta Blockers	Withdrawal can cause HTN	Continue during surgery	Continue during surgery
α2 Antagonists	Withdrawal can cause HTN	Continue during surgery	Continue during surgery
Calcium Channel Blockers	Slight increased risk of bleeding	Continue during surgery	Continue during surgery
ACE Inhibitors	Possible hypotension	Continue during surgery	Continue during surgery
Diuretics	Possible hypovolemia and hypotension	Continue up to day of surgery and hold that morning	Continue up to day of surgery and hold that morning
Statins	Slight risk of myopathy	Continue during surgery	Continue up to day of surgery

Box 16.6 for preoperative chronic drug considerations, and Table 16.10 for a list of anesthetic agents and their side effects.

SPECIFIC PROBLEMS IN DISEASE STATES

The following is a review of a variety of diagnoses, most of which tend to have highly particular and important implications for intraoperative care.

Hyperthyroidism and Hypothyroidism

All elective surgery should be postponed until the hyperthyroid patient is rendered euthyroid via medical treatment. Preoperative assessment should include normal thyroid function tests and a resting heart rate of less than 85 beats/min. Avoid ketamine, pancuronium, indirect-acting adrenergic agonists, and other sympathomimetic agents in hyperthyroid patients.

Mild to moderate hypothyroidism (Box 16.7) is not an absolute contraindication to surgery. Ketamine is the induction agent of choice in these patients. Such patients should be treated with histamine H_2 blockers and metoclopramide, because of slow gastric emptying times. See Table 16.11 for laboratory values in hypothyroidism.

GLAUCOMA

Normal intraocular pressure is maintained between 10 and 20 mmHg. The aqueous humor normally flows in and out of the eye through a drainage system at the angle where the iris and the cornea meet. When the drainage system is blocked, the fluid cannot filter out of the eye at its normal rate, and pressure builds up within the eye. Most anesthetic drugs either lower or have no effect on intraocular pressure. Ketamine and possibly etomidate increase intraocular pressure. In addition, succinylcholine can cause a 5- to 10-mmHg increase in intraocular pressure for 5–10 minutes.

Box 16.6 PREOPERATIVE CHRONIC DRUGS CONSIDERATION

Continue on the Day of the Operation

Antidepressant, antianxiety, and psychiatric medications

Antihypertensive medications, except angiotensin-converting enzyme inhibitors or angiotensin receptor-blocking agents, which may be selectively discontinued on the day of the operation

Antiseizure medications

Asthma medications

Birth control pills

Cardiac medications (e.g. digoxin)

Diuretics, such as triamterene or hydrochlorothiazide, for hypertension

Heartburn or reflux medications

Insulin—all intermediate, combination, and long-acting insulins

- Type 1 diabetics should take a small amount (usually one-third) of their usual morning long-acting insulin (e.g., lente or NPH) on the day of the operation
- Type 2 diabetics should take none or up to one-half of long-acting or combination (70/30 preparations) insulins on the day of the operation
- Patients with an insulin pump should continue only their basal rate on the day of the operation

Narcotic pain medications

Ophthalmic drops

Statins

Steroids, oral or inhaled

Thyroid medications

Cyclooxygenase-2 inhibitors, unless surgeon is concerned about bone healing

Box 16.6 CONTINUED

Discontinue 7 Days Before the Operation

Aspirin, except for vascular patients and patients having cataract surgery

Clopidogrel (Plavix), except for vascular patients and patients having cataract surgery

Herbals and nonvitamin supplements

Hormone replacement therapy

Discontinue 4 Days Before the Operation

Warfarin (Coumadin), except for patients having cataract surgery without a bulbar block

Discontinue 48 Hours Before the Operation

Nonsteroidal anti-inflammatory drugs

Discontinue 24 Hours Before the Operation

Erectile dysfunction medications

Discontinue on the Day of the Operation

Diuretics, except triamterene or hydrochlorothiazide for hypertension, which should be continued

Insulin—all regular insulins

- Type 1 diabetics should take a small amount (usually one-third) of their usual morning long-acting insulin (e.g., lente or NPH) on the day of the operation
- Type 2 diabetics should take none or up to one-half of long-acting or combination (70/30 preparations) insulins on the day of the operation
- Patients with an insulin pump should continue only their basal rate on the day of the operation

Iron

Oral hypoglycemic agents

Topical medications (e.g., creams or ointments)

Vitamins

Special Considerations Before the Operation

Monoamine oxidase inhibitors—patients taking these antidepressant medications need an anesthesia consultation before the operation (preferably 3 weeks before).

Patients should take medications with a small sip of water even if otherwise nothing by mouth (NPO).

UREMIA

Uremia is the terminal clinical manifestation of renal failure, with accumulation in the blood of toxic nitrogenous substances (protein metabolism end products, such as urea and creatinine) that are normally expelled by the healthy kidney. In addition, fluid buildup (edema) and electrolyte/hormone imbalances are commonly seen in uremic patients. Cisatracurium and atracurium are the muscle relaxants of choice in these patients, as renal function is generally impaired. Use fluids cautiously and avoid potassium-containing fluids in anuric patients. Succinylcholine may be used safely only if serum potassium is not elevated (potassium generally increases by 0.5–1 meq/L when succinylcholine is administered). If postoperative hypertension due to fluid overload occurs, postoperative dialysis is required.

INCREASED CEREBROSPINAL FLUID PRESSURE

The skull of an adult is in effect a rigid box that contains brain tissue (1400–1500 g), blood (100–150 mL), cerebrospinal fluid (110–120 mL), and extracellular fluid (less than 100 mL). Thus, an increase in the volume of one component invariably results in an increase in intracranial pressure (ICP) unless the volume of another component decreases (Monroe-Kellie hypothesis). Normal ICP is 10–12 mmHg, and cerebrospinal fluid is produced at 400–500 cc/day. The cranium can absorb an additional 100–150 cc fluid before ICP begins to rise. An increase in ICP has an impact on cerebral perfusion pressure, or CCP (CCP = MAP- [ICP + CVP]), and can cause cerebral herniation (central, cingulate, and uncal herniation). Causes of increased ICP include mass lesions (tumors, abscess), impaired drainage (acquired and congenital hydrocephalus), and volume increases (subarachnoid or subdural hemorrhage, cerebral edema). Perfusion is maintained until the CPP falls below 50 mmHg, with the onset of critical ischemia at 30–40 mmHg.

CHRONIC STEROIDS

Steroid treatment longer than 1 month within the past 6–12 months is considered chronic steroid use. If the standing dose is >10 mg prednisone/day (or equivalent), to avoid adrenal insufficiency, consider:

1. For major surgery: give daily dose with premedications, cortisol 25 mg IV on induction, then 100 mg IV by infusion over the next 24 hours. Resume daily dose postoperatively.
2. For minor surgery: give usual daily dose with premedications and cortisol 25 mg IV on induction. Resume daily dose postoperatively.

It should be noted that the administration of perioperative steroids is a source of great debate currently, and as such clinical practice may differ from what is described above or in classic teaching.

Table 16.10 AGENTS AND THEIR SIDE EFFECTS

DRUG	ROUTE	ADULT (MG)	PEDIATRIC (MG/KG)	ONSET (MIN)	SIDE EFFECTS
Pentobarbital	PO PR IM	150–200	2–4 3 2–6	10–30 15–60 10–15	Hypotension, somnolence, pain at injection site, confusion, lightheadedness, respiratory depression, dependence.
Methohexital (Brevital)	IM PR	150–200	5–10 20–35	5–20 5–20	Hypotension, hiccups, coughing, muscle twitching, myoclonic activity, nausea, vomiting, respiratory depression, sedation, seizures, tachycardia, thrombophlebitis, pain on injection.
Ketamine	IV IM IN PO	0.25–1 mg/kg 2–3 mg/kg	0.25–1 2–3 5–6 6–10	1–2 5–10 5–10 10	See above
Fentanyl	IV OFTC	12.5–100	0.01–0.02 0.015–0.02	1–3 5–15	Miosis Nausea and vomiting
Sufentanyl	IN		0.0015–0.003	5	Respiratory depression and cough suppression
Morphine	IM	5–15	0.05–0.02		Bradycardia and ↓cardiac contractility (more with meperidine)
Meperidine	IM	25–100	1–1.5		Biliary colic (spasm of sphincter of Oddi—less with meperidine) Muscle rigidity Histamine release (only morphine and meperidine)→itchiness, ↓SVR, hypotension & ↑HR Urinary retention Cross the placenta→neonatal depression
Phenergan	IM	12.5–50	0.25–0.1	15–20	Tremor (uncontrolled shaking), drooling, trouble swallowing, problems with balance or walking, high fever, stiff muscles, confusion, sweating, fast or uneven heartbeats, rapid breathing
Diphenhydramine (Benadryl)	PO IV	25–75 10–50			Hypotension, tachycardia, dizziness, urinary retention, seizures
Midazolam (Versed)	IV IM IN PO PR	1–5 2.5–5	0.05 0.1–0.2 0.1–0.3 0.4–1.0 0.25–1.0	2–3 5 10 5–7	Sedation, dizziness, weakness, unsteadiness, physical dependence, respiratory depression, lack of coordination. Hypotension and suppressed breathing (associated with IV administration)
Diazepam (Valium)	PO	2–10	0.1–0.3		
Clonidine	PO	0.3–0.4	0.004	30–60	↓BP, dry mouth, dizziness, fatigue, constipation, anorexia, arrhythmias, local skin reactions with patch.
Dexamethasone	IV		0.15		Delayed wound healing, seizures, osteoporosis, hyperglycemia, diarrhea, nausea, GI bleeding, cushingoid effects
Hydrocortisone (Solu-Cortef)	IV IM PO PR	*Acute adrenal insufficiency*: Adult: 100 mg bolus IV, then 300 mg/day IV 3 divided doses or as a continuous infusion Older children: 1–2 mg/kg/dose IV, then 150–250 mg/day IV in 3–4 divided doses Infants/young children: 1–2 mg/kg/dose IV, then 25–150 mg/day IV in 3–4 divided doses. *Stress coverage for surgery*: 1.5–4 mg/kg/day IV as a continuous infusion beginning at the time of surgery and continuing for 24 hrs. or 40–100 mg/m²/day divided every 6–8 hours.		Immediate Rapid 1–2 hour Slow	Adrenocortical insufficiency (Addison's crisis) with abrupt withdrawal, delayed wound healing, CNS disturbances, osteoporosis, or electrolyte disturbances.

TaBle 16.10 CONTINUED

DRUG	ROUTE	ADULT (MG)	PEDIATRIC (MG/KG)	ONSET (MIN)	SIDE EFFECTS
		Shock: Adult: 500 mg to 2 g IV/IM every 2–6 hours; Ped: 50 mg/kg IV/IM, may repeat in 4 hours. ***Status asthmaticus***: 1–2 mg/day/dose IV every 6 hours for 24 hours, then maintenance of 0.5–1 mg/kg IV every 6 hours.			
Droperidol	IV	0.625–1.25	0.05–0.075	3–10	Extrapyramidal reactions, dysphoric reactions; cerebral vasoconstrictor; ↓BP by alpha blockade and dopaminergic antagonism; laryngospasm; bronchospasm; ↓ seizure threshold; ↑QT interval.
Granisetron	IV	4	0.04		Granisetron: constipation, anemia, headache, fever, abdominal pain, elevated liver enzymes.
Ondansetron	IV		0.1		Ondansetron: headache, dizziness, musculoskeletal pain, drowsiness, sedation, shivers, reversible ↑transaminase, ↑bilirubin, bronchospasm, ↑HR, ↓k+, lightheadedness and diarrhea.
Atropine	IM, IV	0.3–0.6	0.01–0.02		Atropine: tachydysrhythmias, AV dissociation, dry mouth, urinary retention, CNS effects (dizziness, hallucinations, restlessness, fatigue, headache).
Scopolamine	IM, IV	0.3–0.6	0.01–0.02		Scopolamine: excitement, delirium, transient tachycardia, hyperthermia, urinary retention, blurred vision, photophobia.
Glycopyrrolate	IM, IV	0.2–0.3	0.01		Glycopyrrolate: tachycardia, nausea, constipation, confusion, bronchospasm, blurred vision, and dry mouth.
Metoclopramide (Reglan)	PO IV	10–15 10	0.15	30–60 1–3	Metoclopramide: exacerbate depression, extrapyramidal reactions may occur, restlessness, somnolence, diarrhea, weakness, headache, anxiety, leukopenia.
Ranitidine (Zantac)	PO IV	150–300 50	0.25–1.0		Ranitidine: headache, GI disturbance, malaise, insomnia, sedation, arthralgia, hepatotoxicity
Cimetidine (Tagamet)	PO IV	300–800 300	5–10 5–10		Cimetidine: ↓ metabolism of diazepam (inhibits cytochrome P450) diarrhea, rash, myalgia, confusion, neutropenia, gynecomastia
Famotidine (Pepcid)	PO IV	20–40 20	0.15	60–120	Famotidine: Confusion, dizziness, headache, diarrhea
Omeprazole (Prilosec)	PO	20	0.3–0.7	30–60	Omeprazole: headache, diarrhea, nausea-vomiting.
Lansoprazole (Prevacid)	PO	15–30			Lansoprazole: Diarrhea skin rash or itching, abdominal or stomach pain, ↓↑appetite, joint pain, nausea-vomiting

Note:

Sedatives and analgesics should be reduced or withheld in the elderly, newborn/peds (<1 year of age), debilitated, and acutely intoxicated and in those with upper airway obstruction or trauma, central apnea, neurologic deterioration, or severe pulmonary or valvular heart disease.

OBESITY

The BMI (kg/m^2) is widely used to classify obesity: BMI of 18–25 is normal, 26–30 is overweight, 31–35 is obese, over 35 is morbidly obese, and super obesity is a BMI greater than 50. Morbidly obese patients have low life expectancy and high risk of perioperative mortality and morbidity. Obese patients have less water per unit of body weight, they tolerate hypovolemia badly, and they may also compensate poorly for changes of position during anesthesia. They also have an increased risk of hypertension and coronary artery disease.

Increase in neck circumference leads to problems in tracheal intubation and in maintaining the airway with a face mask. The increase of mass effect of chest weight leads

Box 16.7 CAUSES OF HYPOTHYROIDISM

Primary Hypothyroidism (95% of Cases)

Idiopathic hypothyroidism
Hashimoto's thyroiditis
Irradiation of the thyroid subsequent to Graves' disease
Surgical removal of the thyroid
Late-stage invasive fibrous thyroiditis
Iodine deficiency
Drug therapy (e.g., lithium, interferon)
Infiltrative diseases (e.g., sarcoidosis, amyloidosis, scleroderma, hemochromatosis)

Secondary Hypothyroidism (5% of Cases)

Pituitary or hypothalamic neoplasms
Congenital hypopituitarism
Pituitary necrosis (Sheehan's syndrome)

to reduced chest wall compliance and restriction of spontaneous respiration; reduced functional residual capacity, total lung capacity, inspiratory capacity, and expiratory reserve. And increased breathing work and abdominal mass lead to diaphragmatic splinting and increased pulmonary "shunting" with mild hypercapnia and perioperative hypoxia. Avoid sedation in patients with preoperative hypoxia, hypercapnia, or obstructive sleep apnea. From a gastrointestinal perspective, there is an increased risk of hiatal hernia and increased GERD leading to increased risk of pulmonary aspiration of gastric contents. Consider H_2 antagonists, metoclopramide, and sodium citrate in premedication. From an endocrine perspective, there is a fivefold increase in overt diabetes mellitus and an increase in plasma insulin levels, which is linked to high calorie intake. However the insulin binding to cell receptors decreases (insulin resistance).

OBSTRUCTIVE SLEEP APNEA

Obstructive sleep apnea results in total collapse of the airway with intermittent and complete obstruction for more than 10 seconds. Five percent of obese patients suffer from OSA-related hypoventilation, and manifest the "Pickwickian syndrome," comprising obesity, somnolence, polycythemia, pulmonary hypertension, and right heart failure. Consider rapid-sequence induction/intubation in these patients. Initial drug doses are based on actual body weight, while maintenance drug doses should be based on ideal body weight. Do not extubate until the patient is fully emerged (or "awake"). A postoperative semisitting position helps to optimize breathing.

DEPRESSION

Antidepressant drugs increase brain catecholamine activity and anesthetic requirements as well. Use with centrally acting anticholinergic agents may increase postoperative confusion.

CHRONIC OBSTRUCTIVE PULMONARY DISEASE

Chronic bronchitis is defined as daily cough with sputum production for at least 3 months a year for at least 2 consecutive years. A *blue bloater* is a patient who is hypoxemic and cyanosed with cor pulmonale leading to peripheral edema, increased JVP, and hepatomegaly, but with little dyspnea. *Emphysema* is histological enlargement of the air spaces distal to the terminal bronchioles with destructive changes in the alveolar wall. *Pink puffers* have severe dyspnea but have relatively normal gas exchange.

Chronic obstructive pulmonary disease is characterized by expiratory airflow obstruction strongly associated with

Table 16.11 LABORATORY VALUES IN HYPOTHYROIDISM

TSH LEVEL	FREE T4 LEVEL	FREE T3 LEVEL	LIKELY DIAGNOSIS
HIGH	LOW	LOW	Primary hypothyroidism
HIGH (>10:U per mL)	NORMAL	NORMAL	Subclinical hypothyroidism with high risk for future development of overt hypothyroidism
HIGH (6 to 10:U per mL)	NORMAL	NORMAL	Subclinical hypothyroidism with low risk for future development of overt hypothyroidism
HIGH	HIGH	LOW	Congenital absence of T4-T3–converting enzyme; amiodarone (Cordarone) effect on T4-T3 conversion
HIGH	HIGH	HIGH	Peripheral thyroid hormone resistance
LOW	LOW	LOW	Pituitary thyroid deficiency or recent withdrawal of thyroxine after excessive replacement therapy

cigarette smoking and susceptible to acute respiratory failure in the postoperative period. Ventilated patients should be controlled with small to moderate tidal volumes and slow rates to avoid air trapping. The goal should be to maintain normal arterial pH, not necessarily a normal $PaCO_2$.

Lung function tests show an obstructive pattern:

1. ↓FEV1, ↓FVC, ↓FEV1/FVC ratio, ↓ diffusing capacity
2. ↑Residual volume, ↑FRC, ↑total lung capacity(forced expiratory volume in 1 second (FEV1), forced vital capacity (FVC))

HYPERTENSION

Elevated blood pressure on three to six readings over a period of weeks to months characterizes hypertension (Table 16.12). Etiologically, it is divided into essential (idiopathic) and secondary hypertension. Treatment depends on the stage:

Stage I hypertension

1. Monotherapy:

   First choice: dihydropyridine CCB (African American and elderly), ACE inhibitors/ARBs (young and renal disease)

   Alternative: thiazide diuretics (chlorthalidone is preferred over HCTZ)

2. Sequential monotherapy is indicated after failure of initial first-line therapy (failure drug 1→ switch to drug 2→ failure drug 2→ switch to drug 3)
3. Add a second drug if sequential therapy fails.

- Stage II hypertension: Start two-drug combination therapy.

Table 16.12 **CLASSIFICATION OF BLOOD PRESSURE FOR ADULTS**

CATEGORY	SYSTOLIC (MMHG)	DIASTOLIC (MMHG)
Optimal	<120	<80
Normal	<130	<85
High-normal	130–139	85–89
Hypertension		
Stage 1	140–159	90–99
Stage 2	160–179	100–109
Stage 3	>180	>110

The sixth report of the Joint National Committee on Prevention, Detection, Evaluation, and Treatment of High Blood Pressure. *Arch Intern Med.* 1997 Nov 24;157(21):2413–2446.

- Stage III hypertension (urgency and emergency): IV nitroprusside as first-line choice and IV labetolol/nicardipine as alternative choices.

REFERENCES

1. Garcia-Miguel FJ, Serrano-Aguilar PG, Lopez-Bastida J. Preoperative assessment. *Lancet.* 2003;362:1749–1757.
2. Practice advisory for preanesthesia evaluation: An updated report by the American Society of Anesthesiologists Task Force on Preanesthesia Evaluation. *Anesthesiology.* 2012;116:1–17.
3. Fischer S, Bader A, Sweitzer B. Preoperative evaluation. In: Miller RD, ed. *Miller's Anesthesia.* Philadelphia, PA: Churchill Livingstone Elsevier; 2010:1001–1067.
4. King MS. Preoperative evaluation. *Am Fam Physician.* 2000;62: 387–396.
5. Saklad M. Grading of patients for surgical procedures. *Anesthesiology.* 1941;2:281–284.
6. Wolters U, Wolf T, Stutzer H, Schroder T. ASA classification and perioperative variables as predictors of postoperative outcome. *Br J Anaesth.* 1996;77:217–222.
7. Fleisher LA, Beckman JA, Brown KA, et al. ACC/AHA 2007 guidelines on perioperative cardiovascular evaluation and care for noncardiac surgery: executive summary: a report of the American College of Cardiology/American Heart Association Task Force on Practice Guidelines. *Circulation.* 2007;116:1971–1996.
8. Fleisher LA. Cardiac risk stratification for noncardiac surgery: update from the American College of Cardiology/American Heart Association 2007 guidelines. *Cleve Clin J Med.* 2009; 76:S10–S115.
9. Cardiac Risk Index in Noncardiac Surgery (Goldman et al.). Website. http://medcalc3000.com/CardiacRisk_G.htm Published 1998-2013.Accessed June 6, 2014.
10. Goldman L, Caldera D, Nussbaum S, et al. Multifactorial index of cardiac risk in noncardiac surgical procedures. *N Engl J Med.* 1977;297:845–850.
11. Apfelbaum JL, Hagberg CA, Caplan RA, et al. Practice guidelines for management of the difficult airway: an updated report by the American Society of Anesthesiologists Task Force on Management of the Difficult Airway. *Anesthesiology.* 2013; 118:251–270.
12. American Society of Anesthesiologists Task Force on Perioperative Management of Patients with Obstructive Sleep Apnea. Practice guidelines for the perioperative management of patients with obstructive sleep apnea: an updated report by the American Society of Anesthesiologists Task Force on Perioperative Management of Patients with Obstructive Sleep Apnea. *Anesthesiology.* 2014;120:1–19.
13. American Society of Anesthesiologists. Ethical guidelines for the anesthesia care of patients with do-not-resuscitate orders or other directives that limit treatment. http://www.asahq.org/For-Members/Standards-Guidelines-and-Statements.aspx. Approved October 17, 2001. Last affirmed October 22, 2008. Accessed June 14, 2014.
14. Henderson J. Airway assessment. In: Miller RD, ed. *Miller's Anesthesia.* Philadelphia, PA: Churchill Livingstone Elsevier; 2010:1573–1607.

FURTHER READING

Miller R, Pardo M. *Basics of Anesthesia.* 6th ed. Philadelphia, PA: Elsevier; 2011.

QUESTIONS

1. Which of the following clinical factors requires cardiac evaluation prior to noncardiac surgery according to the 2007 ACC/AHA preoperative guidelines?
   A. Atrial fibrillation with rate control
   B. Mild aortic stenosis
   C. Stable angina
   D. NYHA functional class IV
   E. Patient on Plavix

2. Which clinical risk factor is considered to hold the highest positive correlate for postop cardiac complications?
   A. Age > 70
   B. Signs of Heart Failure: ventricular gallop or jugular venous distention
   C. Arrhythmia other than sinus
   D. Emergency surgery
   E. Aortic stenosis

3. Which preoperative finding on airway evaluation is associated with possible difficult intubation?
   A. Short incisors
   B. Mouth opening of 5 cm
   C. Thyromental distance of 7 cm
   D. Overbite
   E. Neck circumference of <16 inches

ANSWERS

1. D. There are four active cardiac conditions that require preoperative evaluation and treatment prior to noncardiac surgery: unstable coronary syndromes, decompensated heart failure, significant arrhythmias, and severe valvular disease. NYHA functional class IV falls under decompensated heart failure.[8]
2. B. According to the Goldman Cardiac Risk Index, there are nine independent risk factors that positively correlate to life-threatening and fatal cardiac complications. Each of the nine is assigned a point value depending on their cardiac risk, with signs of heart failure and previous MI within 6 months being the highest risk factors. Totaling the points will give a percentage of complication applicable to the patient.[9,10]
3. D. There are many components to assessing a patient's airway preoperatively. While the presence of one isolated finding on the airway exam does not always predict a difficult intubation, it is important for the clinician to determine whether multiple risk factors exist, then a plan should be formulated to manage the airway with alternative devices or with the patient awake.[14]

17.

REGIONAL ANESTHESIA

Vadim Ioselevich, Yefim W. Bogomolny, Jibin Sam Mathew, and George W. Williams

GENERAL TOPICS

PREMEDICATION

Light sedation is often appropriate during the placement of a neuraxial block, as the experience can cause anxiety in the patient. A short-acting benzodiazepine (midazolam) can be used for anxiolysis and a short-acting opioid (fentanyl) can be used to help with the discomfort of block placement. It is important to avoid heavy sedation so that the patient can maintain good position to facilitate block placement. It is also vital for the patient to be able to communicate with the anesthesiologist to determine block height, presence of paresthesia during the procedure, and in the case of epidurals to determine the effect of the test dose. Doses of 1.5 mg of midazolam with 75 μg of fentanyl have been shown to decrease the patient's ability to accurately report symptoms of intravenous local anesthetic injection. Once the block is placed, additional sedation can be given as deemed appropriate.

PATIENT POSITIONING

Position during the placement of a neuraxial block is crucial for success. Poor positioning can turn an easy spinal or epidural into a challenging one. The sitting position is used most often by anesthesiologists because it is easier to identify midline and other landmarks in this position. The patient's back should be toward the anesthesiologist at the edge of the bed with the hips square to avoid rotation of the spine. The optimal position is to have the patient's feet on a footstool, the head flexed, arms around a pillow, and to have the patient actively curve the back outward. The lateral decubitus position can also be used. In this position the patient's shoulders and hips are positioned perpendicular to the bed to avoid rotation of the spine. The knees and the head are flexed with the back curved outward in a fetal position. The goal in positioning is to flex the spine and spread the spinous processes apart. This will increase the size of the interlaminar foramen and provide a larger target to reach the epidural or intrathecal space. For patients having surgeries requiring the prone position (rectal, peroneal, or lumbar) a spinal can be performed after first placing the patient prone in the jackknife position. This approach avoids having to reposition the patient after the block is placed.

Jackknife Position

Equipment

Most institutions use sterile disposable trays that contain everything necessary to perform a block, including a prep solution, paper towel, fenestrated drape, gauze sponges, and 1% lidocaine for skin infiltration. Spinal kits contain ampules of local anesthetic for spinal injection, an ampule of epinephrine, sterile syringes, a filter straw, and spinal needles. An epidural kit will have similar supplies with the addition of epidural needles instead of spinal needles, an ampule of saline, an epidural catheter, and a vial of 1.5% lidocaine with 1:200,000 epinephrine for the test dose and a loss of resistance syringe. A combined spinal/epidural kit will also contain a spinal needle designed to fit through the epidural needle.

There are two types of spinal needles: pencil-point (Sprotte and Whitacre) and cutting (Quincke and Pitkin) (Figure 17.1). All the needles have a removable stylet that prevents the needle from getting plugged with skin and adipose tissue, which can be deposited in the subarachnoid space. Pencil-point needles have a solid tip and a noncutting rounded bevel. The opening on these needles is on the side about 2–4 mm proximal to the tip. Cutting needles have a sharp tip, and the opening is at the tip. Quincke has a medium cutting bevel, while Pitkin has a short cutting bevel. The advantages of the pencil-point needles are that they provide a better tactile feel of the layers and ligaments and have a lower incidence of developing a postdural puncture headache (PDPH). The disadvantages are that they require more force to insert and advance and are more

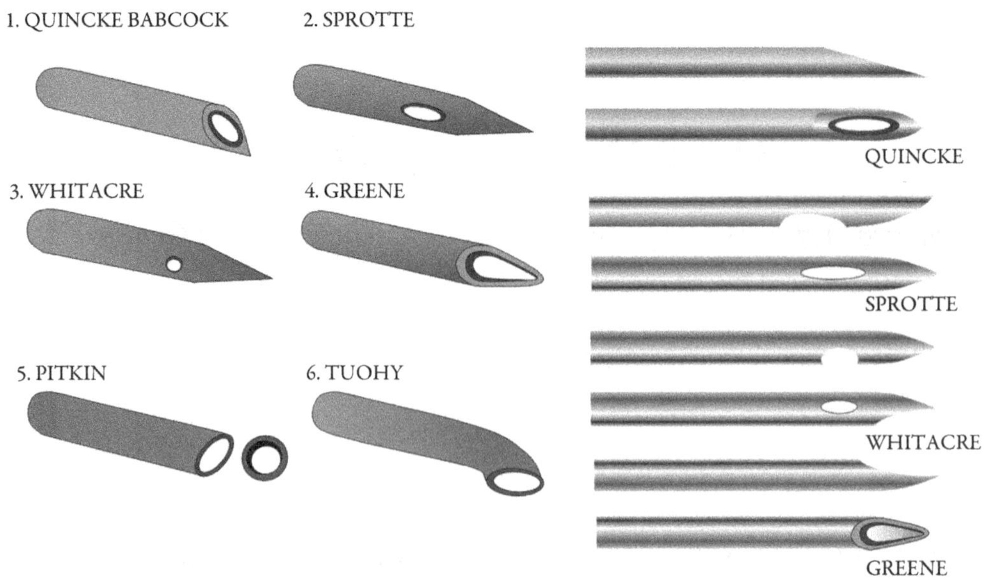

Figure 17.1 Needle diagram. Image courtesy of Ariana Rojas, MD. Adapted from NYSORA.com

likely to get deflected during advancement. Also, because the opening is located 2–4 mm from the end there is a possibility that if the needle is not advanced far enough, some of the medication may spill out of the intrathecal space, leading to an incomplete spinal block. Cutting needles are less likely to be deflected and are easier to advance, but have a higher risk of PDPH. Even with smaller cutting gauge needles the risk of PDPH is higher than with larger bore pencil-point needles (i.e., a 25-g Whitacre has a lower risk of a PDPH than a 27-g Quincke).

There are several different kinds of epidural needles, Tuohy and Hustead needles are the most common. The needles are styleted and are 16–18 gauge and 8–10 cm in length. The tip has a 15- to 30-degree curve and a blunt bevel. The blunt and curved tip decreases the risk of dural puncture and helps thread the catheter into the epidural space. Epidural catheters are typically 20 gauge so that they can fit through the epidural needle. Some catheters have one opening at the end, others have multiple holes on the sides. The flexibility of the catheters also varies. Catheters that are more flexible are less likely to be unintentionally threaded into other structures or spaces outside the epidural space. They are also less likely to kink but are more difficult to thread. Stiffer catheters are easier to advance but are more likely to kink and to be threaded into false spaces.

In addition to the equipment necessary to perform the procedures, it is also essential to be prepared to resuscitate the patient should any unforeseen complications arise. This includes having medications to support blood pressure and heart rate and medications for induction of general anesthesia. Equipment to secure the airway must also be readily available, including laryngoscope, endotracheal tubes, ambu bag and mask, and oral and nasal airways. Intralipid should also be available in case of local anesthetic toxicity.

Monitoring

Injecting local anesthetic into the intrathecal or epidural space can cause a significant drop in blood pressure and affect respiratory mechanics. For this reason monitoring pulse oximetry, blood pressure, and ECG is necessary during the performance of a spinal or epidural blockade.

SPINAL

INDICATIONS

Spinal anesthetic is a useful alternative for surgical anesthesia for surgeries involving the lower extremities; rectal, inguinal, urogenital areas; and the lower abdomen. It can also be used for surgeries on the lower lumbar spine. Surgeries on the upper abdomen can also be done under a spinal block though it may be difficult to achieve an adequate sensory block to keep the patient comfortable without causing a high block and affecting respiratory mechanics or causing significant hemodynamic instability from the extensive sympathetic blockade. Spinals are useful in obstetrics both as surgical blocks for cesarean sections and to help with pain during labor when the patient is close to delivering and there may not be enough time to place an epidural. A spinal with injection of preservative-free morphine (Duramorph) rather than local anesthetic can also be used to help manage postoperative pain. Though most commonly used to manage pain after cesarean delivery, Duramorph can also be used for a variety of surgical procedures from lower extremity procedures to thoracic surgeries.

ABSOLUTE CONTRAINDICATIONS

Patient refusal, infection at the site of the block, coagulopathy, increased intracranial pressure (ICP), and severe hypovolemia are absolute contraindications. The patient's back needs to be examined prior to the block to assure that there is no infection at the site of injection, as the needle going through an infected area can seed the subarachnoid space with microbes. In the setting of elevated ICP, a dural puncture can cause excessive CSF drainage from the puncture site, leading to uncal herniation. In the setting of idiopathic intracranial hypertension (pseudotumor cerebri), however, a spinal anesthetic may be performed. This is because in patients with pseudotumor cerebri, there is no other cause of elevated ICP and drainage of CSF is a mainstay of therapy. Because a spinal causes a decrease in systemic vascular resistance (SVR), performing a block on someone who is hypovolemic significantly increases the risk of hypotension. For this reason, patients with severe hypovolemia need to be sufficiently resuscitated before the block can be placed. It is important to ensure normal coagulation status prior to performing a spinal blockade, because bleeding in the epidural space can compress the spinal cord and nerve roots and lead to paralysis. It is often a surgical emergency. The PT/INR and PTT need to be normal prior to performing the block. Patients who are anticoagulated need to have the anticoagulant or platelet inhibitor held before the block. The American Society of Regional Anesthesia (ASRA) has published guidelines on the timing of how long the various agents need to be held.

RELATIVE CONTRAINDICATIONS

Relative contraindications include sepsis or other infection not affecting the site of the block, neurological disorders or deficits, uncooperative patient or inability to communicate with the patient, severe stenotic valvular disease, significant spinal anatomic deformity, and prolonged surgery or complex surgery associated with a large blood loss. Patients with neurological deficits or disorders need to have a thorough neurological exam prior to placement of the block to document any preexisting deficits. There has been no clinical data to show that performing a block on a patient with a neurological disorder worsens preexisting deficits, however the stress of surgery and other factors may lead to an exacerbation of neurological deficits, and in the setting of a spinal or an epidural it may be more difficult to determine the cause of worsening symptoms. There is also in vitro data showing that local anesthetic is more toxic to demyelinated nerves. Thus caution is needed in patients who have demyelination disorders. In order to have a successful block, the anesthesiologist needs to have cooperation from the patient to assure optimal positioning. It is also important to be able to communicate with the patient so that the patient can alert the anesthesiologist of any parathesia or pain on injection. Both pain on injection and parathesia have been associated with postoperative nerve injury. In the past severe aortic and mitral stenosis have been considered as absolute contraindications. These patients rely on a high afterload for perfusion of the myocardium, and a decrease in SVR can compromise myocardial perfusion. Despite this, with adequate volume resuscitation and careful monitoring of blood pressure, a spinal anesthetic can be safely performed on these patients. Lastly, anatomic deformities or presence of hardware in the back from prior back surgeries can make a spinal anesthetic more challenging to place, and for this reason some practitioners may choose to avoid spinal anesthesia in these patients. In long, complex surgeries there is a risk that the spinal anesthetic will wear off before the surgery is over, and for this reason spinal anesthesia is generally avoided for these surgeries.

SITES OF ACTIONS

The spinal cord starts at the foramen magnum and ends at the L1 vertebral body in adults (L3 in children). It is surround by three meninges (pia mater, arachnoid mater, and dura mater). The CSF is found between the pia and arachnoid mater (the subarachnoid or intrathecal space). The goal of the spinal blockade is to enter the subarachnoid space and inject a local anesthetic with or without other adjuncts. The site of action of the local anesthetic is the nerve roots. The local anesthetic blocks nerve conduction of both anterior and posterior nerve root fibers. Blockade of the anterior root fibers prevents efferent motor and sympathetic conduction, while blockade of the posterior fibers prevents afferent conduction of sensory nerves. The result is complete sensory and motor blockade, which provides excellent operative conditions for the surgeon. Local anesthetic also blocks conduction of sodium and potassium channels in the dorsal and ventral horn. In the dorsal horn, nociceptive impulse generation and propagation is inhibited, while in the ventral horn, propagation of motor impulses is inhibited. Calcium channels in the spinal cord are also blocked by local anesthetic. The blockade of calcium channels makes nociceptive afferent nerve fibers resistant to electrical stimulation. The combined effect of the various mechanisms above is to produce a strong analgesia.

The three main factors that affect the levels and dermatomes that are blocked include baricity, patient position at the time of the block and immediately after, and dose of the anesthetic. The baricity is calculated by dividing the density of the local anesthetic by the density of CSF at 37°C. A baricity of 1 is isobaric, a number greater than 1 is hyperbaric, and a number less than 1 is hypobaric. Baricity is the main determinant of how the local anesthetic spreads after injection. A hyperbaric solution is heavier than the CSF and will follow gravity, while a hypobaric solution is lighter and will rise against gravity. An isobaric solution will stay at the level that it is injected. During the first few minutes after the block is placed, proper patient positioning is important to achieve the desired spread. As an illustration, to perform a successful spinal for a patient undergoing rectal surgery one can position patient in the sitting position, inject a hyperbaric local anesthetic, and let the patient sit up for a few minutes to allow for the local to fall and anesthetize the sacral nerve roots. Alternatively, for the same surgery one can position the patient prone in the jackknife position and inject a hypobaric solution and allow it to rise to cover sacral nerve roots. Depending on the concentration and the solution, a local anesthetic can have different baricities. It is important to choose the local anesthetic with the desired baricity. Hyperbaric local anesthetics are the most commonly used, and when the patient is placed in the supine position the curvature of the spine will cause the local to travel to about the T4/T5 level, which is the lowest point of the back in the supine position. The last determinant of spread is the dose of the local anesthetic. A higher dose will result in blockade of more dermatomal levels. The actual concentration of the local anesthetic does not affect the level of the block, because once the medication is injected, it mixes with a CSF, creating a new concentration. There are also patient factors that may influence the height of the block. The average patient has a CSF volume of about 150 mL, half of which is in the spinal column. In patients with increased abdominal pressure from obesity, pregnancy, or other causes, some of the CSF can be displaced from the spinal column to the cranium, leading to a lower volume of CSF in the spinal column, resulting in a higher-than-anticipated level of blockade. Unfortunately, because the CSF volume is so variable, it is very difficult to predict the exact level of the blockade. Patient height may also play a role; short patients may have a higher level of blockade with the same dose of local anesthetic.

Various additives have been used to prolong the duration of spinal anesthesia. Vasoconstrictors such as epinephrine and phenylephrine prolong blockade by causing vasoconstriction and decreasing systemic absorption of the local anesthetic, thereby prolonging the time the local anesthetic is in contact with the nerve roots. Additionally these adrenergic agonists can provide analgesia when injected into the subarachnoid space independent of local anesthetic. These drugs stimulate α-adrenergic receptors in the dorsal horn and inhibit afferent nociceptive transmission. In large doses, α-adrenergic agonists can also produce flaccid paralysis by causing motor neurons to become hyperpolarized. Opioids can also prolong and intensify a spinal block by targeting opioid receptors that are found on spinal cord neurons in the dorsal horn. Opioids modulate A-δ and C fibers to inhibit afferent nociceptive input via activation presynaptic μ and δ receptors, which inhibit Ca^{2+} influx. The opioids also target postsynaptic μ receptors, which increase the conductance of K^+ in the ascending neurons. The effect is the hyperpolarization of these neurons and decreased likelihood of propagating an action potential. Lipophilic opioids have a fast onset of action and can intensify the surgical block. Hydrophilic opioids like morphine have a long onset time and do not help for surgical anesthesia. The primary role of morphine when given either intrathecally or epidurally is for postoperative pain control. Because it is hydrophilic, it can stay in the subarachnoid or epidural space for a long period of time and provide as much as 24 hours of postoperative pain relief. Clonidine, an α_2-agonist, similar to other α-agonists, causes hyperpolarization of the ventral horn, and enhances the effect of local anesthetic. Acetylcholinesterase inhibitors such as neostigmine inhibit the breakdown of acetylcholine. When injected intrathecally, the increased levels of acetylcholine help provide analgesia.

FACTORS INFLUENCING ONSET, DURATION, AND TERMINATION OF ACTION

The potency of local anesthetic is determined by lipid solubility. The more lipid-soluble drugs require a lower dose to achieve anesthesia and analgesia. The speed of onset is determined by the pK_a of the local anesthetic. The pK_a is the pH at which half of the molecules are ionized and half of the molecules are nonionized, and only the nonionized form is able to cross the cell membrane. Local anesthetics inhibit the sodium channels of neurons from inside the cell by binding the sodium channels in the inactivated state. Local anesthetics are weak bases and have a pK_a higher than the cellular pH. Therefore the lower the pK_a of the local anesthetic, the more of it will be in the nonionized form and the faster the onset of action will be. The uptake of local anesthetic into the nerve roots depends on the size of the nerve and the myelination of the nerve. Myelinated nerves have a higher lipid content and therefore uptake more local anesthetic, leading to faster onset. Smaller nerves require less local anesthetic to be blocked, and are therefore blocked faster than larger nerves. Concentration also plays a role in onset. The site of highest concentration of local anesthetic has the highest uptake, and the uptake decreases as the concentration decreases. The duration of action, on the other hand, is determined by protein binding. Local anesthetics that have a higher fraction of the drug protein-bound have a longer duration of action. In addition to uptake at the nerve root, there is also uptake at the spinal cord. There are two mechanisms by which the spinal cord takes up local anesthetic. One is via diffusion of the local anesthetic from the CSF through the pia mater and into the very superficial layer of the spinal cord. This is a very slow process. The other mechanism is into Virchow-Robin spaces, which is a faster process. These are parts of the pia mater which surround blood vessels that travel from the subarachnoid space into the spinal cord. Local anesthetic is eliminated from the subarachnoid space by vascular absorption both in the subarachnoid space and the epidural space as local anesthetics are able to cross the dura mater. Blood flow can vary depending on the local anesthetic used. Some local anesthetics like tetracaine increase blood flow, while others like lidocaine and bupivacaine decrease blood flow. Because perfusion can vary, the rate of elimination also varies.

EPIDURAL

INDICATIONS

An epidural, like a spinal, can be used for surgical anesthesia for surgeries on the lower extremities, peroneam, and lower abdomen. It is generally chosen over a spinal for longer surgeries where a spinal block may not last. Surgeries on the upper abdomen and thorax have also been performed successfully with an epidural anesthetic; in fact, minimally invasive valve replacements and off-pump coronary bypass grafts have been performed with the use of epidural anesthesia. This practice has not been adopted in the United States because blockade above T5 leads to a significant sympathetic blockade that could lead to hemodynamic instability. More often an epidural is used in combination with a general anesthetic to limit opioid requirements in the OR and to help manage postoperative pain. It is also a mainstay of management of labor pain.

ABSOLUTE CONTRAINDICATIONS

Patient refusal, severe hypovolemia, increased intracranial pressure, infection at the site of the block, and coagulopathy are absolute contraindications to a block for the same reasons as described for spinal anesthesia. It is important to know that bleeding can occur not only at the time of epidural placement but also at the time of catheter removal. For this reason it is important to make sure that the patient is not coagulopathic at the time the catheter is removed. The patient also cannot have an indwelling epidural catheter while being therapeutically anticoagulated. If a patient does require therapeutic anticoagulation, the epidural catheter needs to be removed prior to initiation of anticoagulation.

RELATIVE CONTRAINDICATIONS

An uncooperative patient, inability to communicate with the patient, sepsis, neurological disorders, anatomical deformity, prior spine surgery, and severe valvular abnormalities are all relative contraindications. A cooperative patient is important not only for positioning for the block and avoiding accidental neurological injury but also because after the epidural catheter is placed, a test dose of local anesthetic with epinephrine is typically administered via the catheter to ensure that the catheter is not intravascular or intrathecal. Inability to communicate with the patient would make it difficult to determine the effects of the test dose prior to administering larger doses of local anesthetic via the catheter. In the setting of sepsis, placement of an epidural is safe as long as there is no infection at the site of the block. However because an epidural is a foreign body, in the setting of sepsis it is at risk of becoming colonized by microbes and seeding the epidural space. There are case reports of epidurals being placed safely in patients with neurological disorders, however an epidural may mask exacerbation of symptoms. A thorough neurological exam is critical prior to placement of an epidural in these patients. In those patients with previous spine surgery the placement of the block may be technically challenging or impossible. Also the epidural space may be disrupted and may no longer be continuous. This would lead to a "patchy" or incomplete blockade. In patients with severe valvular abnormalities such as aortic stenosis the epidural has the advantage over a spinal in that it can be dosed slowly and carefully while carefully managing the blood pressure.

SITE OF ACTION

The epidural space starts from the base of the skull and extends to the sacral hiatus. It surrounds the dura mater posteriorly, laterally, and anteriorly. The space is filled with fat tissue, veins, lymphatics, and nerve roots. There is no free fluid in the epidural space. As with a spinal, the nerve roots are the main site of action of local anesthetic injected into the epidural space. Additionally epidurally injected local anesthetics lead to calcium channel blockade at the presynaptic terminals of dorsal root ganglion cells and prevent the release of substance P. Substance P is a neurotransmitter involved in the transmission of pain, and blocking its release prevents the transmission of pain to the brain.

Because there is no free fluid in the epidural space, it is important to select an injection site close to the dermatomal nerve roots that need to be blocked for that particular procedure. As described above, the nerve roots contain sensory, motor, and autonomic fibers, and all three will be blocked with local anesthetic. Because the different nerve fibers vary in size and myelination, they show different sensitivity to local anesthetics. Sympathetic fibers are blocked first, pain/temperature fibers are blocked next, then proprioception fibers, and finally motor fibers. Because of this, the sensory blockade is usually 2 levels higher than the motor blockade and the sympathetic blockade is usually 0–4 segments higher than the sensory blockade. This concept is known as differential blockade.

FACTORS INFLUENCING ONSET, DURATION, AND TERMINATION OF ACTION

The onset of action of an epidural block is about 5–10 minutes, however time to achieve a surgical block and analgesia is longer than that and depends on the local anesthetic used: 2-chloroprocaine has the fastest onset, lidocaine and mepivicaine are intermediate in duration, and bupivacaine and ropivicaine are long lasting. Because the onset of the epidural is much longer than that of a spinal, various things have been tried to speed up onset. One common technique is the alkalization of the local anesthetic by adding a small amount of sodium bicarbonate to the solution, typically 1 mEq per 10 mL of local anesthetic. This works by increasing the percentage of the local anesthetic that is in the nonionized form, making it more readily available to cross the cell membrane and block the sodium channels. This technique works well with chloroprocaine, lidocaine, and mepivicaine. With ropivicaine and bupivacaine, the addition of sodium bicarbonate will cause the local anesthetic to precipitate out of solution unless concentrations of 0.1 mEq per 10 mL of local are used, making this technique much less effective. Mixing of short- and long-acting anesthetics has also been tried to speed up onset while still providing a long-lasting block. This technique has not proven to be effective. However, because an epidural catheter is typically placed at the time of the block and can be redosed as needed, mixing of local anesthetics is unnecessary. Unlike with a spinal block, the concentration of local anesthetic determines the density of the epidural block. For a surgical block a higher concentration of local anesthetic is needed, while for analgesia a lower concentration is preferred, because it may limit the motor blockade and side effects of epidural analgesia. The volume of local anesthetic determines the number of levels that are blocked, or the height of the block. The general rule is that 1–2 mL of local anesthetic is needed per level. In extremes of height this rule may not apply and the volume might have to be adjusted. Patient position does not play a role in the height of the block, though the block may be more dense on the dependent side.

The duration of the block depends on the local anesthetic. Additives like epinephrine and clonidine have been used in the epidural to prolong the duration of action and intensify the block. Epinephrine, as with the spinal, works by causing vasoconstriction and decreasing the elimination of local anesthetic from the epidural space. Clonidine does not appear to work by activating central α-adrenoreceptors. In animals it has been shown to decrease blood flow to the spinal cord at the site of the block and decrease elimination of local anesthetic. It may also be related to hyperpolarization of the nerves. When used as a surgical block, the epidural is typically bolused initially with a volume adequate to reach the height necessary for surgery. After the initial bolus, the goal is to prevent the block from receding by more than two levels to ensure patient comfort for the surgery. To ensure this, the epidural catheter needs to be redosed before the two-segment regression occurs. The volume of the redose is one-third to one-half of the initial dose. The time to redose depends on the local anesthetic; for short-acting local anesthetic the time is 45 minutes, 60–90 minutes for intermediate local anesthetic, and 120 minutes for long-lasting anesthetic. When the epidural is used for analgesia, after the initial bolus the catheter is connected to an epidural pump that continuously infuses local anesthetic to maintain the desired level of the block. Older patients tend to have a higher block height compared with younger patients. There are several suggested reasons for this phenomenon. One is that there is a narrowing of the intervertebral foramina, which decreases how much local anesthetic leaks out of the epidural space. Another possibility is that there is a loss of epidural fat, which allows for more local anesthetic to surround the nerve roots. Lastly there may be a loss of compliance in the epidural space, resulting in increased cephalad spread. Pregnancy has also been associated with increased sensitivity to local anesthetics, which may be related to increased levels of progesterone. The termination of action is related to the elimination of local anesthetic from the epidural space by vascular absorption.

COMBINED SPINAL/EPIDURAL

A combined spinal/epidural (CSE) is performed at the lumbar spine level, typically L3/4 or L4/5. The procedure to place it is almost the same as for an epidural, after reaching the epidural space with the Touhy needle before threading the catheter, a spinal needle is passed through the Touhy needle and punctures the dura, then a dose of local anesthetic is injected into the subarachnoid space, the needle is removed, and the epidural catheter is threaded.

A CSE can be used for surgical anesthesia when the duration of the case is expected to outlast the duration of a spinal anesthetic. The initial dosing is through the spinal needle, and the dose would be the same as for a single-shot spinal. A CSE has an advantage over an epidural because the spinal portion provides a quick onset of the block and surgical conditions rather than waiting for the onset of the epidural. Once the spinal begins to wear off, the epidural can be dosed similar to the way a normal epidural would be dosed, thus providing surgical anesthesia for long cases where a single shot spinal would not last long enough. The disadvantages of a CSE are that it carries a higher risk of PDPH than a lumbar epidural and, because the initial block is from the spinal dose, there is no way to know for sure whether the epidural catheter is in the epidural space until the spinal portion begins to wear off. The CSE technique is also very useful in obstetrics. It can be used for labor analgesia and can provide almost instantaneous pain relief instead of waiting for the onset of the epidural. When used for analgesia, the spinal dose of local anesthetic is significantly lower than that for surgical anesthesia. Alternatively, a small dose of an opioid such as fentanyl can be injected intrathecally instead of a local anesthetic to provide pain relief. Lastly the CSE can be used for cesarean delivery. This technique is useful when there is a possibility that the cesarean section will be prolonged, either because it is a repeat cesarean section or there is concern for placental accreta.

CAUDAL

The caudal space is the sacral extension of the epidural. The sacral hiatus is created as a result of incomplete fusion of S4 and S5 laminae. The sacrococcygeal ligament covers the hiatus and defines the posterior border of the caudal space. In adults the dural sac and the subarachnoid space end at about the S1 level. In infants the dural sac may extend to the S3 level. Therefore there is a higher risk of dural puncture in infants. Once the dural sac terminates, the sacral nerve roots and the filum terminale exit the dura and are contained within the sacral canal.

INDICATIONS AND CONTRAINDICATIONS

The indications and contraindications for a caudal block are similar to those for a lumbar epidural. It may be more preferential in cases where spread of local anesthetic to sacral nerve roots is desirable over spread to lumbar nerve roots. However, unlike with a lumbar epidural, with a caudal block cephalad spread is unpredictable and unreliable. It is primarily used in the pediatric population for postoperative analgesia both as a single shot and as a catheter technique. Pediatric patient age older than 2 is a relative contraindication to the block. This is because children at that age are ambulating and having a motor block postoperatively can create significant anxiety and distress for the child. The risk of significant pain must be weighed against the concern for prolonged motor block postoperatively. The caudal is preferred in pediatric patients because the distance from skin to the epidural space is very short and lumbar or thoracic epidurals carry a higher risk of unintentional dural puncture then a caudal block. A single-shot technique can be used for surgeries on the lower extremities or lower abdomen. A catheter can be placed and threaded to thoracic nerve roots as needed for upper abdominal or thoracic surgeries. The technique is not commonly used in adults because the sacrococcygeal ligament becomes calcified in adults making the performing of the block very difficult or impossible. Furthermore cephalad spread is less reliable in adults then in children.

SITE OF ACTION

The site of action is the sacral and lumbar nerve roots. The sacral nerve roots contain parasympathetic nerve fibers, not sympathetic fibers. As a result, there is often loss of visceromotor function of the distal intestines and bladder. There is also some sympathetic blockade from the lumbar nerve roots. However because the sympathetic chain typically ends at L2, there is usually little vasodilation or hypotension with a caudal block compared with a lumbar epidural.

The factors affecting onset, duration, and termination of action are similar to those for lumbar epidural. The dosing of local anesthetic is also similar.

LOCAL ANESTHETIC SYSTEMIC TOXICITY (LAST)

Systemic toxicity may result from either accidental intravascular injection of local anesthetics or from rapid systemic absorption. Intra-arterial injections are usually associated with regional anesthetic techniques in the neck and (interscalene block, cervical plexus block, stellate ganglion block) are characterized by a rapid onset of symptoms as the local anesthetic directly enters the cerebral circulation. Toxic doses of local anesthetics primarily affect the central nervous system (CNS) and the cardiovascular system (CVS). Local anesthetics differ with regard to their toxicity profile (Box 17.1). Systemic toxic reactions to local anesthetics are manifested by a progressive spectrum of neurological and cardiovascular symptoms and signs as the blood levels rise.[1]

CENTRAL NERVOUS SYSTEM TOXICITY

The CNS is more sensitive to the effects of local anesthetics as compared with the CVS. Initially there is CNS excitation due to the blockade of inhibitory pathways in the cerebral cortex by local anesthetic drug. This can also result from the net stimulation of release of glutamate, an excitatory neurotransmitter. Blockade of inhibitory pathways allows excitatory neurons to function unopposed, which may result in convulsions. A further increase in the dose of local anesthetic leads to inhibition of activity of both the inhibitory and excitatory pathways, which results in a generalized CNS depression. In general, a correlation exists between potency of the local anesthetic and intravenous CNS toxicity.[2]

CARDIOVASCULAR SYSTEM TOXICITY

Local anesthetics act directly on the cardiac myocytes and peripheral vascular smooth muscle cells and indirectly through the autonomic nervous system. The local anesthetics act by decreasing the conduction in Purkinje fibers and cardiomyocytes by prolonging the recovery time. Lipophilic and highly potent local anesthetics such as bupivacaine,

Box 17.1 LAST CLINICAL PICTURE

1. Lightheadedness
2. Tinnitus (classic premonitory sign)
3. Perioral tingling, numbness/metallic taste of tongue (classic premonitory sign)
4. Slurred speech (classic premonitory sign)
5. Seizures
6. Respiratory arrest
7. Cardiovascular depression

tetracaine, and etidocaine are more cardiotoxic than the less lipophilic agents such as procaine, prilocaine, and lidocaine. The cardiovascular (CV)/CNS ratio describes the dose required to produce CV arrhythmias versus that required to produce seizures.[3] This ratio tends to be lower with bupivacaine as compared with lidocaine. The dissociation of bound bupivacaine from the local anesthetic binding site is slower ("fast-in," "slow-out" of the bupivacaine block of the cardiac Na+ channel). Cardiac resuscitation is more difficult after bupivacaine-induced cardiovascular collapse. Acidosis and hypoxia markedly potentiate the cardiotoxicity of bupivacaine.[4]

PREVENTION OF LAST

Prevention of adverse consequences[3, 5] is the cornerstone of improving patient safety while performing regional anesthesia procedures. The following measures can help avert the undesired complications:

1. Using the *lowest effective dose* of local anesthetic.
2. Using *incremental* injection of local anesthetics when performing a block.
3. *Aspirating* the needle or catheter before each injection.
4. *Ultrasound* guidance may reduce the frequency of intravascular injection.
5. Using an *intravascular marker* (e.g., epinephrine) that helps in detecting the systemic entry of the local anesthetic.
6. Continual communication with the patient to detect early signs and symptoms of intravascular or intraneural injection
7. Caution should be exercised in patients with cardiac disease (low cardiac output, conduction abnormalities or ischemia), renal impairment, liver disease, low plasma protein concentration, and acidosis (increases free fraction of local anesthetic), which likely reduces the threshold for LAST.

TREATMENT OF LAST

Treatment of LAST is mainly supportive. The essence of treatment is in maintaining *oxygenation and ventilation* at all times. It is important to understand that hypoxia, hypercarbia, and acidosis decrease the threshold for LAST.

For patients experiencing signs or symptoms of LAST[6]:

- Call for help
- Initial focus
  - Airway management: Ventilate with 100% oxygen.
  - Seizure suppression: Benzodiazepines are preferred. If benzodiazepines are not readily available, small doses of propofol or thiopental are acceptable.
  - Prolonged resuscitation efforts may be necessary
- Infuse 20% Lipid emulsion (LE) (values mentioned are for a 70-kg patient)
  - Bolus 1.5 mL/kg (lean body mass) intravenously longer than 1 minute (approximately 100 mL).
  - Continuous infusion at 0.25 mL/kg/min (approximately 18 mL/min; adjust by roller clamp).
  - Repeat bolus once or twice for persistent CV collapse.
  - Double the infusion rate to 0.5 mL/kg/min if blood pressure remains low.
  - Recommended upper limit is approximately 10 mL/kg LE over the first 30 minutes.
- Alert the nearest facility having cardiopulmonary bypass capability.
- Avoid vasopressin, calcium channel blockers, and beta blockers during resuscitation.

Test Dose

An ideal test dose[1] should be able to detect all instances of accidental intravascular or subarachnoid placement of an epidural catheter. The most common test dose is 3 mL of local anesthetic containing 5 mcg/mL of epinephrine (1:200,000). The dose of local anesthetic should be sufficient that subarachnoid injection will result in clear evidence of spinal anesthesia. Usually 45 mg of lidocaine is used for the epidural test dose. Intravenous injection of 15 mcg of epinephrine typically produces an average 30 beats per minute heart rate increase between 20 and 40 seconds after injection. The inclusion of epinephrine is the primary differentiating factor for the test dose included in standard epidural kits in comparison to using low-dose lidocaine. Heart rate response to epinephrine may not be accurately captured in beta-blocked patients, active labor, advanced age, or general anesthesia. In beta-blocked patients, a systolic blood pressure increase of more than 20 mmHg may be a more reliable indicator of intravascular injection. Many other agents have been used to detect accidental intravascular catheter placement, for example, isoproterenol, air, and fentanyl.

IMPLICATIONS OF ANTICOAGULANTS AND PLATELET INHIBITORS

Anticoagulant and antiplatelet medications have been increasingly used in the prevention and treatment of thromboembolism.

AMERICAN SOCIETY OF REGIONAL ANESTHESIA AND PAIN MEDICINE (ASRA) GUIDELINES

In patients on anticoagulants or platelet inhibitors it is recommended to review the medical records to determine the concurrent use of medications that affect other components of the clotting mechanisms before performing any procedure.[7]

Regional Anesthetic Management of the Patient Receiving Antiplatelet Medications

- NSAIDs, by themselves, represent no significant risk for the development of spinal hematoma in patients having epidural or spinal anesthesia.
- Allow platelet function to recover before neuraxial block after administration of ticlopidine, clopidogrel, and platelet GP IIb/IIIa receptor antagonists. The time to normal platelet aggregation after discontinuation of therapy is
  - 14 days for ticlopidine
  - 5–7 days for clopidogrel
  - 7–10 days for prasugrel
  - For the platelet GP IIb/IIIa inhibitors, the duration ranges from 8 hours for eptifibatide and tirofiban to 48 hours after abciximab administration

Regional Anaesthetic Management of the Patient on Oral Anticoagulants

- Discontinue oral anticoagulation and verify prothrombin time(PT) normalization before neuraxial block.
- Monitor the PT and international normalized ratio (INR) daily.
- Remove indwelling neuraxial catheters when the INR is less than 1.5 in order to assure that adequate levels of all vitamin-K-dependent factors are present.
- There is no definitive recommendation for facilitating removal of neuraxial catheters in patients with INR more than 1.5 but less than 3.0. Removal of neuraxial catheters should be done with caution and neurological status assessed until the INR has been stabilized.
- In patients with an INR more than 3, warfarin should be withheld.

Management of the Patient Receiving Unfractionated Heparin

- In patients receiving thromboprophylaxis with subcutaneous unfractionated heparin (UFH) 5000 U twice daily, there is no contraindication to the use of neuraxial techniques.
- Regional anesthesia and IV heparinization for patients undergoing vascular surgery is acceptable with the following recommendations:
  - Delay IV heparin administration for 1 hour after needle/catheter placement.
  - If systematic anticoagulation therapy is begun with an epidural catheter in place, delay catheter removal for 2–4 hours after heparin discontinuation and after evaluation of coagulation status.
  - Remove indwelling catheters 1 hour before a subsequent heparin administration.
- Serial platelet counts are indicated for patients receiving subcutaneous heparin for 5 days.

Regional Anaesthetic Management of the Patient Receiving Low Molecular Weight Heparin

Administration of antiplatelet or oral anticoagulant medications administered in combination with low molecular weight heparin (LMWH) is not recommended.

Preoperative Management

Perform neuraxial techniques at least 10–12 hours after a thromboprophylaxis dose and 24 hours after a high therapeutic dose of LMWH.

Postoperative Management

- With *twice daily* dosing, administer the first dose of LMWH no earlier than 24 hours after operation, regardless of anesthetic technique, and only in the presence of adequate hemostasis.
  - Remove indwelling catheters before initiation of LMWH thromboprophylaxis.
  - The first dose of LMWH administered 2 hours after catheter removal and 24 hours after needle/catheter placement, whichever is later.
- *Once daily* dosing requires 6–8 hours between needle/catheter placement and the first dose of LMWH. Subsequent dosing should occur no sooner than 24 hours later

Regional Anesthetic Management of the Patient on Thrombolytic and Fibrinolytic Therapy

- Patients receiving fibrinolytic and thrombolytic drugs should be cautioned against receiving spinal or epidural anesthetics except in highly unusual circumstances.

- There is no definitive recommendation for timing of neuraxial catheter removal in patients who unexpectedly receive fibrinolytic and thrombolytic therapy during a neuraxial catheter infusion. The measurement of fibrinogen might be helpful to assess the presence of residual thrombolytic effects.

Dabigatran

Discontinue 7 days before procedure; for shorter time periods, document normal thrombin time (TT). First postoperative dose 24 hours after needle placement and 6 hours post catheter removal (whichever is later).

COMPLICATIONS OF NEURAXIAL BLOCKADE

Several complications have been reported when a central neuraxial blockade is performed, but the incidence of serious complications is rare.

POST DURAL PUNCTURE HEADACHE

Post dural puncture headache is a common complication of spinal anesthesia, with a reported incidence as high as 25% in some studies.[1] Any break/hole in the dura mater, which may follow a spinal anesthetic, an epidural "wet tap," diagnostic lumbar puncture, myelography, or migration of epidural catheter may result in PDPH.

The mechanism of PDPH is thought to be persistent leakage of CSF through the meningeal needle hole at a rate faster than that of CSF production. This CSF leak leads to decreased CSF pressure without an accompanying decrease in intravenous pressure. This pressure difference causes cerebral venous dilation and is likely the cause of the resultant headache during upright position. Gravity causes traction on highly innervated meninges and pain-sensitive intracranial vessels.

The diagnosis of PDPH is clinical, usually presents 48–72 hours after the procedure, typically bilateral, frontal, and occipital extending up to neck and shoulders. Pain may be associated with neck stiffness, photophobia, nausea, vomiting, and cranial nerve symptoms (e.g., diplopia, tinnitus). The hallmark of PDPH is that it is *postural* in nature and often mild or absent when the patient is supine.

FACTORS THAT INCREASE THE INCIDENCE OF PDPH

- PDPH is more common in younger individuals
- Female gender
- Use of large diameter needles
- Use of cutting needles (Quincke vs. Whitacre)
- Needle bevel orientation—The incidence of PDPH is more if the needle bevel is placed perpendicular to the long axis of the neuraxis.
- Pregnancy
  - Multiple dural punctures

Miller RD, Eriksson LI, Fleisher LA, Wiener-Kronish JP, Young WL, eds. *Miller's Anesthesia*. 7th ed. Philadelphia, PA: Elsevier Churchill Livingstone; 2009.

Management

Bed rest, hydration, and analgesics as necessary are the mainstay of conservative treatment. Cerebral vasoconstrictors such as caffeine, sumatriptan, and oral methergine may also produce short-term symptomatic relief.

Epidural blood patch is the most effective treatment, resulting in complete resolution of most of the symptoms. Aseptically withdrawn autologous blood is injected in the same space or one space below. Blood injected into the epidural space compresses the thecal sac and increases subarachnoid pressure, thereby forcing the CSF cephalad.[1]

BACKACHE

Backache is a common complaint after spinal and epidural anesthesia. Compared with spinal anesthesia, back pain following epidural anesthesia is more common and of longer duration. Trauma due to needle insertion, local anesthetic irritation, and ligamentous strain secondary to muscle relaxation are the likely causative factors for the backache following neuraxial anesthesia.

NEUROLOGIC INJURY

Cauda Equina Syndrome

Hyperbaric 5% lidocaine has been implicated as a cause of multiple cases of cauda equina syndrome following subarachnoid injection through small-bore ("microspinal") catheters during continuous spinal anesthesia.[1] The US Food and Drug Administration has subsequently banned the use of these small-gauge catheters for continuous spinal anesthesia. Nerve injury is believed to result from the apparent maldistribution of the local anesthetic within the CSF around the dependent cauda equina nerve roots.

Transient Neurological Symptoms

Transient neurological symptoms (TNSs) are defined as pain or paresthesia in lower back, posterior thighs, or buttocks within 24 hours after spinal anesthesia. It appears to be due to a direct neural inflammatory reaction caused by the local anesthetic. Transient neurologic symptoms after spinal anesthesia develop most frequently after ambulatory procedures, especially in patients placed in the lithotomy or knee arthroscopy positions. All local anesthetics have been shown to cause TNS, although the risk with lidocaine appears to be more. To minimize the risk, alternative local anesthetics may be chosen, especially for patients at risk of developing TNS.[8]

HEMORRHAGIC COMPLICATIONS

Spinal hematoma is a rare but potentially devastating complication of spinal and epidural anesthesia. The incidence of neurologic dysfunction resulting from hemorrhagic complications associated with neuraxial blockade is increasing.[8] Patients who are receiving anticoagulants for thromboembolism prophylaxis and who also have received neuraxial anesthesia should be closely monitored for the prompt recognition of neuraxial hematoma formation. Patients most commonly present with numbness or lower extremity weakness. The diagnosis can be confirmed by radiological imaging (CT or MRI). Prognosis is good if diagnosis and operative decompression for treatment occur within 6 hours of the onset of hematoma formation.[9] In patients receiving anticoagulant medications, the ASRA recommendations regarding the timing of performance of spinal/epidural and placement and withdrawal of epidural catheters must be followed.

INFECTIOUS COMPLICATIONS

Bacterial infection of the central neuraxis may present as meningitis or cord compression secondary to abscess formation. Possible risk factors include underlying sepsis, diabetes, depressed immune status, steroid therapy, localized bacterial colonization or infection, and chronic catheter maintenance. The infectious source for meningitis and epidural abscess may result from distant colonization or localized infection with subsequent hematogenous spread and CNS invasion. The anesthesiologist may also transmit microorganisms directly into the CNS by needle or catheter contamination through a break in aseptic technique or passage through a contiguous infection.[8] Strict asepsis should be adhered to when performing spinal or epidural block. Epidural abscess presents as localized back pain and tenderness with associated fever and leukocytosis. As with epidural hematoma, the presence of progressive neurologic deterioration is cause for immediate surgical decompression. Arachnoiditis, another rare complication of neuraxial anaesthesia may appear as transient nerve root irritation, cauda equina, and conus medullaris syndromes.[10]

TOTAL SPINAL BLOCK

A total spinal block is a rare and life-threatening complication that occurs due to excessive cephalic spread of the local anesthetic. Total spinal anesthesia can happen when there is unintentional intrathecal administration of local anesthetics during epidural or caudal anesthesia. The onset is usually rapid. Total spinal usually manifests as severe hypotension, bradycardia, and respiratory insufficiency.

Risk Factors for Total Spinal Block

- Obesity and pregnancy
  - Engorged epidural veins
  - Increased intra-abdominal pressure
- Fluid in epidural space from epidural infusion: further compresses the subarachnoid space
- Dose, volume, and baricity can affect spread

HEMODYNAMIC DISTURBANCE

Hypotension

The primary cause of hypotension following neuraxial anesthesia is sympathetic blockade. Reduced sympathetic outflow leads to a reduction in peripheral arterial tone, which results in reduction of SVR. The degree to which SVR is reduced is related to the number of spinal segments blocked. The sympathectomy that accompanies the techniques depends on the height of the block, with the sympathectomy typically described as extending for two to six dermatomes above the sensory level with spinal anesthesia and at the same level with epidural anesthesia. After sympathetic block of the lower spinal segments, there is a compensatory increase in sympathetic tone at the unblocked levels. With a higher block, such compensatory vasoconstriction becomes impossible. This explains the correlation between the incidence of hypotension and peak block height. Sympathetic blockade also affects the intrinsic tone of the venous system. Reduction in tone of venous capacitance vessels results in decreased venous return. This reduction in preload is the main reason for the decrease in CO during high spinal anesthesia.

Bradycardia

Bradycardia occurs commonly during spinal anesthesia. In the normal balance of autonomic influences on the heart, sympathetic drive counters a predominant parasympathetic activity due to vagus. With blockade of cardiac accelerator fibers from the upper thoracic levels (T1 to T4), there remains an unopposed vagal influence on the sinoatrial node, resulting in a slowing of the heart rate. This blockade would also obstruct the ability of the carotid baroreceptor to reflexively increase heart rate in the face of hypotension.

THERMOREGULATORY DYSFUNCTION

Autonomic thermoregulation is impaired during regional anesthesia. This typically results in intraoperative core hypothermia. Three principal reasons explain why patients become hypothermic during neuraxial blockade. First, heat is internally redistributed from the core to the peripheral compartment. Second, the loss of thermoregulatory vasoconstriction below the level of the blockade results in increased heat loss from body surfaces in excess of metabolic heat production. Third, epidural and spinal anesthesia decrease the thresholds triggering vasoconstriction and shivering (above the level of the block) by about 0.6°C. Core hypothermia during regional anesthesia may not trigger a perception of cold, as the skin temperature is high.[2]

REFERENCES

1. Barash P, Cullen B, Stoelting R, Cahalan M, Stock M. *Clinical Anesthesia.* 7th ed. Philadelphia, PA: Lippincott Williams & Wilkins; 2013.
2. Miller R, ed. *Miller's Anesthesia.* 7th ed. Philadelphia, PA: Elsevier; 2010.
3. Neal M, Bernards C, Butterworth J, et al. ASRA practice advisory on local anesthetic systemic toxicity. *Reg Anesth Pain Med.* 2010;35(2):152–161.
4. Stoelting R, Hillier S. *Pharmacology and Physiology in Anesthetic Practice.* 4th ed. Philadelphia, PA: Lippincott Williams & Wilkins; 2005.
5. Mercado P, Weinberg G. Local anesthetic systemic toxicity: prevention and treatment. *Anesthesiol Clin.* 2011;29(2):233–242.
6. Neal J, Mulroy M, Weinberg G, American Society of Regional Anesthesia and Pain Medicine. American Society of Regional Anesthesia and Pain Medicine checklist for managing local anesthetic systemic toxicity: 2012 version. *Reg Anesth Pain Med.* 2012;37(1):16–18.
7. Horlocker T, Wedel D, Rowlingson J, Enneking F, American College of Chest Physicians. Executive summary: regional anesthesia in the patient receiving antithrombotic or thrombolytic therapy: American Society of Regional Anesthesia and Pain Medicine Evidence-Based Guidelines (Third Edition). *Reg Anesth Pain Med.* 2010;35(1):102–105.
8. Horlocker T. Complications of regional anesthesia and acute pain management. *Anesthesiol Clin.* 2011;29(2):257–278.
9. Pages-Arroyo E, Pian-Smith M. Neurologic complications of neuraxial anesthesia. *Anesthesiol Clin.* 2013;31(3):571–594.
10. Agarwal A, Kishore K. Complications and controversies of regional anaesthesia: a review. *Indian J Anaesth.* 2009;53(5):543–553.

FURTHER READING

Morgan GE, Mikhail MS, Murray MJ. *Clinical Anesthesiology.* New York, NY: Lange Medical Books/McGraw-Hill; 2006.

Hadzic A. *Textbook of Regional Anesthesia and Acute Pain Management.* New York, NY: McGraw-Hill; 2007.

Barash PG, Cullen BF, Stoelting RK, Cahalan MK, Stock MC. *Clinical Anesthesia.* Philadelphia, PA: Wolters Kluwer/Lippincott Williams & Wilkins; 2009.

Collins A, Gray A. Peripheral nerve blocks. In: Miller R, Pardo M. *Basics of Anesthesia.* 6th ed. Philadelphia, PA: Elsevier; 2011.

Drasner K, Larson M. Spinal and epidural anesthesia. In: Miller R, Pardo M. *Basics of Anesthesia.* 6th ed. Philadelphia, PA: Elsevier; 2011.

QUESTIONS

1. Which of the following is NOT a risk factor for PDPH?
   A. PDPH is more common in younger individuals
   B. Male
   C. Use of large diameter needles
   D. Use of cutting needles
   E. Pregnancy

2. Which of the following can be used for identifying intravascular catheter placement in an epidural test dose?
   A. Isoproterenol
   B. Air
   C. Fentanyl
   D. Epinephrine
   E. All of the above

3. The time to normal platelet aggregation after discontinuation of prasugrel is:
   A. 14 days
   B. 7-10 days
   C. 48 hours
   D. 5-7 days
   E. 8 hours

4. CV/CNS ratio is least for:
   A. Bupivacaine
   B. Ropivacaine
   C. Etidocaine
   D. Lignocaine
   E. Mepivacaine

ANSWERS

1. B. Females are at a higher risk of developing PDPH.[2]
2. E. Epinephrine is most commonly used for this purpose, but all others can also be used.[1]
3. B. It is important to allow platelet function to recover before neuraxial block after administration of ticlopidine, clopidogrel, and platelet GP IIb/IIIa receptor antagonists. The time to normal platelet aggregation after discontinuation of therapy is 14 days for ticlopidine, 5–7 days for clopidogrel, and 7–10 days for prasugrel. It is a reasonable expectation to require an examinee to recall the duration of action of such drugs, as this knowledge is applied in daily neuraxial practice.[8]
4. B. Cardiotoxicity of local anesthetics can be compared using the CV/CNS dose ratio. The lower the number the more cardiotoxic the drug (e.g., the CV/CNS for bupivacaine is approximately 3, versus 7 for lidocaine).[2]

18.

GENERAL ANESTHESIA

Matthew D. James, Aimee Gretchen Kakascik, Young Su, Shilpa Dabhade, and George W. Williams

INTRODUCTION

Anesthesia has always been concerned with providing the right amount. Too little anesthesia leads to patient discomfort and awareness; too much anesthesia results in death. Arthur Earnest Guedel classified the depth of anesthesia into stages in 1937. These stages were seen under diethyl ether anesthesia without muscular blockade.

Stage I starts with the beginning of the inhalational induction to the initial loss of consciousness.

Stage II is the loss of consciousness to the onset of loss of controlled breathing. Automatic respirations occur with possible coughing, breath holding, and irregular respiratory pattern. The eyelid reflex disappears, but the patient may still cough, vomit, and laryngospasm.

Stage III starts with the automatic respirations and ends with the cessation of breathing. This stage has four planes.

1. Plane I has involuntary breathing, and loss of conjunctival, lid, and swallowing reflex.
2. Plane II has the beginning of paralysis of the intercostal muscles, loss of laryngeal and corneal reflex, regular deep breathing, and loss of reaction to skin stimulation.
3. Plane III has complete intercostal muscle paralysis with only diaphragmatic breathing. The pupils are dilated and have loss of light reflex. Surgery can be performed in this stage without movement.
4. Plane IV has intercostal and diaphragmatic paralysis. The patient will be apneic with no central drive to breathe.

Stage IV is the presence of apnea and cardiovascular collapse. In this stage the pupils are dilated and fixed and the skeletal muscles are relaxed. Death ensues.

Joseph F. Artusio divided Stage I of Guedel's anesthetic depth classification into three planes in 1954.[1,2]

1. In Plane I there is no amnesia or analgesia.
2. In Plane II there is amnesia with partial analgesia.
3. In Plane III there is complete analgesia and amnesia.

One of the greatest fears of patients undergoing anesthesia is awareness. Awareness is when the patient can recall events that occurred while he or she was receiving anesthesia. Studies have shown that the incidence is from 0.1% to 1.1% depending on the type of anesthesia used and different at-risk patient groups. The highest risk groups include cardiac surgery, trauma, cesarean section, airway endoscopic surgery, and pediatric surgery patients. Awareness results from differences in requirement and the amount of anesthetic delivered. If the patient does not require an abnormal amount of anesthesia but the delivery of anesthesia is not potent enough then the patient will have awareness. An example is a healthy patient who does not receive enough anesthetic agent because the vaporizer is empty. A patient may have awareness even when the patient does not need as much anesthetic as normal and has very little anesthetic given to him or her. This can be observed in the pregnant patient with uterine rupture. She needs fewer anesthetics due to pregnancy and also can tolerate less anesthesia due to the blood loss and hemodynamic instability associated with uterine rupture. The anesthesiologist would administer fewer agents in this situation, and awareness could occur. In addition, awareness could occur in the patient who requires more anesthesia than normal and is only delivered as much anesthesia as would normally be required by most patients. This could happen with a patient with chronic alcohol abuse undergoing surgery while not inebriated.

Awareness can be reduced by recognizing patients at risk for intraoperative awareness and preventing inadequate delivery of anesthetics. Monitors can also be used to help determine the depth of anesthesia. The BIS (bispectral index) monitor (Aspect Medical Systems, Inc.) has been used to help prevent awareness. The monitor records EEG signals and interprets these signals into a number. A range is given under which most patients will have amnesia. Awareness may occur outside of this range, and with artifact awareness is still possible. Awareness during anesthesia is detrimental to the patient and can lead to post-traumatic stress disorder. The anesthesiologist can suffer from litigation as well.[3]

There are many techniques for the administration of anesthesia. The inhalational technique involves an inhalational agent such as sevoflurane and possibly nitrous oxide. Older inhalational agents such as halothane and ether are not used in practice much anymore due to side effects. Other inhalational agents such as desflurane are too irritating to the airway to use for inhalational induction. The inhalational technique is good for those with a needle phobia, such as children. It is also a good technique for preserving spontaneous respirations in patients with difficult airways such as an anterior thoracic mass. Deep anesthesia is needed to intubate with inhaled anesthetics alone. Hypotension, hypoventilation, and airway obstruction can occur during the time it takes to get to this point.

A combined inhalational and intravenous anesthetic technique may be helpful to allow for intubation without hypotension. Also, if airway obstruction occurs it will be difficult to increase the anesthetic depth with inhalational agents alone due to no gas exchange occurring. Lidocaine can be given intravenously or topically to allow for intubation. Propofol or another amnestic agent can be given to help increase the depth of anesthesia also. Nondepolarizing or depolarizing muscle relaxants can be given in addition.

A total intravenous anesthetic can be used when inhalational agents are not desired, as with malignant hyperthermia patients. An amnestic agent such as propofol, etomidate, or ketamine can be given along with an opioid and/or a muscle relaxant to achieve intubation. The infusion is then continued throughout the procedure. Some disadvantages are rapid loss of vascular tone, loss of airway, and difficult ventilation due to "chest wall rigidity" from the opioid administration.[4]

Loss of an airway is very concerning for the anesthesiologist. Steps must be taken to prevent such an event. One must first try to identify potentially difficult airways so that a plan to prevent airway loss can be made before induction. The American Society of Anesthesiologists (ASA) recommends 11 steps to determine whether an airway will be difficult. An airway may be difficult if the upper incisors are long, the patient has an overbite, the patient cannot protrude mandible, the inter-incisor distance is less than 3 cm, the uvula cannot be visualized, the palate is high-arched, the mandible is immobile or has a mass invading it, the thyromental distance is less than 5 cm, and the neck is short and thick and immobile. The patient should be able to touch the chin to the chest and extend the neck.[5]

Mallampati classification is another method of assessing the airway and giving it a score as to what is visualized when the patient opens the mouth as wide as possible and protrudes the tongue. In class I, everything is seen: soft palate, fauces, uvula, and pillars. In class II, only a portion of the uvula can be visualized but the soft palate and fauces are still seen. In class III, only the soft palate and the base of the uvula are seen. In class IV, only the hard palate is visualized.

Other notable components to the airway exam include presence of facial hair, obesity, and large neck circumference of greater than 60 cm or 17 inches in men and 16 inches in women.[6]

There are also patients with congenital and acquired pathologies with associated difficult airways. In children this is most often observed in patients with Treacher-Collins, Pierre Robin, and Down syndromes. Difficult airways are also encountered in patients with ankylosis, degenerative arthritis, subglottic stenosis, lingual or tonsillar hypertrophy, and pituitary tumors associated with excess growth hormone release.[7]

If the airway appears problematic from your examination and history, it would be prudent to suggest an awake intubation. This can be performed by fiber-optic bronchoscopy, direct laryngoscopy, blind orotracheal or nasotracheal intubation, retrograde wire intubation, a light wand or illuminated stylet, rigid bronchoscopy, or a percutaneous tracheostomy/cricothyrotomy. The patient may not agree to awake intubation despite the risks or may not be able to comprehend the risks or is combative and in need of emergency surgery or airway control. In this case the patient should be preoxygenated and an induction of anesthesia begun while striving to maintain spontaneous respirations. A nondepolarizing or depolarizing muscle relaxant can be used to facilitate intubation, but it may make awakening the patient more difficult especially with the longer-acting muscle relaxants such as rocuronium and vecuronium. This is the often referred to "burning your bridge" problem with muscle relaxation. Succinylcholine is preferred for difficult airways if not contraindicated, that is, in malignant hyperthermia, burns older than 24 hours, immobilization, muscle damage due to trauma or underlying myopathy, and hyperkalemia. Succinylcholine has the fastest onset at 1 minute and only lasts for 5 to 10 minutes. If intubation or mask ventilation is still not possible after succinylcholine administration, attempts should still be made to obtain an airway and the patient not allowed to recover from the muscle relaxant without intervention. Rocuronium or vecuronium can be used with intubating doses of 1.2 mg/kg and 0.2 mg/kg if succinylcholine is contraindicated. The muscle relaxant will last for 1 to 2 hours after administration. Sugammadex can reverse this block, but it is not yet approved for use in the United States.[8]

If mask ventilation is possible, an intubation or airway securement should proceed with one or more of the previously listed options or the patient should be awakened and surgery canceled. If mask ventilation is not possible a supraglottic airway should be used and, if successful, the patient should be awakened, or another method of intubation chosen. If the supraglottic device fails (especially common with devices not allowing a greater than 20 cmH_2O peak inspiratory pressure), then a combitube, transtracheal jet ventilation, or rigid bronchoscopy should be attempted. If all else fails, a surgical airway is needed.[9]

There are several devices available to assist with difficult intubations. The simplest device is the gum elastic bougie, which is an intubating stylet. The bougie is inserted under direct laryngoscopy and then the endotracheal tube is passed over it. It is easier to place than an endotracheal tube, because it is smaller and has a soft tip with which one can feel the tracheal rings as it passes into the airway. When the cords cannot be visualized, the epiglottis can be lifted with the bougie and passed into the trachea. Alternatively, it can be used with the GlideScope, which provides indirect visualization of the airway.

Another device for failed intubation is the combitube. The combitube is inserted into the esophagus, and the esophageal balloon is inflated to occlude the esophagus. A second tube connected to the device is then able to deliver oxygen to the lungs and prevent air entry into the stomach. The combitube can cause esophageal rupture and injury; therefore, it is mainly for emergency intubations where direct laryngoscopy has failed.[8]

The flexible fiberoptic laryngoscope can be used for difficult airways while the patient is awake or anesthetized. The nasal approach allows a direct path to the trachea, but this route may be contraindicated by trauma or risk of bleeding and obstructing visualization, as in pregnant patients with engorged mucous membranes. The oral route may be used, but the patient may bite down on the scope or the gag reflex may be elicited. The scope is advanced while the distal end is manipulated to guide around structures. Once the scope passes through the vocal cords into the trachea, the endotracheal tube is advanced over the scope. If this is difficult, the scope can be inserted through a laryngeal mask airway (LMA) or a retrograde wire can be threaded into the channel of the scope to guide positioning. Indirect rigid laryngoscopy can also be used to lift the soft tissues and to visualize placement of the fiberoptic scope. Rigid indirect laryngoscopes include Airtraq, TruView, Glidescope, McGrath, and others, which project the image onto a screen.[10]

Retrograde intubation involves inserting a flexible guide wire through an 18-gauge sheath in the larynx. The wire is advanced until it exits the mouth or nose. Once the guide wire is in position, a catheter is threaded over it. Finally the endotracheal tube is advanced over the catheter. Some risks with this type of blind intubation are bleeding, subcutaneous emphysema, pneumomediastinum, and infection. This technique should be avoided, especially if other techniques of intubation are available, in cases of coagulopathy, lack of neck landmarks, laryngeal disease, and local infection, namely Ludwig's angina.[10]

A light stylet may also be used for blind nasotracheal or orotrachal intubation. There are multiple devices, such as the light wand, that use a bright light at the tip of a stylet to intubate. The lighted tip is inserted into the endotracheal tube and then the apparatus is inserted into the airway. The neck is observed for illumination that is midline with a small intense glow. If the lighted stylet is not in the trachea but the esophagus, the light will be much dimmer and less intense. There are risks with this blind technique including: damage to the airway structures and obstructing the airway by pushing a foreign body if present deeper into the trachea.[10]

The LMA is recommended in the ASA algorithm for difficult airways (Figures 18.1 and 18.2) (more details on the difficult airway algorithm in Chapter 16). The LMA is a supraglottic airway that can be used for ventilation of the patient while waiting for a more secure airway such as tracheostomy placement. An endotracheal tube can be placed in the airway through the opening in the LMA blindly or with a fiberoptic bronchoscope. An LMA Fastrach is an intubating LMA that is specialized for inserting an endotracheal tube through it. The LMA Fastrach has an elevating bar with which the glottis opening can be aligned.

The LMA ProSeal may be inserted using the index finger or the thumb. The LMA ProSeal may also be inserted using the LMA ProSeal introducer. If the mask is inserted incorrectly it may enter the vestibule of the larynx, causing obstruction to ventilation. The mask should be reinserted.

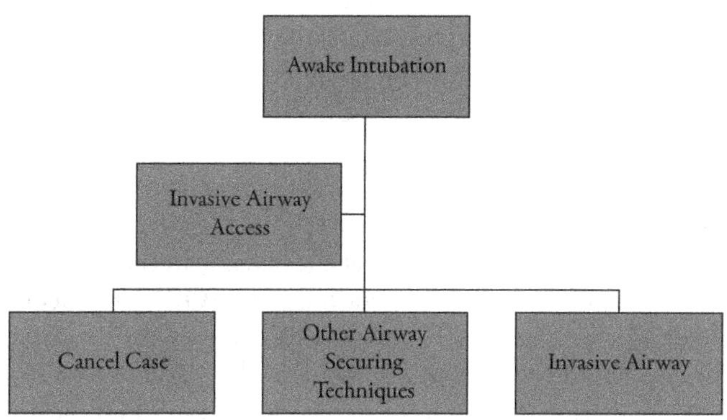

Figure 18.1 Simplified ASA algorithm for awake airway.

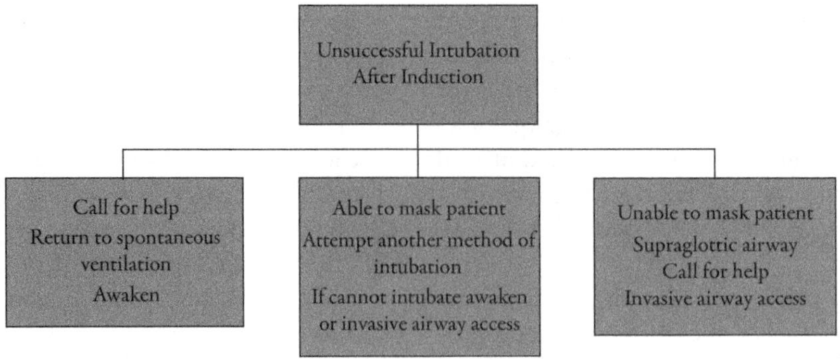

Figure 18.2 Simplified ASA algorithm for difficult airway.

To verify correct placement, a small amount (1–2 mL) of lubricant gel is placed in the proximal end of the drain tube. If the mask is in proper position, there should be a slight up-down bobbing movement of the lubricant. If there is no movement, or the lubricant is pushed out, the mask may be incorrectly positioned.

TRANSCUTANEOUS OR SURGICAL AIRWAY

The anesthesiologist may encounter a tracheostomy in a few different settings: a patient presenting for surgery with a tracheostomy in situ, a patient with prolonged intubation presenting for creation of tracheostomy, a pediatric patient with known anatomical variation predisposing to difficulty breathing for creation of tracheostomy, or a patient requiring emergency tracheostomy as the culmination of management using the difficult airway algorithm.[7] A patient with a tracheostomy in situ may be induced by simply connecting the tracheostomy tube to the anesthesia breathing circuit—an accordion extension tube is usually used to allow some flexibility in the connection and to allow space for the tubing. The patient may need to be positioned in a "sniffing" position to gain access to the ostomy site. Due to the presence of a large leak around an uncuffed tracheostomy tube, the inhalation induction of anesthesia may be prolonged, and the ability to adequately ventilate may be impaired. A throat pack may be used to alleviate a leak and maintain ventilation. If a large leak is present from the breathing circuit then the practitioner should be aware that the readings for respiratory parameters on the ventilator, and therefore those recorded on the medical record, will not be accurate.

A planned tracheostomy is a frequent surgical procedure in both adult and pediatric centers for a variety of reasons. These cases may be done at the bedside in the intensive care unit (ICU) or in the operating room (OR). The special challenge for the anesthesiologist in these cases is to have the breathing tube mostly untaped and accessible to withdraw when the surgeon has entered the airway and indicates verbally that they are ready to insert the new tracheostomy tube. Once the tracheostomy is inserted and the endotracheal tube has been removed, the anesthesiologist must rapidly confirm the presence of an appropriately placed airway circuit via the detection of exhaled CO_2, chest rise, fogging of the tube, and breath sounds in the chest.

Finally, a tracheostomy may be an emergency procedure for securing the airway in a patient that unexpectedly could not be ventilated or intubated. In patients with a pathological airway obstruction (see section on cricothyroidotomy below), or in a case in which sudden airway collapse/occlusion may be expected with the induction of anesthesia, a capable surgeon should be present with a rigid bronchoscope and the equipment to perform a tracheostomy.

Cricothyroidotomy is an alternative to tracheostomy for the purpose of temporary oxygenation until the airway may be secured. Cricothyroidotomy may be required in the following scenarios: in a patient who cannot be ventilated or intubated, in the absence of a surgeon who can perform a tracheostomy, in a patient with increased airway resistance (airway edema postoperatively from surgical procedures to the neck or with angioneurotic edema), or in a patient with pathological airway obstruction (i.e., epiglottitis, retropharyngeal abscess, tumor, trauma/foreign body), where it may be dangerous to manipulate the airway.[9] Commercially available kits exist for cricothyroidotomy. However, if no such kit is available, other supplies that are regularly available to the anesthesiologist may be used: an appropriately sized intravenous catheter (16- to 14-gauge for an adult), attached to a slip-tip 3-mL syringe (with plunger removed), attached to an ETT connector from a 7.0-mm endotracheal tube. This apparatus may be connected to a breathing circuit for hand or mechanical ventilation, or one can be used to employ jet ventilation.

Transtracheal jet ventilation is an emergency and temporary technique to provide oxygenation and some ventilation to a patient who cannot be intubated or ventilated and when there is no a surgeon present who is capable of performing a tracheostomy. Usually performed via a cricothyroidotomy, an angiocatheter is connected to an apparatus that delivers high-pressure bursts of oxygen to the airway.[11] Preferably a high-pressure and adjustable system is used to give 1- to 1.5-second breaths at 20 to 25 psi, for a rate of about 12 breaths per minute.[12] When using a high-resistance angiocatheter, the usual low-pressure systems such as an ambu bag or common-gas outlet will not adequately expand the chest.[3] With any high-pressure ventilatory system there is significant risk of barotrauma, specifically subcutaneous emphysema or pneumomediastinum from rupture of a pulmonary bleb or bronchus, or from incorrect placement of the ventilating catheter. Jet ventilation may also be useful in the patient with a large bronchopleural fistula, where conventional positive pressure ventilation may not be effective.

ENDOBRONCHIAL INTUBATION

Separation of the lungs and one-lung ventilation has many absolute and relative indications. Absolute indications include isolation to prevent contamination of the healthy lung from infection or hemorrhage, control of ventilation to avoid bronchopleural fistula or bronchocutaneous fistula or unilateral cyst/bullae or in the setting of unilateral bronchial trauma/disruption, to facilitate unilateral lung lavage, and to facilitate thoracscopic surgery (not usually necessary in pediatrics). Relative indications include facilitating thoracic exposure for lung lobectomy or pneumonectomy, or repair of aortic aneurysms, or for esophageal repair.[13]

An endobronchial blocker is placed into the bronchus of the lung that is to be nonventilated and then its cuff is inflated until occlusion. If the blocker has a central lumen then it may be used for suctioning the distal airway or to insufflate oxygen. The disadvantage of this type of device is that it may become easily dislodged. A Fogarty catheter is a type of arterial embolectomy catheter that is frequently used as a bronchial blocker. It has a malleable wire stylet, and is placed with a fiber-optic bronchoscope, and may be placed alongside the endotracheal tube or through an endotracheal tube with a y-joint connector. A drawback of the Fogarty catheter is the low-volume, high-pressure balloon design that may exert significant pressure on the bronchial mucosa and may be easily dislodged into the trachea.[14] The Arndt endobronchial blocker (Cook Critical Care, Bloomington, IN) has the advantage of a wire snare that allows it to be attached to the bronchoscope for more direct placement of the balloon. There are other endobronchial blockers with directional tips and with high-volume, low-pressure balloons. The Univent (Fugi Systems Corp., Japan) is a single-lumen endotracheal tube with a built-in side channel and bronchial blocker. Disadvantages of the Univent tube are that the blocker may be difficult to direct into the desired bronchus, and the larger size and irregular shape of the tube may make it difficult to pass through the vocal cords.[15]

Double-lumen endotracheal tubes are the most common means of accomplishing one-lung ventilation. Double-lumen tubes are essentially two tubes bonded together such that one lumen is placed into a mainstem bronchus and the other lumen opens into the distal trachea. Lung separation is accomplished by inflating two cuffs—one proximal to each tube opening. The first double-lumen endotracheal tube, called the Carlens tube, had a carinal hook. Today's tubes are Roberstshaw tubes without the carinal hook and with a fixed bend distally to aid in advancement into the desired bronchus. Double-lumen tubes are available in right-sided versions, but left-sided tubes are usually used. A cuff inflated high in the right mainstem bronchus may compromise ventilation of the right upper lobe. A usual left-sided Robertshaw tube is inserted with a stylet under direct laryngoscopy, with the tip of the tube pointed anteriorly until it passes the vocal cords, then it is turned 90 degrees to the left and advanced into the assumed position. After the stylet is removed, the tube position should be assessed with auscultation to ensure the ability to inflate both lungs first, and then to perform ventilation of each lung separately. Then tube placement should be confirmed with a fiber-optic bronchoscope passed initially through the tracheal lumen.[16] A bronchial blocker may be preferred to a double-lumen endotracheal tube in cases where exchanging the tube at the end of the case is required for postoperative ventilatory support and there was a difficult intubation or severe airway edema is suspected.[17] At the end of the operative case a double-lumen tube may need to be replaced. The ICU staff will be unfamiliar with the double-lumen tube, it may be displaced, and it is difficult to suction the airway in the usual ICU fashion. During tube exchange one should visualize the exchange if possible with a direct laryngoscopy or using a video-laryngoscope. If a tube exchanger is used, then a direct laryngoscopy should still be preformed to reduce the trauma to airway structures.

INTUBATION AND TUBE CHANGE ADJUNCTS

There are several commercially available products that may be used as an aid in intubation or as stylets for endotracheal tube exchange. Lighted stylets allow transillumination of the airway. As the stylet is passed through the larynx it shows a more focal light presence, but when in the esophagus the light is relatively dim or diffuse. A lighted stylet may be difficult to remove, and the oropharyngeal and laryngeal structures may be traumatized inordinately if the endotracheal tube is passed without direct visualization.[18]

The term *bougie* encompasses a variety of solid or hollow semimalleable stylets. When the larynx is not visualized during direct or video-laryngoscopy, a bougie may be inserted blindly such that the breathing tube may be then advanced over the bougie and into the trachea. The Eschmann introducer (Eschmann Health Care, Kent, England) was introduced in 1949 and is made of woven polyester (sometimes called the gum elastic bougie). It has a tip with a 40-degree bend 3.5 cm from one end that allows it to be placed under the epiglottis and up into the trachea without direct visualization. Confirmation of tracheal placement may first be recognized by the tactile sensation of the bougie tip "clicking" on rings of cartilage as it advances down the trachea. There are other bougies that have lumens for flexible stylets or for insufflation of oxygen. A bougie may be used as a stylet for endotracheal tube exchange.[19]

Tracheal extubation over a long, hollow, semirigid catheter with a small internal diameter (may be referred to as a *jet stylet*) may greatly reduce the risk of inadequate ventilation and failed reintubation in cases of a known difficult airway or when postsurgical changes may complicate further laryngoscopy. There are many types of stylets/tubes available for this technique. Hollow tubes may be used for insufflating oxygen or for jet ventilation. A stylet/catheter that is too small or thin-walled may kink and impede advancement of the breathing tube. Placement of a new tracheal tube should always involve direct laryngoscopy when possible to reduce the chance of damage to the surrounding structures. Care must be taken with the insertion of any type of rigid device into the airway to not apply excessive force for risk of mucosal laceration or perforation. A tube exchanger left in the airway is very irritating and the patient will most likely remove the catheter unless the patient is sedated or topically anesthetized or restrained.

ENDOTRACHEAL TUBE TYPES

The first endotracheal tubes used in the 1870s by Sir William Macewen were made out of steel and brass. Then flexible metal tubes, by F. Kuhn, and red mineralized rubber tubes, by I. W. Magill, were developed. The cuffed endotracheal tube was introduced in 1928 by A. Guedel and R. M. Waters. In 1941, an opening at the end of the endotracheal tube, called the Murphy eye, was developed as an alternate means of gas flow in case of obstruction of the distal tip. The double-lumen tube was first used by Carlens in 1949.[20]

Most current endotracheal tubes are made out of polyvinyl chloride (PVC). Other tubes have been made out of silicone, Teflon, nylon, metal, and even ceramic. Common features of modern breathing tubes include a high-volume, low-pressure cuff, a bevel with opening facing left and a Murphy eye facing right, a radio-opaque line, depth markers, and a standard 15-mm connector to the breathing circuit (the interior diameter of the tube will be labeled/embossed on the underside of the removable tube connector). To cause less mucosal trauma, some tube tips may be more rounded versus pointed. Some tube tips may have a curved or bird's beak shape (Flex-tip by Parker Medical, Englewood, CO, USA) to facilitate passage over an introducer or through the nose with less catching on tissues. Endotracheal tubes are generally selected based on internal diameter size based on patient age and size and sex, with adjustments made for specific anatomical variations or surgical requirements or specific tube designs.

There are several specific endotracheal tube types that may be indicated for certain surgical procedures or techniques. Mallinckrodt (Mallinckrodt Co., St Louis, MO, USA) makes an extralong microlaryngoscopy tube (MLT) for laryngeal surgery. Multiple companies make wire-reinforced tubes (also called anode, armored, or spiral-embedded) intended to reduce kinking or collapse. The Ring-Adair-Elwin (RAE) tube is made in both oral and nasal varieties, and both cuffed or uncuffed, and is useful for directing the tube and breathing circuit away from surgical field. In order to reduce the risk of airway thermal injury or fire, there are a few types of endotracheal tubes used specifically for laser surgery cases. These include foil-wrapped tubes, flexible metal tubes, and metal-impregnated tubes. If airway fire or cuff rupture is a risk, then the cuff may be filled with sterile saline, and some tubes have more than one cuff. The Portex line (Smiths Medical) of tubes have a port that allows suctioning of secretions from the supraglottic area. The Endotrol (Mallinckrodt) tube has a pull-ring attached to a cord that travels to the distal end of the tube to allow flexion of the tube tip. Endotracheal tubes with an internal coating of silver may reduce ventilator-associated pneumonia in the ICU.

Traditionally, cuffed endotracheal tubes were used in adults and children over 6–8 years of age. Due to the pediatric airway being narrower below the glottis, and in order to maximize tube size, uncuffed tubes were placed in small children. It is now commonly accepted that cuffed endotracheal tubes may be used in children and infants with the advantage of reducing repeat laryngoscopies and intubations without increased incidence of croup.[21]

Maintaining appropriate endotracheal tube cuff pressure can be critically important to minimize mucosal injury or to ensure lung protection or isolation. A high-volume, low-pressure cuff is desirable when the tube is expected to be in place for longer than 24 hours. Inflating to the point of air leak at 15–20 cmH_2O pressure in the distal airway should be the goal when adding air to the cuff.[22] Any less and you may not have an adequate seal to prevent aspiration, for gas scavenging, for efficient use of modern low-flow circuits, or for reaching desired tidal volumes and having accurate readings for end-tidal gas and respiratory parameter measurements.

There are several devices available to manage endotracheal tube cuff pressure. The Lanz valve (Covidien) is built into some tubes to automatically maintain intracuff pressure at approximately 30 cmH_2O to help reduce the risk of tracheal damage during long-term intubations. Other devices can attach to the pilot balloon and act as a pressure regulator/indicator, including the Cufflator (Posey Medical) and the disposable Pressure-Easy (Smiths Medical). It should be noted that nitrous oxide may diffuse into the cuff and increase cuff pressure over time.

AMERICAN SOCIETY OF ANESTHESIOLOGISTS MONITORING

1. Monitored Anesthesia Care and Sedation: ASA Guidelines for Sedation, Sedation Guidelines for Non-Anesthesiologists

The ASA publishes standards for monitoring of patients undergoing anesthesia and sedation, and separately offers practice guidelines for sedation and analgesia by nonanesthesiologist providers.

The ASA Basic Standards for Anesthetic Monitoring were adopted in 1986 and last amended in 2010[23]:

1. STANDARD I

Qualified anesthesia personnel shall be present in the room throughout the conduct of all general anesthetics, regional anesthetics, and monitored anesthesia care.

1.1 Objective—

Because of the rapid changes in patient status during anesthesia, qualified anesthesia personnel shall be continuously present to monitor the patient and provide anesthesia care. In the event there is a direct known hazard, e.g., radiation, to the anesthesia personnel which might require intermittent remote observation of the patient, some provision for monitoring the patient must be made. In the event that an emergency requires the temporary absence of the person primarily responsible for the anesthetic, the best judgment of the anesthesiologist will be exercised in comparing the emergency with the anesthetized patient's condition and in the selection of the person left responsible for the anesthetic during the temporary absence.

2. STANDARD II

During all anesthetics, the patient's oxygenation, ventilation, circulation, and temperature shall be continually evaluated.

2.1 Oxygenation—

2.1.1 Objective—To ensure adequate oxygen concentration in the inspired gas and the blood during all anesthetics.

2.2 Methods—

2.2.1 Inspired gas: During every administration of general anesthesia using an anesthesia machine, the concentration of oxygen in the patient breathing system shall be measured by an oxygen analyzer with a low oxygen concentration limit alarm in use.*

2.2.2 Blood oxygenation: During all anesthetics, a quantitative method of assessing oxygenation such as pulse oximetry shall be employed.* When the pulse oximeter is utilized, the variable pitch pulse tone and the low threshold alarm shall be audible to the anesthesiologist or the anesthesia care team personnel.* Adequate illumination and exposure of the patient are necessary to assess color.*

3. VENTILATION

3.1 Objective—

To ensure adequate ventilation of the patient during all anesthetics.

3.2 Methods—

3.2.1 Every patient receiving general anesthesia shall have the adequacy of ventilation continually evaluated. Qualitative clinical signs such as chest excursion, observation of the reservoir breathing bag, and auscultation of breath sounds are useful. Continual monitoring for the presence of expired carbon dioxide shall be performed unless invalidated by the nature of the patient, procedure, or equipment. Quantitative monitoring of the volume of expired gas is strongly encouraged.*

3.2.2 When an endotracheal tube or laryngeal mask is inserted, its correct positioning must be verified by clinical assessment and by identification of carbon dioxide in the expired gas. Continual end-tidal carbon dioxide analysis, in use from the time of endotracheal tube/laryngeal mask placement, until extubation/removal or initiating transfer to a postoperative care location, shall be performed using a quantitative method such as capnography, capnometry, or mass spectroscopy.* When capnography or capnometry is utilized, the end-tidal CO2 alarm shall be audible to the anesthesiologist or the anesthesia care team personnel.*

3.2.3 When ventilation is controlled by a mechanical ventilator, there shall be in continuous use a device that is capable of detecting disconnection of components of the breathing system. The device must give an audible signal when its alarm threshold is exceeded.

3.2.4 During regional anesthesia (with no sedation) or local anesthesia (with no sedation), the adequacy of ventilation shall be evaluated by continual observation of qualitative clinical signs. During moderate or deep sedation the adequacy of ventilation shall be evaluated by continual observation of qualitative clinical signs and monitoring for the presence of exhaled carbon dioxide unless precluded or invalidated by the nature of the patient, procedure, or equipment.

4. CIRCULATION

4.1 Objective—

To ensure the adequacy of the patient's circulatory function during all anesthetics.

4.2 Methods—

4.2.1 Every patient receiving anesthesia shall have the electrocardiogram continuously displayed from the beginning of anesthesia until preparing to leave the anesthetizing location.*

4.2.2 Every patient receiving anesthesia shall have arterial blood pressure and heart rate determined and evaluated at least every five minutes.*

4.2.3 Every patient receiving general anesthesia shall have, in addition to the above, circulatory function continually evaluated by at least one of the following: palpation of a pulse, auscultation of heart sounds, monitoring of a tracing of intra-arterial pressure, ultrasound peripheral pulse monitoring, or pulse plethysmography or oximetry.

5. BODY TEMPERATURE

5.1 Objective—

To aid in the maintenance of appropriate body temperature during all anesthetics.

5.2 Methods—

Every patient receiving anesthesia shall have temperature monitored when clinically significant changes in body temperature are intended, anticipated, or suspected.

† Note that "continual" is defined as "repeated regularly and frequently in steady rapid succession" whereas "continuous" means "prolonged without any interruption at any time."

* Under extenuating circumstances, the responsible anesthesiologist may waive the requirements marked with an asterisk (*); it is recommended that when this is done, it should be so stated (including the reasons) in a note in the patient's medical record.

These standards for basic anesthetic monitoring are to be applied to monitored anesthesia care (MAC) cases. Monitored anesthesia care refers to a specific anesthesia service for a diagnostic or therapeutic procedure that may include varying levels of sedation, analgesia, and anxiolysis as necessary. The provider of MAC must be prepared and qualified to convert to general anesthesia when necessary.[24]

The ASA Practice Guidelines for Sedation and Analgesia by Non-Anesthesiologist Providers were initially adopted in 1995 and then revised in 2002 and published in *Anesthesiology*.[25] These guidelines are for patients undergoing both moderate and deep sedation:

1. Preprocedure evaluation

   Relevant history (major organ systems, sedation–anesthesia history, medications, allergies, last oral intake)

   Focused physical examination (to include heart, lungs, airway)

   Laboratory testing guided by underlying conditions and possible effect on patient management

   Findings confirmed immediately before sedation

2. Patient counseling

   Risks, benefits, limitations, and alternatives

3. Preprocedure fasting

   Elective procedures—sufficient time for gastric emptying

   Urgent or emergent situations—potential for pulmonary aspiration considered in determining target level of sedation, delay of procedure, protection of trachea by intubation

   See ASA Guidelines for Preoperative Fasting

4. Monitoring

   (Data to be recorded at appropriate intervals before, during, and after procedure) Pulse oximetry

   Response to verbal commands when practical

   Pulmonary ventilation (observation, auscultation)

   Exhaled carbon dioxide monitoring considered when patients separated from caregiver

   Blood pressure and heart rate at 5-min intervals unless contraindicated

   Electrocardiograph for patients with significant cardiovascular disease

   For deep sedation: Response to verbal commands or more profound stimuli unless contraindicated

   Exhaled carbon dioxide monitoring considered for all patients

   Electrocardiograph for all patients

5. Personnel

   Designated individual, other than the practitioner performing the procedure, present to monitor the patient throughout the procedure

   This individual may assist with minor interruptible tasks once patient is stable

   For deep sedation:

The monitoring individual may not assist with other tasks

6. Training

   Pharmacology of sedative and analgesic agents

   Pharmacology of available antagonists

   Basic life support skills—present

   Advanced life support skills (ACLS)—within 5 min

   For deep sedation:

   Advanced life support skills in the procedure room

7. Emergency Equipment

   Suction, appropriately sized airway equipment, means of positive-pressure ventilation

   Intravenous equipment, pharmacologic antagonists, and basic resuscitative medications

   Defibrillator immediately available for patients with cardiovascular disease

   For deep sedation: Defibrillator immediately available for all patients

8. Supplemental Oxygen

   Oxygen delivery equipment available

   Oxygen administered if hypoxemia occurs

   For deep sedation:

   Oxygen administered to all patients unless contraindicated

9. Choice of Agents

   Sedatives to decrease anxiety, promote somnolence

   Analgesics to relieve pain

10. Dose Titration

    Medications given incrementally with sufficient time between doses to assess effects

    Appropriate dose reduction if both sedatives and analgesics used

    Repeat doses of oral medications not recommended

11. Use of anesthetic induction agents (methohexital, propofol)

    Regardless of route of administration and intended level of sedation, patients should receive care consistent with deep sedation, including ability to rescue from unintended general anesthesia

12. Intravenous Access

    Sedatives administered intravenously—maintain intravenous access

    Sedatives administered by other routes—case-by-case decision

    Individual with intravenous skills immediately available

13. Reversal Agents

    Naloxone and flumazenil available whenever opioids or benzodiazepines administered

14. Recovery

    Observation until patients no longer at risk for cardiorespiratory depression

    Appropriate discharge criteria to minimize risk of respiratory or cardiovascular depression after discharge

15. Special Situation

    Severe underlying medical problems—consult with appropriate specialist if possible

    Risk of severe cardiovascular or respiratory compromise or need for complete unresponsiveness to obtain adequate operating conditions—consult anesthesiologist

INTRAVENOUS FLUID THERAPY DURING ANESTHESIA

Fluid management is of vital importance to the anesthesiologist. Fluid replacement therapy must first consider the patient's regular requirements for water, sodium and potassium, and dextrose. In the surgical patient, one must factor in losses of fluid, intraoperative fluid shifts, and the patient's ability to mobilize the fluid that is given. There are many choices of intravenous fluids including crystalloids, colloids, and hypertonic solutions, each with specific indications.

The most commonly used formula for water replacement is known as the "4-2-1" formula: 4 mL/kg/h for the first 10 kg of patient weight then an additional 2 mL/kg/h for the weight of 11–20 kg, then 1 mL/kg/h for additional kilograms. Therefore, a patient who weighs 70 kg would get a maintenance fluid rate of crystalloids at 110 mL/h. Average daily intake of sodium and potassium for the 70-kg adult are, respectively, 75 mEq/L and 40 mEq/L. Combining these two calculations, we conclude a 70-kg adult will get 2500 mL of fluid/day that will need to contain sodium of about 30 mEq/L and potassium of about 15–20 mEq/L. It is important to note that the kidneys can manage a wider range of sodium than potassium intake. An alternative way to understand fluid requirements it to consider the average adult will have about 100–200 mL/day gastrointestinal losses, 500–1000 mL/day insensible losses, and about 1000 mL/day urinary losses.[26]

Of great concern for the anesthesiologist is to prevent hypoglycemia in the anesthetized patient. Glucose is usually administered in the form of dextrose-containing solutions. Because the usual stress response to surgery results in a rise in serum glucose, only infants and patients that have taken insulin or oral hypoglycemic drugs should need supplemental dextrose. There is strong evidence that in critically ill patients, tight control of plasma glucose between 80 and 110 mg/dL is associated with reduced morbidity and mortality.[26] Iatrogenic hyperglycemia may induce osmotic diuresis.

Surgical fluid losses from the extracellular compartment include direct blood loss, wound drainage, burn edema, ascites, pleural fluid, and gastrointestinal secretions. Many of these fluids are rich in plasma proteins and electrolytes, and may require more accurate replacement. Chronic upper gastrointestinal loss may result in hypochloremic metabolic alkalosis that may be treated with 0.9% normal saline, whereas lower gastrointestinal loss may result in hyperchloremic metabolic acidosis that is best treated with a bicarbonate- or lactate-containing solution. Patients with impaired cardiac or renal function may need more precise volume and electrolyte replacement.[26]

Fluid shifts during surgery can create a major need for additional intravenous fluids beyond those calculated for replacement of deficit and blood loss. Extravasation of fluid into surgically manipulated tissues or into cavities after ascitic or pleural fluid drainage must be considered. It is generally taught that 4–10 mL/kg/h may be needed depending on the severity of the tissue trauma or the degree of exposure of mucosal and serosal surfaces in the surgical field. Intraoperative fluid replacement strategies will continue to be debated, with some studies showing better clinical outcomes from fluid restriction and some studies claiming the opposite.[26]

Crystalloids are aqueous solutions with small molecule solutes that will cross semipermeable membranes such as cell and capillary membranes. Commonly used crystalloid solutions are 0.9% normal saline and so-called balanced salt solutions such as Lactated Ringer's and Plasmalyte (Baxter Healthcare).

Colloid solutions contain large solutes that will not freely cross semipermeable membranes. A colloid solution may only be beneficial in the setting of an intact capillary bed. In fact, the administration of colloids may cause harm in states of capillary leak by inducing pulmonary edema, ascites, or osmotic diuresis. Five percent albumin exerts a colloid oncotic pressure similar to that of human plasma, while 25% albumin may translocate significant volume from the interstitial fluid volume to the plasma volume.[26] Hydroxyethyl starch solutions (there are a variety of preparations) are expensive and may induce a coagulopathy with doses exceeding 20 mL/kg/day.

Describing a replacement fluid as hypertonic has to do with its osmotic pressure as compared with that of plasma. Hypertonic saline (usually 3% sodium) causes hypernatremia that is largely restricted to the extracellular fluid volume compartment. It is most often used in the neurosurgery patient, where there are several proposed mechanisms for the reduction in cerebral edema and intracranial pressure. The main effect is to draw water from parenchyma into the intravascular compartment, but it may also significantly favor the reabsorption of cerebrospinal fluid and improve cerebral capillary perfusion by dehydrating endothelial cells.[26]

ANESTHETIC COMPLICATIONS

Assessing perioperative or periprocedure morbidity and mortality as complications related to anesthesia is a difficult task. There is difficulty in obtaining data on complications, and there is great variability in the methodology used both to perform preoperative risk assessment and to assign the contribution of anesthesia care to patient outcome. Here we consider perioperative mortality and specific complications including postoperative nerve injury, awareness and recall, eye injury, and dental injury. Overall it is generally recognized that anesthesia safety has vastly improved over the years.[27]

Reports of anesthesia-related mortality will vary widely depending on date of service, location of service, characteristics of service provider, and a multitude of patient characteristics such as age, ASA risk classification, and length of follow-up (i.e., death within 24 hours vs. 48 hours). Most studies conducted within the last 20 years show an anesthesia-related death rate of 1 in 10,000 to 1 in 100,000.[27]

The most common nerve injury that produces anesthesia malpractice claims is ulnar neuropathy, with an incidence of between 3.7 and 50 per 10,000 patients.[27] Lower extremity neuropathy specifically after surgery in the lithotomy position has been observed in 2.7 per 10,000 patients.[28] Awareness with recall has been documented in 15–40 per 10,000 patients.[27] Eye injuries are a common complication after anesthesia and range from the painful corneal abrasion to more the serious vision deficit due to ischemic optic neuropathy and central retinal artery occlusion. Eye injury after nonocular surgery was observed in 5.6 per 10,000 patients.[29] Dental injuries that required dental intervention were observed in 1 in 4537 patients.[30]

COMPLICATIONS OF ANESTHESIA

General anesthesia depresses the protective airway reflexes, and as such puts patients at risk for intraoperative pulmonary aspiration or for aspiration during recovery. Central nervous system depressant medications such as inhalation anesthetics, barbiturates, and opioids suppress swallowing and laryngospasm. While laryngospasm is commonly thought of as a negative occurrence, in principle it is a perturbation of protective reflexes designed to prevent inappropriate material from entering the airway.

The immediate sequelae of aspiration includes cough, mild tracheal irritation, or transient laryngospasm. Aspiration of large volume predisposes to infection, small airway obstruction, and pulmonary edema. Aspiration of "sterile" blood causes minor airway obstruction but is rapidly cleared by mucociliary transport, resorption, and phagocytosis. On the other hand, massive blood clots can obstruct the airway and impair oxygenation. Over time, this results in fibrinous changes in air spaces leading to pulmonary hemochromatosis due to iron accumulation in phagocytic cells. If purulent matter or tissue is aspirated it can cause secondary bacterial infection (again, in time).

Diffuse reflex bronchospasm and airway obstruction leading to hypoxemia with distal atelectasis are characteristic features related to chemical pneumonitis, which commonly occurs due to aspiration of acidic gastric contents resulting from vomiting or regurgitation. Accumulation of gas in the stomach during general anesthesia increases the frequency of postoperative vomiting (this gas can easily accumulate when peak pressures associated with ventilation exceed 20 cmH_2O).

Morbidity increases directly with volume and inversely with the pH of acidic aspirate. When partially digested food is aspirated, the severity of pneumonitis is increased as well as prolonged. Food particles obstruct the airways mechanically and form a nidus for secondary bacterial infection. Significant aspiration of gastric contents is associated with rapid progression to acute respiratory distress syndrome (ARDS) and pulmonary edema. ARDS involves degeneration of epithelium, interstitial and alveolar edema, and hemorrhage into air spaces. These pathophysiologic changes cause obstruction of the airways resulting in lower surfactant function, hyaline membrane formation, and emphysematous changes. This further leads to ventilation perfusion (V/Q) mismatch and reduced lung compliance (and therefore, increased ventilator requirements).

Multiple factors are responsible for aspiration of gastric contents. Residual effects of laryngeal nerve blocks or topical local anesthetics used to reduce lower airway irritation additionally reduce postoperative airway protection. Reflexes may also be impaired by residual neuromuscular paralysis. A train of four T4/T1 ratio of > 0.9 should be achieved before reflexes can be considered completely competent. Hypotension, acidemia, or hypoxemia cause vomiting and altered consciousness thereby increasing aspiration risk, which also may occur when reversal of neuromuscular blockade is omitted.

Due to limited treatment options for aspiration, strict vigilance for preventing it is critical and most efficacious. This includes avoidance of particulate antacids and administration of nonparticulate antacids such as sodium citrate. Sodium citrate increases the pH of gastric fluid without excessively increasing volume and should be used preoperatively for patients at high risk. Histamine type 2 receptor blockers such as cimetidine or ranitidine reduce the gastric volume and increase gastric pH. Additionally, metoclopramide increases gastroesophageal sphincter tone and promotes gastric emptying. If vomiting occurs during intubation, prompt lateral head positioning and suctioning of the airway is mandatory (assuming intact cervical spine integrity) if gastric secretions are found in the pharynx.

Head elevation in unconscious patients can create a gravitational gradient from pharynx to lung and should be avoided. Trendelenburg position favors regurgitation but helps in airway clearance if regurgitation or vomiting occurs. As such, in the event of aspiration, head down/ Trendelenburg is a more ideal position in general. One should carefully monitor the upper airway for secretions or vomitus and suction if appropriate. Cuff deflation should be avoided until extubation, as the rigid endotracheal tube interferes with swallowing and other protective reflexes. When extubating, suction the pharynx completely and extubate at end inspiration (*following* positive airway pressure if needed) to aid in expulsion of material trapped below the cords but above the inflated cuff.

If there is a suspicion that significant aspiration has occurred, the patient should be admitted with pulse oximetry and temperature monitoring (in addition to standard vital signs), complete blood count with differential, and blood gases along with chest radiograph, if appropriate. Monitoring for development of aspiration pneumonitis is recommended for 24 to 48 hours; recall that the chest x-ray can lag behind the clinical picture of lung injury patients by 24 to 48 hours. Chest physiotherapy, incentive spirometry, and adequately treating preexisting pulmonary comorbidities with medications aid in reducing infection and shunting.

If there is evidence of hypoxemia, consolidation, or pulmonary edema, prompt antibiotic treatment should be started based on *culture results* and/or gram staining. The presence of equivocal cultures mandates the use of broad spectrum antibiotics for anaerobic and gram negative coverage if clinically appropriate, but antibiotics should not be started prophylactically for all occurrences of suspected aspiration. Support the patient with supplemental oxygen, positive end expiratory pressure (PEEP) or continuous positive airway pressure (CPAP) as needed, keeping in mind that mechanical ventilation is often necessary (this is usually evident early in the admission). Adequate hydration is necessary in case of fluid losses into the lung and diffuse vasodilation secondary to an inflammation response when it occurs.

AIRWAY TRAUMA

Endotracheal intubation (ETI) is a rapid, simple, safe, and nonsurgical technique that achieves all the goals of airway management, namely, maintains airway patency, protects the lungs from aspiration, and permits leak-free ventilation during mechanical ventilation, and remains the gold-standard procedure for airway management. When ETI is difficult or has failed, other devices can be used both for elective airway management as well as for emergency airway management. These devices include the LMA and the combitube. Endotracheal intubation–related complications are more likely in infants, children, and adult women, as these patients have a relatively small larynx and trachea and are more prone to airway edema; additionally, complications are more likely during emergency situations. The knowledge, technical skills, and crisis management capabilities of the anesthesiologists play a vital role in the occurrence and outcome of complications during airway management.

Tracheal and Esophageal Injuries

The shape of the standard endotracheal tube (ETT) results in maximal pressure being exerted on the posterior aspect of the larynx. Sterilization of plastic tubes with ethylene oxide (uncommon in the United States) may lead to production of toxic ethylene glycol if adequate time for drying has not been allowed. Cuff-related injuries might occur with the use of high-pressure cuffs or inappropriate use of low-pressure cuffs. Injury to the lips, teeth, tongue, nose, pharynx, larynx, trachea, and bronchi can occur during laryngoscopy and intubation, but the most frequent sites of injury are larynx, pharynx, and esophagus.

Esophageal perforation can occur with attempts at intubation, especially in patients with a difficult airway or multiple attempts. Subcutaneous emphysema may be noticed soon after intubation. Later, neck pain, difficulty in swallowing, neck erythema, and edema may occur. Mediastinitis leading to sepsis may result in death or serious morbidity. Placement of a nasogastric tube has also been associated with esophageal perforation. Tracheal laceration may occur due to overinflation of the ETT cuff, multiple intubation attempts, use of stylets (especially when the stylet protrudes beyond the end of the ETT), malpositioning of the tube tip, and tube repositioning without cuff deflation. Placement of double-lumen ETTs has also been associated with tracheobronchial rupture. When any perforation occurs, a search must be made for such perforations, including by bronchoscopy. Nitrous oxide should be discontinued when pneumothorax or pneumomediastinum is suspected.

Epistaxis is a common problem, caused by the tip of the ETT traumatizing nasal and pharyngeal mucosa. Nasal intubation is relatively contraindicated in patients with coagulopathy. Prolonged nasal intubation can lead to pressure necrosis of the nostrils and septum. Nasal septal abscesses, retropharyngeal abscesses, and paranasal sinusitis can occur after intubation. Macroglossia is seen with prolonged compression by an ETT leading to ischemia and venous congestion.

Laryngeal Trauma

In the subglottic larynx, an anterior branch of the recurrent laryngeal nerve enters between the cricoid and the thyroid cartilage, innervating the intrinsic muscles of the larynx. An inflated cuff at this location can compress the nerve between the cuff and the overlying thyroid cartilage, causing injury. Recurrent nerve injury can be prevented by avoidance of overinflation of the ETT cuff, and prevention of excessive tube migration during anesthesia. Ulcerations or erosions of the larynx are common even after a short duration of intubation. *Granuloma of the vocal cords* may develop from an ulcer but usually heal spontaneously. Prolonged anterior displacement of the mandible, as in the jaw thrust maneuver, has been implicated in lingual nerve injury. Tongue cyanosis and swelling can also occur after the use of an LMA.

VASCULAR COMPLICATIONS

Intra-Arterial Injections

With unintentional intra-arterial injection, many patients complain of immediate discomfort (often within seconds), ranging from local irritation to intense pain distal to the site of injection. Altered motor function (involuntary muscle contractures and muscle weakness) and cutaneous manifestations (flushing, mottling) also occur. Patients may complain that inserting the cannula was more painful than expected. Most cases of accidental intra-arterial cannulation involve radial artery branches of the forearm and hand and are often due to vascular anomalies. The drugs that cause the most severe injury are barbiturates and benzodizapines. The key signs that indicate inadvertent intra-arterial injection include backflow of bright red blood into an IV catheter, pulsatile movement of blood in the IV tubing, and backflow of blood into the IV tubing even when the fluid bag is at a level higher than the catheter insertion site.

Thrombophlebitis

Thrombophlebitis is an inflammation of a vein, usually in the legs, that becomes swollen due to a blood clot. Superficial thrombophlebitis affects veins closer to the surface of skin. If it is not treated, deep vein thrombosis can develop, leading to pulmonary embolism. Pregnancy, obesity, and hormone therapy (including some birth control pills), are the risk factors for blood clots. Symptoms that suggest thrombophlebitis are pain, warmth, tenderness, swelling, redness of the affected area, and palpable cord-like veins.

Sheared Catheter

Shearing/rupture is a recognized complication of central venous, epidural, and subarachnoid catheters. Causes include the force of introducer needle during insertion, high pressure within the catheter caused by bolus infusions, fracturing of the external portion by the patient's body movements (mostly infants) or during removal of a stuck catheter (mostly by fibrin sheath formation around the catheter), and weakening of the central venous catheter tip by movements of the tricuspid valve and right ventricular motion. Metal forceps or clamps should not be used to remove catheters. If pain or parasthesia develops during catheter removal in the intrathecal space, stop removal and consult neurosurgery with radiologic evaluation to locate the retained catheter.

Cardiac/Vascular Perforations

Patients with congenital heart disease undergo various cardiac diagnostic procedures. Cardiac perforation can occur during the course of angiocardiography or cardiac catheterization. Acute perforation is defined as event within 24 hours after implantation. Delayed perforation is defined by the event that presents at least 1 month after pacemaker/ICD implantation. The presenting symptoms and signs include chest pain, dyspnea, hypotension, syncope, inappropriate ICD shocks, muscle or diaphragm stimulation, abdominal pain, pericardial effusion, or cardiac tamponade.

Pulmonary Artery Rupture

Swan-Ganz catheters are commonly used (though decreasing in frequency) for hemodynamic monitoring in the ORs and ICUs. The incidence of Swan-Ganz catheter-associated pulmonary artery rupture is 0.031%, and an urgent thoracotomy should be performed if hemothorax is present at any point. Hemoptysis is the leading symptom after pulmonary artery rupture.

NEUROLOGICAL INJURIES

Pressure Injuries of Mask

Pressure from a mask or mask strap may result in a pressure injury to underlying nerves. The mask should be removed from the face periodically and readjusted to make certain that continuous pressure is not applied to one area. Face masks should be completely free of residual cleansing agents, as these can cause serious mucosal, skin, or eye injury (conjunctivitis, burning, irritation) and tongue swelling (allergic glossitis).

Peripheral Neuropathies

Brachial plexus neuropathy: Shoulder braces when placed tightly at the base of the neck can injure the roots of the brachial plexus, as can the exaggerated rotation of the head away from an extended arm.

Axillary nerve trauma from humeral head: Abduction of the arm on an arm board to >90 degrees may thrust the head of the humerus into the axillary neurovascular bundle, causing it to stretch.

Radial nerve injury: The radial nerve can be compressed against the underlying bone on the lateral aspect of the arm. Excessive cycling of the noninvasive blood pressure cuff and restrictive towels used to tuck the arms can potentially cause injury to the radial nerve.

Median nerve compression: Median nerve compression can occur due to iatrogenic trauma during intravascular access in the antecubital fossa. Forced elbow extension while positioning the arms can stretch the median nerve.

Ulnar neuropathy: Patient characteristics like male sex, high body mass index (>38), and prolonged postoperative bed rest are associated with ulnar neuropathies.

Nerve Injury Due to Tourniquet

The radial nerve is the most common nerve affected by use of a tourniquet. Inability to detect pain, heat, cold, or pressure over the skin along the source of the nerve and a sluggishness or inability to move large or small muscles on command are the symptoms of nerve injury. Use of a tourniquet for longer than 2 hours and with pressure greater than 350 mmHg in a lower extremity and greater than 250 mmHg in an upper extremity increases the risk of compression neurapraxia. Remember that the nerve has a central blood supply, so if the pressure exerted on the nerve exceeds blood pressure, then the nerve is by definition ischemic, leading to injuries when this is too prolonged. Padding should be used beneath tourniquets and over pressure points, and extreme joint positions, particularly of the shoulder and head, should be avoided. Tourniquet times must also be carefully monitored.

Intraneural Injections

Peripheral nerve injury is a rare complication of regional anesthesia. Mechanical needle trauma and intraneural injection leading to nerve edema, hematoma, and ischemia and local anesthetic neurotoxicity are some of the mechanisms of post-block-related nerve injury.

Retractors

Cervical retractors used during anterior cervical discectomy cause significant increase in cuff pressure of the tracheal tube.

Burns

The patient plate electrode should have good contact with dry, shaved skin. The contact surface area should be at least 70 cm^2 and should be away from bony prominences, scar tissue, and metal implants. Incorrect placement of the patient plate electrode is the most common cause of accidental diathermy burns. However, careless surgical technique can also cause local tissue burns. Monopolar surgical diathermy uses high-frequency alternating current, which can generate local temperatures of up to 1000°C. Current passes from the active electrode, held by the surgeon (high current density), through the body, returning via the patient plate electrode (low current density) to the generator. If the patient plate electrode is incorrectly placed, the return pathway is interrupted. In that case, any points of contact between metal and skin (e.g., ECG electrodes) will provide an alternate return pathway, resulting in burns. Monopolar diathermy can lead to large currents persisting beyond the operative site, causing tissue burns.

If the active electrode touches skin, the local concentration of high-density currents will cause skin burns. Any pools of alcohol-based skin preparation fluids can heat up and even ignite during diathermy use. Bipolar diathermy is safer, as current passes only between the two points of the diathermy forceps. It should be used on appendage surgery (e.g., digits and penis).

Bronchospasm

Bronchospasm is the spasmodic contraction of the bronchial smooth muscles. This can occur during anesthesia in isolation or as a complication of a serious condition such as anaphylaxis. The risk of perioperative bronchospasm increases with history of chronic bronchitis, asthma and atopy, tobacco exposure, and upper respiratory tract infection. But many patients presenting with perioperative bronchospasm do not have underlying chronic obstructive lung disease or asthma. The triggers for inducing bronchospasm include viral respiratory infection, environmental allergen, and chemical and mechanical irritation. During induction, the main cause is tracheal irritation during intubation. The airway manipulation and surgical stimulus under light anesthesia triggers bronchospasm as well as laryngospasm. Severe anaphylactic reaction caused by drugs (antibiotics, neuromuscular blockers), blood products (red blood cells, fresh frozen plasma) and other allergens (latex) are the agents commonly responsible for bronchospasm during maintenance of anesthesia. Intravenous anesthetics like thiopental, muscle relaxants like atracurium, mivacurium, d-tubocurarine, and other intravenous drugs like beta blockers, prostaglandin inhibitors (NSAIDs), and cholinesterase inhibitors (neostigmine) are implicated.

Laryngospasm

Laryngospasm, a protective reflex mediated by the vagus nerve, is the most frequent cause of postextubation airway obstruction. This can result in hypoventilation, inability to ventilate the lungs, and hypoxia. Laryngospasm can usually be overcome by providing gentle positive pressure in the oropharynx with 100% O_2. Prolonged laryngospasm may be relieved with a small dose of succinylcholine (e.g., 0.1 mg/kg). Because suctioning of the oropharynx does not adequately remove secretions around the vocal cords, it is best to extubate patients during a positive pressure breath or during patient expectoration.

Negative-Pressure Pulmonary Edema

When airway obstruction occurs after extubation, such as in the case of laryngospasm, negative-pressure pulmonary edema may occur in the spontaneously breathing patient. As a result of inspiratory effort against the closed glottis, these patients generate negative intrapleural pressure. The condition is seen within minutes after extubation. Management involves removing the obstruction, supporting the patient with oxygen, monitoring the patient closely, and reducing the afterload.

Anaphylaxis

During anaphylaxis (type I immediate hypersensitivity reaction, mentioned earlier in the chapter), an antigen enters a patient during anesthesia via a parenteral route, that is, intramuscularly or intravenously. This antigen binds two IgE antibodies on the surface of basophils and mast cells. This causes the release of stored mediators like histamine, tryptase, eosinophilic chemotactic factor of anaphylaxis (ECF-A), leukotrienes, prostaglandins, and kinins. These released mediators produce the characteristic symptoms of bronchospasm, wheezing, laryngeal edema in the respiratory system, increased capillary permeability in cardiovascular system, and urticaria in the cutaneous system. Patients are exposed to a variety of foreign substances such as drugs (i.e., antibiotics, anesthetic agents, neuromuscular blocking agents), blood products, and polypeptides like protamine, aprotinin, and latex (natural rubber). It is imperative that anesthesiologists rapidly recognize the warning signs of anaphylaxis, the most life-threatening form of an allergic reaction, and treat it in a timely manner.

Latex Allergy

Healthcare workers are found to have an increasing number of allergic reactions to latex-containing products. This may include contact dermatitis, which is a delayed, type IV T-cell-mediated reaction or sometimes a serious Type I IgE-mediated reaction such asthma, conjunctivitis, rhinitis, contact urticaria, or full-blown anaphylactic shock. In addition to healthcare workers, children with spina bifida, urogenital anomalies, or certain food allergies like bananas, avocados, and kiwi fruit, have been recognized as people with an increased risk of anaphylaxis to latex. A history of atopy and asthma also poses significant risk of latex allergy.

Hypothermia and Shivering

Postoperative *hypothermia* is one of the most important complications in the postanesthesia care unit (PACU). Average PACU stay is prolonged by 40–90 minutes for hypothermic patients; this is secondary to the fact that hypothermia is essentially an anesthetic and further degrees of hypothermia result in further degrees of sedation. During anesthesia, several mechanisms contribute to heat loss. Body heat is redistributed and also lost by *evaporation* during skin preparation. *Radiation* and *convection* from the skin and wound and humidification of dry gases in the airway are also responsible for heat loss. Radiation is the primary mechanism of heat loss in the OR, because the degree of loss correlates with the difference in ambient temperatures to the fourth power. *Conduction* of heat from the body to the table occurs. Furthermore, cold intravenous fluids and low ambient temperature accelerate temperature reduction. Paralysis and anesthesia impair shivering and thermoregulatory vasoconstriction. Regional anesthesia causes residual vasodilation and paralysis, which impedes heat generation and retention. Thus rewarming is slower after regional anesthesia. Minimal alveolar concentration of inhalation anesthetics decreases by 5%–7% per 1°C cooling. This accentuates residual sedation. Cardiac rhythm generation and impulse conduction are also affected. On ECG, the PR, QRS, or QT intervals lengthen and J waves appear. Below 28°C, spontaneous ventricular fibrillation occurs. Hypothalamic regulation generates *shivering* to increase endogenous heat production during emergence. Shivering interferes with pulse oximetry and ECG monitoring and increases the risk of incidental trauma. Oxygen consumption and CO_2 production increase by up to 200% (really bad if a patient has poor cardiac function or low oxygen reserve).

Hyperthermia

Some patients can exhibit hyperthermia from aggressive intraoperative heat preservation or close draping. Causes include drug or transfusion reaction, aspiration, retained secretions, and atelectasis due to loss of lung volume. Drug such as atropine (muscaranic blocking agents) interfere with cooling.

OCULAR INJURIES

Corneal Abrasions

Corneal abrasions are commonly seen due to direct mechanical trauma from high-riding oxygen face masks, laryngoscopes, sterile drapes, nasal cannulas, low-hanging identification badges, or patient attempts to rub the eyes with a "pulse-oximetered" finger. Eyes should be closed and securely taped immediately after induction of anesthesia. Preservative-free eye ointment is preferred, as preservative can cause corneal epithelial sloughing and conjunctival hyperemia. General anesthetics also abolish Bell's phenomenon (when eyes roll to the back of the head upon losing consciousness) and cause a significant decrease in tear production, further risking corneal exposure. The cornea may also be traumatized by inadvertent pressure, or by chemicals such as the sterile prep. Abrasion causes photophobia, tearing, decreased visual acuity, and pain. Although corneal abrasion usually heals spontaneously within 72 hours without scarring, severe injury can cause cataract formation and impair vision.

Postoperative Visual Loss

Visual loss after anesthesia is a rare but devastating injury as perioperative retinal artery occlusion results in permanent loss of vision in most cases. The incidence is on the rise, particularly in the setting of spinal fusion, cardiac, and head and neck surgery. This discussion is confined to visual loss that follows nonocular surgery. Spine and cardiac surgery appear to be associated with a higher incidence of perioperative visual loss than other operative procedures.

Central retinal artery occlusion (CRAO) is most commonly related to external compression of the eye due to improper patient positioning that is typical during spine surgery performed with the patient in prone position. External compression by a horse shoe head rest raises the intraocular pressure sufficient to stop flow in the central retinal artery. Pressure within the orbit can also be increased after retrobulbar hemorrhage, which is associated with vascular injuries during sinus or nasal surgery. Retinal microemboli are common during open-heart surgery. In osteogenesis imperfecta, sclera and cornea are unusually thin, and exophthalmos is common as a result of bony facial abnormalities. Thus the eye is more vulnerable to damage from external pressure. The anesthesiologist must take steps to avoid globe compression. Anesthetic masks should be carefully placed to avoid pressure on the eye. In patients positioned prone for surgery, it is mandatory to check the position of the head and the eyes intermittently by palpation or visualization.

A foam headrest should be used with the eyes properly placed in the opening of the headrest.

Cortical Blindness

Initially, total cortical blindness is usually accompanied by signs of stroke in the parieto-occipital region. The patient may suffer agnosia (an inability to interpret sensory stimuli). About 80% of cases of cortical blindness postoperatively have followed cardiac or other thoracic surgery. Patients at high risk of cortical blindness include those with coronary artery disease, congenital heart disease, liver failure, postpartum pulmonary embolism, and hypercholesterolemia.

ENVIRONMENTAL FACTORS

Anesthetic gases are used in a variety of treatment and research procedures throughout the medical industry. When these materials escape into the work environment they are referred to as *waste anesthetic gases* (WAGs). Every time an inhaled anesthetic is delivered, trace amounts of waste gases enter the OR atmosphere. The OR personnel are thus exposed to these waste gases chronically. High concentrations of WAGs can cause a narcotic effect, resulting in reduced mental performance, audiovisual ability, and manual dexterity. Chronic exposure to WAGs may increase the risk, causing other health effects including reduced fertility, spontaneous abortion, an increase in birth defects, and neurological, renal, and liver disease. Mask inductions, the use of LMAs, uncuffed endotracheal tubes, and circuit disconnects or leaks all contribute to OR contamination. Pediatric anesthesia results in more exposure to anesthetic gases, as mask inductions and uncuffed endotracheal tubes are common in standard practice. Malfunctions of the scavenging system, including disconnects, result in higher contamination levels than levels due to inhaled inductions. More often, scavenging system disconnects are due to human error rather than equipment failure. Patients continue to exhale trace amounts of N_2O for 5 to 8 hours after arrival in the PACU. Thus, transfer to the PACU does not eliminate the risk of exposure to waste gases.

In the OR, a minimum of 15 air exchanges per hour with at least 3 air exchanges of outdoor air per hour is recommended. In the recovery room at least six air exchanges are required with a minimum of two exchanges of outdoor air per hour. Additional methods for controlling WAGs include work practices that minimize gas leakage, such as making sure the waste gas disposal lines are connected, waiting until the circuit is connected to the patient before turning on the nitrous oxide or vaporizer, making sure the mask fits the patient, switching off the nitrous oxide and vaporizer when not in use, and finally, maintaining oxygen flow until the scavenging system is flushed.

Studies conducted in the late 1960s concluded that the incidence of congenital anomalies in children of male and female anesthesiologists was higher than in the control groups of physicians. Also, a meta-analysis of six of these studies linked the exposure to anesthetic gases to hepatic disease in males and cervical cancer, liver disease, and kidney disease in females. No definitive evidence has shown that trace concentrations of volatile anesthetics in the ambient air of the OR present a health hazard.

RADIATION/LASERS

Operating room personnel are routinely exposed to both ionizing radiation primarily from x-rays and nonionizing radiation from lasers. If the radiation exposure is severe enough, tissues may be destroyed or chromosomal changes may induce malignant growth. In the case of nonionizing radiation, the heat produced by the absorbed radiation may damage tissues. Ionizing radiation has become a health hazard in recent times with new advances in endovascular surgery, where procedures performed in the radiology suite expose anesthesia personnel to the radiation. Occupational exposure to radiation comes from primarily from x-rays scattered by the patient and surrounding equipment. A distance of 6 feet from the patient provides the same protection as 2.5 mm of lead. A distance of 3 feet from the patient is recommended to minimize occupational exposure. Physical separation is the best protection, because the intensity of scattered radiation is inversely proportional to the square of the distance from the source. Aprons with an equivalent of 0.25 to 0.5 mm of lead sheet are effective in blocking most scattered radiation. The lens of the eye still bears the risk of injury, as it remains uncovered.

Laser stands for "light amplification by stimulated emission of radiation." A surgical laser produces intense focused electromagnetic radiation to cut or destroy tissues. Eye injuries can occur due to burns to the cornea and retina, destruction of the optic nerve, and cataract formation. Protective eye goggles are recommended, however it should be confirmed that patient monitors can be seen and interpreted correctly. The vapor and cellular debris produced during laser surgery is called plume. Under experimental conditions, intact DNA from human papilloma virus (HPV) has been detected in the vapor from both laser-treated plantar warts and genital condylomata. Human immunodeficiency virus (HIV) proviral DNA has been found in laser smoke produced by vaporizing cultures of HIV-positive cells.

It is necessary to stress the importance of adequate evacuation and filtration of such vapors by a scavenging system. A case report of laryngeal papillomas in a laser surgeon suggest that it may have been caused by inhaled virus particles, hence the need to scavenge all vaporized debris.

REFERENCES

1. Guedel A. *Inhalation Anesthesia*. 2nd ed. New York, NY: Macmillan; 1951.

2. Artusio J. Di-ethyl ether analgesia: a detailed description of the first stage of ether analgesia in man. *J Pharmacol Exp Ther.* 1954;111:343–334.
3. Miller R, ed. *Miller's Anesthesia*. 7th ed. Philadelphia, PA: Elsevier; 2010:1237–1241.
4. Miller R, ed. *Miller's Anesthesia*. 7th ed. Philadelphia, PA: Elsevier; 2010:1578–1579.
5. Bready L, Noorily S, Dillman D. *Decision Making in Anesthesiology: An Algorithmic Approach*. Philadelphia, PA: Mosby/Elsevier; 2007:20.
6. Miller R, ed. *Miller's Anesthesia*. 7th ed. Philadelphia, PA: Elsevier; 2010:1007.
7. ASA Practice Guidelines for Management of the Difficult Airway. American Society of Anesthesiologists website. http://www.asahq.org/~/media/Sites/ASAHQ/Files/Public/Resources/standards-guidelines/practice-guidelines-for-management-of-the-difficult-airway.pdf. Accessed March 26, 2015.
8. Miller R, ed. *Miller's Anesthesia*. 7th ed. Philadelphia, PA: Elsevier; 2010:2285–2286.
9. Bready L, Noorily S, Dillman D. *Decision Making in Anesthesiology: An Algorithmic Approach*. Philadelphia, PA: Mosby/Elsevier; 2007:20–27.
10. Miller R, ed. *Miller's Anesthesia*. 7th ed. Philadelphia, PA: Elsevier; 2010:1591–1599.
11. Mecca RS. Postoperative recovery. In: Barash PG, Cullen BF, Stoelting RK, eds. *Clinical Anesthesia*. 5th ed. Philadelphia, PA: Lippincott Williams & Wilkins; 2006:1390.
12. Rosenblatt W. Airway management. In: Barash P, Cullen B, Stoelting R, eds. *Clinical Anesthesia*. 5th ed. Philadelphia, PA: Lippincott Williams & Wilkins; 2006:638.
13. Cohen E, Neustein S, Eisenkraft J. Anesthesia for thoracic surgery. In: Barash P, Cullen B, Stoelting R, eds. *Clinical Anesthesia*. 5th ed. Philadelphia, PA: Lippincott Williams & Wilkins; 2006:824.
14. Cohen E, Neustein SM, Eisenkraft JB. Anesthesia for thoracic surgery. In: Barash P, Cullen B, Stoelting R, eds. *Clinical Anesthesia*. 5th ed. Philadelphia, PA: Lippincott Williams & Wilkins; 2006:831.
15. Cohen E, Neustein S, Eisenkraft J. Anesthesia for thoracic surgery. In: Barash P, Cullen B, Stoelting R, eds. *Clinical Anesthesia*. 5th ed. Philadelphia, PA: Lippincott Williams & Wilkins; 2006:825.
16. Cohen E, Neustein S, Eisenkraft J. Anesthesia for thoracic surgery. In: Barash PG, Cullen B, Stoelting R, eds. *Clinical Anesthesia*. 5th ed. Philadelphia, PA: Lippincott Williams & Wilkins; 2006:826–827.
17. Cohen E, Neustein S, Eisenkraft J. Anesthesia for thoracic surgery. In: Barash P, Cullen B, Stoelting R, eds. *Clinical Anesthesia*. 5th ed. Philadelphia, PA: Lippincott Williams & Wilkins; 2006:825.
18. Rosenblatt W. Airway management. In: Barash P, Cullen B, Stoelting R, eds. *Clinical Anesthesia*. 5th ed. Philadelphia, PA: Lippincott Williams & Wilkins; 2006:636.
19. Rosenblatt W. Airway management. In: Barash PG, Cullen B, Stoelting R, eds. *Clinical Anesthesia*. 5th ed. Philadelphia, PA: Lippincott Williams & Wilkins, 2006:637.
20. Larson M. History of anesthetic practice. In: Miller R, ed. *Miller's Anesthesia*. 6th ed. Philadelphia, PA: Elsevier Churchill Livingstone; 2005:37–38.
21. Gal T. Airway management. In: Miller R, ed. *Miller's Anesthesia*. 6th ed. Philadelphia, PA: Elsevier Churchill Livingstone; 2005:1630.
22. Gal T. Airway management. In: Miller R, ed. *Miller's Anesthesia*. 6th ed. Philadelphia, PA: Elsevier Churchill Livingstone; 2005:1630.
23. ASA Standards for Basic Anesthetic Monitoring. https://www.asahq.org/For-Members/~/media/For%20Members/documents/Standards%20Guidelines%20Stmts/Basic%20Anesthetic%20Monitoring%202011.ashx.
24. ASA Position Statement on MAC. https://www.asahq.org/For-Members/~/media/For%20Members/Standards%20and%20Guidelines/2014/POSITION%20ON%20MONITORED%20ANESTHESIA%20CARE.pdf.
25. ASA Practice Guidelines for Sedation and Analgesia by Non-Anesthesiologists. https://ecommerce.asahq.org/p-180-practice-guidelines-for-sedation-and-analgesia-by-non-anesthesiologists.aspx.
26. Prough D, Wolf S, Funston J, Svensen C. Acid-base, fluids, and electrolytes. In: Barash P, Cullen B, Stoelting R, eds. *Clinical Anesthesia*. 5th ed. Philadelphia, PA: Lippincott Williams & Wilkins; 2006:181–187.
27. Posner K, Cheney F, Kroll D. Professional liability, quality improvement, and anesthetic risk. In: Barash P, Cullen B, Stoelting R, eds. *Clinical Anesthesia*. 5th ed. Philadelphia, PA: Lippincott Williams & Wilkins; 2006:106–107.
28. Warner M, Martin J, Schroeder D, Offord K, Chute C. Lower extremity motor neuropathy associated with surgery performed on patients in a lithotomy position. *Anesthesiology*. 1994;81:6.
29. Roth S, Thisted R, Erickson J, Black S, Schreider B. Eye injuries after nonocular surgery. *Anesthesiology*. 1996;85:1020.
30. Warner M, Benenfeld S, Warner M, Schoeder D, Maxson P. Perianesthetic dental injuries: frequency, outcomes, and risk factors. *Anesthesiology*. 1999;90:302.
31. Donlon J, Doyle D, Feldman M. Anesthesia for eye, ear, nose, and throat surgery. In: Miller R, ed. *Miller's Anesthesia*. 6th ed. Philadelphia, PA: Elsevier Churchill Livingstone; 2005:2537.

FURTHER READING

Mecca RS. Postoperative recovery. In: Barash PG, Cullen BF, Stoelting RK, eds. *Clinical Anesthesia*. 5th ed. Philadelphia, PA: Lippincott Williams & Wilkins; 2006.

Rosenblatt W. Airway management. In: Barash P, Cullen B, Stoelting R. *Clinical Anesthesia*. 5th ed. Philadelphia, PA: Lippincott Williams & Wilkins; 2006.

Prough D, Wolf S, Funston J, Svensen C. Acid-base, fluids, and electrolytes. In: Barash P, Cullen B, Stoelting R, eds. *Clinical Anesthesia*. 5th ed. Philadelphia, PA: Lippincott Williams & Wilkins; 2006.

Posner K, Cheney F, Kroll D. Professional liability, quality improvement, and anesthetic risk. In: Barash P, Cullen B, Stoelting R, eds. *Clinical Anesthesia*. 5th ed. Philadelphia, PA: Lippincott Williams & Wilkins; 2006.

QUESTIONS

1. A 30-year-old male is scheduled for a laparoscopic cholecystectomy. He is worried about intraoperative awareness. Which of the following is NOT true about consciousness in the operating room?
    - A. The incidence of awareness with explicit recall is 0.13%.
    - B. Awareness is associated with post-traumatic stress disorder.
    - C. The BIS (bispectral index) monitor has been proven to be better than the PSI (patient state index) with intravenous and inhaled anesthetics.
    - D. The BIS levels are elevated with ketamine.
    - E. State entropy modules have similar performance to the BIS.

2. You have placed a ProSeal laryngeal mask airway in a patient. Which is NOT a normal result of the initial check of function of the ProSeal laryngeal mask airway?

A. The water-soluble gel placed in the drainage tube does not move with positive pressure ventilation.
B. The water-soluble gel placed in the drainage tube does not move with pressure applied to the sternum.
C. The water-soluble gel placed in the drainage tube does not move with airway pressure of 20 cmH2O.
D. The water-soluble gel placed in the drainage tube does not move with brief pressure on the esophagus.
E. All of the above.

3. You have a patient with a known difficult airway for an emergency surgery. You plan on having cannula cricothyrotomy set up as one of your backup techniques for ventilation. Which is correct concerning the use of cannula cricothyrotomy?

A. The hospital pipeline cannot be used.
B. Barotrauma is less likely with initial inflation pressures of less than 55 psi.
C. 14-gauge intravenous cannulas may be used.
D. The mouth should be sealed to prevent ventilation leak.
E. All of the above.

4. Induction of anesthesia was historically performed by the inhalation of gaseous anesthetics. Which are problems associated with inhalational induction?

A. Seizure activity with sevoflurane.
B. Sudden airway obstruction.
C. The respiratory and cardiac effects of anesthesia occur rapidly.
D. A and B.
E. All of the above.

5. Awareness is due to imbalances in the amount normally needed and the amount given. Which scenario demonstrates a high requirement–normal delivery situation of awareness under anesthesia?

A. Awareness in a 24-year-old female after an emergency cesarean section under general anesthesia for fetal distress.
B. A 44-year-old red-headed female with a history of seizure disorder has awareness after a knee arthroscopy under general anesthesia for chronic knee pain.
C. A 5-year-old boy with an intravenous infiltration of propofol for sedation for a magnetic resonance imaging scan of the brain for headache has awareness during the scan.
D. A 14-year-old male has awareness after an emergency exploratory laparoscopy for bowel perforation from a bicycle handle bar injury.
E. A 55-year-old male has awareness after a hip-replacement surgery in which the sevoflurane vaporizer was not filled and the agent was not delivered.

6. Which device should not be used in a difficult airway scenario in which you are unable to intubate and oxygenation cannot be achieved with face mask and hand ventilation?

A. Laryngeal mask airway classic
B. Esophageal obturator device
C. Cricothyrotomy
D. Combitube
E. ProSeal laryngeal mask airway

7. All of the following are conditions that may lead to a cricothyroidotomy EXCEPT:

A. Acute epiglottitis
B. Angioneurotic edema
C. Postoperative edema
D. Retropharyngeal abscess
E. Anterior mediastinal mass

8. A pediatrician who is certified in the administration of deep sedation is providing a deep sedation for a 17-year-old autistic patient, who is otherwise healthy, to facilitate an MRI of the brain and spine. Which of the following is mandated by the ASA Practice Guidelines for Sedation and Analgesia by Non-Anesthesiologist Providers?

A. Supplemental oxygen must be provided.
B. ECG monitoring is not required.
C. $ETCO_2$ monitoring is required.
D. Someone with ACLS training must be available to respond within 5 minutes.
E. There does not need to be a defibrillator immediately available.

9. All of the following are common features of standard endotracheal tubes EXCEPT:

A. Radio-opaque line
B. Murphy Eye
C. High-pressure, low-volume cuff
D. Depth markers
E. 15-mm connector

10. Which one of the following is mandated by the ASA Basic Standards for Anesthetic Monitoring?

A. Supplemental oxygen must be provided to every patient.
B. When an ETT is placed, its position must be checked by the presence of expired CO_2.
C. During MAC the anesthesia provider may leave the room for brief periods.
D. The patient's blood pressure shall be evaluated at least every 3 minutes.

E. During deep sedation the adequacy of ventilation shall be evaluated continuously.

11. What is the maintenance intravenous fluid rate for a 65-kg adult?
A. 65 mL/h
B. 80 mL/h
C. 105 mL/h
D. 120 mL/h
E. 130 mL/h

12. The most common injury to the eye that occurs under general anesthesia is:
A. Corneal abrasion
B. Retinal artery occlusion
C. Eyelid laceration
D. Conjunctivitis
E. Uveitis

ANSWERS

1. C. The estimated incidence of awareness with explicit recall is 0.13% according to a study by Sebel. Studies have shown up to a 50% incidence of post-traumatic stress disorder. The BIS and PSI were found to be similar in validation studies. Nitrous oxide and ketamine may raise BIS values. The state entropy modules perform similarly to the BIS in studies.

FURTHER READING

Miller R, ed. *Miller's Anesthesia*. 7th ed. Philadelphia, PA: Churchill Livingstone Elsevier; 2010:Vol. 1, 1237–1239.

2. D. Gel placed in the drainage tube should move slightly when pressure is applied to the sternal notch in a quick, repetitive fashion. This action places pressure on the esophagus causing the gel to move in the drainage tube. The rest of the answers are correct for confirming placement.

FURTHER READING

Miller R, ed. *Miller's Anesthesia*. 7th ed. Philadelphia, PA: Churchill Livingstone Elsevier; 2010:Vol. 2, 1584.

3. B. For cannula cricothyrotomy, effective ventilation requires a high-pressure oxygen source such as the hospital pipeline. An adjustable Luer-Lok device should be connected to the source. Initial inflation pressure of less than 4 kPa or 55 psi has been shown to decrease the incidence of barotrauma. Standard intravenous cannulas cannot be used because of the tendency to kink and obstruct airflow. Only kink-resistant cannulas can be used. The oxygen must have passive exhalation, which is through the mouth and nose, so the airway must be open and exhalation must be confirmed. Sometimes a laryngeal mask airway is placed to keep the upper airway open.

FURTHER READING

Miller R, ed. *Miller's Anesthesia*. 7th ed. Philadelphia, PA: Churchill Livingstone Elsevier; 2010:Vol. 2, 1604.

4. D. A rapid inhalational induction with sevoflurane can induce seizure activity. Inhaled induction can result in apnea with airway obstruction. Usually an inhalational induction allows a gradual increase in the depth of anesthesia with less dramatic decreases in blood pressure and maintenance of spontaneous ventilation.

FURTHER READING

Miller R, ed. *Miller's Anesthesia*. 7th ed. Philadelphia, PA: Churchill Livingstone Elsevier; 2010:Vol. 2, 1578.

5. B. A high requirement for anesthesia usually includes tolerance to benzodiazepines, barbituates, opioids, or alcohol. Certain families have a higher incidence of awareness due to some genetic component. Redheads have also been shown to require more anesthesia than usual. B is the case where the tolerance was from seizure medications and pain medications along with genetic predisposition. The anesthesia was delivered normally with no reduction in amount for a normal individual. A is a case of low requirement due to the pregnant state and low delivery due to the general desire to prevent too much anesthesia from harming the fetus, which is already in distress. C involves a normal individual who received an inadequate delivery of anesthetic due to the infiltration of the amnestic agent. D had a low anesthesia requirement due to the traumatic nature of the event with hypovolemia. He also had a low delivery during the resuscitation and repair of the bowel due to his cardiovascular system not being able to tolerate the trauma and the anesthesia to produce amnesia. E is another incidence of a normal requirement with low delivery of the sevoflurane agent leading to awareness.

FURTHER READING

Miller R, ed. *Miller's Anesthesia*. 7th ed. Philadelphia, PA: Churchill Livingstone Elsevier; 2010:Vol. 1, 1239–1240.

6. A. The LMA often fails in situations of "cannot intubate, cannot ventilate." A supraglottic device is recommended such as the Combitube, ProSeal LMA, or Laryngeal Tube Sonda. If these are not available, cricothyrotomy is preferred to tracheostomy. The LMA classic lacks the appropriate seal to deliver the high pressures often needed in this situation.

FURTHER READING

Miller, R., ed. *Miller's Anesthesia*. 7th ed. Philadelphia, PA: Churchill Livingstone Elsevier; 2010:Vol. 2, 1581, 1606–1607.

7. E. The first four conditions have been described as indications for a cricothyroidotomy if the patient cannot be intubated or adequately ventilated and there is no capable surgeon to perform an emergency tracheostomy. An anterior mediastinal mass may place the patient at risk of collapse of the distal airway, but that situation would not likely be improved by a cricothyroidotomy.[30]

8. A. Section 8 of the ASA Practice Guidelines for Sedation and Analgesia by Non-Anesthesiologist Providers mandates that oxygen be administered to all patients unless contraindicated, and there is no contraindication in this patient. ECG monitoring is required in section 4. $ETCO_2$ monitoring is not required in section 4, but it is to be considered. Section 6 mandates that someone with advanced life support training be present in the procedure room.

9. C. Most standard endotracheal tubes today have a high-volume, low-pressure cuff intended to provide a good seal within the trachea while minimizing mucosal injury.[26] However, a high-volume, low-pressure cuff may not be as protective in preventing aspiration.

10. B. Section 3.2.2 in the Basic Standards for Anesthetic Monitoring describes that an endotracheal tube must have its position checked by both clinical assessment and by the identification of expired carbon dioxide (ASA standards). Supplemental oxygen is required to be given to every patient. Even during MAC the sole anesthesia provider may not leave the room except for emergencies. The patient's blood pressure is to be evaluated at least every 5 minutes. The standards are very specific about *continuous* versus *continual* monitoring on several accounts, and during deep sedation provided by an anesthesiologist only a continual evaluation of ventilation is required.

11. C. According to the "4-2-1" rule of intravenous fluid replacement therapy, the 65-kg patient would receive 105 mL/h.[26]

12. A. The most common eye injury under anesthesia is a corneal abrasion. Patient's eyes must be covered at all times. Tear production is reduced under general anesthesia. Treatment of a corneal abrasion consists of antibiotic eye ointment and covering for at least 48 hours. If pain lasts more than 24 hours then an ophthalmologist should be consulted. Retinal artery thrombosis is usually caused when there is direct pressure to the eye and is a serious complication but rarely occurs.[31]

19.

THE POSTOPERATIVE PERIOD

Kenneth N. Hiller, Esi M. Rhett, and George W. Williams

OPIOIDS

Opioids are all substances, both natural and synthetic, that bind to opioid receptors (including antagonists).[1] The relationship between opioid dose and effect depends on both pharmacokinetic and pharmacodynamic variables. Pharmacokinetics, or "what the body does to the drug," determines the relationship between drug dose and its concentration at the effect site. Pharmacodynamics, or "what the drug does to the body," determines the concentration of the drug at its site of action and the intensity of its effects.[1]

Receptor theory states that drugs have two independent characteristics at receptor sites. The first is affinity, which is the ability to bind a receptor and produce a stable complex. The second is efficacy, represented by its dose-effect curve, resulting from the drug–receptor interaction. Efficacy can range from no effect (zero) to maximal possible effect (the plateau of a dose-effect curve). See Figure 19.1.

The range in magnitude of the effect produced by a drug-receptor combination relative to the maximum possible effect is different from potency. Potency, which is related to receptor affinity, refers to the dose required to produce a given effect.

Drug receptor dualism theory explains the complex clinical effects of opioids that result from binding three classic receptors. Selective peripheral opioid receptor antagonists take advantage of this receptor structure. Alvimopan is a synthetic high molecular weight zwitterion (a molecule with both positive and negative regions of charge) that is a highly potent competitive μ antagonist used for opioid-induced constipation and acute postoperative ileus. Its poor oral bioavailability restricts its activity predominantly to the gut, where it gets metabolized.[2] See Table 19.1.

Pharmacokinetic parameters include distribution volumes, clearances, and half-lives. Distribution volumes do not represent actual volumes or anatomic regions in the body. They are estimated based on the volume of water into which a particular drug appears to be distributed. Clearances quantify the volume of plasma from which a drug is completely cleared per unit of time. Half-lives represent the time required for the concentration to decrease by 50% after drug administration has ceased. Half-life varies *directly* with volume of distribution and *inversely* with clearance.[3]

In general, opioids are metabolized by the hepatic microsomal cytochrome P450 system, although hepatic conjugation and subsequent excretion by the kidney are important for some drugs. For certain opioids, the specific metabolic pathway involved has important clinical implications in terms of active metabolites (morphine, meperidine) or an ultrashort duration of action (remifentanil).[1]

Phase I drug metabolism is the conversion of lipophilic drugs from an active hydrophobic form to a hydrophilic form through a series of enzymatic reactions that include oxidation, reduction, or hydrolysis. Phase II drug metabolism involves conjugation of a drug metabolite with an endogenous hydrophilic molecule to produce a more water-soluble compound that is easier to eliminate.[4] Biotransformation is the chemical modification made by an organism on a chemical compound; phase I and II reactions are examples of biotransformation. See Figure 19.2.

In general, opioids are highly lipid soluble weak bases that are highly protein bound and largely ionized at physiologic pH. Opioid physicochemical properties significantly affect their clinical behavior. The lipid-soluble, relatively unbound, unionized (low pKa) opioids alfentanil and remifentanil have shorter latency-to-peak effect after bolus injection due to their rapid transfer across cell membranes combined with their small volumes of distribution. Only the nonionized form of opioids cross the cell membrane. The physiologic implication of low pKa, a lower rate of ionization, means that the opioid more rapidly enters the highly lipid tissues of the central nervous system, allowing for more rapid clinical onset. See Table 19.2.

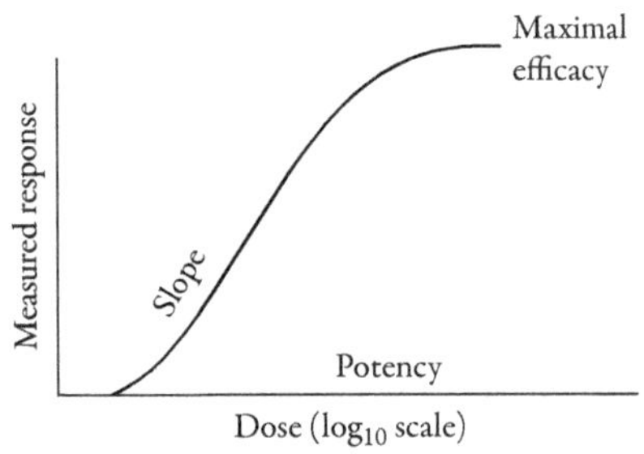

Figure 19.1 Dose-effect curve.

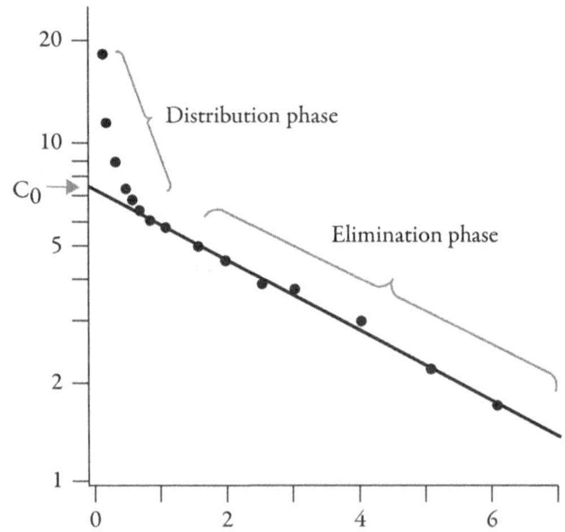

Figure 19.2 Plasma drug concentration versus time after a single intravenous dose.

LOCAL ANESTHETICS

Amide and ester local anesthetics block the transmission of nerve impulses by binding voltage-gated sodium channels. This disrupts action potential propagation along nerve fibers.

Local anesthetics are bases with pKa above physiologic pH. This favors formation of the ionized/protonated form. At physiologic pH, local anesthetics in solution are in equilibrium between a protonated, cationic form and a lipid-soluble, neutral form. The larger the pKa, the greater the extent of dissociation at any given pH. Only the nonionized form of a drug crosses the cell membrane.

The degree of nerve blockade depends on the concentration and volume of the local anesthetic. A minimal concentration is required to produce complete nerve blockade for a given local anesthetic. The rapid onset time and short-lived duration of action of 2-chloroprocaine illustrates this point. Its rapid onset time is secondary not to its pKa of 9, but rather to the high concentration that can be safely given due to its low potential for systemic toxicity. Absorption rates of local anesthetics are as follows:

Intercostal > caudal > epidural > topical > brachial plexus

Amide and ester local anesthetics are named according to the moiety that connects a lipid-soluble, aromatic benzene ring to an intermediate chain. Amide and ester local anesthetics differ in their metabolism, allergic potential, chemical stability, and structure (see Figure 14.1).

Esters are hydrolyzed by plasma cholinesterase, while hepatic microsomal enzymes degrade amides. Ester local anesthetics, derivatives of para-aminobenzoic acid (PABA), have a higher incidence of allergic reactions. Allergic reactions to amide local anesthetics are extremely rare.

Ropivacaine is an amide local anesthetic with pharmacokinetic and pharmacodynamic properties similar to racemic bupivacaine. Ropivacaine, though, has less potential for cardiac and central nervous system toxicity (local anesthetic systemic toxicity) and is associated with less motor blockade. Bupivacaine-induced cardiotoxicity studies suggest that cardiotonic effects predominate over "lipid sink"/sequestration in providing cardiovascular recovery.[5] See Table 19.3.[6]

Table 19.1 A SUMMARY OF SELECTED FEATURES OF OPIOID RECEPTORS

	MU (μ)	DELTA (δ)	KAPPA (κ)
Endogenous ligand	β-Endorphin	Leu-enkephalin	Dynorphin
	Endomorphin	Met-enkephalin	
Agonist prototype	Morphine	Deltorphin	Buprenorphine
	Fentanyl		Pentazocine
Antagonist	Naloxone	Naloxone	Naloxone
Supraspinal analgesia	Yes	Yes	Yes
Spinal analgesia	Yes	Yes	Yes
Respiratory depression	Yes	No	Yes
Gastrointestinal effects	Yes	No	Yes
Sedation	Yes	No	Yes

From: Bailey PL, Egan TD, Stanley TH. Intravenous opioid anesthetics. In: Miller RD, ed. *Anesthesia*. 5th ed. New York: Churchill Livingstone; 2000:312.

NONSTEROIDAL ANTI-INFLAMMATORY DRUGS

Arachidonic acid is converted to prostaglandin by either the cyclooxygenase (COX) or the lipoxygenase pathway in the periphery and central nervous system. The therapeutic

Table 19.2 SELECTED PHYSICOCHEMICAL AND PHARMACOKINETIC FEATURES OF OPIOID RECEPTORS

	MORPHINE	FENTANYL	SUFENTANIL	ALFENTANIL	REMIFENTANIL
pKa	8.0	8.4	8.0	6.5	7.1
% Nonionized at pH 7.4	23	<10	20	90	67?
Octanol/H_2O partition coefficient	1.4	813	1778	145	17.9
% Bound to plasma protein	20–40	84	93	92	80
% Diffusible fraction	16.8	1.5	1.6	8.0	13.3
Vd (L/kg)	3–5	3–5	2.5–3.0	0.4–1.0	0.2–0.3

From: Bailey PL, Egan TD, Stanley TH. Intravenous opioid anesthetics. In: Miller RD, ed. *Anesthesia*. 5th ed. New York: Churchill Livingstone; 2000:312.

effects of nonsteroidal anti-inflammatory drugs (NSAIDs) are primarily related to COX-2 inhibition, whereas some of their most frequent adverse effects may be caused by COX-1 inhibition (see Figure 19.3). Physiologic functions include the mediation of the inflammatory response, transduction of pain signals (gain), and a central pyretic effect.[7] The NSAIDs and acetaminophen alone can be sufficient for the management of mild pain and are a useful adjunct in the management of moderate to severe pain. The latest American Society of Anesthesiologists guidelines for acute pain management in the perioperative setting encourage their use whenever possible.[7]

Long-term NSAID administration can trigger bronchoconstriction, inhibit platelet aggregation (increasing the likelihood for bleeding), and lead to gastric ulcer formation. The COX-2 inhibitors have no effect on platelet function, while nonselective NSAIDs reversibly inhibit the COX-1 receptor, affecting platelet function for 3 days following discontinuation. The cerebrovascular safety of nonselective NSAIDs has been questioned in several studies, suggesting that nonselective NSAIDs should be used with caution in patients at high risk for cerebrovascular disease.[7] Aspirin and all other NSAIDs can transiently decrease renal function in selected patients.[7]

The NSAIDs are classified as salicylates, oxicam derivatives, fenamates, propionic acid derivatives, acetic acid derivatives, and COX-2 inhibitors. The NSAIDs provide anti-inflammatory and analgesic properties sufficient for mild to moderate postoperative pain. See Table 19.4.

Table 19.3 PHYSICOCHEMICAL PROPERTIES OF LOCAL ANESTHETICS

LOCAL ANESTHETIC	PK	% IONIZED (AT PH 7.4)	PARTITION COEFFICIENT (LIPID SOLUBILITY)	% PROTEIN BINDING
Amides				
Bupivacaine	8.1	83	3,420	95
Etidocaine	7.7	66	7,317	94
Lidocaine	7.9	76	366	64
Mepivacaine	7.6	61	130	77
Prilocaine	7.9	76	129	55
Ropivacaine	8.1	83	775	94
Esters				
Chloroprocaine	8.7	95	810	N/A
Procaine	8.9	97	100	6
Tetracaine	8.5	93	5,822	94

From: Liu SS. Local anesthetics and analgesics. In: Ashburn MA, Rice U, eds. *The Management of Pain*. New York, Churchill Livingstone, 1997:141.

ACETAMINOPHEN

Acetaminophen, on the other hand, provides analgesic and antipyretic effects with minimal anti-inflammatory properties. Its antipyretic effects are thought to be from a direct effect on the hypothalamic heat-regulating center

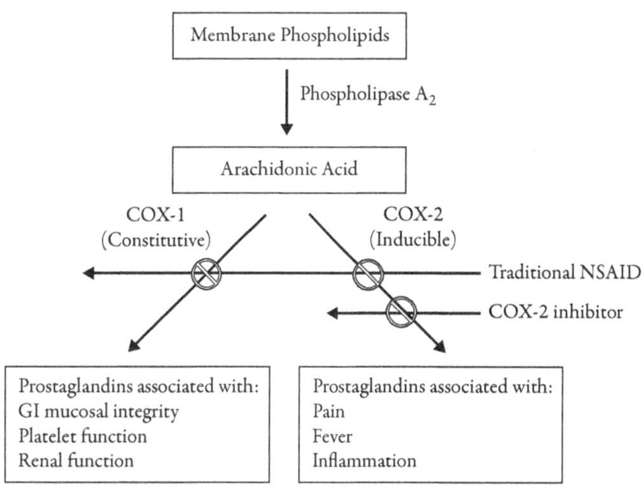

Figure 19.3 NSAID inhibition of arachidonic acid.

Table 19.4 NSAID DRUG CLASSIFICATION WITH CORRESPONDING GENERIC NAMES

NSAID CLASSIFICATION	GENERIC NAME
Salicylates	Aspirin
Oxicam derivatives	Meloxicam, piroxicam
Fenamates	Diclofenac, ketorolac
Propionic acid derivatives	Ibuprofen, ketoprofen, naproxen
Acetic acid derivatives	Etodolac, indomethacin
COX-2 selective	Celecoxib

From: Brogan S, Mandyam S, Drennan DA. Non-opioid analgesics. In: Hemmings HC, Egan TD, eds. *Pharmacology and Physiology for Anesthesia.* Philadelphia, PA: Saunders; 2013.

via endogenous pyrogen inhibition, while the mechanism of action of its analgesic effects is poorly understood.[7] Acetaminophen has minimal gastrointestinal effects and no effect on the cardiovascular and respiratory systems, platelets, or coagulation. In 2009, an FDA advisory panel recommended lowering the maximum daily dose of acetaminophen to 2600 mg and decreasing the maximum single dose to 650 mg. Acetaminophen toxicity may lead to hepatic necrosis, renal tubular necrosis, hypoglycemic coma, and fulminant hepatic failure. N-acetylcysteine is the first-line treatment for acetaminophen toxicity and works even in the setting of activated charcoal administration.

NEUROPATHIC PAIN MANAGEMENT

Neuropathic pain results from a lesion or disease affecting the somatosensory system. Neuropathic pain syndromes include postherpetic neuralgia (PHN), diabetic painful neuropathy (DPN), spinal cord injury (SCI), fibromyalgia, human immunodeficiency virus (HIV) neuropathy, and complex regional pain syndrome (CRPS). See Tables 19.5–19.7.[8]

Table 19.5 NEUROPATHIC PAIN PHARMACOLOGIC THERAPY DRUG CLASS WITH GENERIC NAME

DRUG CLASS	GENERIC NAME
Tricyclic antidepressants	Amitriptylline, nortriptylline, desipramine
Anticonvulsants	Gabapentin, pregabalin, lamotrigine, oxcarbazepine, topiramate, valproic acid
Selective serotonin reuptake inhibitors	Paroxetine, fluoxetine
Serotonin-norepinephrine reuptake inhibitors	Duloxetine, milnacipran
Topical agents	Lidocaine patch, capsaicin patch
Opioid agonist + monoaminergic agent	Tramadol
NMDA antagonist	Low-dose ketamine infusion

From: Benzon HT. Update on the pharmacologic management of chronic pain. Refresher Course Lectures, American Society of Anesthesiologists, 2012.

Transcutaneous Electrical Nerve Stimulation: The transcutaneous electrical nerve stimulation (TENS) unit makes possible the application of electrical stimulation across the skin to the peripheral nerves. This technique may be added to a multimodal regimen for pain control but may not be used as a sole technique. The resulting modulation of pain is not well understood, but may be caused by modulation of nociceptive impulses in C fibers though stimulation of large myelinated A fibers. It may also be a modulation of release of endogenous endorphins like enkephalins. Contraindications include demand-type cardiac pacemakers, pregnancy, placement over the carotid sinus or eyes (may induce a reflex bradycardia and loss

Table 19.6 EVIDENCE-BASED PHARMACOLOGIC THERAPY FOR VARIOUS NEUROPATHIC PAIN SYNDROMES

POSTHERPETIC NEURALGIA (PHN)	DIABETETIC PERIPHERAL NEUROPATHY (DPN)	SPINAL CORD INJURY (SCI)	FIBROMYALGIA	HIV NEUROPATHY	COMPLEX REGIONAL PAIN SYNDROME (CRPS)
Pregabalin	Pregabalin	Pregabalin	Duloxetine	Lamotrigine	Gabapentin
Gabapentin	Gabapentin	Gabapentin	Pregabalin	Gabapentin	Ketamine infusion
Opioid	Duloxetine	IV lidocaine	Milnacipran		
Antidepressants	Antidepressants		Tramadol		
Tramadol					
Lidoderm, capsaicin patch					

From: Benzon HT. Update on the pharmacologic management of chronic pain. Refresher Course Lectures, American Society of Anesthesiologists, 2012.

Table 19.7 COMMON SIDE EFFECTS ASSOCIATED WITH ANTICONVULSANTS AND ANTIDEPRESSANTS

Gabapentin & pregabalin	Dizziness, somnolence, fatigue, weight gain, peripheral edema
Lamotrigine	Rash, Stevens Johnson syndrome
Oxcarbazepine	Hyponatremia, low thyroid concentrations
Topiramate	Weight loss, cognitive effects
Valproic acid	Tremor
Tricyclic antidepressants	Cholinergic effects (dry mouth, sedation, urinary retention)
Milnacipran	Nausea, headache, constipation

From: Benzon HT. Update on the pharmacologic management of chronic pain. Refresher Course Lectures, American Society of Anesthesiologists, 2012.

of consciousness), or placement across the chest (may send a current through the heart).[9]

Cryotherapy: Cryotherapy, or "cold therapy" is an effective pain reliever due to reduction of edema by promoting vasoconstriction, decreasing inflammation by decreasing cellular metabolism, muscle spasm, and metabolic activity. It is used as an adjunct to physical therapy and is often used with physical therapy as part of a regimen, namely, applying heat to warm up the muscles, physical therapy, then applying cold to decrease inflammation and pain. Contraindications to cryotherapy include insensate and ischemic skin, peripheral vascular disease, Reynaud's phenomenon, cold urticaria, cryoglobinemia, paroxysmal cold hemoglobinuria. [9]

Acupuncture: A traditional Chinese therapy, acupuncture involves insertion of special needles into the skin at specific points to achieve a desired result. Acupuncture analgesia is mainly caused by the activation of the endogenous antinociceptive system to modulate transmission of pain.[9]

Hypnosis: Hypnosis is defined as a "natural state of aroused attentive focal concentration coupled with a relative suspension of peripheral awareness." Hypnosis is used in a multimodal technique and as an adjunct for chronic pain.[9]

NEUROLOGIC CONSEQUENCES OF ANESTHESIA

Postoperative cognitive dysfunction and delirium are more common in the elderly population, as higher rates (5%–50%) of mood disorders (depression, dementia) may complicate effective management. Visual and hearing impairments, preexisting impairments, and stress of surgery from fever, pain, nausea, and loss of routine also contribute. Younger patients also display cognitive dysfunction that typically resolves in 3 months, but dysfunction resolves more slowly in the elderly. Cognitive dysfunction may be related to central cholinergic depletion caused by narcotics, sedatives, and anticholinergics.

It is important to remember to rule out physiologic or pharmacologic causes of impaired sensorium before attributing symptoms to postoperative delirium or confusion, which can be life threatening. For example, hyperosmolarity from hyperglycemia or hypo- and hypernatremia as well as hypoxia and hypercarbia must be considered. Dialysis patients and dehydrated patients often experience cerebral fluid shifts after dialysis or rapid correction of fluid status. Doses of benzodiazepines, anticholinergics, or narcotics often have a greater effect in the elderly.

Failure to emerge from anesthesia should cause one to go through a memorized differential diagnosis that will be needed in the operating room and the oral examination room.[9]

- Neurologic—vessel occlusion or embolism, intracranial bleeding, subclinical seizure
- Pharmacologic—inadequate reversal of neuromuscular blockade, opioid overdose, persistence of volatile anesthetic
- Physiologic—hypoglycemia, hypothermia, hypercarbia, hypoxemia

RESPIRATORY CONSEQUENCES OF ANESTHESIA AND OF SURGICAL INCISIONS

Effects on lung volumes and compliance post anesthesia can be significant. Placing patients in the supine position will decrease functional residual capacity (FRC) by up to 20%. Induction of general anesthesia will further reduce the FRC by 15%–20%. That is a potential reduction by up to 40% caused by the posterior diaphragm moving cephalad, increased blood volume in the lung, and changes in chest wall shape. This decrease in FRC may be sustained for several hours post anesthesia.

Anesthesia effects airway resistance postoperatively. The volatile anesthetics have potent bronchodilating properties, so this counteracts the increase in airway resistance seen with the decrease in FRC. Increased airway resistance is usually caused by pathological factors, such as bronchospasm, secretions, or blood, or by equipment malfunction, small endotracheal tubes, or circuit obstruction.

Postoperative patients may experience increased work of breathing caused by resistance from the endotracheal tube (ETT) and decreased lung and chest wall compliance. In order to emphasize this concept, recall Poiseuille's law; for example, shortening the ETT length by cutting several centimeters off of the end may reduce the work of breathing in a patient. Sometimes this may lead to increased airway resistance. Increased work of breathing is counteracted by controlled mechanical ventilation. Keep this in mind at the end of a case when allowing spontaneous ventilation in a very sick patient.

CARDIOVASCULAR CONSEQUENCES OF GENERAL ANESTHESIA

Volatile anesthetics in general cause a dose-dependent inhibition of calcium release into the sarcoplasmic reticulum of cardiac myocytes. These negative inotropic effects result in less forceful cardiac contractions and decreased blood pressure and cardiac output. Nitrous oxide, in contrast, will directly depress myocardial contractility in vitro, but because of in vivo catecholamine release, arterial blood pressure, cardiac output, and heart rate are unchanged or slightly increased. This myocardial depression may become more dramatic in patients who are hypovolemic, have coronary artery disease, or have a systemic illness like sepsis.

Isoflurane has the least amount of cardiac depression, which explains its popularity in cardiac surgeries. A rapid increase in isoflurane leads to a transient increase in heart rate and blood pressure due to the increase in plasma levels of norephinephrine. This effect may be masked by other anesthetic agents or by patient and surgical factors.[10]

CARDIOVASCULAR CONSEQUENCES OF REGIONAL ANESTHESIA

Neuraxial blocks will interrupt the vasomotor tone, which is carried by sympathetic fibers arising from thoracic level 5 to lumbar level 1 (T5-L1); when a block is initiated in these areas, the result is vasodilation of venous capacitance vessels, pooling of blood, and a decrease in arterial blood pressure.[10] These effects can be minimized by giving intravenous fluids 500–1000 mL and prophylactic doses of pressors in patients who would be sensitive to the effects of severe hypotension, namely, those with coronary artery disease.

NAUSEA AND VOMITING

In the brain, vomiting originates in the reticular formation of the medulla at the olivary nuclei.

Well-known risk factors include female gender, nonsmokers, obesity, young age, history of postoperative nausea or motion sickness, anesthetic agents (volatiles, nitrous oxide), pain, type of surgery (urogenital, middle ear, abdominal). See Table 19.8 for drugs that can be used to control postoperative nausea and vomiting.

Table 19.8 DRUGS FOR THE TREATMENT OF PONV

AGENT	DOSAGE
Propofol	10–20mg IV
Metoclopramide	10–20mg IV
Ondansetron	4 mg IV
Droperidol	0.63–1.25 mg (check EKG for prolonged QT)
Ranitidine	150 mg PO or 50 mg IV
Scopolamine	1.5 mg transdermal patch
Dexamethasone	4 mg IV, (up to 10 mg can be given)
Cimetidine	300 mg IV or PO

HISTAMINE ANTAGONISTS

Histamine receptors are located in the chemoreceptor trigger zone in the central nervous system, mediating the control of emesis. There are four subtypes of histamine receptors. Antagonism of the H1 receptor has a significant role in both preventing and treating perioperative nausea and vomiting. **Promethazine** (Phenergan; common dose 12.5–25 mg IV or 12.5–50 mg IM) has equal antihistamine and anticholinergic properties. It is effective in controlling nausea and vomiting, but care should be taken in administration to patients with glaucoma or prostatic hypertrophy secondary to its anticholinergic effects. Promethazine has also been attributed to causing skin necrosis, necessitating surgical intervention, even subsequent amputation, when administered rapidly. Recommendations have been made to dilute the desired dose and administer as a slow infusion. **Diphenhydramine** (common dose 31.25–62.5 mg IV), also an H1 antagonist, has very little anticholinergic action. It is most commonly used to combat motion sickness. Both medications are effective in preventing postoperative nausea and vomiting (PONV), but their side effects can be significant and may limit usefulness in some clinical situations. Common side effects include sedation, urinary retention, dry mouth, blurred vision, and extrapyramidal symptoms.

Antagonism of H2 receptors counters the histamine-induced secretion of acidic gastric fluid. It does not, however, alter the existing pH or promote gastric emptying. Commonly used medications in this class are **cimetidine** (common dose 300 mg IV or PO), **famotidine** (common dose 20 mg IV) and **ranitidine** (common dose 150 mg PO or 50 mg IV). These medications are traditionally used in the preoperative period to minimize complications of potential aspiration. Their role in preventing or treating PONV is minimal.

DOPAMINE ANTAGONISTS

Dopamine receptors also reside in the chemoreceptor trigger zone, where the transmission of dopamine can trigger the vomiting reflex. **Metoclopramide** (Reglan) (common dose 10–20 mg IV) is a dopamine antagonist with prokinetic properties commonly used to treat gastroparesis. Large doses (200 mg every 6 hours), although not commonly administered in today's practice, are often associated with extrapyramidal symptoms. These side effects could be effectively countered with antihistamines or benzodiazepines. On the other hand, the smaller doses currently in practice, 10 mg IV, are credited with improving gastroparesis and reducing nausea and vomiting.

Droperidol (common dose 0.625–1.25 mg IV) specifically antagonizes the second subtype of dopamine receptors (D2). It is highly effective even with small doses but has a relatively short half-life of 3 hours. For this reason it may be best given toward the end of surgery. Reported side effects include sedation, anxiety or restlessness, akathisia, and dystonia. Droperidol has fallen out of favor as an antiemetic after being associated with prolongation of the QT interval, leading to possible arrhythmias including torsades de pointes. For this reason, the FDA issued a "black box" warning in 2001. The warning established the relationship between droperidol and prolongation of the QT interval. It recommended that all patients should undergo a 12-lead EKG before administration. In the presence of existing prolonged QT (QTc >440 milliseconds in males and >450 milliseconds in females), droperidol should not be administered. If the potential benefit is determined to outweigh the risk of serious arrhythmias, EKG monitoring should be instituted prior to treatment and for 2–3 hours after treatment. Caution is advised in patients thought be at risk for developing an increased QT, with factors including presence of congestive heart failure, bradycardia, use of a diuretic, cardiac hypertrophy, hypokalemia, hypomagnesemia, or concomitant drugs known to increase the QT interval. Other risk factors may include age over 65 years, alcohol abuse, and use of agents such as benzodiazepines, volatile anesthetics, and IV opiates. It is pertinent to remember that general anesthesia itself has an association with QT prolongation, which some texts consider a "much stronger overall effect" than the sole effect of droperidol.[11] Ondansetron, although not a dopamine antagonist, has also been associated with increasing the QT interval. The clinical significance of an increased QT interval is still debated. In the UK, increases in this interval less than 30 milliseconds are considered irrelevant.

Perphenazone (common dose 2.5–5 mg IM or IV) and **prochlorperazine** (Compazine) (common dose 6.25–12.5 mg IM or IV) are dopamine antagonists most commonly used as potent neuroleptics, although both have implications in treating PONV.

ANTICHOLINERGIC AGENTS

Scopolamine (common dose 1.5-mg patch) is a centrally acting anticholinergic. Its antimuscarinic effects on the gastrointestinal system include decreased secretions, decreased lower esophageal sphincter tone, and increased intestinal relaxation. As a tertiary amine, it is able to cross the placenta and the blood-brain barrier. This accounts for the unpleasant side effects experienced by some patients: blurred vision (18%), dry mouth (8%), dizziness (2%), agitation (1%).[11] Scopolamine's relatively short plasma half-life has led to the necessity of administration through a transdermal patch. The patch is best applied the night before surgery and left in place for 24 hours after surgery. Application as briefly as 1 hour before cesarean section can prevent PONV while minimizing exposure to the fetus. The transdermal patch administers medication for up to 72 hours.

SEROTONIN ANTAGONISTS

Serotonin antagonists that specifically block the 5-HT3 receptors were first used to combat chemotherapy-induced nausea and vomiting. The 5-HT3 receptors are found in multiple sites involved in the emesis pathway including vagal afferents, the area postrema, the solitary tract nucleus, and the chemoreceptor trigger zone. Their efficacy in preventing nausea with minimal side effects soon made these antiemetics a popular choice in preventing perioperative nausea and vomiting. **Ondansetron** (Zofran) (common dose 4 mg IV) has a short time to onset and a half-life of approximately 4 hours. When given close to the end of surgery, ondansetron is highly effective in the prevention of nausea. Ondanestron is metabolized by CYP2D6; a dysmorphism of the cytochrome P450 enzyme can lead to both decreased efficacy and ultrarapid metabolism, making it less useful in this subset of the population. **Dolasetron** (common dose 12.5–50 mg IV) has active liver metabolites, which increase its effective half-life to nearly 8 hours, twice that of ondansetron. **Granisetron** (common dose 1 mg IV) also has an effective half-life of 8 hours. **Palonosetron** (common dose 0.075 mg IV) has the longest half-life of all the serotonin antagonists, at nearly 40 hours, making it an ideal choice for delayed PONV.

OTHER TYPES OF THERAPY

Dexamethasone (common dose 8 mg IV) acts in the central inhibition of the solitary tract nucleus, aiding in the prevention of nausea and vomiting. It has a slow onset of action, therefore is best given at the beginning of a surgical case. Traditionally, doses of 8–10 mg IV have been used, but smaller doses (2.5–5 mg IV) appear to be equally effective.

Neurokinin Antagonist

Substance P is a neuropeptide found in the central nervous system and spinal cord associated with inflammatory processes and pain modulation. Substance P binds to the neurokinin 1 (NK-1) receptors, which are also found in vagal afferents in gastrointestinal tract and in the vomiting reflex center in the CNS. Although there are several emetic pathways, substance P and the NK-1 receptor appear to be involved in the final common pathway that controls vomiting. **Aprepitant** (Emend) (common dose 40 mg PO) is a commercially available NK-1 antagonist that has an increased efficacy in preventing vomiting, although equal efficacy in preventing nausea, compared with ondansetron. Its routine use is limited by cost, although the expense may be warranted following surgeries when vomiting could be detrimental (i.e., neurosurgical procedures, upper GI surgery, wired jaw, ophthalmic surgeries).

Multimodal Therapy

Assessing the need for antiemetic therapy in the perioperative patient includes assessing baseline risk (patient, surgical, anesthetic factors) and the potential risk reduction with intervention. Patients at low risk for postoperative nausea and vomiting have little benefit from routine prophylaxis; their risk may be reduced from a baseline of 10% modestly down to 7%. For patients with significant risk of perioperative nausea and vomiting, prophylaxis can have a greater impact on prevention, and multimodal therapy may be necessary to reduce risk to an acceptable level.

A large multicenter trial was created to assess the individual and combined effects of multimodal therapy. The IMPACT trial, "International Multicenter Protocol to Assess the single and combined benefits of antiemetic interventions in a Controlled clinical Trial of a 2×2×2×2×2×2 factorial design (IMPACT)," illustrated that all interventions acted independently of each other and these interventions are independent of patient's risk (Miller's Anesthesia). In essence, each intervention reduces the risk the same amount and the reductions are additive. A patient with a baseline risk of 80% receives a single intervention with a risk reduction value of 74%. The new risk assessment of 59% (0.80*0.74) can be further reduced by receiving another intervention with an equal risk reduction of 74%. After four such interventions, the final risk of postoperative nausea and vomiting can be reduced to 24% (0.80*0.74*0.74*0.74*0.74 = 0.24).

In the event that prophylaxis is not effective, rescue therapy should be initiated. The previously described antiemetics are effective as therapeutic, in addition to preventative, interventions. Patient discomfort and overall satisfaction guides the practice to regularly attempt prevention rather than the "wait and see" approach. In selecting the appropriate rescue intervention, it is recommended to administer a medication from a class not previously used. Giving "more of the same," is rarely effective. The 5-HT3 antagonists are advantageous as rescue therapy considering the short onset of action and few side effects. Patients with a history of delayed, or post-discharge, nausea and vomiting need special consideration and administration of a long acting antiemetic.

Adjuvants Therapy

Adjuvant therapies are emerging as cost-effective and efficacious strategies to combat perioperative nausea and vomiting. Acupuncture and acupressure are now commonly accepted as beneficial adjuvants in modern medicine. The P6 point, the sixth point on the pericardial meridian on the volar side of the wrist, can effectively treat nausea. Studies have shown equal risk reduction in treating nausea and vomiting compared with conventional medications.

Ginger is commonly regarded as a useful therapy for nausea, but current studies do not support this claim. Although the liberal administration of crystalloid may contribute to a decrease in postoperative nausea and vomiting, the mechanism is likely indirect by offsetting the need for large PO intake after surgery.

NEUROMUSCULAR CONSEQUENCES

RESIDUAL PARALYSIS

Paralytics are commonly used for muscle relaxation during surgical procedures, and residual neuromuscular blockade is not uncommon in the postoperative period. Factors that can contribute to this residual paralysis are the assessment of depth of neuromuscular block, the method of monitoring, and the approach to reversal. The standard in objective measurement of return of neuromuscular function is mechanomyography, although this is rarely used in clinical situations. Traditionally, a train of four ratio (TOFR) of >0.6 was thought to be adequate for recovery of function based on consistent return of baseline respiratory rate, tidal volume, forced expiratory volume, and forced vital capacity.[12] It is now known that impairment of several parameters can be present even at a TOFR as high as 0.8–0.9, including the hypoxic ventilatory response, strength of upper airway musculature, coordination of swallowing, and upper esophageal sphincter tone. These findings correlate with the increased risk of upper airway collapse leading to airway obstruction, hypoxemia, atelectasis, pneumonia, and aspiration. Careful selection of neuromuscular blocker, adequate monitoring of depth of blockade, and vigilance in the postoperative period can reduce the incidence of complications.

POSTOPERATIVE MYALGIA

Succinylcholine has a well-established association with postoperative myalgia, although the exact mechanism is unclear. It occurs "most often after minor surgery, especially in women and in ambulatory rather than bedridden patients."[11] Studies have not been able to prevent the myalgia with preoperative anti-inflammatory medications, suggesting the process is not solely inflammatory. Pretreatment with pregabalin and gabapentin decreased postoperative pain scores and fentanyl consumption.[13] Administering a "defasiculating dose" of nondepolarizing neuromuscular blocker before the administration of succinylcholine clearly prevents fasiculations and may attenuate myalgia.

REFERENCES

1. Ogura T, Egan TD. Opioid agonists and antagonists. In: Hemmings HC, Egan TD, eds. *Pharmacology and Physiology for Anesthesia*. Philadelphia, PA: Saunders; 2013.
2. Mehta V. Peripheral opioid antagonism. *Anaesthesia*. 2009;64:1277–1282.
3. Obara S, Egan TD. Pharmacokinetic and pharmacodynamics principles for intravenous anesthetics. In: Hemmings HC, Egan TD, eds. *Pharmacology and Physiology for Anesthesia*. Philadelphia, PA: Saunders; 2013.
4. Perry TE, Collard CD. Drug metabolism and pharmacogenetics. In: Hemmings HC, Egan TD, eds. *Pharmacology and Physiology for Anesthesia*. Philadelphia, PA: Saunders; 2013.
5. Fettiplace MR, Akpa BS, Ripper R, et al. Resuscitation with lipid emulsion. *Anesthesiology*. 2014;120:915–925.
6. Suzuki S, Kokofer A, Gerner P. Local anesthetics. In: Hemmings HC, Egan TD, eds. *Pharmacology and Physiology for Anesthesia*. Philadelphia, PA: Saunders; 2013.
7. Brogan S, Mandyam S, Drennan DA. Non-opioid analgesics. In: Hemmings HC, Egan TD, eds. *Pharmacology and Physiology for Anesthesia*. Philadelphia, PA: Saunders; 2013.
8. Benzon, HT. Update on the pharmacologic management of chronic pain. Refresher Course Lectures, American Society of Anesthesiologists, 2012.
9. Benzon H, Rathmell J, Wu C, Turk D, Argoff C, Hurley R. *Practical Management of Pain*. 5th ed. Philadelphia, PA: Elsevier; 2013:763–764, 752, 785
10. Butterworth I, Mackey D, Wasnick J. *Clinical Anesthesiology*. 5th ed. Philadelphia, PA: McGraw-Hill; 2013.
11. Miller R. *Miller's Anesthesia*. 7th ed. Philadelphia, PA: Elsevier; 2010.
12. Hemmings H, Egan T. *Pharmacology and Physiology for Anesthesia: Foundations and Clinical Application*. Philadelphia, PA: Saunders; 2013.
13. Pandey C, Karna S, Tandon M, Pandey V, Singh A. Comparative evaluation of prophylactic use of pregabalin, gabapentin and diclofenac sodium for prevention of succinylcholine-induced myalgia: a randomized, double-blinded study. *J Postgrad Med*. 2014;60(1):16–20.

FURTHER READING

Lin Y. Accupuncture. In: Yao F, Malhotra V, Fonet M. *Yao and Artusio's Anesthesiology: Problem-Oriented Patient Management*. Philadelphia, PA: Lippincott Williams & Wilkins; 2006.

Mecca R. Postoperative Recovery. In: Barash P, Cullen B, Stoelting R. *Clinical Anesthesia*. 5th ed. Philadelphia, PA: Lippincott Williams & Wilkins; 2006.

QUESTIONS

1. The relationship between drug dose and its concentration at the effect site is known as:
   A. Drug receptor dualism
   B. Efficacy
   C. Pharmacokinetics
   D. Pharmacodynamics
   E. Potency

2. Which of the following best describes the early rapid decline in opioid plasma drug concentration?
   A. Affinity
   B. Distribution phase
   C. Elimination half-life
   D. Elimination phase
   E. Biotransformation

3. In general, which opioid physicochemical property MOST results in shorter latency-to-peak effect following bolus injection?
   A. High water-solubility
   B. High protein binding
   C. High ionization
   D. Large volume of distribution
   E. High lipid-solubility

4. Amide and ester local anesthetics do not differ in:
   A. Binding site
   B. Metabolism
   C. Allergic potential
   D. Chemical stability
   E. Structure

5. All of the following are possible side effects of long-term, nonselective nonsteroidal anti-inflammatory drugs (NSAIDs) EXCEPT:
   A. Bronchospasm
   B. Inhibition of platelet aggregation
   C. Gastrointestinal irritation
   D. Thrombotic events
   E. Increased creatinine clearance

6. Evidence-based pharmacologic treatment for neuropathic pain does not include:
   A. Tricyclic antidepressants
   B. Certain anticonvulsants
   C. Selective norepinephrine reuptake inhibitors
   D. Methadone
   E. Topical agents

7. Which single medication would be BEST for your patient who has a history of postdischarge nausea and vomiting?
   A. Ondansetron
   B. Transdermal scopolamine
   C. Dexamethasone
   D. Promethazine
   E. Droperidol

8. Which of the following parameters can best signify residual muscle weakness in the postanesthesia care unit?
   A. Tidal volume
   B. Forced Expiratory Volume

C. Forced Inspiratory Volume
D. Forced Vital Capacity
E. Hand grip

9. Which of the following factors would lead to the greatest apparent risk reduction in postoperative nausea and vomiting?
A. Class of antiemetic
B. Dose of antiemetic
C. Type of surgery
D. Preoperative risk assessment
E. Preoperative administration

ANSWERS

1. C. "What the body does to a drug" determines its concentration at the effect site.

   Pharmacodynamics, or "what the drug does to the body," determines the intensity of effect of a given concentration of drug. Efficacy refers to the measured response from a drug-receptor interaction. Potency, on the other hand, is the dose required to produce a given effect. Drug receptor dualism theory explains the complex clinical effects of opioids that result from binding multiple, distinct receptors.

2. B. Pharmacokinetics can be separated into distinct categories of absorption, distribution, metabolism, and elimination.[3] The early rapid decline in opioid plasma drug concentration occurs secondary to distribution. Affinity is the ability of a drug to bind a receptor and produce a stable complex. Elimination half-life is the time it takes for blood levels of drug to decrease to half of what it was at equilibrium. At five half-lives, 97% of a single dose of a drug is eliminated from the body. The elimination phase accounts for the decline in plasma drug concentration over time following the distribution phase. Biotransformation is the chemical modification of a chemical compound by an organism.

3. E. High lipid-solubility facilitates passage of a substance across the cell membrane and results in shorter latency-to-peak effect. The other choices result in longer latency-to-peak effects.

4. A. Amide and ester local anesthetics both bind voltage-gated sodium channels.

   Their metabolism, allergic potential, chemical stability, and structures differ. Amide compounds undergo enzymatic degradation in the liver, whereas ester compounds are hydrolyzed in plasma by esterase enzymes. Cocaine, an ester, is an exception, as it is metabolized predominantly by the liver. The metabolites of esters include PABA, which can occasionally induce allergic reactions. Allergies to amides are extremely rare. Amides are extremely stable, whereas esters are relatively unstable.[6]

5. E. Nonselective NSAIDs would not be expected to improve renal function. They can, however, inhibit bronchodilation, inhibit platelet activation, cause gastrointestinal upset, and increase the risk of serious cardiovascular events.

6. D. Studies have shown efficacy of opioids for neuropathic pain, but the unpredictable half-life, varying rate of metabolism between individuals, and potential for cardiac arrhythmias make methadone a less-than-ideal choice. Tricyclic antidepressants, certain anticonvulsants, selective norepinephrine reuptake inhibitors, and topical agents all have a role in evidence-based treatment of various neuropathic pain syndromes.

7. B. Patients with postdischarge nausea and vomiting often exhibit no clinical signs of nausea in the postanesthesia care unit, manifesting symptoms only after leaving the hospital. For this patient population, selecting an antiemetic that has a long duration of action, or effective half-life, is essential. Ondansetron, dexamethasone, and promethazine are effective in prevention of postoperative nausea and vomiting, but their usefulness is limited by the relative short duration of actions. In addition, promethazine can be quite sedating and prevents timely discharge of ambulatory patients. Transdermal scopolamine can be worn for up to 72 hours after application, making it an ideal choice for postdischarge nausea and vomiting.

FURTHER READING

Miller RD. *Miller's Anesthesia*. 7th ed. Philadelphia, PA: Elsevier; 2010.

8. C. Residual neuromuscular blockade can be present in a significant portion of patients after surgical procedures. Although respiratory function can appear normal with baseline respiratory rate, tidal volume, forced expiratory volume, and forced vital capacity, there may be substantial weakness in the upper airway muscles that usually prevent airway collapse. For this reason, the forced *inspiratory* volume will be reduced with residual muscle weakness, illustrating the airway's tendency for collapse.

FURTHER READING

Hemmings HC, Egan TD. *Pharmacology and Physiology for Anesthesia: Foundations and Clinical Application*. Philadelphia, PA: Saunders; 2013.

9. D. Reducing the risk of postoperative nausea and vomiting is multifactorial. A patient's preoperative risk assessment has the largest contribution in the apparent reduction of that risk. For example, a patient with multiple risk factors and a preoperative risk assessment of 80% can reduce that risk to 59% with one

intervention. A patient with no risk factors and a baseline risk of 10% will only further reduce their risk to 7% with intervention. The class of antiemetic does not greatly influence the risk reduction. The IMPACT trial showed that there is equal efficacy of ondansetron, dexamethasone, and droperidol.[11] Increasing the dose of a single medication does not further reduce risk; adding a different class of antiemetic would. The type of surgery does influence a patient's risk assessment, but it is only one of many factors to consider. Antiemetics are useful as both prophylactic and therapeutic medications, so timing of administration is not essential to overall risk reduction.

FURTHER READING

Miller, R.D. (2009) *Miller's Anesthesia.* 7th ed. Philadelphia, PA: Elsevier; 2010.

SECTION V

ORGAN-BASED BASIC AND CLINICAL SCIENCES

20.

CENTRAL NERVOUS SYSTEM

Andrew Allison and Jennifer D. Wu

BRAIN PHYSIOLOGY

The human brain is an organ that weighs about 1400 grams, or 2% of total body weight. It has a high metabolic rate and receives 15% of cardiac output. The brain consumes 20% of total body oxygen. The brain consists mainly of two types of tissue: gray matter and white matter.

The brain, cerebral blood vessels, and cerebral spinal fluid exist in a fixed space within the cranium, and a complex system exists to maintain a balance between these elements.

The brain can be divided into two functional areas: the cerebral cortex and the subcortical areas. The cerebral cortex is composed mainly of gray matter. The subcortical areas, which are mostly white matter, include the basal ganglia, hippocampus, internal capsule, cerebellum, brain stem, and reticular activating system.[1]

THE CEREBRAL CORTEX

The cerebral cortex can be organized by hemispheres (left and right cerebral hemispheres), lobes (frontal, parietal, temporal, occipital), or Brodmann areas. The gray matter that makes up the cerebral cortex has a relatively higher metabolic rate, making it particularly susceptible to hypoxic injury.[2,3] The Brodmann areas are based on the cellular structure.

By understanding the functional organization of the brain, one can recognize the relationship between brain lesions and clinical findings (Table 20.1). For example, the left hemisphere controls language in 90% of people and the language areas include Broca's area, Wernicke's area, and the primary auditory cortex. Damage to one or more of these areas may result in the clinical finding of aphasia. Major forms in which aphasia may be manifested include expressive (nonfluent), receptive (fluent), and global.

SUBCORTICAL AREAS: BASAL GANGLIA, HIPPOCAMPUS, INTERNAL CAPSULE, CEREBELLUM, BRAIN STEM, RETICULAR ACTIVATING SYSTEM

As is found with the cerebral cortex, regions in the subcortical areas are responsible for certain functions. The basal ganglia regulate posture and voluntary movements. The hippocampus makes up part of the limbic system, which is responsible for learning, emotion, aggression, and sexual behavior. The internal capsule is a white matter area that contains tracts that run from the cortex to the spinal cord. This includes information that is carried from the motor cortex to the spinal cord. The role of the cerebellum is to control gait, stance, balance, and muscle tone.[4]

The brain stem lies between the brain and spinal cord and consists of the midbrain, pons, and medulla oblongata. It contains the nerve fibers that run between the brain and spinal cord. The midbrain contains centers of auditory and visual reflexes and the origin of cranial nerves III (oculomotor) and IV (trochlear). The pons contains the pneumotaxic center, which is a respiratory center. The pons also contains the origins of cranial nerves V (trigeminal), VI (abducens), and VII (facial). The medulla oblongata has the respiratory center, cardioinhibitory center, and vasomotor center. It also houses the origins of cranial nerves VIII (vestibulocochlear), IX (glossopharyngeal), X (vagus), XI (spinal accessory), and XII (hypoglossal). Recall that stimulation of cranial nerve (CN) IX elicits the "gag" reflex and CN X innervates the trachea and vocal cords.

The reticular activating system (RAS) is located primarily in the midbrain, with portions in the pons, medulla, hypothalamus, and spinal cord. It is responsible for arousal and alertness.

The hippocampus and cerebellum are the areas most sensitive to hypoxic injury.

Table 20.1 COMMON BRAIN LESIONS: NAMES, LOCATIONS, AND CLINICAL SYMPTOMS

TYPE	NAMING	FLUENCY	AUDITORY COMPREHENSION	REPETITION	LOCATIONS OF LESION	
Broca's		+/–	–	+	–	Broca's Area (Area 44 and 45)
Wernicke's	–	+	–	–	Wernicke's Area (Area 22)	
Global	–	–	–	–	Large left hemispheric lesions	
Conduction	+/–	+	+	–	Arcuate fasciculus	

Adapted from Waxman SG. Higher cortical functions. In: Waxman SG, ed. *Clinical Neuroanatomy.* 27th ed. New York, NY: McGraw-Hill; 2013:ch. 21. Higher cortical functions of aphasias with impaired repletion.

CEREBRAL BLOOD FLOW

Careful regulation of cerebral blood flow (CBF) is critical for the constant delivery of oxygen and glucose to the brain. Cerebral vascular resistance (CVR) and cerebral perfusion pressure (CPP) determine CBF. Cerebral blood flow is inversely proportional to CVR and directly proportional to CPP. Blood flow to the brain is influenced by cerebral metabolism, autoregulation, and chemical regulation. Outside factors that affect CBF include intravenous anesthetics, inhalation agents, and vasoactive drugs.[1]

Average CBF under normal conditions is 50 mL blood per 100 g tissue per minute. Blood flow that is lower than 25 mL/100 g/min can cause cerebral impairment, while an isoelectric EEG may occur at flows less than 20 mL/100 g/min. These concepts are commonly tested.

Physiologic Variables

Perfusion Pressure

Cerebral perfusion pressure is defined as the difference between mean arterial pressure (MAP) and intracranial pressure (ICP) or central venous pressure (CVP), whichever value is higher.

$$CPP = MAP - ICP$$

Normal CPP is 80–100 mmHg, and normal ICP is less than 10 mmHg. Therefore, in a healthy adult the cerebral pressure is mainly dependent on the MAP. Decreases in CPP are detrimental to the brain. A CPP less than 50 mmHg will result in electroencephalogram (EEG) slowing, and a sustained CPP less than 25 mmHg may cause permanent brain damage.

pH

Acute changes in systemic pH do not alter CBF because bicarbonate and hydrogen ions do not cross the blood brain barrier.

$PaCO_2$

Changes in $PaCO_2$ alter CBF, and this change is directly proportional when $PaCO_2$ is in the range of 20 to 80 mmHg. Cerebral blood flow decreases by 1 mL/100 g/min for each 1 mmHg decrease in $PaCO_2$ down to a $PaCO_2$ of about 20 mmHg. This relationship is important in anesthesia because changes in mechanical ventilation can be used to manipulate the CBF. The decrease in CBF achieved by hyperventilation can be maintained for about 6 hours. After this time period, equilibration of extracellular pH in the brain takes place and the decrease in CBF is no longer maintained.[1]

Changes in PaO_2 in the physiologic range do not have significant impact on CBF. However, cerebral vasodilation and increase in CBF occurs rapidly when the PaO_2 is less than 60 mmHg.

$CMRO_2$

The cerebral metabolic rate of oxygen consumption ($CMRO_2$) is the rate of oxygen consumed per 100 grams of brain tissue per minute. The average $CMRO_2$ is 3.5 mL of oxygen per 100 grams of brain tissue per minute. About 60% of this oxygen consumption is used to support neuronal electrical activity, and 40% is used to maintain cellular integrity.[1]

Increases in brain activity cause a proportional change in $CMRO_2$ and in CBF. This proportional increase is called flow-metabolism coupling. Factors that affect flow-metabolism coupling are complex and not completely understood.

Brain activity such as stimulation and arousal cause an increase in $CMRO_2$, while epileptic seizures can cause a dramatic increase. The $CMRO_2$ is reduced during sleep and can be regionally reduced following brain injury.

External factors that influence $CMRO_2$ include intravenous anesthetic agents, inhalation agents, and temperature.

Intravenous anesthetic agents, with the exception of ketamine, decrease $CMRO_2$. The decrease in $CMRO_2$ caused by these agents is typically dose related until EEG suppression occurs.

Inhalation agents, with the exception of nitrous oxide, cause a decrease in $CMRO_2$ in a dose-related manner. However, inhalation agents cause vasodilation. At a half MAC, the net result is a decrease in CBF (undersupply). At one MAC, the net result is unchanged CBF. At greater than one MAC, CBF increases even though $CMRO_2$ has decreased (oversupply).

Temperature changes result in changes in CBF and $CMRO_2$. Each degree Celsius decrease in temperature causes a decrease in $CMRO_2$ by 6%.

Inverse Steal

Inverse steal is also known as the "Robin Hood" effect. It occurs when blood is shunted from adequately perfused areas of the brain to ischemia areas. This takes place when the patient is hyperventilated and becomes hypocarbic. The opposite phenomenon is cerebral steal, or luxury perfusion. Dilation of normal vessels by administration of a systemic vasodilator or by hypercapnia caused by hypoventilation can steal blood from the ischemic areas of the brain that need oxygen.

Gray Versus White Matter

The CBF is highest for gray matter at a rate of 80 mL of oxygen per 100 grams brain tissue per minute. The white matter receives 20 mL of oxygen per 100 grams brain tissue per minute.[2] This is why gray matter is more sensitive to ischemic changes and why loss of gray–white differentiation occurs on CT scan following hypoxic ischemic injury (see section, "The Cerebral Cortex").

Autoregulation

Cerebral autoregulation exists to maintain relatively constant blood supply to the brain throughout a wide range of mean arterial pressures. In a normotensive, healthy adult, autoregulation is maintained during MAPs of approximately 50–150 mmHg. A decrease in CPP will cause cerebral vasodilation and an increase in CPP will result in vasoconstriction. Low CPP beyond the lower limits of autoregulation may cause ischemia, and high CPP above the upper limits of autoregulation can cause deleterious effects such as disruption of the blood-brain barrier (BBB), hemorrhage, and edema.

CEREBROSPINAL FLUID

INTRODUCTION

Cerebrospinal fluid (CSF) is one component of the intracranial contents along with brain tissue and the cerebral blood volume. It is essentially continuous with extracellular fluid (ECF) and has many functions. The CSF acts as a protective cushion, provides nutrition for the neural tissues' electrophysiologic and basal cellular functions, regulates the chemical environment so that neurons can function optimally, serves as a vehicle for transport and excretion of cellular waste, and can transport intracerebral neurotransmitters.[7] This section examines the different aspects of CSF, its relation to the BBB, and how different anesthetics affect CSF.

COMPOSITION

The CSF is a clear aqueous solution composed primarily of sodium, chloride, and magnesium. Potassium, calcium, and bicarbonate as well as proteins, glucose, and amino acids are also present but at much smaller concentrations.[7] The specific gravity of CSF is 1.003 to 1.007. The pH is slightly acidic relative to blood (~7.31) with a pCO_2 of 50 to 51.[5] The pH is tightly regulated in order to optimize cellular conditions and is more a function of CO_2 concentrations rather than H+ concentration. This is because the BBB is freely permeable to CO_2 and not H+. The CSF content is precisely regulated by the BBB in order to provide neurons with the proper environment for neuronal function. As such, protein is present in much smaller amounts (0.5% the concentration of plasma protein). Glucose is regulated as well through active transport. The glucose concentration level remains constant (60% that of plasma) until plasma glucose levels rise above 270 to 360 mg/dL.[5]

FORMATION

The CSF is formed at two sites: choroid plexuses located in the third and lateral ventricles, and extrachoroidal sites located in the ependyma and pia mater. The choroid plexuses are groups of specialized cells that have looser tight junctions to allow for passive transport of fluid. Active transport does however play a role in choroid function. Between 40% and 70% of CSF is formed at these sites, while 30% to 60% is formed at the extrachoroidal sites.[7] The rate of formation is between 0.35 and 0.4 mL/min with a total 500 to 600 mL of CSF produced daily and a turnover time of 5 to 7 hours. The total volume is 140 to 150 mL in adults. As mentioned earlier, CSF is continuous with ECF. The ECF contributes another 300 to 350 mL of fluid to the overall intracranial fluid content.[7] The CSF production is controlled by several mechanisms. Cerebral perfusion pressure contributes somewhat with constant production until the CPP drops below 70 mmHg. Adrenergic and cholinergic neurotransmitters as well as intracerebral CO_2 levels play a role by effecting blood flow. Temperature is also an important variable. For every 1°C drop in temperature, CSF production decreases by 11%.[7]

CIRCULATION

The CSF flows in a fashion comparable to blood. It passes from the lateral ventricles, third ventricle, and ependyma to the fourth ventricle. It then passes through the basal cisterns into the subarachnoid space. Ultimately, CSF is reabsorbed into plasma through arachnoid villi and granulations into the superior sagittal sinus and dural venous sinusoids. Absorption is limited by venous sinus pressure and the inherent resistance created by villi endothelium.[7] The rate of absorption remains constant until the ICP reaches approximately 30 mmHg, at which point the resistance to absorption declines by increasing fluid channel density.[2] When ICP is elevated the first protective mechanism is displacement into the subarachnoid space of the spinal cord, followed by increased absorption, decreased production, and lastly displacement of intracranial venous blood.[2,6] It is noteworthy, however, that despite elevated ICP the rate of formation of CSF is minimally affected until CPP is compromised.[7]

BLOOD-BRAIN BARRIER

The "blood-brain barrier" is a term that essentially illustrates that the endothelium separating blood from CSF and tissue has relatively small tight junctions (one-eighth the size of normal endothelial tight junctions)[6] restricting movement of substances between the two compartments. This allows for tight control of CSF and ECF composition. Some substances do cross passively through the blood-brain barrier (BBB) such as water, electrolytes, and CO_2, while others pass via facilitated transport (i.e., glucose). Protein permeability is limited, but does increase with age. Anesthetics do not alter the BBB, but acute HTN can breach the barrier and acutely alter its permeability.[6]

ANESTHETIC AND ADJUVANT DRUG EFFECTS

Many different medications affect CSF. The mechanisms of some are known while others (i.e., anesthetics) remain uncertain. Volatile anesthetics have different effects on CSF dynamics depending on the agent. For example, in situations where elevated ICP is an issue, enflurane is considered the worst of anesthetics due to its effects on CSF.[6] It increases formation and decreases absorption, ultimately exacerbating the elevated ICP. Halothane also decreases absorption but reduces formation overall, producing a slight increase in ICP. Isoflurane has no effect on formation and increases absorption at high doses, lowering ICP. Sevoflurane has the same effect as halothane, but the overall effect on ICP is unknown. Desflurane has minimal to no effects on formation or absorption of CSF or ICP. Nitrous oxide has no effect on CSF.[7] Intravenous anesthetics in general produce little to no effect on CSF dynamics. Of note, however, etomidate and thiopental reduce formation and increase absorption at high doses, while ketamine reduces absorption with no effect on formation.[7] Narcotics have little to no effect on formation. However, they do increase absorption at low doses, thus lowering ICP. Many other drugs are useful in neuroanesthesia because of their effects on CSF dynamics. Diuretics reduce CSF formation by limiting sodium secretion. Steroids reduce CSF formation and increase absorption. Dexamethasone seems to have the largest effect, with decreases up to 50% in CSF formation.[7] Although considered a diuretic, mannitol deserves separate mention. Mannitol is a sugar that passes through the BBB and ultimately is excreted in the renal tubules, where it acts as an osmotic diuretic reducing overall body water. It has a direct effect on CSF, however, by reducing formation. It also draws fluid from the ECF into CSF and facilitates CSF absorption by increasing bulk flow. Ultimately, by reducing total body water, it will favor outward flow of CSF.[9]

SPINAL CORD

ORGANIZATION

In general the spinal cord (SC) is organized into tracts that transmit impulses between the periphery and the cortex. To illustrate, sensory first-order neurons have bifurcated axons that innervate tissues and synapse in the dorsal horn of the SC central gray matter with second-order neurons. These neurons travel in the contralateral corticospinal tracts and synapse in the thalamus (which modulates sensory and motor conduction). Third-order neurons then carry the impulse from the thalamus through the internal capsule and corona radiata and to the sensory cortex. Motor neurons have the same basic orientation, however they carry impulses in the opposite direction.[10] There are two tracts that carry sensory data: the dorsal columns and the spinothalamic tracts. The dorsal columns are located in the posteriomedial portion of the SC and carry touch/pressure/vibration sensations. Within this these tracts, sacral stimuli are located medial and cervical stimuli are lateral. Blood supply to this region is unique in that two posterior spinal arteries only supply the posterior one-third of the SC. The spinothalamic tracts (lateral and ventral) carry pain/temperature sensations and are located in the anteriomedial portion of the SC. Sacral stimuli are lateral while cervical stimuli are medial. These tracts are supplied by a single anterior spinal artery, which covers the anterior two-thirds of the SC. Motor tracts are located in two areas: the lateral and the anterior corticospinal tracts. The lateral motor tracts are just lateral to the dorsal columns. The anterior corticospinal tracts are just lateral to the anterior midline.[10]

EVOKED POTENTIALS

Fundamentally, evoked potentials (EPs) record the effect of a stimulus. They help by providing information about the tract relevant to that stimulus. When a tract is impaired anywhere along its path, a change in the EP can be recorded and quantified. The potential is a series of peaks, troughs, and pauses. The data is broken down into amplitudes (the height from the peak of a wave to the adjacent trough), latency (the time from stimulation to peak potential), and polarity (direction of deflection). Generally, a 50% amplitude decrease and 10% latency increase are clinically relevant. However, patterns of smaller changes can be useful as potential signs of tract disruption.[11]

Somatosensory EPs (SSEPs) measure cortical sensory responses to peripheral stimulation. The dorsal columns are the relevant tracts. Commonly measured nerves are the median (C6-T1), ulnar (C8-T1), common peroneal (L4-S1), and posterior tibial (L4-S2).[11] Potentials are recorded over the cortex. A single potential is very small; thus, multiple potentials are summated and averaged to generate acceptable data.[12] Due to the location of the dorsal columns, this modality is most used during spinal surgery. The idea is to detect direct insults to the SC or interruption in blood flow (e.g., from a retractor) so that changes can be made acutely to improve the outcome. However, there is some utility in surgery on the cortex. An example is the placement of a temporary clip during cerebral aneurysm clipping. Upon placing the temporary clip, a sudden loss of signal indicates permanent damage, while a slower decline in signal indicates the potential for recovery upon removal of the clip. Another example is during carotid surgery. The medial cerebral artery supplies the sensory cortex. When the operative carotid is impaired during surgery, the SSEP signal can be used to detect adequacy of collateral flow.[11] Brain-stem auditory EPs (BAEP) and visual EPs (VEPs) are similar in principle to SSEPs. The stimulI are clicking sounds and light flashes respectively. These modalities are useful in brain stem/posterior fossa surgeries due to the origin of the respective cranial nerves (VII and II) in the brain stem or when the specific nerves are in question (i.e., acoustic neuromas and pituitary masses).

Motor EPs (MEPs) measure muscle activity after direct cortical stimulation of the motor cortex. The stimulus is delivered transcranially and the response is usually measured at either the thenar eminence or the abductor hallicus muscle. Unlike with SSEPs, latency has been shown to be less clinically reliable. A 50% decrease in amplitude is still the set point for relevance. As mentioned, the motor tracts are located in different areas of the SC with different blood supply than the dorsal columns. Therefore this modality can be used to monitor different regions of the SC. This can give a more universal view of the SC in concert with SSEPs.[12] Also, just like SSEPs, MEPs can be useful in cortex surgery to monitor the function of the motor cortex when in question.[13] Spontaneous electromyography (EMG) is another modality similar to MEPs. Muscle activity is monitored that is relevant for a given tract. The difference is that there is no delivered stimulus. When a nerve is locally irritated a potential is created with resultant muscle activity. In this case, muscle activity indicates nerve dysfunction. One caveat, however, is that acute transection of a nerve will often fail to elicit a response. Despite this drawback, this modality is still considered clinically useful and is applied most often to monitor cranial nerves. The facial nerve is the most commonly monitored tract, however the vocals cords can indicate CN X function and the trapezius and sternocleidomastoid muscles can indicate CN XI function. This is most useful in skull base, cavernous sinus, and posterior fossa surgeries.[7]

ANESTHETIC EFFECTS

Both IV and inhalational anesthetics attenuate EP signals. However, volatiles are much more potent in this regard (signals are undetectable at 1–1.5 MAC). Reducing the volatile agent to one-half MAC with IV supplementation is considered acceptable.[7] Different modalities have different responses to anesthetics. For example BAEPs are much less sensitive to anesthetic effect due to the fact there are fewer synapses along the relevant tract. On the other hand, MEPs tend to be the most sensitive. Total Intravenous Anesthetic (TIVA) is the preferred technique when MEPs are utilized. In addition, MEPs and EMG preclude the usage of muscle relaxants. Opioids and anxiolytics have no effects on EPs. And, of note, ketamine and etomidate have been noted to enhance EPs, however, evidence for clinical relevance is lacking.[12]

SPINAL REFLEXES

The stimulus-response arc does not always involve the cortex as is the case with reflexes. Here the stimulus is relayed by α motor nerves in the SC, which produces an immediate motor response. Although the primary tract is local, the reflex is modulated by descending pathways. When monitored, this mechanism can be used to indicate SC function at the level of the reflex and above. Although reflexes tend to fade with repeated stimulation due to descending pathway modification, reflex arcs are more sensitive to physiologic changes than SSEPs. In the setting of spinal cord injury, autonomic dysreflexia can be seen, which is described in Figure 20.1. The only effective treatment is deepening the anesthetic and/or removing the stimulus.

CEREBRAL ISCHEMIA

PATHOPHYSIOLOGY

In general, ischemia is an imbalance between cellular requirements and delivery of energy substrate. Cells require both glucose and oxygen to support function. Anaerobic metabolism does occur. However, this mechanism is limited due to reduced ATP yield and the accumulation of acidic byproducts.[6] Neural tissue requires energy for both basal cellular and electrophysiologic function. Delivery is dependent on CBF, which is directly related to CPP and inversely related to CVR. In short, CBF = CPP/CVR. Furthermore, as previously discussed, CPP = MAP − ICP (or CVP, whichever is higher). These distinctions are

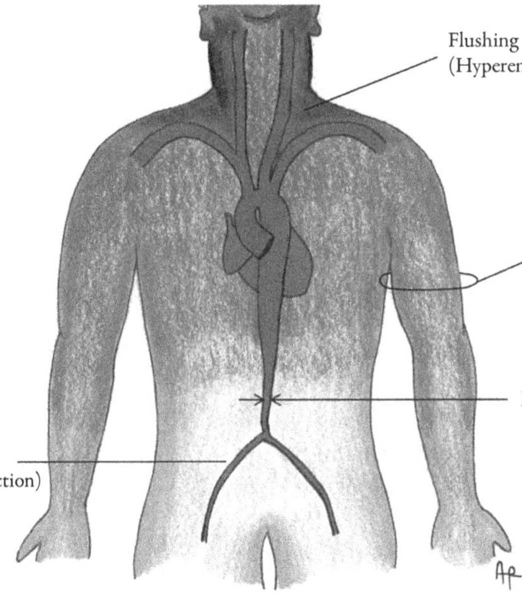

Figure 20.1 Physiology of autonomic dysreflexia. Illustrated by Ariana Rojas, MD.

important when considering cerebral protection (see section "Cerebral Protection").

Cerebral ischemia occurs when CBF is impaired by a variety of causes. These causes are either global or focal in nature. Global ischemia is defined as a complete cessation of CBF, best exemplified by cardiac arrest. In this circumstance, CBF is impaired equally among the different tissues. This is in contrast to what Miller et al. term "incomplete ischemia," which confers some partial protection of cerebral tissue through variable amounts of collateral and residual blood flow.[6] Incomplete, or focal, ischemia is when blood flow to tissues is impaired to varying degrees. With severe hypotension, for example, some tissues may receive more blood flow than others depending on their energy needs. Despite the fact that brain CPP is invariably reduced, some tissues will be protected by CVR adjustments at the cost of CBF to other cerebral tissues. Another example is a stroke, or cerebrovascular accident (CVA). In this situation, CBF is regionally impaired by vascular occlusion, such as a clot, atherosclerosis, or air embolism, or by hemorrhage. With intracranial hemorrhages, a concern is that over time the breakdown products of hemoglobin can irritate the intact vasculature and lead to regional vasospasm.[8] This can cause tissue ischemia by limiting CBF to the tissues supplied by the spastic vasculature.

When CBF to cerebral tissue is impaired, electrophysiologic function is affected as illustrated by EEG tracings. As CBF is progressively reduced, EEG tracings will first become flattened, then isoelectric (which indicates no electrophysiologic function.) Typically at CBF of ~20 mL/100 g/min EEG tracings will flatten. At <15 mL/100 g/min the tracings will become isoelectric. As CBF continues to decline, neural tissue will progressively deteriorate, with evidence of immediate and irreversible membrane failure at <6 mL/100 g/min. This implies that the tissues are not receiving enough CBF to maintain basic cellular function. Because CBF is dependent on CPP, slowed EEG tracings are seen with a CPP of <50 mmHg, isoelectric at 25–40 mmHg, and evidence of tissue injury at <25 mmHg.[14]

BRAIN TUMORS

In discussing cerebral ischemia, some mention of brain tumors is relevant. Tumors can cause ischemia by a number ways, both globally and focally. An intracranial tumor can become large enough or can obstruct the outflow of CSF and corrupt the ICP. This can affect overall CBF by limiting the CPP. Generally brain tumors have reduced CBF in comparison to normal cerebral tissue (i.e., meningiomas). Some tumors, however, have increased CBF (i.e., meningiomas). Autoregulation of that blood flow is variably present within the tumor. This can lead to a "steal phenomenon," where blood is preferentially shunted to the tumor at the expense of surrounding normal cerebral tissue.[6] Also, edema is often present in adjacent tissues. This may be of vasogenic origin by disruption of vascular membranes with resultant leakage of protein, obstruction of CSF flow, or obstruction of venous flow.[6]

TRAUMA

In neurological trauma, within the context of ischemia, the goal is to maintain cerebral blood flow, perfusion pressure, and ultimately tissue oxygenation to limit damage. Focally, there are several mechanisms by which trauma can compromise tissue. A cerebral contusion damages tissues by blunt force. In addition, the vasculature within the contusion is damaged, leading to local hemorrhage, edema, and reduced tissue oxygenation. As mentioned, extravasated blood can lead to vasospasm. Also, intracranial hemorrhages (intracerebral, subdural, or epidural) can compress blood flow to adjacent tissues.[8] The next section focuses on tissue protection in a variety of circumstances. Briefly, to protect tissue oxygenation the goal is to maintain CPP by supporting the MAP, limiting cerebral edema, and controlling ICP. There is some controversy about what MAP is considered adequate to maintain CPP while limiting edema formation. Currently it is recommended to limit the MAP to 50–70 mmHg.[9] In addition, to control against excess CPP, mannitol or hypertonic 3% saline can be used to reduce tissue edema. This can also help to control the ICP, thus maximizing tissue perfusion. To control against elevated ICP, CSF can be removed directly from the cranium. Hyperventilation can be used acutely to reduce the cerebral blood volume by causing vasoconstriction. The thought is that this will reduce the overall intracranial volume and alleviate the elevated ICP. Aggressive hyperventilation may result in cerebral infarction and should not be sustained more than a few minutes. See the section "Cerebral Protection" for further discussion.

GLUCOSE

Along with oxygen, glucose is required for cellular energy production.[6] Without glucose, cerebral tissues will not have the fuel required to carry out normal function. Similar in concept to reduced CBF and CPP, EEG patterns begin to drop at glucose concentrations of ~40 mg/dL.[6] The injurious effects of hypoglycemia are not difficult to understand. However, there is substantial attention paid to hyperglycemia as well. Many studies focus on the detrimental impact of hyperglycemia when cerebral ischemia is present. Hyperglycemia worsens ischemic tissue injury presumably through increased acidosis from anaerobic metabolism.[6] However, treatment of hyperglycemia is a bit complicated. Many studies have shown worsened outcomes when the goal is tight glucose control (i.e., glucose 80–120 mg/dL).[15] Currently the recommendation is to withhold treatment of hyperglycemia when the glucose concentration is <150 mg/dL.[6]

CEREBRAL PROTECTION

GENERAL

Cerebral tissue damage occurs when either the tissue is injured directly (i.e., cerebral contusion) or there is an imbalance between metabolic substrate requirement and substrate delivery (i.e., cerebral ischemia). With this in mind, in order to protect cerebral tissue at risk, there are two strategies that often work together synergistically: (1) to return or enhance CBF to damaged tissues, and (2) to reduce the CMR of the damaged or at-risk tissues and thus the need for substrate. Maintaining adequate CBF either by relieving an obstruction, maximizing collateral flow, or manipulating physiologic parameters will ensure that tissues at risk will have the energy needed to minimize progressive injury and begin repair. Reducing the CMR will lower the energy needed thus providing an abundance of available energy substrate.

MAINTAINING ENERGY DELIVERY

As mentioned, protecting cerebral tissues from further injury requires maintenance of CBF to damaged tissues, often by manipulation of physiologic parameters. It is helpful to keep in mind the different parameters involved. To briefly review, CBF = CPP/CVR, where CPP = MAP – ICP (or CVP, if higher).

Avoiding hypotension is obvious when trying to maintain CBF. However, there is not sufficient evidence to support specific guidelines for how high to maintain the MAP. With a stroke, to maintain sufficient collateral flow to the ischemic region, MAPs of 70 to 80 mmHg are currently recommended. This range allows for sufficient flow while reducing tissue edema that can occur when flow is restored to ischemic tissues. With cerebral vasospasm, higher levels are advocated (SBP 180-220 mmHg).[6] With traumatic brain injury, due to the elevated risk of cerebral edema, MAPs of 60 mmHg are sufficient.[7,8] Furthermore, maintaining lower MAPs will reduce the cardiopulmonary risk that keeping MAPs above 70 mmHg for prolonged periods of time will entail.[8]

Theoretically, altering the arterial CO_2 tension will change the CVR and alter the CPP. CO_2 levels have a direct effect on the caliber of the cerebral vasculature. Ischemic tissue vasculature will already be dilated maximally to maintain CBF. Hypercapnia will dilate other tissue vasculature, effectively shunting blood away from stressed tissues. On the other hand, hypocapnia will reduce overall CBF, which is undesirable. Current recommendations are to maintain normocapnia.[6]

Another component of the CPP is the ICP. When the ICP becomes elevated beyond the internal compensatory mechanisms the CPP becomes compromised. There are many modalities for reducing ICP. The CSF can be directly removed with an indwelling catheter. This will reduce the intracranial content volume and reduce pressure. Despite recommendations that during cerebral ischemia arterial CO_2 should be kept at normal levels, hyperventilation with resultant hypocapnia can reduce CBF and intracranial blood volume acutely. Because CBF is reduced (especially < $PaCO_2$ 25 mmHg) this should be reserved for dire circumstances where CPP is greatly compromised by elevated ICPs and cerebral herniation is a concern. Furthermore, this effect is time limited. The elevated intracranial pH that occurs with hypocapnea will be autocorrected resulting in normal CBF within

6–18 hours.[8] Pharmacologic intervention can also be helpful. Diuretics will draw water from cerebral tissues and reduce intracranial volume. Loop and osmotic diuretics are the most frequently used. Mannitol is a commonly used osmotic diuretic that does cross the BBB. The increased intracranial osmolarity will draw ECF into the vascular space and decrease tissue volume. Over time, the fluid will be secreted along with the mannitol in the urine. The fact that it crosses the BBB infers that slow administration is preferred so as not to cause sudden hyperosmolarity, which would lead to acute increases in cerebral fluid volume and ICP.[8] Steroids are also used in limited circumstances. They are effective at reducing tissue swelling around tumors and have some role in spinal cord injury but are not advised for traumatic brain injury patients due to a lack of evidence for any benefit and some suggestion that there may be deleterious effects.[8]

As mentioned before, glucose is a crucial component for cellular survival. As such, hypoglycemia leads to tissue injury. Furthermore, it was once believed that a hyperglycemic environment could theoretically be beneficial by providing at-risk tissues with excess energy substrate. Now the evidence has shown that preischemic hyperglycemia is detrimental. This is believed to be due to increased lactate formation from anaerobic metabolism leading to worsened intracellular acidosis that is harmful to neurons.[6] Despite the harmful nature of hyperglycemia, there is much evidence that "tight control" increases morbidity and mortality due the attendant risk of hypoglycemia. As such it is generally recommended to avoid glucose-containing fluids and treat hyperglycemia only when it becomes exceedingly high (180–220 mg/dL glucose).[6,15]

REDUCING CEREBRAL TISSUE METABOLISM

If the delivery of required energy substrate to damaged or at risk tissues is sufficient, then reducing the CMR, thus creating an abundance of energy relative to cellular need, will further help to preserve tissue function. There are many ways to accomplish this, some proactive and others preventive.

Hypothermia is the only known way to reduce basal cellular energy need. Other methods only reduce electrophysiologic functional need. The CMR will drop 5%–7%/1°C. Despite this benefit, there are side effects that confer risk: coagulation dysfunction, dysrhythmias, and increased infection.[6] Mild hypothermia (32°C–34°C) has been an area of interest intraoperatively. This range reduces CMR while minimizing the risk of side-effects. Currently, the evidence regarding clinical benefit is contradictory. Maintaining hypothermia is not recommended for routine use for focal ischemia.[6,8] On the other hand, there is evidence of clinical benefit for hypothermia in post–cardiac arrest patients. Mild hypothermia has shown improved neurologic outcome and is recommended for cardiac arrest patients if instituted within a short period of time following arrest.[6,8]

While hypothermia confers cerebral protection by reducing CMR, the opposite is true for hyperthermia. Hyperthermia greatly increases CMR. If cerebral tissue is compromised, a fever will worsen the situation. Preventing elevations in temperature is very important in protecting damaged or compromised tissues.[6] Similarly, seizures, which are essentially uncoordinated and unregulated electrophysiologic impulses, increase CMR. Any form of cerebral tissue damage, whether by trauma or surgical incision, will create the possibility for seizures, even subclinical. As such, anticonvulsants are recommended to decrease seizure activity.[8]

Anesthetics, like hypothermia, reduce CMR. However, they only reduce electrophysiologic energy requirements. Basal cellular energy requirements are unaffected. There is significant variability among the different anesthetic agents in their overall effects on cerebral physiology; however, the idea of reducing CMR to protect damaged or endangered tissues is the same. This principle, however, does not apply to systemic ischemia, such as that facilitated by cardiac arrest, where the mainstay of treatment is recovery of cardiopulmonary function.

While intravenous anesthetics, in general, cause reduced CMR and reduced CBF, there are notable exceptions. Despite a reduction in CBF, there is a greater effect on CMR conferring protection to tissues at risk. One exception is ketamine. Ketamine actually increases both CMR and CBF. In addition, it is generally known to provoke seizure potentials in patients who are at risk for seziures.[6] Recently, ketamine has been use in the neurocritical care setting as a treatment of status epilepticus. This has rarely been used in the operating room; and for the purposes of the ABA, ketamine is considered contraindicated for use in patients with risk for seizures. In summary, ketamine is not an ideal anesthetic for neurosurgical procedures. Another exception is etomidate. Although etomidate acts in similar physiologic fashion to other induction agents, there is evidence of worsened tissue hypoxia associated with its use. Methohexital also has similar effects to other induction agents but potentiates seizure foci and has been used to activate them during mapping procedures.[7] Narcotics are variably effective. Additionally, morphine and fentanyl decrease CMR. Morphine, however, does not affect CBF, while fentanyl does. Remifentanyl and alfentanyl have no effect on CMR. Lastly, lidocaine substantially lowers CMF, however, unlike the induction agents, the MAP, and by extension CPP, is maintained.[6]

Inhalational anesthetics have the same protective effect as IV agents. However, unlike IV agents, they typically increase CBF (to varying degrees.) This has been widely termed "uncoupling" in the past, implying that CBF is not altered by changing CMR.[6] In contrast, Miller et al. assert that CBF remains somewhat coupled to CMR during inhalational anesthesia, and that this leads to "luxury perfusion." In fact, changes in CBF are dose related. The CBF is reduced at 0.5 MAC, unchanged at 1 MAC, and increased at >1 MAC. The implication is that, although inhalational anesthetics are inherent vasodilators, coupling remains substantially intact.[6] Similar to IV anesthetics, the reduction in CMR is dose related, the endpoint being an isoelectric EEG at which point no further reduction in CMR can be achieved. Of note, enflurane is a potential epileptogenic, which is potentiated by hypocapnea. Halothane increases CBF the most by far. Isoflurane produces modest increases in CBF at 1 MAC, while sevoflurane and desflurane reduce CBF at 1 MAC to lesser degrees. It is noteworthy that the inherent vasodilatory properties of the volatiles along with their effects on CBF can increase ICP when intracranial compliance is compromised. If increased ICP is a significant issue, then a total intravenous anesthetic should be considered. Nitrous oxide is a little different from the volatile agents. Nitrous oxide causes increased CBF and ICP, which can be attenuated by concomitant IV anesthetic. This effect is additive to a substantial degree with inhalational agents.[7] The use of N_2O in neurosurgery, however, is limited due to its ability to expand air emboli.

REFERENCES

1. Patel P, Drummond J. Cerebral physiology and the effects on anesthetic drugs. In: Miller R., ed. *Miller's Anesthesia*. 7th ed. Philadelphia, PA: Elsevier; 2010.
2. Butterworth I, Mackey D, Wasnick J. *Clinical Anesthesiology*. 7th ed. Philadelphia, PA: McGraw-Hill; 2013.
3. Barash P, Cullen B, Stoelting R, Cahalan M, Stock M. *Clinical Anesthesia*. 6th ed. Philadelphia, PA: Lippincott Williams & Wilkins; 2009.
4. Lomen-Hoerth C, Messing R, Lomen-Hoerth C, Messing R. Nervous system disorders. In: McPhee S, Hammer G, McPhee S, Hammer G, eds. *Pathophysiology of Disease*. 6th ed. New York, NY: McGraw-Hill; 2010.
5. Waxman S. Higher cortical functions. In: Waxman S. *Clinical Neuroanatomy*. 27th ed. New York, NY: McGraw-Hill; 2013.
6. Miller R, ed. *Miller's Anesthesia*. 7th ed. Philadelphia, PA: Elsevier; 2010:ch. 13.
7. Cottrell J, Young W. *Cottrell and Young's Neuroanesthesia*. 5th ed. Philadelphia, PA: Mosby Elsevier; 2010:60–70.
8. Miller R, ed. *Miller's Anesthesia*. 7th ed. Philadelphia, PA: Elsevier; 2010:2046–2071.
9. Barash P, Cullen B, Stoelting R, Cahalan M, Stock M. *Clinical Anesthesia*. 6th ed. Philadelphia, PA: Lippincott Williams & Wilkins; 2009:1023–1024.
10. Morgan M, Edward G, Mikhail M, Murry M. *Clinical Anesthesiology*. 4th ed. Philadelphia, PA: McGraw-Hill; 2006:363–366.
11. Cottrell J, Young W. *Cottrell and Young's Neuroanesthesia*. 5th ed. Philadelphia, PA: Mosby Elsevier; 2010:115–117.
12. Barash P, Cullen B, Stoelting R, Cahalan M, Stock M. *Clinical Anesthesia*. 6th ed. Philadelphia, PA: Lippincott Williams & Wilkins; 2009:1010–1011.
13. Morgan M, Edward G, Mikhail M, Murry M. *Clinical Anesthesiology*. 4th ed. Philadelphia, PA: McGraw-Hill; 2006:120–125.
14. Morgan M, Edward G, Mikhail M, Murry M. *Clinical Anesthesiology*. 4th ed. Philadelphia, PA: McGraw-Hill; 2006:615.
15. Barash P, Cullen B, Stoelting R, Cahalan M, Stock M. *Clinical Anesthesia*. 6th ed. Philadelphia, PA: Lippincott Williams & Wilkins; 2009:1016.

FURTHER READING

Miller R, ed. *Miller's Anesthesia*. 7th ed. Philadelphia, PA: Elsevier; 2010:ch 13, 63.

QUESTIONS

1. Which of the following decreases cerebral blood flow?
   A. Mean arterial pressure of 80 mmHg in a healthy patient.
   B. PaO_2 of 50 mmHg
   C. Nitroglycerin
   D. Etomidate
   E. Ketamine

2. In a patient with a blood pressure of 150/90, intracranial pressure of 10, and central venous pressure of 8, calculate the cerebral perfusion pressure.
   A. 100
   B. 102
   C. 92
   D. 60
   E. 62

3. What is the function of the reticular activating system?
   A. Awareness and the transition from sleep to wakefulness
   B. Balance and coordination
   C. Problem solving
   D. Control of breathing
   E. Control of voluntary motor movements

4. Select the CORRECT statement regarding cerebral blood flow.
   A. PaO_2 of 40 mmHg causes a decrease in cerebral blood flow.
   B. Inhalation agents always cause an increase in cerebral blood flow.
   C. Epileptic seizures and coma increase cerebral blood flow.
   D. Hypothermia does not influence cerebral blood flow.
   E. For each 1-mmHg increase in $PaCO_2$, cerebral blood flow increases by 1–2 mL/100 g/min
   F. For each 1-mmHg increase in $PaCO_2$, cerebral blood flow decreases by 1–2 mL/100 g/min

5. Changes in ventilation may alter regional blood flow in the brain. The expected result of mild hyperventilation in a patient with ischemic regions of the brain would be:
   A. Hypoventilation causes vasodilation in normal areas of the brain and deprives ischemic areas of oxygen.
   B. Inverse steal is also known as luxury perfusion.
   C. Administration of intravenous nitroglycerin causes inverse steal.
   D. Hyperventilation causes blood to be shunted from normally perfused areas of the brain to ischemic areas.

6. Which of the following values is incorrect? Example: The brain consumes a significant amount of oxygen during normal metabolism. Which of the following DOES NOT describe cerebral oxygen physiology?
   A. $CMRO_2$ of 3.5 mL/100 g/min
   B. CBF to gray matter is 80 mL per 100 g brain tissue per minute
   C. The brain receives 15% of cardiac output
   D. The brain consumes 20% of total body oxygen
   E. Cerebral blood flow of 15 mL/100 g/min

7. Which of the following is the first compensatory mechanism that occurs following an increase in intracranial volume?
   A. CSF translocation to the spinal space
   B. Increased CSF reabsorption
   C. Decreased CSF production
   D. Reduced intracranial blood volume
   E. Reduced intracranial extracellular fluid volume

8. A lesion in the lumbar spine results in loss of sensation to touch on the right lower extremity and sensation to nociception and temperature in the left lower extremity. What is the likely diagnosis?
   A. Complete transection
   B. Central cord syndrome
   C. Anterior spinal syndrome
   D. Brown-Sequard syndrome
   E. Cauda equina syndrome

9. During the performance of a cerebral aneurysm clipping the surgeon announces that she will place a temporary clip to stem aneurysm flow. While titrating barbiturate, what EEG tracing is preferable under these circumstances?
   A. Predominant beta waves
   B. EEG silence
   C. Burst suppression
   D. Predominant delta waves
   E. Barbiturate spindles

10. Which is not a component of the management of cerebral vasospasm?
   A. Maintaining MAPs above the patient's baseline blood pressure
   B. Maintaining high-normal hematocrits
   C. IV calcium channel blockers
   D. Volume expansion
   E. Localized injection of calcium channel blocker

11. What is the estimated average CBF of a patient whose body temperature is 34°C?
   A. 62 mL/100 g/min
   B. 52 mL/100 g/min
   C. 42 mL/100 g/min
   D. 32 mL/100 g/min
   E. 22 mL/100 g/min

12. Which of the following agents will not decrease the amplitude of SSEP signals?
   A. Isoflurane
   B. Propofol
   C. Thiopental
   D. Nitrous oxide
   E. Etomidate

ANSWERS

1. D. Intravenous administration of etomidate causes a decrease in cerebral blood flow by decreasing the cerebral metabolic rate. Choice A is incorrect because 80 mmHg is a mean arterial pressure within the range of autoregulation. The autoregulation curve is generally agreed to be maintained between mean arterial pressures of 60 and 150 mmHg. Choice B is incorrect because cerebral blood flow will increase, not decrease, when PaO_2 is below 60 mmHg. Choice C is incorrect because systemic vasodilators such as nitroglycerin increase cerebral blood flow by vasodilating the cerebral vessels. Choice E is incorrect because ketamine increases cerebral metabolic rate, which causes an increase in cerebral blood flow.
2. A. The equation needed to solve this problem is as follows:

   $$CPP = MAP - ICP$$

   To solve this problem, the mean arterial pressure (MAP) must first be calculated. The MAP is equal to one-third of the systolic blood pressure plus two-thirds of the diastolic blood pressure, for a MAP of 110. When intracranial pressure (ICP) is subtracted from the MAP, this gives us a cerebral perfusion pressure of 100. Because the intracranial pressure is higher than central venous pressure, we do not need the central venous pressure value to calculate the answer.
3. A. The reticular activating system is responsible for awareness. Answer B refers to the function of the cerebellum. Answer C describes the function of the frontal lobe of the cerebral cortex. Answer D refers to a

function of the pons. Answer E refers to a function of the basal ganglia.

4. E. E is correct. Cerebral blood flow changes with $PaCO_2$. Answer A is incorrect because a decrease in PaO_2 below 60 mmHg causes an increase in cerebral blood flow. Answer B is incorrect. Inhalation agents cause a decrease in cerebral metabolic rate and a dose-dependent increase in cerebral blood flow. A net increase in cerebral blood flow occurs when the inhalation agent is at one MAC or greater, while at lower levels the net cerebral blood flow is decreased or unchanged. Answer C is incorrect because states of stimulation, arousal, and seizure increase the cerebral metabolic rate and therefore cerebral blood flow, while the states of sleep and coma cause decreases in cerebral metabolic rate and cerebral blood flow. Answer D is incorrect because hypothermia decreases cerebral metabolic rate and cerebral blood flow. Cerebral metabolic rate decreases by 6% for each one-degree-Celsius decrease in temperature. Answer F is incorrect because an increase in $PaCO_2$ causes an increase, not decrease, in cerebral blood flow.
5. D. Inverse steal is also known as the Robin Hood effect and occurs when blood is shunted toward ischemic areas of the brain that need oxygen. This can be achieved when the anesthesiologist mildly hyperventilates the patient, causing mild hypocapnia. It can also occur when the cerebral metabolic rate is decreased by the administration of intravenous anesthetic agents (with the exception of ketamine). Answers A, B, and C all describe cerebral steal, which is also known as luxury perfusion. In instances of cerebral steal, blood flows preferentially to normal areas of the brain and is shunted away from the ischemic areas, further depriving them of oxygen. This occurs during hypoventilation that leads to hypercarbia and when vasodilators, such as nitroglycerin, are administered.
6. E. E is the false statement. The average cerebral blood flow to the brain under normal circumstances is 50 mL per 100 g brain tissue per minute. Answers A, B, C, and D are correct statements.
7. A. When the intracranial pressure (ICP) begins to rise, from any cause, the first mechanism by which this change is combated is translocation of the CSF to the spinal subarachnoid space. The other mechanisms listed will follow as the pressure continues to rise. This trend follows the principle of the Monro-Kellie hypothesis. The ultimate goal is to prevent cerebral herniation. A general principle that indicates that compensatory mechanisms have reached their limit is if the ICP rises 4 mmHg with injection of 1 mL of fluid into the intracranial space, cerebral herniation is imminent. (See *Miller's Anesthesia*, 7th ed., Chapter 63, or Morgan, Mikhail, and Murray's *Clinical Anesthesiology*, Chapter 25, for more information.)
8. D. Brown-Sequard syndrome is due to trauma that damages half of the spinal cord to varying degrees. This will produce the symptoms described in the stem. A complete transection would cause a complete loss of sensation and motor function below the lesion. Central cord syndrome can occur after trauma and is thought to be due to bleeding into the cord itself. The result is paresis that is greater in the upper versus the lower extremities as well as bladder dysfunction and variable degrees of sensory loss. Anterior cord syndrome is due to disruption of the anterior spinal artery, which effects spinal cord function within its perfusion area. Cauda equina syndrome is due to injury below the spinal cord conus and results in perineal sensation loss, bowel and bladder function loss, and lower extremity weakness. (See Barash's *Clinical Anesthesia*, 6th ed., Chapter 39, for more information.)
9. C. Burst suppression is characterized by intervals of activity punctuated by short periods of silence. This tracing implies return of function shortly after cessation of drug administration. Electroencephalographic silence, or complete isoelectric EEG, implies complete cessation of electrophysiological function, which will protect the tissue from ischemia. However, recovery of function is less predictable under these circumstances. Delta waves are the predominant pattern under deep anesthesia. However, this pattern does not confer ischemic protection. Barbiturate spindles are seen after modest boluses of barbiturates but do not imply temporary cessation of function needed to protect against ischemia. Beta waves are seen in the completely awake state. (See *Miller's Anesthesia*, 7th ed., Chapter 46, and Barash's *Clinical Anesthesia*, 6th ed., Chapter 39, for more information.)
10. B. Historically, treatment of vasospasm has been described as "triple H therapy" (hypertension, hypervolemia, and hemodilution). The efficacy of this approach has been questioned recently. However, maintaining elevated MAPs is still a mainstay of treatment to maintain CPP to the ischemic areas. Volume expansion is still practiced, albeit much more limited, to maintain adequate cardiac output and to prevent the hematocrit from becoming too high and thus increasing the systemic vascular resistance via excess blood viscosity. Calcium channel blockers are widely used as prophylaxis and treatment of vasospasm both through IV infusions and radiographically guided localized injections. (See *Miller's Anesthesia*, 7th ed., Chapter 63, for more information.)
11. D. Although there is wide fluctuation of CBF throughout the different cerebral tissues, the average CBF is 50 mL/100 g/min. The CBF (and CMR) drop 5%–7% per degree Celsius of body temperature. The patient in question has a temperature roughly 3°C below normal.

Thus, the CBF will be 18 mL/100 g/min below the normal average CBF. (See Morgan, Mikhail, and Murray's *Clinical Anesthesiology*, Chapter 25, for more information.)

12. E. Different anesthetics have different effects on SSEP signals. Typically the volatile agents, propofol, barbiturates, and opioids all reduce amplitude and increase latency progressively with increasing dosages. Nitrous oxide is unique in that in reduces amplitude without effecting latency. Etomidate does increase latency, but it also increases amplitude. (See *Miller's Anesthesia*, 7th ed., Chapter 46, and Morgan, Mikhail, and Murray's *Clinical Anesthesiology*, Chapter 25, for more information.)

21.

PERIPHERAL AND AUTONOMIC NERVOUS SYSTEMS

Shruti Deshpande, Muhammad B. Rafique, and Naveen Vanga

INTRODUCTION

A neuron is the fundamental structure in the entire nervous system. The neuron acts as a conductor of information from the central nervous system (CNS) to rest of the body and vice versa in the form of impulses called action potentials. Neurons communication with other neurons, glands, or muscle cells across junctions called synapses. Typically, different types of neurotransmitters—acetylcholine (ACh), epinephrine, and norepinephrine—serve as messengers across synapses called chemical synapses. Sometimes the communication between cells in the CNS is through electric current, crossing electrical synapses.

NEUROMUSCULAR JUNCTION

The neuromuscular junction is the synapse between the prejunctional motor nerve fiber coming from the ventral horn of spinal cord and the postjunctional skeletal muscle fiber. There is gap of 20 nm between these two structures called the junctional or synaptic cleft. The motor endplate, formed by the postjunctional skeletal muscle fiber, is highly corrugated and folded on itself with deep invagination of junctional clefts called primary and secondary clefts. There is dense population of ACh receptors located on the shoulders of these muscular clefts. The deeper parts of the clefts contain sodium channels on their membrane.

NEUROMUSCULAR SYNAPTIC TRANSMISSION

Acetylcholine is the most important neurotransmitter acting at the neuromuscular junction. It also acts as an important neurotransmitter at all autonomic ganglia, at many autonomically innervated organs, and at many synapses in the CNS. It is formed from acetyl Coenzyme A (acetyl CoA) and choline in presence of the enzyme choline acetyl transferase. It is synthesized and stored by the prejunctional nerve fiber in small, uniform-sized packages called synaptic vesicles. The ACh is stored with ATP and proteoglycan for subsequent release. The transport of ACh from cytoplasm into the vesicle is assisted by the vesicle associated transporter (VAT). Vesamicol can block VAT-assisted transport of ACh into vesicles.

When the motor neuron is stimulated, an action potential is propagated down the neuron by depolarization of each adjacent neuronal segment to the threshold. The Ca++ channels on the prejunctional motor neurons are sensitive to this depolarization, which widely opens them. This opening increases Ca++ permeability, and Ca++ flows down its electrochemical gradient into the nerve terminal.

With the entry of Ca++, the synaptic vesicles filled with ACh move toward the synaptic cleft, fuse with the plasma membrane, and release ACh into the synaptic cleft. The release of ACh is by the process of exocytosis. This process of fusion of vesicles to the surface membrane and ACh release can be blocked by botulinum toxin.

Acetylcholine diffuses across the synaptic cleft and binds to alpha subunit of the nicotinic ACh receptors on the motor endplate. The binding of ACh to ligand-gated ACh nicotinic receptors causes conformational change in the receptor. These receptors contain Na+ K+ channels. Conformational change in the receptors leads to the opening of these Na+K+ channels, which increases the permeability of the postjunctional motor endplate to both of these ions. The Na+ flows into the endplate and K+ moves out, according to their respective electrochemical gradients. Thus these ions try to maintain endplate potential at its equilibrium potential. But the endplate depolarizes further beyond this equilibrium point to −50 mV, as there are many other ion channels that influence membrane potential. This is known as endplate potential (EPP), which is local endplate membrane depolarization that spreads by local currents to adjacent muscle fibers, which are depolarized to their threshold and fire action potentials. Action potentials run down the muscle membrane to initiate muscle contraction.

The action of ACh at the nicotinic receptor ceases by degradation of ACh due to enzyme cholinesterase on the motor endplate. Endplate potentials cease to develop with degradation of ACh to acetyl CoA and choline. Drugs like neostigmine, physostigimine, and edrophonium bind with and inhibit the action of acetylcholinesterase. These drugs increase the action of ACh by increasing its concentration at the synaptic cleft. About half of the choline is taken up by the prejunctional motor nerve membrane by the action of Na+ choline cotransporters to be used again. Hexamethonium can block Na+—dependent choline transporter (CHT) and prevent its reuptake by the nerve cell.

BASIC STRUCTURE OF CHOLINERGIC RECEPTORS

Acetylcholine receptors (AChRs) are broadly classified into nicotinic receptors and muscarinic receptors.

NICOTINIC ACETYLCHOLINE RECEPTORS

Nicotinic ACh receptors (nAChRs) are ligand-gated ion channels that are mainly present in neuromuscular junctions. These receptors mediate fast synaptic transmission of neurotransmitters. These are further divided into two types according to their location: neuronal type and muscle type. Muscle-type nicotinic receptors are found at neuromuscular junctions, and the action of ACh at the neuromuscular junction mediates muscular contraction and is responsible for muscle tone, already discussed above. These types of nicotinic receptors are synthesized in the muscle cells and are anchored to the endplate membrane by a protein known as rapsyn. They are densely populated on the motor endplate membrane. Neuronal-type nicotinic receptors are mainly present at synapses between CNS neurons, autonomic ganglia, and other parts of the nervous system, and are involved in cognitive function, learning and memory, arousal, reward, motor control, and analgesia. These are activated by the binding of ACh to the receptors and in turn cause the movement of cations through the opening of an ion channel, with the influx of calcium ions affecting the release of neurotransmitters, similar to the muscle-type nicotinic receptors.

Each nicotinic receptor is a pentamer of subunit proteins that are arranged like staves of a barrel in cylindrical fashion with a central ion channel. The pentamer consists of different combinations of individual subunits according to different types of receptor. The adult or mature type contains two alpha subunits and one each of the beta, delta, and epsilon subunits. The fetal type of ACh receptor has a gamma subunit instead of an epsilon subunit.

The alpha subunit in the receptor has ligand sites on either side for attachment of ACh. The ion channel within the receptor gets opened only after two molecules of ACh attach to two binding sites on the alpha subunits. Neuromuscular blocking agents also bind to the receptor at the same site, blocking the action of ACh and muscular contraction.

Other Types of Nicotinic Acetylcholine Receptors

Extrajunctional Nicotinic Receptors

These are present in very limited number, as their synthesis is inhibited by neural activity. But they proliferate when there is less motor nerve activity, such as in trauma or skeletal muscle denervation.

Prejunctional Nicotinic Receptors

These are present on the motor nerve endings and influence the release of neurotransmitters.

MUSCARINIC ACETYLCHOLINE RECEPTORS

These types of ACh receptors are more complex than nicotinic receptors. The muscarinic ACh receptors are G-protein-coupled receptors found mainly at autonomic ganglia, organs innervated by the parasympathetic division of the autonomic nervous system, and in the CNS. There are five subtypes of muscarinic AChRs, according to their location and binding studies (Figure 21.1). These are M1, M2, M3, M4, and M5. G-protein has three subunits: alpha, beta, and gamma. A conformational change in the muscarinic receptor causes release of guanosine diphosphate (GDP) from the alpha subunits and binding of guanosine triphosphate (GTP) in its place. This activates the G-protein-coupled receptors. The action of the G-protein-coupled receptors is terminated by the GTPase enzyme through hydrolysis of the GTP from the alpha subunits.

M1, M4, M5 receptors: These are mainly found in the CNS and involve complex CNS functions such as memory, arousal, attention, and analgesia.

M2 receptors: These receptors are present in the heart. When ACh binds to these receptors on the heart, it gets activated and lowers the heart rate by lowering the conduction velocity at the SA and AV nodes.

M3 receptors: These receptors are present at the smooth muscles in the bronchus, bladder, and exocrine glands. Activation of M3 receptors causes different responses at various organs.

After binding of ACH to the muscarinic receptor, transmission of a signal to the effector cell is not simple and fast

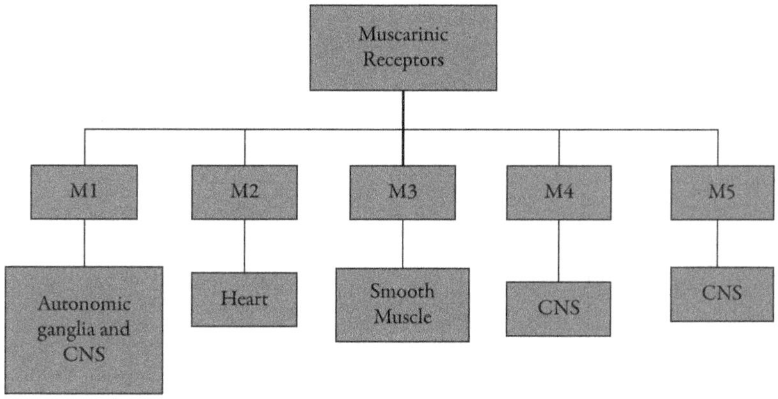

Figure 21.1 Muscarinic receptors.

as with a nicotinic receptor. M1 and M3 are coupled to the enzyme phospholipase C (PL C) through G-protein. The activation of these receptors causes an increase in activity of the enzyme phospholipase C on phosphatidylinositol polyphosphate in the plasma membrane, splitting it into inositol 1, 4, 5 triphosphate (IP3) and diacylglycerol (DAG). The DAG mediates the regulation of enzyme activity through activation of protein kinase C. The IP3 enters into cell membrane and activates the IP3 receptors on the endoplasmic reticulum (ER). This increases the release of Ca from the ER, which increases the cytosolic Ca. This increase in cytosolic Ca causes contraction of smooth muscles and glands. Thus, M1 and M3 mediate excitatory responses in effector cells.

M2 mediates the inhibitory response of the nodal cells of the heart. This is done by inhibiting adenylyl cyclase through G-protein. The reduced cyclic AMP (cAMP) causes reduced action of cAMP-dependent protein kinase. It also activates K channels in the plasma membrane, leading to increased K+ conductance. Increased conductance of K into the cell increases the resting membrane potential of the myocardial and other cell membranes, leading to inhibition. All these actions lead to reduced heart rate and contraction strength.

AUTONOMIC NERVOUS SYSTEM

The autonomic nervous system can be divided into three divisions: (1) sympathetic or adrenergic system, (2) parasympathetic or cholinergic system, and (3) enteric system (Figure 21.2).

Sympathetic system: The preganglionic fibers emerge from the thoracic and the upper two lumbar levels (T1 through L2). The preganglionic fiber releases ACh, and the postganglionic fiber releases norepinephrine as a neurotransmitter. Norepinephrine acts on adrenergic receptors on the effector organs to produce action.

Parasympathetic system: The preganglionic fibers of this system emerge with cranial nerves III, VII, IX, and X and at spinal cord levels S2–S4. Its pre- and postganglionic fiber secretes ACh as a neurotransmitter. The ACh released from the parasympathetic postganglionic fibers mediates action of effector cells through muscarinic receptors.

Enteric nervous system: This is an independent system that innervates the whole of the gut. Thus the gut can function autonomously, even when the sympathetic and parasympathetic supply is disconnected.

ADRENERGIC RECEPTORS AND THE AUTONOMIC NERVOUS SYSTEM

The response of the sympathetic nervous system is mediated through the adrenergic receptors, which can be divided broadly into alpha (α) and beta (β) receptors. Agonists or antagonists acting on these receptors determine the final response of the effector cell.

Alpha Receptors

Alpha receptors are further classified into two subtypes, alpha 1 and alpha 2, according to their function after activation.

The alpha 1 receptors are located postsynaptically at sympathetic neuroeffector junctions of many organs. The alpha1 receptors are abundantly found on all vascular smooth muscle, although densities vary throughout the body; gastrointestinal and urinary sphincters; the dilator muscle of the iris; and the errector pili muscle of hair follicles. These receptors are more responsive to norepinephrine than epinephrine. Activation of alpha 1 receptors leads to stimulatory response of the effector cell. On vessels, activation of alpha1 causes increased vascular smooth muscular tone, reducing blood flow to downstream organs. It increases tone of gastrointestinal and urinary sphincters, reducing the passage of contents past them. Increased tone of the dilator of the iris causes pupils to dilate. And

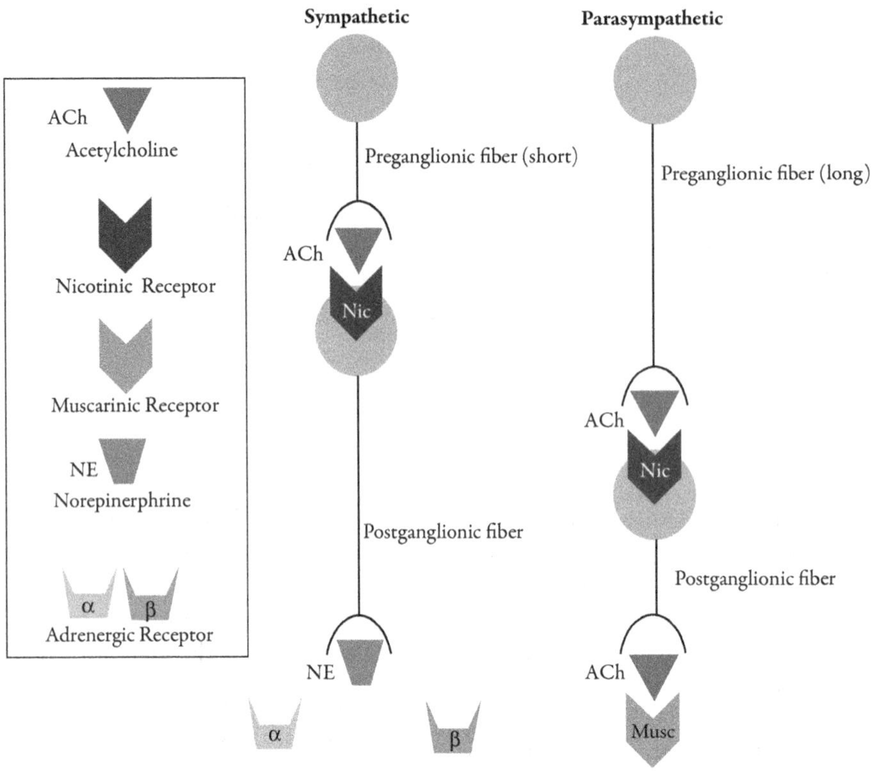

Figure 21.2 Autonomic nervous system.

increased tone of erector pilli due to alpha1 stimulation pulls on the hair follicle, causing hair to "stand on end."

Alpha 2 receptors are located postsynaptically and also exist presynaptically associated with nerve terminals. Activation of alpha 2 receptors leads to inhibitory response of the effector cell. Activation of these receptors inhibits the release of norepinephrine. Released norepinephrine acts on the presynaptic alpha 2 receptors to reduce its own release from the nerve terminal; it is a negative feedback mechanism.

Beta Receptors

Activation of beta receptors triggers a sympathomimetic (adrenergic) response. These receptors are further classified into three types according to their affinities to adrenergic agonists and antagonists, different locations, and functions: beta 1, beta 2, and beta 3.

Beta 1 receptors (beta 1) are present mainly in the heart and the kidneys. In the heart, activation of beta 1 receptors increases the chronotropy (heart rate), inotropy (force of contraction), and AV-node conduction velocity. In the kidneys, beta 1 is located on the juxtaglomerular apparatus. Activation of beta 1 here causes renin release.

The beta 2 receptors are mainly present in the respiratory and reproductive systems. Other sites for beta 2 include blood vessels, GIT, skeletal muscle, liver, and mast cells. Activation of these receptors results in vasodilatation, bronchodilation, relaxation of the GIT, glycogenolysis in the liver, tremor in skeletal muscle, and inhibition of histamine release from mast cells. In the uterus, stimulation of beta 2 causes relaxation of uterine smooth muscles.

The beta 3 receptors are located on adipose tissues, and activation of beta 3 receptors promotes lipolysis.

SKELETAL MUSCLE CONTRACTIONS

To learn the physiology of skeletal muscle contraction, we need to know the basic structures and components of skeletal muscles.

STRUCTURE OF SKELETAL MUSCLE

Skeletal muscle is formed of large numbers of muscle cells in groups called fascicles. Each muscle cell is usually called a muscle fiber. Muscle fibers are very large, multinucleated, and up to several millimeters in length. Each muscle cell is made up of large number of cylindrical contractile strands called myofibrils. Myofibrils are divided into segments called sarcomeres.

Sarcomeres are the basic contractile units of a muscle (Figure 21.3). Each sarcomere is made up of a number of proteins, including alpha actinin, which is the major constituent of the Z line, and actin and myosin, which are the major components of the thin and thick filaments, respectively. There are two parts of myosin: a tail that forms the core of the thick filament and the head, which projects out

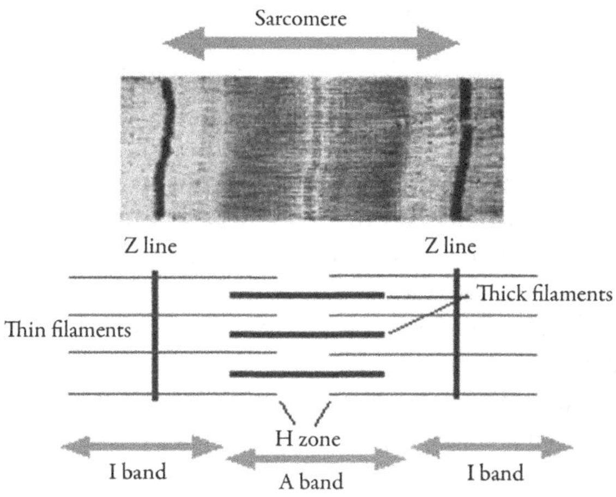

Figure 21.3 Sarcomere.

from the thick filament. These heads are also termed as cross-bridges.

Sarcomeres have alternate dark (called "A" bands) and light (called as "I" bands) bands. The I bands contain only thin (actin) filaments, whereas the A bands contain thick (myosin) filaments. The peripheral part of the A band has overlapping actin and myosin filaments. There is a middle zone called the "H" zone, which has only myosin filaments in it. Actin is attached to the Z line, and myosin is anchored to the "M" line in the middle of the sarcomere. There are two accessory proteins bound to the actin filaments: tropomyosin and troponin. Troponin is a complex of three proteins, troponin C (Ca2+–binding), troponin I (inhibitory), and troponin T (tropomyosin-binding). Tropomyosin is attached to troponin.

Other structures in the sarcomere are mitochondria, lipids, glycogen, T-tubules, and the sarcoplasmic reticulum. T-tubules are responsible for conduction of electrical signals from the cell surface, and the sarcoplasmic reticulum is responsible for the intracellular storage and release of calcium required for contraction to occur.

PHYSIOLOGY OF SKELETAL MUSCLE CONTRACTION

The binding of actin with the globular heads of myosin brings about the muscular contraction. When the motor nerve stimulates the muscle fiber, the depolarization impulse travels through the T-tubule and reaches the sarcoplasmic/endoplasmic reticulum. This stimulates the release of Ca++ from the sarcoplasmic reticulum.

When the intracellular Ca++ concentration increases above the threshold, it gets attached to troponin C, forming a troponin calcium complex. This brings about a conformational change in the tropomyosin-actin complex, allowing actin to bind with myosin. The actin-myosin complex allows the S1 unit on the head of the myosin to move in the unstrained position (strained in relaxed position), causing muscle contraction. At this step the ADP and Pi molecules are released from the myosin heads.

The contraction of each sarcomere in each muscle fiber is required for the contraction of the muscle. The relaxation of muscle also requires energy. When ATP binds to the S1 unit, it gets broken down to ADP and Pi. The S1 unit bound to ADP and Pi moves to the "strained" or "relaxed" position.

If calcium influx is continuous in the cytosol due to continued motor nerve stimulation, all the steps above will keep repeating, resulting in muscular contraction. This is called contraction cycling.

When nerve stimulation fails to produce muscle depolarization or an action potential fails to reach the myoneural junction, calcium is actively pumped back into the sarcoplasmic reticulum, and muscle relaxation happens.

ENERGY SOURCE AND RELEASE

Energy for muscular contraction is obtained from the ATP molecule. There are two enzymes that provide the short-term supplies of ATP: creatine kinase and adenylate kinase (myokinase) catalyze a reversible reaction to produce creatine phosphate by creatine phosphorylation with the help of ATP.

$$\text{Creatine} + \text{ATP} \xrightarrow{\textit{Creatine Kinase}} \text{Creatine Phosphate} + \text{ADP}$$

Thus, creatine phosphate acts as a storage battery, ready to regenerate ATP when ADP accumulates.

Adenylyl cyclase can combine two molecules of ADP to form one ATP and one adenosine monophosphate. Thus energy is supplied for muscle contraction in the muscle cell.

PAIN MECHANISMS AND PATHWAYS

The transduction and perception of pain involves fundamental biological events at multiple levels of the nervous system. Pain is an important defense mechanism by which the CNS warns the body of potential or actual injury.

NOCICEPTORS

The pain pathway is initiated where the pain is first felt—the nociceptor, or primary afferent nociceptor. These are primary sensory neurons that are activated by the noxious stimuli that can produce tissue damage. Nociceptors transform these noxious stimuli into electrical signals.

Nociceptors are distributed all over the body from head to toe including skin, viscera, muscles, joints, and meninges. Free nerve endings of primary afferent Aδ (thinly myelinated and fast conducting) and C (unmyelinated slow conducting) fibers serve as nociceptors. These nociceptors are stimulated by mechanical (e.g., squeezing the tissue), thermal (heat or cold), or chemical stimuli and inflammatory mediators like bradykinin, serotonin, prostaglandins, cytokines, and H+ released from damaged skin. Inflammatory mediators can also reduce the activation threshold of nociceptors, causing primary sensitization, which needs less stimulation for the activation of nociceptors.

Each nerve fiber carries specific sensory information to the CNS.

> Primary afferent Aδ fibers: Lightly myelinated and fast-conducting Aδ fibers carry rapid, sharp pain and are responsible for the initial reflex response to acute pain. They respond to mechanical and thermal stimuli.
>
> Primary afferent C fibers: Unmyelinated and slowest-conducting C fibers are polymodal, responding to chemical, mechanical, and thermal stimuli. Slow and burning pain activates the C fibers.

Nociceptors release certain neuropeptides (substance P [SP], calcitonin gene-related peptide [CGRP]) from their sensory endings to send efferent information to the various target tissues.

PROCESSING OF PAIN IN THE SPINAL CORD

The spinal cord is the first location in the CNS where the nociceptor nerve fibers synapse. The dorsal horn region in the spinal cord is the place where all these first-order afferent nociceptor fibers synapse with the secondary afferent neurons. The dorsal horn is further divided into ten layers called Rexed laminae. Nociceptive specific neurons in Rexed lamina I (posteromarginal nucleus, or zone) and lamina V (reticular nucleus) receive the information from Aδ, and laminae II (substantia gelatinosa) and III of the dorsal horn receive information from C fibers through excitatory neurotransmitters including glutamate and substance P.

The second-order afferent neurons (or interneurons) have their cell bodies in the dorsal horn of the spinal cord. The interneurons play an important role in modulation of the pain pathway. The sensory information is further carried by the axons of these neurons, which ascend up in the spinal cord to the thalamus directly via the spinothalamic tract or indirectly via the spinoreticular tract in the anterolateral system.

The Spinothalamic Tract

The second-order neurons in the dorsal horn, after synapsing with the Aδ fibers, cross the midline to the contralateral side of the spinal cord in the anterior white commissure and ascend in the contralateral spinothalamic tract to nuclei within the thalamus. The third-order neurons in the thalamic nuclei ascend further up in the CNS to terminate in the somatosensory cortex. Some of the neurons terminate in the periaqueductal gray matter. The spinothalamic tract usually carries the information for pain localization.

The Spinoreticular Tract

Type C fibers synapse with interneurons in lamina II and III, which terminate on the second-order neurons in lamina V-VIII. Some of the axons of these second-order neurons ascend on the same side of the spinal cord in the ipsilateral spinoreticular tract, and some cross the midline to travel in the contralateral spinoreticular tract. The spinoreticular tract carries sensory information to the thalamus indirectly via synapses in the reticular formation. Finally it terminates at the cortex. This pathway is involved in the emotional aspects of pain.

PROCESSING OF PAIN IN THE BRAIN

The ventral posterior lateral, the ventral posterior inferior, and the intralaminar thalamic nuclei house the cell bodies of the third-order neurons. The nerve fibers from ventral posterior lateral nuclei ascend in the posterior limb of the internal capsule and in the corona radiata to terminate in the postcentral gyrus (primary somatosensory cortex, S-I) and somatosensory area II of the parietal lobe of the cerebral cortex.

The somatosensory cortex of the brain is the main area for localization of pain. Acute pain can activate other areas like the primary and the secondary somatosensory (S1 and S2), insular, anterior cingulate, and prefrontal cortices, and the thalamus. These areas are all important in pain perception.

WIND-UP PHENOMENON

With repetitive type C fiber stimulation, excitatory postsynaptic potentials are built up in the dorsal horn neurons. The cyclic or repetitive electrical firing of type C, producing a short-term increase in responses of the spinal cord neurons, is called the wind-up phenomenon. The wind-up phenomenon increases pain intensity and duration.

Another theory behind the wind-up phenomenon is the continued presence of substance P in the dorsal horn released from the type C fibers. The peptides are removed slowly and can diffuse slowly. Continued depolarization causes cellular changes like neural sprouting and activation of NMDA receptors. This in turn leads to prolonged Ca++ influx, which can physically and functionally change the neuron.

PAIN MODULATION

There are two circuits mentioned for pain modulation that play a role in reducing the incoming pain. These are gate control theory and the ascending/descending pain transmission system.

Gate Control Theory

This theory suggests that nonnociceptive stimuli can close the gate for nociceptive stimuli that travel toward brain, and thus prevent pain sensation. The inhibitory neurons inhibiting pain transmission are activated by the long cutaneous sensory inputs. This explains why rubbing at the painful site decreases pain, and it is the rationale behind transcutaneous electrical nerve stimulation therapy for pain relief.

Ascending and Descending Pain-Suppression Mechanism

There are opiate receptors present at the presynaptic ends of the neurons carrying pain sensation at the dorsal horn of spinal cord. Stimulation of these receptors causes hyperpolarization of the neuron and ceases the transmission of pain by inhibition of firing and the release of substance P, a neurotransmitter involved in pain transmission. Descending pathways to inhibit pain include a circuit that consists of the periaqueductal gray (PAG) matter in the upper brain stem, the locus coeruleus (LC), the nucleus raphe magnus (NRM), and the nucleus reticularis gigantocellularis (Rgc).

In humans, we have endogenous opiates such as the endorphins and enkephalins, which activate opiate receptors, which suppresses pain pathways.

OPIOID RECEPTORS

All opioid receptors are G-protein-coupled receptors and activate inhibitory G-proteins. Opioid receptors are distributed widely in the brain, and are found in the spinal cord and digestive tract.

The activation of opioid receptors by agonists inhibits adenylyl cyclase, decreasing the concentration of cAMP. This causes the closure of the Ca^{++} channels and an increase in the influx of K^{+} ions in the cell, which leads to hyperpolarization of the membrane, resulting in reduced excitability. There are three originally classified subtypes: Mu (μ), kappa (κ), and delta (δ) opioid receptors.

Mu (μ) receptors are further classified into two types, μ1and μ2, according to their action. Each receptor has a specific action after it is combined with its full agonist and has a specific location in CNS and the periphery (Table 21.1).

Table 21.1 OPIOID RECEPTOR TYPE AND ASSOCIATED ACTION

OPIOID RECEPTOR	EFFECT
Mu 1	Analgesia, euphoria, low abuse potential, miosis
Mu 2	Analgesia (spinal), physical dependence, marked constipation and ventilatory depression
Kappa	Analgesia (supraspinal, spinal), euphoria, low abuse potential, miosis, sedation, dysphoria
Delta	Analgesia (supraspinal and spinal), physical dependence, minimal constipation and ventilatory depression

CENTRAL AND PERIPHERAL TEMPERATURE SYSTEMS

Temperature is normally tightly regulated through a complex control system and involves positive and negative feedback systems. The hypothalamus is the dominant thermoregulatory site. Thermoregulatory information is processed in three phases: afferent thermal sensing, central regulation, and efferent responses.

Afferent input occurs from thermal receptive cells throughout most of the body. A∂ nerve fibers primarily conduct cold signals, whereas warm signals are mainly transmitted by unmyelinated C fibers. This explains the inability to discriminate between sharp pain and intense heat. The principle temperature-sensing elements both in skin and the dorsal root ganglia are the transient receptor potential (TRP) vanilloid (V) and menthol (M) receptors. These receptors change their activity over a 10°C range with a sensitivity up to a thousandth of a degree. The receptors TRPV1–4 are heat activated, and TRPM1 and TRPA8 are cold responsive. The cutaneous information is then transmitted via the anterior spinothalamic tracts of the spinal cord to the hypothalamus.

TEMPERATURE-REGULATING CENTERS

The center of the thermoregulation is the hypothalamus, which integrates thermal sensory information and coordinates various autonomic functions that will allow the body to autoregulate itself to maintain homothermic levels. Thermal information ascends through the spinothalamic tracts but has been demonstrated to ascend through the afferent somatosensory pathway as well. It is postulated that no single spinal tract is responsible for thermal transmission but rather the anterior spinal cord region cohesively conveys various thermal signals. As a result, the entire anterior cord must be ablated to eliminate thermoregulatory responses. Approximately 80% of this thermal input is derived from the core body temperature. The other contributors of thermal input include the spinal cord, deep abdominal and thoracic tissues, and the skin surface.

HEAT PRODUCTION AND CONSERVATION

Any changes in temperature beyond the homeostatic threshold will activate effector mechanism response by increasing metabolic heat production. Efferent responses to thermal changes include sweating, peripheral cutaneous vasoconstriction, and brown fat metabolism. The thermoregulatory system has integrated secondary mechanisms including shivering, blood pressure, and osmotic control to further compensate for thermal variations. Core temperatures that exceed the hyperthermic threshold produce cutaneous vasodilation and sweating. Core temperatures below the threshold will provoke an autonomic effector response of vasoconstriction first followed by nonshivering thermogenesis, and ultimately shivering. These temperature changes trigger effector responses that mediate appropriate increases in environmental heat loss or increases in metabolic heat production. Behavioral changes can also be activated to compensate for situations that the body cannot control. Examples include clothing changes, modifying the environment's temperature, manipulating body positions to supress heat loss, or increasing the body's skin surface apposition, among others.

The sympathetic postganglionic cholinergic (parasympathetic) nerves regulate sweating, the principle mechanism by which the body dissipates heat. Sweating can also occur in response to anxiety, pain, hypercarbia, noxious stimuli in the presence of inadequate anesthesia, or a vagal reaction. Nonshivering thermogenesis increases in intensity linearly to the degree of mean body temperature departure from threshold. Heat production is nearly doubled in infants, however increases only slightly in adults. Skeletal muscle and brown fat tissue are the major site sources of energy in adults. Shivering can increase metabolic heat production 50% to 100% in adults as along it is sustained. The shivering mechanism does not develop until 3–5 years of age. Infants have a greater surface area to body weight ratio, which results in the loss of body heat more readily. Cold stress triggers infants and newborns to increase norepinephrine production, which enhances metabolism of brown fat and produces pulmonary and peripheral vasoconstriction.

MECHANISMS OF HEAT LOSS

A patient exposed to the cold operating room environment is at risk for hypothermia due to anesthetic-induced changes in the body's regulatory heat mechanisms. The various forms of heat loss that occur from patient to environment are categorized as radiation, evaporation, conduction, and convection.

- Radiative heat losses occur any time an object is above absolute zero. It is dependent on cutaneous blood flow and the body's exposed surfaces to the environment. This accounts for up to 60% of heat loss and is the major source of heat loss in most surgical patients.
- Evaporation is the process of a liquid converting into a solid into vapor and is responsible for 20% of heat loss. Energy is needed to vaporize liquid from mucosal and serosal surfaces, skin, and lungs, and heat loss results from the process. Evaporative heat loss is dependent on exposed body surface area and the relative humidity of the environment. Major open wound exposure accounts for significant heat loss. Sweating increases cutaneous evaporative loss significantly, but it is rare during anesthesia. Heat loss through the respiratory system is generally negligible. Infants may lose a higher fraction of their metabolic heat from transpiration of water, as they generally have thinner skin.
- Conductive heat loss is heat transferred from a warm to a cool object. This heat loss accounts for 5% of human heat loss, and the amount of heat transferred depends on the temperature gradient between two objects, the surface area in contact, and the conductive heat transfer coefficient of the materials.
- Convective heat loss occurs with the transfer of heat from a body to moving medium such as air or liquid. The air layer adjacent to the skin is heated by conduction from the body but carries the heat away from the body in the ambient air currents. Convection accounts for approximately 15% of anesthetic heat loss.

SITES FOR BODY TEMPERATURE MEASUREMENT

Body temperature is not uniformly homogeneous. The deep thoracic and abdominal region and the CNS are considered the core, and core temperatures range from 2°C to 4°C warmer than the rest of the body. Core temperature is the best single indicator of thermal status in humans. Core temperature monitoring sites include the tympanic membrane, distal portion of the esophagus, nasopharynx, and the pulmonary artery, which is the gold standard. Monitoring these regions provides timely reactions to core temperature changes and also allows detection of malignant hyperthermia. These regions are composed of highly perfused tissues whose temperature is uniform and high in comparison to the rest of the body. Oral, axillary, rectal, and bladder sites can also be used to measure core body temperatures accurately. Unlike the tightly regulated core temperature, skin temperature varies markedly as a function of environmental exposure and is not considered accurate.

COMPLICATIONS OF HYPOTHERMIA

There are three common complications associated with hypothermia—an increase in morbid myocardial events, an increase in the risk of surgical wound infections and prolonged hospitalizations, and increased blood loss and transfusion requirements.

Hypothermia through increases myocardial oxygen demand through increases in heart rate, blood pressure, oxygen consumption, shunting and cathecholamine release and easily predisposes patients to morbid myocardial events. Hypothermia contributes to wound infections by impairing immune function and through thermoregulatory vasoconstriction, which reduces oxygen delivery to surgical sites. Mild hypothermia interferes with coagulation by impairing the enzymes in the coagulation cascade. Platelet function is also reduced in hypothermia, with local temperatures contributing more so than the core.

In the postoperative period, mild hypothermia can delay the recovery of patients through decreased metabolism of drugs and delay of mentation. Increased oxygen consumption results from shivering and nonshivering thermogenesis. Shivering can cause up to a fivefold increase in oxygen consumption. Postanesthetic shivering is a thermoregulatory response to intraoperative hypothermia, which is always preceded by core hypothermia and arteriovenous shunt vasoconstriction. There are also harmful effects that result from the physiology of rewarming. Vasoconstriction can exacerbate hypertension. This worsens the effects of pulmonary shunt on arterial oxygen content and also increases in cardiac output demand, which could be detrimental to some patients.

FURTHER READING

Barash P, Cullen B, Stoelting R, Cahalan M, Stock M. *Clinical Anesthesia*. 6th ed. Philadelphia, PA: Lippincott Williams & Wilkins; 2009.

Greenberg S, Murphy G, Vender J. Standard monitoring techniques. In: Barash P, Cullen B, Stoelting R, Cahalan M, Stock M, eds. *Clinical Anesthesia*. 6th ed. Philadelphia, PA: Lippincott Williams & Wilkins; 2009.

Johnson J, Grecu L, Lawson N. Autonomic nervous system. In: Barash P, Cullen B, Stoelting R, Cahalan M, Stock M, eds. *Clinical Anesthesia*. 6th ed. Philadelphia, PA: Lippincott Williams & Wilkins; 2009.

Kampine J, Stowe D, Pagel P. Cardiovascular anatomy and physiology. In: Barash P, Cullen B, Stoelting R, Cahalan M, Stock M, eds. *Clinical Anesthesia*. 6th ed. Philadelphia, PA: Lippincott Williams & Wilkins; 2009.

QUESTIONS

1. Which anticholinergic drug has least central nervous effect?
   A. Atropine
   B. Scopolamine
   C. Glycopyrolate
   D. Ipratropium bromide

2. Acetylycholine is released into the synaptic cleft by nerve terminal due to influx of:
   A. Na^+
   B. Ca^{2+}
   C. K^+
   D. Mg^{2+}

3. Botulinum toxin decreases ACh at the synaptic cleft by:
   A. synaptosome-associated proteins (SNAPs) and vesicle-associated membrane proteins (VAMPs) assisted fusion of vesicles to the surface membrane with ACh release
   B. Na+–dependent CHT blockade
   C. VAT-assisted transport of ACh into vesicles blockade
   D. Voltage-sensitive Ca2+ channels blockade

4. The norepineprine binding at beta adrenoceptors results in:
   A. Activation of Gs-coupling protein to activate adenylyl cyclase and increase cAMP.
   B. Activation of Gq-coupling protein, which leads to formation of IP3 and DAG
   C. Dissociation of the inhibitory G protein Gi to inhibit adenylyl cyclase and decrease cyclic adenosine monophosphate
   D. No effect

5. A 54-year-old male presented to the ER with his right eye closed. The past medical history includes a lung resection for cancer. Examination is significant for right pupil constriction. What is the mechanism of these symptoms?
   A. Interruption of parasympathetic innervation of face
   B. Interruption of preganglionic sympathetic innervation of face
   C. Interruption of postganglionic sympathetic innervation of face
   D. Direct trauma of the right eye

6. What drug is used to distinguish pre- versus postganglionic Horner syndrome?
   A. Phenylephrine
   B. Atropine
   C. Lidocaine
   D. Hydroxyamphetamine

ANSWERS

1. C. Acetylcholine is released by preganglionic neurons, parasympathetic postganglionic neurons, and some postganglionic sympathetic neurons. These neurons are called cholinergic neurons, and their receptors are cholinergic receptors. There are two types of cholinergic receptors, nicotinic and muscarinic. The muscarinic receptors are in the sinoatrial node (SA node) and smooth muscles and are blocked by atropine and atropine-like drugs (glycopyrolate, ipratropium, and scopolamine) possessing an ester linkage. In anesthesia, the clinical effects of these drugs are relevant due to their respiratory, cardiovascular, CNS, and gastrointestinal actions, shown in Table 21.2. Atropine and scopolamine are tertiary amines and readily cross the blood-brain barrier and produce CNS effects. Glycopyrolate is a quaternary amine and does not cross the blood-brain barrier, and so is devoid of CNS effects. Ipratropium is used only in inhaled form with beta agonists and does not have CNS effects.

Table 21.2 CLINICAL EFFECTS OF ATROPINE AND ATROPINE-LIKE DRUGS

	ATROPINE	GLYCOPYROLATE	IPRATROPIUM	SCOPOLAMINE
Tachycardia	marked	moderate	none	minimal
Bronchodilation	moderate	moderate	moderate	minimal
Sedation	minimal	none	none	marked
Secretions (both GI and respiratory)	moderate	marked	none	marked

2. B. Acetylcholine (ACh) is synthesized in the nerve terminal from choline and acetyl CoA by the enzyme choline acetyltransferase (ChAT); the choline used is transported from the extracellular space into the nerve terminal through a Na^+–dependent choline transporter (CHT). Once synthesized, ACh is stored in clear synaptic vesicles with peptides and adenosine triphosphate (ATP), and transport from the cytoplasm to vesicles is assisted by vesicle-associated transporter (VAT) in cholinergic neuron terminals. The ACh is released into the synaptic cleft due to the influx of Ca^{2+} caused by the opening of voltage-gated calcium channels; this causes fusion of vesicles to surface membranes, and ACh is expelled. Different chemicals/drugs can interfere with ACh synthesis and release.
3. A. Different chemicals/drugs can interfere with ACh synthesis and release:
   - Hexamethonium—can block Na+-dependent CHT and prevent
   - Vesamicol—can block VAT-assisted transport of ACh into vesicles.
   - Botulinum toxin—can block synaptosome-associated proteins (SNAPs)- and vesicle-associated membrane proteins (VAMPs)-assisted fusion of vesicles to the surface membrane and ACh release.

Once released, ACh is rapidly hydrolyzed to acetate and choline by the enzyme acetylcholinesterase. Drugs like neostigmine, physostigimine and edrophonium bind with acetylcholinestrase and increase ACh concentrations at the synaptic cleft.

4. Norepinephrine is the principal neurotransmitter for the sympathetic nervous system at the postganglionic level and at the effector organs with few exceptions (sweat glands and skeletal muscle blood vessels) and its receptors are called noradrenergic. The adrenal medulla is a sympathetic ganglion that releases norepinephrine and epinephrine into the blood stream. The adrenoceptors (i.e., adrenergic receptors) are alpha 1, alpha 2, beta 1, beta 2, and beta 3. The alpha 1 and beta 1 receptors are stimulatory in nature in general, and the alpha 2 and beta 2 receptors are inhibitory in nature. Adrenoceptors are G-protein-coupled receptors (GPCR). An agonist binding at these receptors depends on receptor subtype.
   - Agonist binding to alpha 1-adrenoceptors activates Gq-coupling protein, which leads to formation of IP3 and DAG and an increase in intracellular Ca2+.
   - Agonist binding to alpha 2-adrenoceptors causes dissociation of the inhibitory G-protein Gi to inhibit adenylyl cyclase and decrease cyclic adenosine monophosphate.
   - Agonist binding to beta adrenoceptors activates the Gs-coupling protein to activate adenylyl cyclase and increase cAMP.
5. C. Anhidrosis (decreased sweating), ptosis (drooping eyelid), and miosis (pupil constriction) are classic presentation of Horner syndrome. It results from sympathetic innervations of face (preganglionic or postganglionic) interruption. It can be due to injury to nerves, injury to carotid artery, brain stem stroke, or lung tumor causing injury to the sympathetic chain. Horner syndrome is usually unilateral. The nature of the lesion, preganglionic (e.g. brain stem stroke) versus postganglionic (injury to sympathetic fibers supplying face) can be determined. If the postganglionic sympathetic fibers are damaged, the nerve terminals are degenerated and will result in loss of stored catecholamine. On the other hand, if preganglionic fibers are damaged, the postganglionic noradrenergic nerve fibers will be intact and catecholamine stores at the nerve ending will be present.
6. D. Administration of a drug that can cause catecholamine store release, for example, hydroxyamphetamine, to the affected eye will show no response in case of a postganglionic lesion, but will dilate the constricted pupil in case of a preganglionic lesion. Phenylephrine, an alpha adrenoceptor agonist will dilate the pupil regardless of the lesion site, as it binds directly to alpha 1 receptors on the iris radial muscle.

22.

FUNCTIONAL NEUROANATOMY

Bilal Rana, Varsha D. Allampalli, and George W. Williams

INTRODUCTION

The nervous system is anatomically and functionally divided into the central nervous system and the peripheral nervous system. The central nervous system consists of the brain, cranial nerves, and spinal cord. The peripheral nervous system acts as a bridge between the rest of the body and the central nervous system. It consists of spinal nerves and the autonomic nervous system, which is further divided into the sympathetic and parasympathetic nervous systems. The peripheral nervous system has a vital role in controlling breathing, heart rate, digestion, and secretion of hormones.

The brain controls the vital functions of many organs in the body and receives and interprets information coming from the peripheral nervous system and all the sensory organs. It assembles all the information and sends orders to other organs to respond accordingly. It also stores information in the form of memory. The brain is composed of the cerebrum, cerebellum, and brain stem. The cranium and skull bones, along with its coverings, envelop the brain in a fixed space (a box). The brain contains *potential* spaces within it called ventricles and cisterns, all of which are filled with cerebrospinal fluid (CSF). Much as a sandwich bag can be overfilled or minimally filled depending on the pressure gradient being used to fill it, the ventricles and cisterns indirectly reflect the pressure in the skull.

There are three fluid-filled layers of covering lying between brain and cranium that aid in protecting the brain and spinal cord from injury. From outside in these are the dura mater, arachnoid mater, and pia mater. The dura mater is the outermost layer, which originates from the foramen magnum and terminates between S1 and S4. There is a potential space surrounding the dura mater called the epidural space, in which epidural anesthesia is given. Closely adherent to dura from within is the arachnoid membrane. It is very delicate but prevents drug permeability from the epidural to the subarachnoid space. The innermost layer is the pia mater, which is adherently attached to the brain and spinal cord. It is an extremely vascular layer and extends below the conus medularis of the spinal cord to form the filum terminale. The Filum terminale is covered with the dural sac, which continues to attach to the posterior wall of coccyx.

THE VENTRICULAR SYSTEM

The ventricular system consists of two lateral ventricles, the third ventricle, the cerebral aqueduct, the fourth ventricle, and the spinal canal. The ventricles contain CSF, which acts as a buffer for the central nervous system. The ventricular system is interconnected; any blockade in the outflow of CSF causes increase in back pressure and increased intracranial pressure (ICP), leading to hydrocephalus. There are two lateral ventricles located in the cerebral hemispheres. Each lateral ventricle has a body and three horns—the anterior, posterior, and inferior horns. The anterior or frontal horns of the lateral ventricles continue inferiorly to form the third ventricle. The third ventricle is situated in the midline between two diencephalons (thalamus and hypothalamus). It inferiorly continues as the aqueduct of sylvius or the cerebral aqueduct. The optic recess, hypophyseal recess, and pineal recess are all anatomically related to the third ventricle and are important radiological landmarks. Next, the cerebral aqueduct of sylvius is the canal that connects third and the fourth ventricles. It is situated in center of the mid brain. Finally, the fourth ventricle is located in the pons and to some degree in the medulla. It is connected to the subarachnoid space laterally via the foramen of Luschka (*L* for *l*ateral), medially via the foramen of Magendie (*M* for *m*edial or *m*iddle), and inferiorly continues as the central canal of the spinal cord. The anatomy described with regard to the ventricular system is reflected in the "Mickey Mouse" diagram (Figure 22.1).

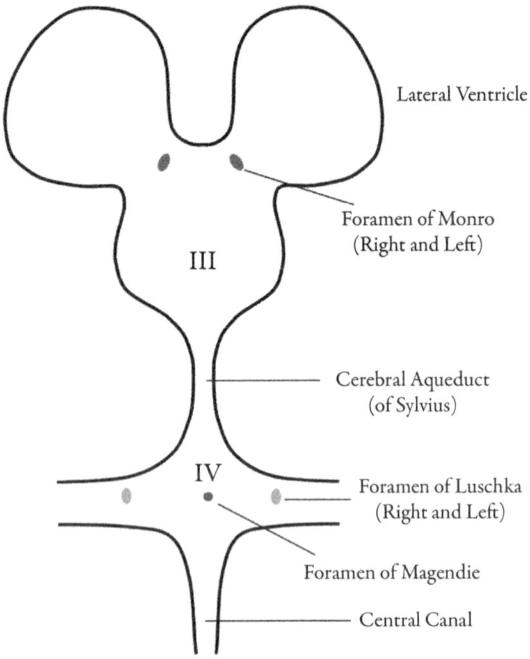

Figure 22.1 The ventricular system could be imagined (in coronal section, not to scale) as the face of Mickey Mouse with two lateral ventricles as two big ears, a pair of foramina of Monro as a set of eyes, the third ventricle as the mouth, the fourth ventricle as the body, and the cerebral aqueduct as the neck.

CEREBROSPINAL FLUID

Cerebrospinal fluid is excreted by the choroid plexus, which lines the lateral ventricles, third ventricle, and fourth ventricle. It flows through the interconnected ventricular system and drains in the dural venous sinuses via the arachnoid villi. The CSF is clear and basic fluid; its composition is similar to plasma fluid with some characteristic differences. See Table 22.1.

Flow of Cerebrospinal fluid

The CSF flows from the lateral ventricles into the third ventricle through the foramen of Monro. From the third ventricle it enters into fourth ventricle via the cerebral aqueduct. In the fourth ventricle it continues with subarachnoid space through two lateral foramens of Luschka and a medial foramen of Magendie. Inferiorly, it continues to flow in the narrow central spinal canal in the spinal cord. In the subarachnoid space, the excess fluid gets reabsorbed into venous sinuses through arachnoid villi or granulations.

Table 22.1 COMPONENTS OF PLASMA AND CSF

	PLASMA	CSF
Na+ (mmol/dL)	138	138
HCO3- (mmol/dL)	23	23
CA2+ (mg/dL)	10	11
K+ (mmol/dL)	4.5	2.8
Glucose (mg/dL)	100	70
Protein (mg/dL)	7000	35
pH	7.41	7.33

The average total volume of CSF is 100–150 mL. it is formed at the rate of 20 mL/h or 500 mL/day.

THE CEREBRUM

The cerebrum is the largest and developmentally most advanced part of brain, where higher functions like touch, smell, vision, and hearing are interpreted. It also controls higher intellectual functions like speech, emotions, ability to learn, and fine motor movement.

The cerebrum is divided into two cerebral hemispheres (right and left) by the great longitudinal fissure. The right and left cerebral hemispheres are further divided into different anatomical area called gyri (bulges) by deep sulci (depressions). (See Figure 22.2). The two hemispheres are *connected* by the corpus callosum at the bottom, which sends information from the right to the left hemisphere and vice versa. The cerebral cortex is composed of pairs of frontal, parietal, temporal, and occipital lobes. Various lobes are differentiated anatomically by the different fissures (see Figure 22.2 and Figure 22.3). Each lobe is further divided into different areas according to the specific functions it performs. The lobes of the brain function through a complex relationship with each other; additionally, the right side of the body (all the way up the face) is controlled by left hemisphere, and the left side is controlled by right hemisphere. More advanced and higher intellectual functions like spoken and written language are controlled by one of the two hemispheres, which is considered as a dominant one.

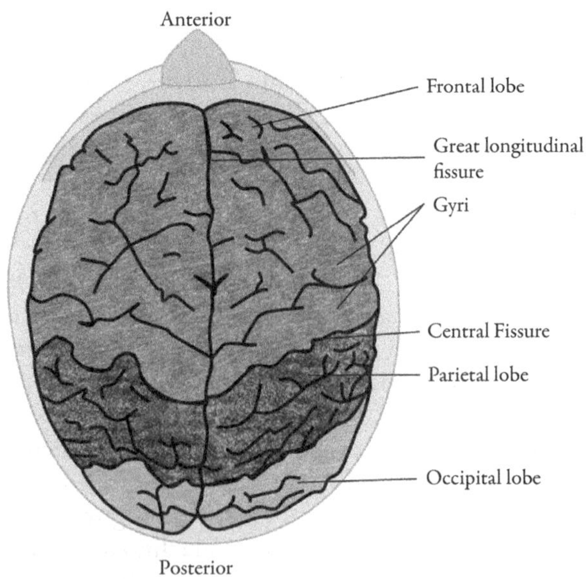

Figure 22.2 Superior view of the brain.

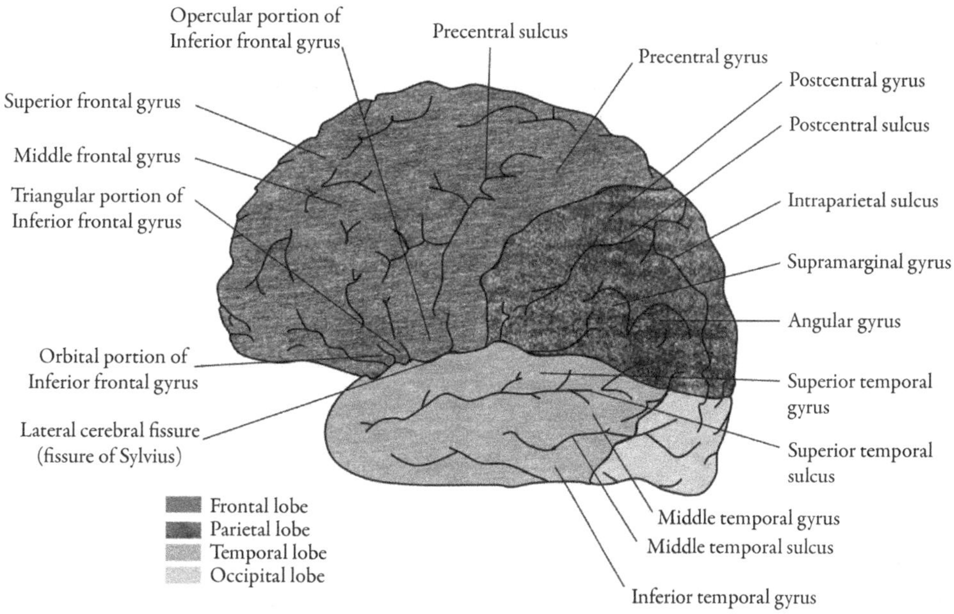

Figure 22.3 Cerebral cortex with major gyri and sulci labeled.

THE CEREBELLUM

The cerebellum is a part of brain residing in the posterior cranial fossa behind the mid brain stem and inferior to the cerebrum (see Figure 22.2). The cerebellum consists of two hemispheres joined together with a midline portion called the vermis. The cerebellum is connected to other important parts of brain with large bundles of nerve fibers called peduncles. The superior peduncle attaches the cerebellum to the mid brain, the middle peduncle attaches the cerebellum to the pons, and the inferior peduncle attaches the cerebellum to the medulla. The cerebellum fine-tunes motor activity or movement (e.g., playing piano, painting). It also helps to maintain posture, balance, and equilibrium by controlling the tone of the muscles. Additionally, the cerebellum helps in coordination of movements and ability to perform rapid and repetitive actions. In the cerebellum, left-sided lesions produce deficits on the same side of the body.

BRAIN STEM

The brain stem is the lower extension of the brain that lies in front of cerebellum and is the connection between the brain and the spinal cord (see Figure 22.4) It comprises three structures: the medulla oblongata, the pons, and the mid brain. The main function of the brain stem is to serve as a relay station and pass messages to and fro between the cerebral cortex and the body. The medulla oblongata is the conical shaped part of the brain stem that connects to the pons superiorly and the spinal cord inferiorly (see Figure 22.2). The medulla has many critical centers that control breathing, blood pressure, heart rate, and swallowing (so if a neurosurgical approach encroaches on this region, the extubation and/or feeding plan may be affected). The pons is the bridge between the medulla and the mid brain (see Figure 22.4). It contains large nerve fibers, many nuclei, and ascending and descending fibers. It coordinates for eye and facial movements, facial sensation, hearing, and balance. The mid brain is an important part of the brain stem, containing the center for ocular motion. It is connected to the cerebellum through the superior peduncles. The brain stem and part of the thalamus contain the reticular activating system, which controls level of wakefulness and sleep patterns. It also makes us aware and attentive to the surrounding environment.

RESPIRATORY CENTERS

There are two respiratory centers: medullary and pontine.

Medullary Respiratory Center

In the medullary respiratory center there are two key components. First, the ventral respiratory group (VRG)

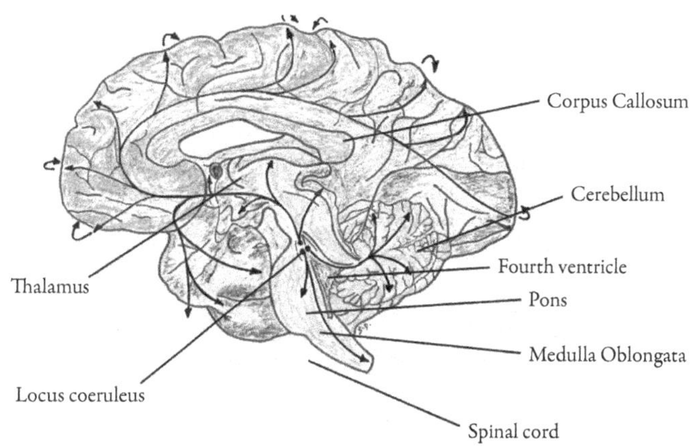

Figure 22.4 Anatomy and general neurologic pathways emphasizing the importance of the brain stem.

regulates and stimulates the rhythmic spontaneous ventilation such as resting and tidal breathing. It contains both inspiratory and expiratory neurons. Second, the dorsal respiratory group (DRG) responds to extraordinary situations to alter the ventilatory pattern in response to different physiological needs of the body for oxygen, carbon dioxide, and acid-base balance. The neurons from the DRG stimulate neurons in the VRG that are responsive to sensory information from chemo- and mechanoreceptors. In short, medullary centers send impulses that rhythmically stimulate contraction of the diaphragm.

Pontine Respiratory Center

The pontine respiratory center is made up of a group of neurons located within the reticular activating system in the pons. It receives signals from higher brain centers and peripheral receptors. These neurons send inhibitory signals to the medullary respiratory center to limit inspiratory duration. Thus, it reduces the duration of respiratory cycle, in turn increasing respiratory frequency. The reticular activating system is a group of interconnected nuclei and nerve fibers that extends from the mid brain to the medulla oblongata. The nuclei in the reticular formation are arranged as follows:

> Parvocellular region: These include smaller sized nuclei in the lateral part of the reticular formation whose function is to receive afferent fibers from the brain stem and other distant regions.
>
> Magnocellular region: This contains different groups of large-sized cells in the medial two-thirds of the reticular formation. The cells in this region give rise to efferent projection of the reticular formation.
>
> Raphe nucleus: This is a group of cells that lie along or adjacent to the midline of the upper medulla, pons, and mid brain. These cells produce serotonin, which is distributed to wide regions of the brain and spinal cord.

Additionally, there are two components of the reticular formation:

> Ascending reticular system: The neurons in this system project to the midline group of the thalamus, which is related to wakefulness. From here, the information is sent to the cerebral cortex. Thus this system is important for human alertness and the sleep-wake cycle.
>
> Descending reticular system: This system receives information from the hypothalamus. This system helps us to stand erect. Thus it helps maintain equilibrium and posture, as well as autonomic nervous system activity and motor movements. Some of the nuclei in this system are involved in reflex activity like coughing, chewing, swallowing, and vomiting. Some of the interneurons in the reticular activating system interact with the cranial nerves responsible for eye movement.

CARDIOVASCULAR CENTER

Cardiovascular equilibrium is maintained due to interaction between peripheral centers (carotid and aortic body) and central medullary cardiovascular centers. The carotid body is located just distal to the bifurcation of the common carotid artery, and the aortic body is present near the origin of the subclavian artery. These are innervated by cranial nerves IX (carotid body) and X (aortic body) respectively. Increases in blood pressure above threshold levels stimulate these peripheral centers, which in turn stimulate medullary centers to depress their activity. This helps to maintain normal cardiovascular equilibrium by reducing blood pressure and heart rate via cranial nerves IX and X.

Two centers that affect cardiovascular function are located in the upper and lower medulla. Stimulation of upper medullary center (called the "presser center") causes an increase in blood pressure and heart rate. In contrast, stimulation of the lower medullary center (called the "depressor center") reduces blood pressure and heart rate.

VOMITING CENTER

The floor of the fourth ventricle above medulla hosts the vomiting center, called the chemoreceptor trigger zone (CTZ) or area postrema. The CTZ is not protected by the blood-brain barrier; therefore, any medication or substance in the blood capable of producing vomiting can directly reach the CTZ and can cause vomiting. The mechanism of vomiting is well illustrated in Figure 22.5.

COUGHING CENTER

The tracheal and laryngeal lining is innervated by free nerve endings associated with the internal laryngeal branch of cranial nerve X (vagus). Irritation or stimulation of the tracheal and laryngeal lining stimulates these free nerve endings. These nerve impulses are carried up by the solitary tract and the same pathway is followed as in the mechanism of vomiting (discussed in the section "Vomiting Center").

BASAL GANGLIA

The basal ganglia are a set of deep-seated nuclei in the brain and are composed of six nuclei. These are distributed in the different parts of the brain like the forebrain, mid brain, and cerebellum. The caudate nucleus, putamen, and nucleus accumbens (together called the ventral striatum) and the globus pallidus are present in the forebrain. They are collectively called the corpus striatum. The putamen and the

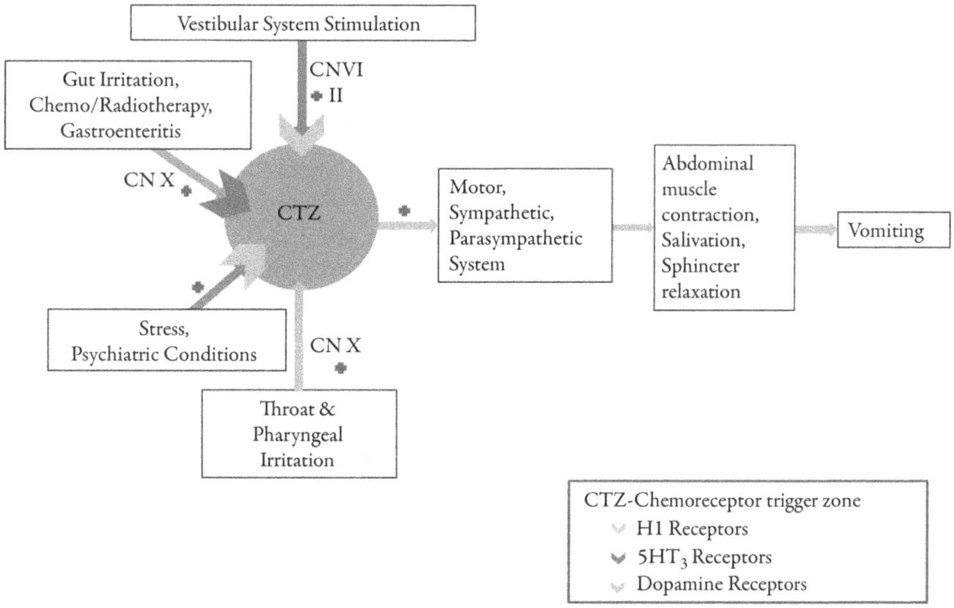

Figure 22.5 The mechanism of vomiting.

globus pallidus together are called the lentiform nucleus or lenticular nucleus. The other two nuclei are the subthalamic nucleus and the substantia nigra. As the name suggests, the subthalamic nucleus is located just below the thalamus. The substantia nigra is a midbrain structure composed of two distinct parts: the pars compacta and the pars reticulata. The substantia nigra is located between the red nucleus and the crus cerebri (cerebral peduncle) on the ventral part of the mid brain. There are many excitatory and inhibitory connections from various parts of brain and other and parts of the basal ganglia that project on the striatum. The striatum in turn has outputs to the globus pallidus, the subthalamic nucleus, and back to the motor cortex 6, 4, 8. In general, injury to the basal ganglia results in a more somnolent neurological examination.

CEREBRAL CIRCULATION

The brain is one of the most highly perfused organs of the body. It receives about 18% of the total blood volume. This is accomplished through two large arterial systems: the left and right internal carotid arteries (ICA) and the left and right vertebral arteries. The two arteries communicate with each other via the "Circle of Willis." These two arterial systems form a part of the anterior and posterior circulation of the brain, respectively (see Figure 22.6).

Anterior Circulation

The anterior circulation is formed by the left and right internal carotid arteries and their branches. It supplies the lateral surfaces and anterior two-thirds of medial surfaces of the cerebral cortices including the corpus callosum, basal ganglia, and anterior diencephalon (recall, this means the thalamus and hypothalamus).

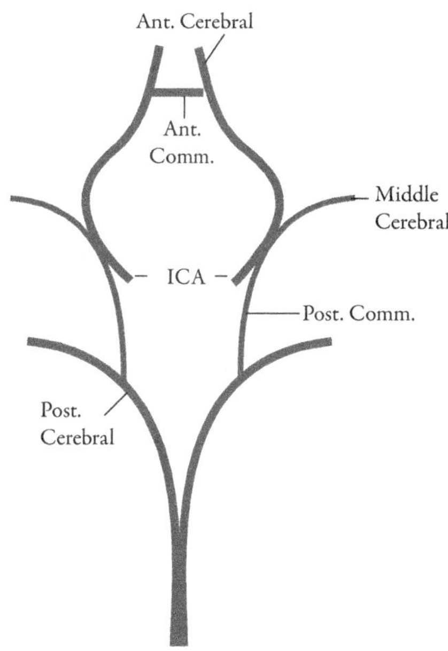

Figure 22.6 The Circle of Willis.

1. Internal carotid artery (ICA): Common carotid arteries *bifurcate at the level of thyroid cartilage* into the external carotid artery and ICA. The ICA supplies about 75% of the total blood supply to the brain.
2. Anterior cerebral artery (ACA): The ACA is one of the terminal branches of the ICA and supplies the medial surface of the hemisphere including the corpus callosum, and frontal, parietal, and cingulate cortices. The right and left anterior cerebral arteries are connected through the anterior communicating artery, which forms the anterior part of the Circle

of Willis. This is a common location for aneurysms to occur.

3. Middle cerebral artery (MCA): The MCA is the largest terminal branch of the ICA and runs medial to lateral. It mainly supplies much of the lateral surface of the brain. An infarction in this territory is so large a hemicraniectomy is frequently required. There are several branches that normally refer to the point of bifurcation, for example, M1 occlusion is before the first bifurcation (meaning a larger territory), and so on.
4. Anterior choroidal artery: This forms a part of the anterior circulation that supplies the base of the brain. During its course it also supplies the optic tract, cerebral peduncle, lateral geniculate, posterior limb of the internal capsule, tail of the caudate, and choroidal plexus of the lateral ventricle.
5. Ophthalmic artery: This branches from the ICA when ICA emerges from the cavernous sinus. It is divided into two more branches: orbital and ocular divisions.
6. Anterior communicating artery: As discussed earlier, two anterior cerebral arteries intercommunicate via the anterior communicating artery under the optic chiasm.

Posterior Circulation

The posterior circulation is formed by the vertebral and basilar arteries and their branches, which include the posterior cerebral arteries and the posterior communicating arteries. It supplies 25% of the total blood supply received by the brain. It forms the posterior part of the arterial Circle of Willis along with the anterior circulation. It supplies blood to the upper cervical spinal cord, cerebellum, brain stem, most of the diencephalon, and inferior and posterior surfaces of the temporal and occipital lobes of the cerebral hemispheres.

1. Vertebral artery: Right vertebral artery is the branch of the left subclavian artery, which in turn is the branch of the brachiocephalic artery from the arch of the aorta. The left subclavian artery directly gives rise to the left vertebral artery.
2. Basilar artery: Two vertebral arteries join to form the basilar artery at the caudal part of the pons. It supplies blood to the pons, the mid brain, and the anterior surface of the cerebellum. At the upper border of the pons, it bifurcates to give the right and left posterior cerebral arteries. An infarction here can result in "locked in" syndrome.
3. Posterior cerebral artery (PCA): The PCA gives posterior communicating arteries to complete the posterior circulation in the Circle of Willis. The PCA provides blood to many vital parts of brain, like the rostral midbrain, posterior thalamus, occipital visual cortex, and others.
4. Posterior communicating artery: The right and left posterior communicating arteries join the PCA with the internal carotid arteries or the middle cerebral arteries to complete the Circle of Willis posteriorly.

VENOUS DRAINAGE

The cerebral veins are thin, valveless vessels devoid of a muscular layer (compared with the intima, media, and adventitia, or the arterial side). There are found on the surface of the brain as well as deep in the brain substance. They drain blood into larger channels called the cranial venous sinuses. The major cerebral veins include:

Superficial cerebral vein: It drains the superficial surface of the cerebral cortex and empties it into the superior sagittal sinus.

Middle cerebral veins: These veins drain the major part of the lateral and inferior surfaces, where they empty into the cavernous sinus.

Inferior cerebral veins: Drain the lateral occipital gyrus and open directly into the transverse sinus.

Basal vein (of Rosenthal): Drains the base of the brain and empties into the cerebral vein.

Internal cerebral vein (of Galen): Deeper parts of the cerebral hemisphere are drained by these veins. These veins unite to form a single great cerebral vein and finally open into the straight sinus.

The venous sinuses are larger vessels present in the dura that carry blood from the brain finally into the internal jugular vein and subclavian vein. There are paired and unpaired venous sinuses (see Table 22.2).

Table 22.2 VENOUS SINUSES

PAIRED LATERAL VENOUS SINUSES	UNPAIRED MIDLINE VENOUS SINUSES
– Transverse	– Straight sinus
– Sigmoid	– Confluence of sinuses
– Cavernous	– Confluence of sinuses
– Intercavernous	– Occipital
– Superior petrosal	– Basilar plexus
– Inferior petrosal	

THE VERTEBRAL COLUMN

The vertebral column is made up of 7 cervical, 12 thoracic, and 5 lumbar vertebrae; the sacrum (5 fused sacral vertebrae), and the coccyx (4 fused coccygeal vertebrae). It has for anteroposterior curvatures: cervical and lumbar both convex anteriorly and thoracic and sacral concave anteriorly, which is also called primary curvature, as it exists from embryonic development. Cervical and lumbar curvatures are the *secondary* curves, which appear later in fetal life and are exaggerated in infancy.

The vertebral column is made up of 33 total vertebrae. Each vertebra has: (1) the vertebral body; (2) the vertebral arch with its spinous, articular, and transverse processes; and (3) the vertebral foramen between the body and arch, which contains the spinal cord. The body of each vertebra is separated with a vertebral disc. There are other important structures in the vertebra: vertebral pedicles attach the arch to the body on both sides. The right and left laminae are the parts of arch that join posteriorly to form the spinous processes. The transverse process emerges at the junction of the lamina and pedicle. The notches formed between the laminae of adjacent vertebrae are called intervertebral foramen. The spinal ganglia and the ventral root of the spinal nerves come out of this foramen (ripe for impingement or pain syndromes). Articular processes have facets to attach adjacent vertebrae.

VARIATIONS IN VERTEBRAL CONFIGURATION

Vertebrae have regional variations and special characteristics according to adjacent structures and attachments.

Cervical vertebrae: Each of these seven cervical vertebrae in the neck has a foramen transversarium, which is an opening in the transverse process. These foramina serve as a conduit for the vertebral artery, starting at C6 and continuing to C1, where they form the basilar artery. *Atlas*, the first cervical vertebra, is a ring-shaped vertebra without body and spinous process. It has two lateral masses with superior and inferior facets to attach to the occipital condyle and the second cervical vertebra, *axis*. Axis has an odontoid process, which fits into atlas and acts as a pivot for atlas (which, when broken, necessitates halo placement or fusion).

Thoracic vertebrae: A typical thoracic vertebra (T2-T8) has a kidney shaped body, demifacets at the junction of body, and pedicles for attachment of ribs. There are costal facets on the transverse vertebrae T1-T10 for the tubercles of the ribs. T1, T11, and T12 are transitional vertebrae that have structural similarity with the preceding and succeeding vertebra respectively. The spinous processes are long, slender, and slanting with tips lying opposite to the body of subjacent vertebra. The articular facet surface is within the coronal plane.

Lumbar vertebrae: There are five lumbar vertebrae in between thoracic vertebrae and the sacrum, the fifth being the largest. They have a kidney-shaped body and quadrangular, thick, and straight spinous processes. The fifth vertebra forms the lumbosacral angle with the sacrum. The lumbar facet surface is in the sagittal plane.

Sacral vertebrae: These are five fused vertebrae in the lower back. The sacrum has articular facets superiorly for the fifth lumbar vertebra, laterally for the hipbones, and inferiorly for the coccyx. The sacrum has a modified fused spinous process called the median crest. It has paired sacral foramina for the ventral and dorsal primary rami of spinal nerves on its ventral and dorsal surfaces respectively. There is a sacral hiatus formed between two sacral cornua at the lowest part of the sacrum. It is an anatomical landmark for caudal anesthesia, which blocks sacral spinal nerves extradurally.

Coccygeal segment: Four to five vertebrae that are fused in the coccyx.

SPINAL CORD

The spinal cord is 40–50 cm long and 1–1.5 cm thick. The spinal cord is housed in the vertebral canal made up of vertebral foramina when all the vertebrae are in anatomical position. The spinal cord is divided into 32 segments: 8 cervical, 12 thoracic, 5 lumbar, 5 sacral, and several coccygeal spinal cord segments. It extends superiorly from the medulla oblongata at the upper border of the C1 and terminates in a conical lower part called the conus medularis at the level of the junction of the first and second lumbar vertebrae. The level of termination varies in the pediatric and adult patient and also with the extension/flexion of the spine. The spinal cord in its transverse section shows central butterfly-shaped gray matter with peripheral white matter. Gray matter on each side is joined by the central gray commissure, which is traversed by a central canal. The gray matter is divided into horns (anterior or ventral, intermediate or lateral, posterior or dorsal) on each half of the spinal cord.

The dorsal horn is composed of sensory neurons receiving and processing sensory information. It sends all the processed information to the mid brain and diencephalon. The intermediate or lateral horn of gray matter consists of autonomic neurons that innervate the visceral and pelvic organs. The ventral horn is made up of motor neurons that innervate skeletal muscles. The white matter is divided into right and left parts by the anterior deep median fissure and the posterior median groove. Each half of the white matter is composed of myelinated and unmyelinated nerve fibers and further divided into three anatomical columns or funiculi: (1) dorsal (posterior), (2) ventral (anterior), and (3) lateral. These columns are organized with the ascending system

Table 22.3 ASCENDING TRACTS

TRACTS	COLUMNS	FUNCTION
Gracile and cuneate fasciculi	Dorsal/posterior column	Tactile sensation, two-point discrimination, vibration, pressure, position, proprioception, and movement sensation.
Lateral spinothalamic tract	Lateral column	Pain, temperature, and crude touch from somatic and visceral structures.
Dorsal and ventral spinocerebellar tracts	Lateral column	Unconscious proprioception from muscles and joints of lower extremities to cerebellum.
Anterior spinothalamic tract	Ventral/anterior column	Pain, temperature, and touch.
Spino-olivary tract	Ventral/anterior column	Carries information from golgi tendon organs to cerebellum.
Spinoreticular	Lateral column	Afferent information to reticular formation and influence level of consciousness

Table 22.4 DESCENDING TRACTS

TRACTS	COLUMNS	FUNCTION
Lateral corticospinal tract and Rubrospinal tract	Lateral column	Associated with voluntary movement
Reticulospinal Vestibulospinal Anterior corticospinal	Ventral column	Mediate balance and postural movements

peripherally and the descending system centrally near the gray matter. The ascending system has important tracts that transmit sensory information from various parts of the body to higher levels of the CNS. See Table 22.3 for details.

The tracts in the descending system originate from different cortical areas and brain stem nuclei. Motor activity–related information is carried through descending pathways. See Table 22.4 for more detail.

Spinal Nerves

There are 31 pairs of spinal nerves emerging from the intervertebral foramina. Dorsal and ventral roots unite to form mixed spinal nerves. Anterior or ventral is the efferent motor root spinal nerve; the posterior or dorsal root carries afferent sensory fibers. Each spinal nerve is named according to the spinal segment it emerges from and numbered according to the number of vertebra above which it exits from the spinal cord in the cervical region and below in the thoracic region (hence the C8 root without the C8 vertebral body).

Spinal nerves have the following branches:

Posterior ramus: innervates the posterior portion of the trunk. It carries visceral motor, somatic motor, and somatic sensory fibers from and to the skin and muscles of the back.

Anterior ramus: serves the anterior part of the trunk and the upper and lower extremities.

Rami communicantes: consists of autonomic nerves that carry visceral motor and sensory information to and from the visceral organs.

Each spinal nerve innervates a specific region of the skin called the dermatome and a specific muscular fiber called the myotome. Knowledge of the segmental innervation of the cutaneous area and the muscles is essential to diagnose the level of a spinal injury.

Blood Supply

Each vertebral artery gives two branches: the anterior spinal artery and the posterior spinal artery. Both the anterior spinal artery joins to form a single artery in the anterior median fissure of the spinal cord. The posterior spinal artery supplies the posterior one-third and the anterior spinal artery supplies the anterior two-thirds of the spinal cord. The anterior and posterior spinal arteries narrow and form an anastomotic network with radicular arteries coming from cervical, trunk, intercostal, and iliac arteries. They supply most of the lower levels of the spinal cord below the cervical region. The largest of the anterior radicular arteries is known as the artery of Adamkiewicz, or the anterior radicularis magna (ARM) artery, which is a direct branch from the aorta and usually arises between L1 and L2.

Thus there are three main arteries supplying blood to spinal cord: one anterior and two posterior spinal arteries along with anastomotic branches of various radicular arteries.

Sacral Nerves

The sacral plexus is formed by the union of the anterior rami of spinal nerves S1-S4. These nerve fibers are then joined by spinal nerve roots of L4 and L5, forming the lumbosacral trunk. The lumbosacral trunk descends down to supply the pelvic and perineal muscles and organs.

Branches

There are five major peripheral nerves of the sacral plexus. The anterior rami of spinal nerves S1-S4 (lumbosacral trunk) divides into several chords which combines together to form these five major branches of sacral plexus.

1. Sciatic Nerve (L4, L5, S1, S2, S3): It is one of the largest branches of the sacral plexus. It is divided into tibial and common peroneal (fibular) nerves.
   a) Tibial portion: innervates all the muscles in the posterior compartment of the thigh, muscles in the posterior compartment of the leg, and muscles in the sole of foot. It also gives sensory supply to the skin on the posterolateral and medial surfaces of the foot as well as the sole of the foot.
   b) Common peroneal (fibular) branch: innervates the short head of the biceps femoris, all muscles in the anterior and lateral compartments of the leg, and the extensor digitorum brevis. Its sensory supply goes to the skin on the anterolateral surface of the leg and the dorsal aspect of the foot.
2. Superior Gluteal Nerve (L4, L5, S1): It has only motor function and innervates the gluteus minimus, gluteus medius, and tensor fascia latae.
3. Inferior Gluteal Nerve (L5, S1, S2): It is also a motor nerve, innervating the gluteus maximus.
4. Posterior Femoral Cutaneous (S1, S2, S3): It is sensory nerve and provides innervation to the skin on the posterior surface of the thigh and leg. It also innervates the skin of the perineum.
5. Pudendal Nerve (S2, S3, S4): It has both motor and sensory innervations. It provides motor innervation to skeletal muscles in the perineum, the external urethral sphincter, the external anal sphincter, and the levator ani. The sensory function of this nerve is to supply the penis and the clitoris and most of the skin of the perineum.

MENINGES

Meninges are the protective sheath around the central nervous system. The sheath consists of three layers: the dura mater, the arachnoid mater, and the pia mater. The primary function of the meninges and the CSF is to cushion the brain and the spinal cord. The spinal meninges are in continuation with the cranial meninges.

DURA MATER

The dura mater is the outermost and thickest layer of meninges. The cranial dura has several reflections within the cranial cavity to form rigid membranes. The falx cerebri is the layer that separates the right and the left cerebral hemispheres, and the tentorium cerebelli is in between the occipital lobes of the cerebrum and the upper surface of the cerebellum. The mid brain passes through a notch in the anterior edge of the tentorium. The cranial dura extends as the spinal dura from the foramen magnum. It is imperative to understand the anatomy of the cranial dura mater especially in relation to the herniations that occur in the context of increased ICP. Increased ICP causes cingulate, central, uncal, cerebrotonsillar, reverse, and transcalvarial (in the context of a skull fracture) types of herniation (see Figure 22.7). Caudally, the spinal dura mater ends at approximately S2, where it fuses with the filum terminale. Laterally, it covers the spinal nerve roots and becomes continuous with the connective tissue of the epineurium at the intervertebral foramina.

The dura mater is made up of randomly arranged collagen fibers and elastin fibers arranged longitudinally and circumferentially. It is mostly acellular except for a layer of cells that is in between the dura mater and the arachnoid mater. It is interesting to note that the inner edge of the dura mater is highly vascular, and this makes it an important route of drug clearance from both the epidural space and the subarachnoid space.[1]

EPIDURAL SPACE

The epidural space lies between the meninges and the bones of the skull or vertebral canal. The intracranial epidural space is not of clinical significance to the practice of anesthesiology outside of the management of traumatic brain injury. In the spinal cord, the epidural space is bounded cranially by

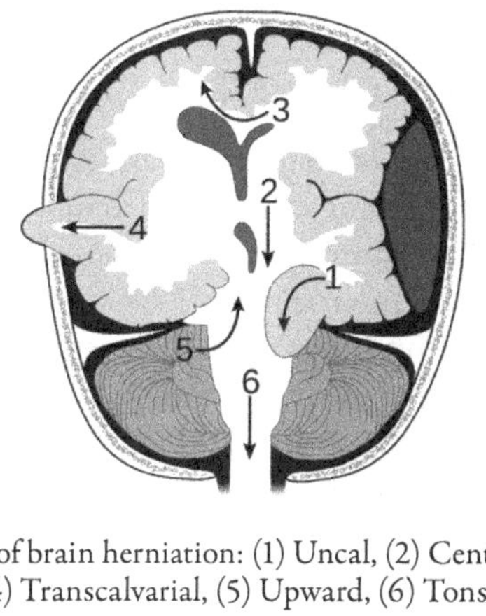

Figure 22.7 Types of brain herniation: (1) Uncal, (2) Central, (3) Cingulate, (4) Transcalvarial, (5) Upward, (6) Tonsillar.

the foramen magnum, caudally by the sacrococcygeal ligament covering the sacral hiatus, anteriorly by the posterior longitudinal ligament, laterally by the vertebral pedicles, and posteriorly by both the ligamentum flavum and the vertebral lamina. The epidural space communicates with the paravertebral space by way of the intervertebral foramina. The epidural space is composed of a series of discontinuous compartments that become continuous when air or liquid is injected into it. The epidural space contains fat, lymphatics, segmental arteries running between the aorta and the spinal cord, and a network of valveless veins (Batson plexus) that is present mainly in the anterior and lateral portions of the epidural space.[2]

EPIDURAL FAT

Epidural fat is located in the posterior and the lateral parts of the epidural space. It appears to have clinically important effects on the pharmacology of epidurally and intrathecally administered drugs like opioids and local anesthetics. The net transfer of an opioid from the epidural space to the intrathecal space is greatest for the least lipid-soluble opioid (morphine) and least for highly lipid soluble opioids (fentanyl, sufentanil). Therefore, increasing the lipid solubility results in opioid sequestration in epidural fat, thence reducing the bioavailability of the drug in the underlying subarachnoid space and spinal tissue.[1] Similarly a highly lipid soluble local anesthetic like etidocaine (10 times more potent than lidocaine in blocking nerve conduction) is almost equipotent with lidocaine in the epidural space. This is because of its greater sequestration into the epidural fat, which eventually reduces the amount of the drug available to produce block in the spinal nerve roots and spinal cord.

SUBDURAL SPACE

This is a potential space between the dura and arachnoid mater. It contains small amounts of serous fluid, which enables the dura and arachnoid to slide over each other. Accidental injection of the local anesthetic into the subdural space during spinal anesthesia may explain the failed spinal anesthetic and the rare "total spinal" after epidural anesthesia.

ARACHNOID MATER

The arachnoid mater is a delicate, avascular membrane. It is composed of overlapping layers of flattened cells with connective tissue fibers running between the cellular layers. The arachnoid cells are interconnected by frequent tight junctions and occluding junctions. These specialized cellular connections are most likely responsible for the fact that the arachnoid mater is the principal barrier to drugs crossing in and out of the CSF and is estimated to account for 90% of the resistance to drug migration. In the region where the spinal nerve roots traverse the dura and arachnoid membranes, the arachnoid mater herniates through the dura mater into the epidural space to form arachnoid granulations. Cranial and spinal arachnoid granulations serve as an exit for various drugs in the central nervous system.[1]

SUBARACHNOID SPACE

The subarachnoid space lies between the arachnoid mater and the pia mater and contains the CSF. The subarachnoid space is relatively narrow over the surface of the cerebral hemisphere, but it becomes much wider in areas at the base of the brain. These widened spaces are the subarachnoid cisterns. The term subarachnoid hemorrhage (SAH) refers to extravasation of blood into the subarachnoid space.

The spinal CSF is in continuum with the cranial CSF. The spinal nerve roots and rootlets pass through the subarachnoid space.

PIA MATER

Pia mater is adherent to the spinal cord and is composed of a thin layer of connective tissue cells interspersed with collagen. It is connected to the arachnoid mater by trabeculae. In multiple areas the pia mater is fenestrated, so that the spinal cord is in direct communication with the subarachnoid space. The pia mater extends to the tip of the spinal cord, where it becomes the *filum terminale*, which anchors the spinal cord to the sacrum. Dentate ligaments formed by the pia mater are thin connective tissue bands extending from the side of the spinal cord through the arachnoid mater to the dura mater. These ligaments serve to suspend the spinal cord within the meninges.

AUTONOMIC NERVOUS SYSTEM

The autonomic nervous system (ANS)[1-3] is mainly concerned with involuntary regulation of cardiac muscle, smooth muscle, and glandular and visceral functions. Autonomic nervous system activity refers to visceral reflexes that function below the conscious level. The ANS helps to maintain homeostasis and organizes "fight or flight" responses. Autonomic reflex activity in the spinal cord accounts for some aspects of autonomic regulation. However supraspinal centers such as brain stem nuclei and the hypothalamus play a major role in its modulation.

The ANS is divided into two major anatomically distinct divisions that have opposing actions: the sympathetic (thoracolumbar) and parasympathetic (craniosacral) divisions. The peripheral efferent portions of the ANS are made up of two neurons: preganglionic and postganglionic (Figure 22.8).

SYMPATHETIC NERVOUS SYSTEM

The sympathetic nervous system (SNS) originates from the spinal cord in the thoracolumbar region, from the first

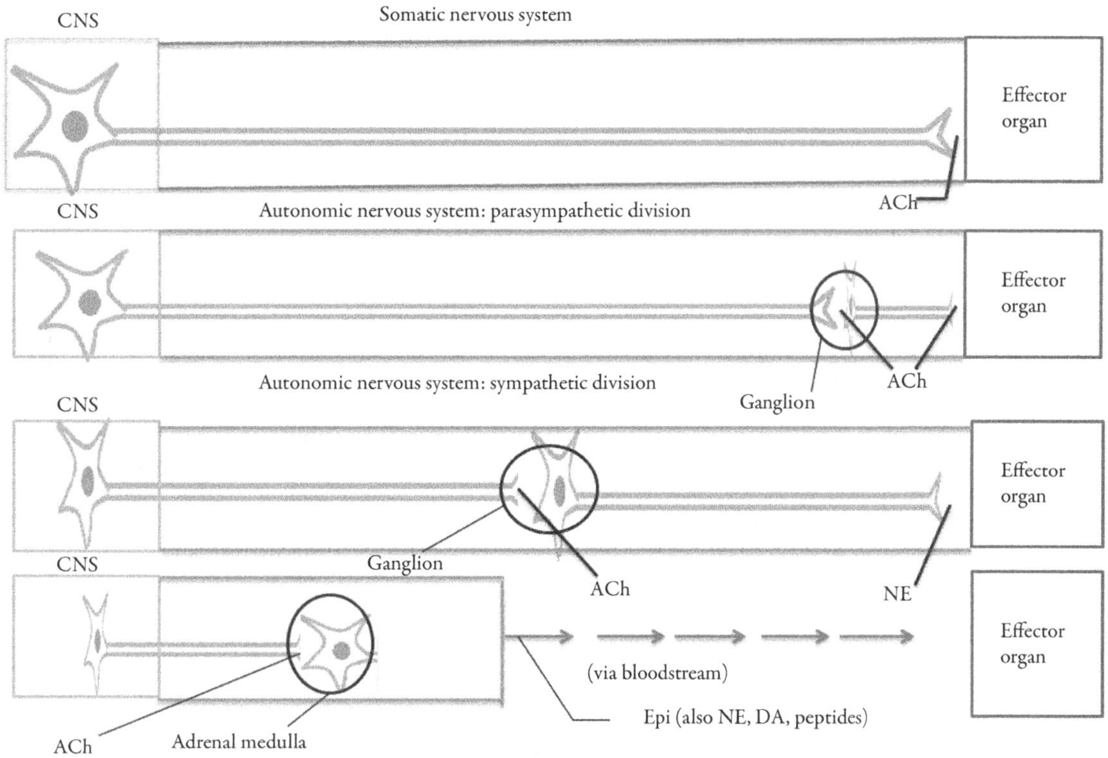

Figure 22.8 Sympathetic and parasympathetic divisions of the autonomic nervous system. Adapted from *Ganong's Review of Medical Physiology*, 24th ed., Fig. 13–1.

thoracic through the second or third lumbar segment. The preganglionic sympathetic neurons have cell bodies within the intermediolateral columns of the spinal gray matter. Sympathetic ganglia are generally close to the central nervous system, but they are distant from the effector organs; therefore, postganglionic fibers run a long course before innervating the effector organs. The axons of the sympathetic preganglionic neurons leave the spinal cord at the same level at which their cell bodies are located and exit via the ventral root along with axons of α (alpha)- and γ (gamma)-motor neurons and enter the ganglion through the *white (myelinated) ramus*. The 22 paired ganglia lie along either side of the vertebral column. Nerve trunks connect these ganglia to each other, and *gray rami communicantes* connect the ganglia to the spinal nerves. In the neck the preganglionic fibers from the first four or five thoracic spinal segments form three special paired ganglia. These are the superior cervical, middle cervical, and cervicothoracic ganglia. The last is known as the stellate ganglion and is actually formed by the fusion of the inferior cervical and first thoracic SNS ganglia. These ganglia provide sympathetic innervation of the head, neck, upper extremities, heart, and lungs. Some preganglionic neurons pass through the paravertebral ganglion chain and end on postganglionic neurons located in prevertebral (or collateral) ganglia close to the viscera, including the celiac, superior mesenteric, and inferior mesenteric ganglia. There are also preganglionic neurons whose axons terminate directly on the effector organ, the adrenal gland.

PARASYMPATHETIC NERVOUS SYSTEM

The parasympathetic nervous system (PNS) is sometimes called the craniosacral division of the ANS because of the location of its preganglionic neurons in several cranial nerve nuclei (III, VII, IX, and X) and in the intermediolateral column of the sacral spinal cord. The PNS preganglionic fibers pass directly to the organ that is innervated. The postganglionic cell bodies are situated near or within the innervated viscera. The cell bodies in the Edinger-Westphal nucleus of the oculomotor nerve project to the ciliary ganglia to innervate the sphincter (constrictor) muscle of the iris and the ciliary muscle. Neurons in the superior salivatory nucleus of the facial nerve project to the sphenopalatine ganglia to innervate the lacrimal glands and the submandibular ganglia to innervate the submandibular and submaxillary glands. The cell bodies in the inferior salivatory nucleus of the glossopharyngeal nerve project to the otic ganglion to innervate the parotid salivary gland. The vagus is the most important of the parasympathetic nerves and supplies the heart, tracheobronchial tree, liver, spleen, kidney, and entire gastrointestinal tract except for the distal part of the colon. The second through fourth sacral segments contribute the nervierigentes, or the pelvic splanchnic nerves. They synapse in terminal ganglia associated with the rectum and genitourinary organs.

FUNCTIONAL NEUROANATOMY OF CRANIAL NERVES

A basic understanding of the functional anatomy is essential for all anesthesiologists.[4]

Optic Nerve (I)

The optic pathway transmits visual impulses from the retina to the brain. The axons of the ganglion cells of the retina pass caudally in the optic nerve and optic tract to end in the lateral geniculate body in the thalamus. The fibers from each nasal hemiretina decussate in the optic chiasm. In the geniculate body, the fibers from the nasal half of one retina and the temporal half of the other synapse on the cells whose axons give rise to the geniculocalcarine tract. This tract projects to the occipital lobe of the cerebral cortex.

Oculomotor (III), Trochlear (IV), and Abducens (VI) Nerves

These nerves innervate the extrinsic ocular muscles (displayed in Figure 22.9).

- Oculomotor (III):
  - Superior division: levator palpebrae superioris, superior rectus
  - Inferior division: medial rectus, inferior rectus, inferior oblique
- Trochlear (IV): superior oblique
- Abducens (VI): lateral rectus

Through its parasympathetic components, the oculomotor nerve also causes constriction of the pupil (miosis) and has a role in accommodation of the lens. Because of its long intracranial course, the abducens nerve is often the first cranial nerve to be affected by intracranial disease.

Trigeminal Nerve (V)

Cranial nerve (CN) V is a mixed nerve that has both sensory and motor components. The trigeminal nerve divides into three main branches in the middle cranial fossa. These divisions—the ophthalmic, maxillary, and mandibular nerves—provide sensation to the eye and forehead, midface and upper jaw, and lower jaw, respectively.

Blockade of the second and third divisions of the trigeminal nerve, as well as blockade of the peripheral branches,

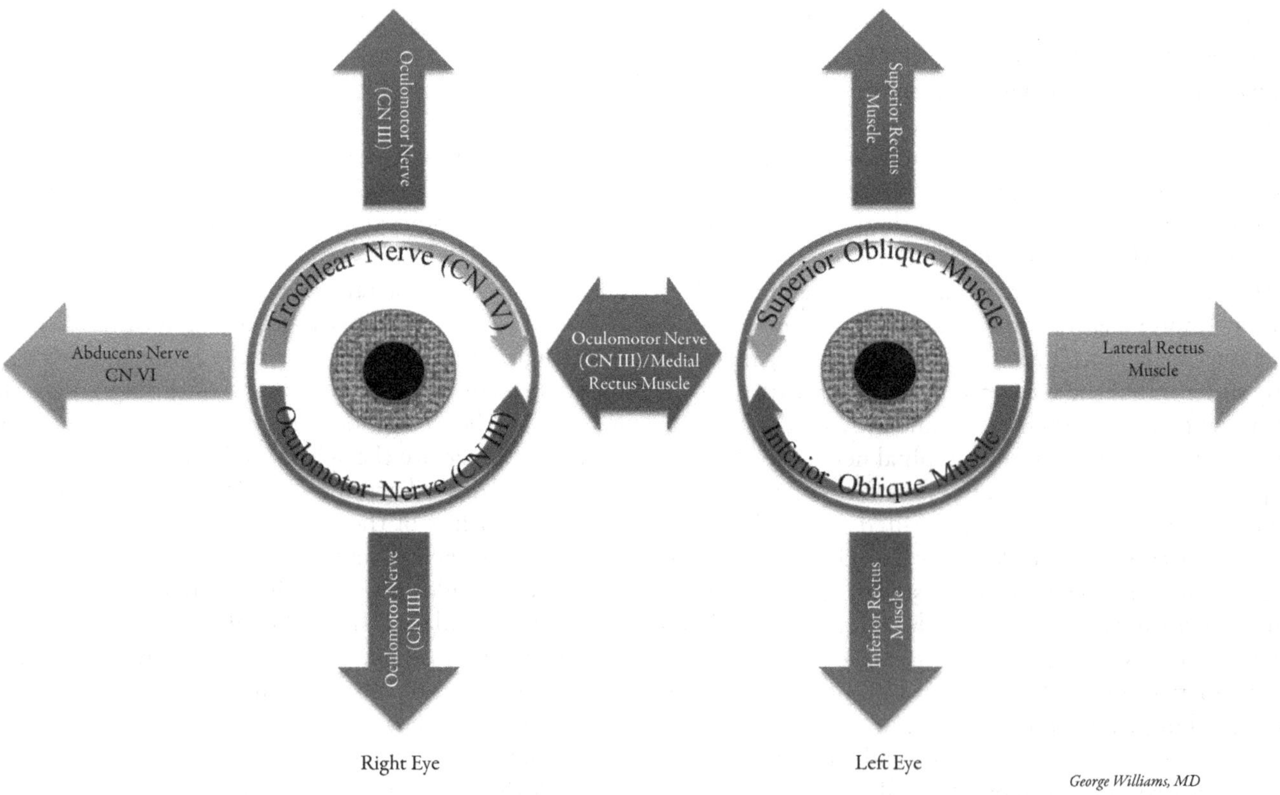

Figure 22.9 Combined cranial nerve (right eye) and ocular muscle (left eye) diagram. As shown, CN IV and CN IV each only innervate one muscle and thereby one function of the eye. All other muscles are associated with CN III.

is occasionally useful in the diagnosis and management of pain syndromes.

Opthalmic Nerve (V_1)

The ophthalmic branch (V_1) divides into three sensory nerves as it passes through the superior orbital fissure: the frontal, lacrimal, and nasociliary nerves. The supraorbital and supratrochlear nerves are terminal branches of the frontal nerve that supplies the upper eyelid, forehead, and scalp. Indications for blocking these nerves include frontal craniotomy, skin lesion removal of the eyebrow and medial part of the forehead, and placement of frontal ventroperitoneal shunts.

Maxillary Nerve (V_2)

The maxillary nerve exits the cranium through the foramen rotundum and enters the pterygopalatine fossa. The infraorbital nerve is a terminal branch of the maxillary nerve. It emerges from the infraorbital foramen that supplies the nose, lower eyelid, and upper lip.

Infraorbital nerve blocks are indicated for surgery of cleft lip, laceration of upper lip, endoscopic surgery of sinus, surgery of nasal septum, and transsphenoidal hypophysectomy.

Mandibular Nerve (V_3)

The mandibular nerve exits the cranium through the foramen ovale to enter the infratemporal fossa. The lingual nerve provides general sensation to the anterior two-thirds of the tongue.

The inferior alveolar nerve enters the mandibular canal through the mandibular foramen to innervate the lower teeth and gums. The mental nerve is the terminal branch of the mandibular nerve (V_3) that supplies the lower lip and chin. Main indications for mental nerve blocks are with surgery involving lower incisor and canine teeth; bilateral blocks allow pain-free procedures on the lower lip. The mandibular nerve also supplies the muscles of mastication, tensor palati and tensor tympani, mylohyoid, and the anterior belly of the digastric muscle.

Facial Nerve (VII)

The facial nerve supplies the muscles of facial expression. Its other functions include:

- Taste sensation from the anterior portion of the tongue and oral cavity;
- Parasympathetic secretomotor function of the salivary, lacrimal, nasal, and palatine glands.

The facial nerve originates from cerebellopontine angle. In upper motor neuron (UMN) lesions of the facial nerve, the forehead and orbicularis oculi muscles are largely spared. This is because there is bilateral cortical representation of the upper facial muscles, and so if corticonuclear fibers on one side of the brain are interrupted (e.g., in the internal capsule) those of the other side are unaffected. For the lower facial muscles there is only contralateral representation.

Facial nerve monitoring is used during middle ear, mastoid, and inner ear procedures to identify the facial nerve and reduce the incidence of iatrogenic facial nerve injury.

Glossopharyngeal Nerve (IX)

The glossopharyngeal nerve provides sensory innervation to the posterior third of the tongue, the vallecula, the anterior surface of the epiglottis (lingual branch), the walls of the pharynx (pharyngeal branch), and the tonsils (tonsillar branch). The gag reflex is mediated by the glossopharyngeal (afferent limb) and the vagus (efferent limb). The glossopharyngeal nerve can be anesthetized using either intraoral or extraoral (peristyloid) approaches. The glossopharyngeal nerve can be blocked intraorally by injecting local anesthetic into the base of each posterior tonsillar pillar. Careful aspiration before injection is mandatory because of the proximity of the internal carotid artery. Caution should be used in a patient with a full stomach because these blocks abolish protective airway reflexes.

Vagus (X)

The vagus, the most extensively distributed of all cranial nerves, arises from the medulla and leaves the posterior cranial fossa through the jugular foramen. It descends in the carotid sheath posteriorly behind the internal jugular vein and internal/common carotid arteries and gives pharyngeal branches and the superior laryngeal nerve, which has internal (sensory innervations above vocal cords) and external (cricothyroid) branches.

The recurrent laryngeal nerves arise in the superior mediastinum and provide sensory innervation to the infraglottic part of the trachea and vocal folds. Blockade facilitates passing of the endotracheal tube into the trachea during awake intubation.

The arteries of the thyroid gland are closely related to the laryngeal branches of the vagus. The superior laryngeal artery is related to the external laryngeal nerve near the origin of the artery, and the recurrent laryngeal nerve is related to the inferior thyroid artery close to the gland. This is relevant to thyroid surgery. Damage to the recurrent laryngeal nerves at this point nearly always affects fibers innervating the vocal cord abductors before those affecting adductors. This has important clinical implications, since if abduction is lost, the cords will be adducted, which can result in stridor.

Vagal Reflexes

Baroreceptors are stretch receptors that respond to changes in pressure. They are located in the carotid sinuses, which are situated at the origin of the internal carotid arteries near the bifurcation of the common carotid arteries, and in the aortic arch. The receptors are located in the adventitia of the vessels. The afferent nerve fibers from the carotid sinus form a branch of the glossopharyngeal nerve, the carotid sinus nerve. The fibers from the aortic arch form a branch of the vagus nerve, the aortic depressor nerve.

Distention of the blood vessels stimulates the baroreceptors, and they discharge at an increased rate when the pressure in these structures rises. Increased baroreceptor discharge inhibits the discharge of sympathetic nerves and excites the vagal innervation of the heart. These neural changes produce vasodilation, venodilation, hypotension, bradycardia, and a decrease in cardiac output. In chronic hypertension, the baroreceptor reflex mechanism is "reset" to maintain an elevated rather than a normal blood pressure. The baroreceptor reflex plays an important role during acute blood loss and shock, and does not work when mean blood pressure is less than 50 mmHg.

CHEMORECEPTOR REFLEX

There is a carotid body near the carotid bifurcation on each side, and there are usually two or more aortic bodies near the arch of the aorta. Each carotid and aortic body (glomus) contains two types of cells, type I and type II cells, surrounded by fenestrated sinusoidal capillaries. Type-I glomus cells have O_2-sensitive K^+ channels, whose conductance is reduced in proportion to the degree of hypoxia to which they are exposed. This reduces the K^+ efflux, depolarizing the cell and causing Ca^{2+} influx, primarily via L-type Ca^{2+} channels. The Ca^{2+} influx triggers action potentials and transmitter release, with consequent excitation of the afferent nerve endings. At an arterial partial oxygen pressure (PaO_2) of less than 50 mmHg or in conditions of acidosis, the chemoreceptors send their impulses along the sinus nerve of Hering (a branch of the glossopharyngeal nerve) and the 10th cranial nerve to the chemosensitive area of the medulla. This area responds by stimulating the respiratory centers and thereby increasing ventilatory drive. The parasympathetic system is also activated, which results in reduction of the heart rate and myocardial contractility.

BEZOLD-JARISCH REFLEX

Activation of chemosensitive vagal C fibers in the cardiopulmonary region (e.g., juxtacapillary region of alveoli, ventricles, atria, great veins, and pulmonary artery) causes profound bradycardia, hypotension, and a brief period of apnea followed by rapid shallow breathing. This response pattern is called the Bezold-Jarisch reflex. This reflex is usually in the clinical setting of myocardial ischemia or infarction, thrombolysis, or revascularization and syncope.

OCULOCARDIAC REFLEX

The oculocardiac reflex was first described by Aschner and Dagnini in 1908. Pressure on the globe or traction on the extraocular muscles results in bradycardia, atrioventricular block, ventricular ectopy, or asystole. It is especially seen with traction on the medial rectus muscle, but can occur with stimulation of any of the orbital contents, including the periosteum. The response is exacerbated by hypercapnia or hypoxemia or inappropriate depth of anesthesia.

The afferent limb is via the trigeminal nerve, and the efferent limb is via the vagal nerve. The afferent limb is from the orbital contents → ciliary ganglion → ophthalmic division of the trigeminal nerve → sensory nucleus of the trigeminal near the fourth ventricle. The efferent limb is via the vagus nerve to the heart.

PAIN AND NOCICEPTION

Pain is defined by the International Association for the Study of Pain (IASP) as "an unpleasant sensory and emotional experience associated with actual or potential tissue damage or described in terms of such damage". The ability of the somatosensory system to detect noxious and potentially tissue-damaging stimuli is an important protective mechanism that involves multiple interacting peripheral and central mechanisms. The neural processes underlying the encoding and processing of noxious stimuli are defined as "nociception."[5]

NOCICEPTIVE PATHWAY

Peripheral transmission of pain involves *transduction*, which is production of electrical signals at the stimulated nerve endings, followed by *transmission*, which is propagation of those signals through the peripheral nervous system.

Peripheral Nociceptors

Nociceptors are physiologically specialized peripheral sensory neurons that respond to noxious stimuli. These are free, unencapsulated peripheral nerve endings found in most tissues of the body including skin, deep somatic tissue (e.g., muscles and joints), and the viscera. The C polymodal nociceptors are the most numerous type and respond to a wide range of mechanical, thermal, and chemical noxious stimuli. They are slowly conducting (<3 m/s) and associated with prolonged "burning" pain. The more rapidly conducting (5–30 m/s) Aδ nociceptors are associated with a more brief "sharp" pain. They are myelinated and respond to mechanical and thermal stimuli.[6] Polymodal nociceptors are slow to adapt to strong pressure and display heat sensitization.

Noxious stimuli are transduced by peripheral nociceptors and transmitted by Aδ and C nerve fibers from peripheral visceral and somatic sites to the dorsal horn of the spinal cord, where integration of peripheral nociceptive and descending modulatory input (i.e., serotonin, norepinephrine, gamma amino-butyric acid, enkephalin) occurs.

Afferent Pathways

Pain impulses are transmitted by two ascending systems. The presence of two pain pathways explains the existence of two components of pain: fast, sharp, and well-localized sensation, which is conducted by Aδ fibers, and a duller slower onset and often poorly localized sensation, which is conducted by C fibers.[7] The first-order neurons originating in the periphery as Aδ and polymodal C fibers synapse on second-order neurons in the dorsal horn primarily within laminae I, II, and V, where they release excitatory amino acids and neuropeptides. In addition, descending axons from the brain stem synapse in the dorsal horn and modulate nociceptive transmission. Second-order neurons consist of nociceptive-specific and wide dynamic-range (WDR) neurons. Nociceptive-specific neurons are located primarily in lamina I, respond only to noxious stimuli, and are thought to be involved in the sensory-discriminative aspects of pain. The WDR neurons are predominately located in laminae IV, V, and VI. The WDR neurons receive both noxious and nonnoxious afferent input and are involved with the affective–motivational component of pain. Axons of both nociceptive-specific and WDR neurons ascend in the spinal cord via the dorsal column–medial lemniscus and the anterior lateral spinothalamic tract to synapse on third-order neurons in the contralateral thalamus, which then project to the somatosensory cortex, where nociceptive input is perceived as pain.

Multiple parallel ascending pathways from the spinal cord to the mid brain, forebrain, and cortex play a role in experiencing various characteristics of the overall pain experience. The spinoreticular and spinomesencephalic tracts are important for integrating nociceptive information with arousal, homeostatic, and autonomic responses, as well as projecting to central areas mediating the emotional or affective component of pain.

Modulation

Modulation of pain transmission involves altering afferent neural transmission along the pain pathway. The dorsal horn of the spinal cord is the most common site for modulation of the pain pathway, and modulation can involve either inhibition or augmentation of the pain signals.

Peripheral Modulation

Tissue damage, such as that associated with infection, inflammation, or ischemia, produces disruption of cells, degranulation of mast cells, secretion by inflammatory cells, and induction of enzymes such as cyclo-oxygenase-2 (COX-2). Ranges of chemical mediators (bradykinin, serotonin, histamine, prostaglandin, leukotriene, cytokines, and nerve growth factor) act either directly via ligand-gated ion channels or via metabotropic receptors to activate and/or sensitize nociceptors. Peripheral sensitization of polymodal C fibers and high-threshold mechanoreceptors by these chemicals leads to primary hyperalgesia, which by definition is an exaggerated response to pain at the site of injury. Voltage-gated sodium channels and the capsaicin receptor (transient receptor potential channel V1-TRPV1) are intimately involved in activation and sensitization of peripheral nociceptors.

Central Sensitization

The term *central sensitization* is used to describe the phenomena of wind-up, long-term potentiation, and secondary hyperalgesia.

Progressive increase in action potential output from the dorsal horn cell is seen with each stimulus, and this rapid increase in responsiveness during the course of a train of inputs has been termed "wind-up." It refers to a process involving WDR neurons in the deeper levels of the dorsal horn. It is produced by repeated low-frequency activation of C-fibers, causing a progressive increase in electrophysiological response. The N-methyl-D-aspartate (NMDA) receptor is closely involved in this sensitization process.[8]

Long-term potentiation (LTP) at individual synapses, thought to be important in learning and memory in hippocampus, may also be the mechanism of hyperalgesia and central sensitization. Long-term potentiation is induced by higher frequency stimuli, but the enhanced response outlasts the conditioning stimulus.

Secondary hyperalgesia occurs in undamaged tissue adjacent to the area of actual tissue damage. It is thought to be due to an increased receptive field and reduced threshold of WDR neurons in the dorsal horn.

Neurochemical mediators of central sensitization include substance P, calcitonin gene-related peptide (CGRP), vasoactive intestinal polypeptide (VIP), cholecystokinin, angiotensin, L-glutamate, and L-aspartate. These substances trigger changes in membrane excitability by interacting with G-protein-coupled receptors by a final common pathway, which leads to increased intracellular calcium concentration; for example, glutamate and aspartate activate the NMDA receptor. Stimulation of NMDA receptors causes intraneuronal elevation of Ca^{2+}, which stimulates nitric oxide synthase (NOS) and the production of nitric oxide (NO). Nitric oxide, a gaseous molecule, stimulates the formation of cGMP in neighboring neurons. Depending on the expression of cGMP-controlled ion channels in target neurons, NO may be excitatory or inhibitory. Nitric oxide has been implicated in the development of hyperexcitability, resulting in hyperalgesia or allodynia.

Inhibitory Mechanisms

Inhibitory mechanisms can be either segmental or supraspinal. *Segmental inhibition* consists of activation of large afferent fibers subserving epicritic sensation (fine touch) inhibitory WDR neurons and spinothalamic activity. Glycine and gamma amino-butyric acid (GABA) are amino acids that function as inhibitory neurotransmitters. Segmental inhibition appears to be mediated by $GABA_B$ receptor activity.

Supraspinal inhibition occurs whereby several supraspinal structures send fibers down the spinal cord to inhibit pain at the level of the dorsal horn. These include the periaqueductal gray, reticular formation, and nucleus raphe magnus (NRM).[9] Axons from these structures act presynaptically on the primary afferent neurons and postsynaptically on second-order neurons (or interneurons). These inhibitory pathways use monoamines, such as noradrenaline and serotonin, as neurotransmitters and terminate on nociceptive neurons in the spinal cord as well as on spinal inhibitory interneurons that store and release opioids. Noradrenaline mediates this action through $\alpha 2$ receptors. The endogenous opiate system acts via enkephalins and β-endorphins. These mainly act presynaptically, whereas exogenous opiates act postsynaptically.

REFERENCES

1. Barash P, Cullen B, Stoelting R, Cahalan M, Stock M. *Clinical Anesthesia*. 7th ed. Philadelphia, PA: Lippincott Williams & Wilkins; 2013.
2. Miller R, ed. *Miller's Anesthesia*. 7th ed. Philadelphia, PA: Elsevier; 2010.
3. Barrett K, Barman S, Boitano S, Brooks H. *Ganong's Review of Medical Physiology*. 24th ed. Philadelphia, PA: McGraw-Hill; 2012.
4. Monkhouse S. *Cranial Nerves: Functional Anatomy*. New York, NY: Cambridge University Press; 2005.
5. Sorkin L. Basic pharmacology and physiology of acute pain processing. *Anesthesiol Clin*. 1997;15(2):235–249.
6. Bridgestock C, Rae C. Anatomy, physiology and pharmacology of pain. *Ann Intensive Care*. 2013;14(11):480–483.
7. Loeser J, Treede R-D. The Kyoto protocol of IASP Basic Pain Terminology. *Pain*. 2008;137(3):473–477.
8. Sandkühler J. Models and mechanisms of hyperalgesia and allodynia. *Physiol Rev*. 2009;89(2):707–758.
9. Tracey I, Mantyh P. The cerebral signature for pain perception and its modulation. *Neuron*. 2007;55(3):377–391.

FURTHER READING

Basic Human Anatomy: A Regional Study of Human Structure. Dartmouth College website. http://www.dartmouth.edu/~humananatomy/index.html. Accessed: April 1, 2015.

Exam 3 Review: Chapter 22: ANS Control of Breathing. Internet Information Services website. http://apbrwww5.apsu.edu/thompsonj/Anatomy%20&%20Physiology/2020/2020%20Exam%20Reviews/Exam%203/CH22%20ANS%20Control%20of%20Breathing.htm. Accessed April 1, 2015.

Jacobson S, Marcus E. *Neuroanatomy for the Neuroscientist*. New York, NY: Springer; 2015.

Neuroscience on the Web Series: CMSD 620 Neuroanatomy of Speech, Swallowing, and Language. California State University Chico website. http://www.csuchico.edu/~pmccaffrey/syllabi/CMSD%20320/362unit6.html. Accessed April 1, 2015.

Siegel A, Sapru H. *Essential Neuroscience*. 3rd ed. Philadelphia, PA: Lippincott Williams & Wilkins; 2015.

Smith G, Aitkenhead A, Moppett I, Thompson J. *Smith and Aitkenhead's Textbook of Anaesthesia*. E book. 6th ed. New York: Churchill Livingstone/Elsevier; 2013.

Snell R. *Clinical Neuroanatomy*. 7th ed. Philadelphia, PA: Lippincott Williams & Wilkins; 2009.

QUESTIONS

1. The carotid baroreceptor sends afferent impulses to which nucleus primarily?
   - A. Nucleus accumbens
   - B. Paramedian nucleus
   - C. Nucleus tractus solitarius
   - D. Nucleus basalis of Meynert
   - E. B and C

2. At what level of the transverse foramina do the vertebral arteries enter?
   - A. C3 to C2
   - B. C7 to C1
   - C. C6 to C1
   - D. L4 to T7
   - E. T8 to C7

3. Relative to the lumbar articular facets, the thoracic articular facets are oriented in which plane of anatomy?
   - A. Coronal
   - B. Oblique
   - C. Sagittal
   - D. Axial
   - E. Transverse

4. Where is the apex of the basilar artery located?
   - A. Anterior fossa
   - B. Posterior fossa
   - C. Anterolateral to the pons
   - D. Supratentorial compartment

5. At what point of the brain stem does the basilar artery bifurcate to form the posterior cerebral arteries?
   - A. Medulla
   - B. Upper pons

C. Mid brain
D. Lower pons
E. No bifurcation, as it directly feeds into the Circle of Willis

6. At which level does the dura mater end in neonates?
A. L1
B. L3-L4
C. S1-S2
D. S3-S4
E. S2

7. The oculocardiac reflex may be triggered by stimulating which of the following structures?
A. Extraocular muscles
B. Conjunctiva
C. Periosteum
D. Sclera
E. All of the above

8. The stellate ganglion is formed by
A. Fusion of the inferior cervical and first thoracic SNS ganglia
B. Superior cervical ganglia
C. Middle cervical ganglia
D. First thoracic ganglia
E. Fusion of superior and middle cervical

ANSWERS

1. E. Both B and C are correct. While efferent impulses are carried through the sympathetic and vagus nerves, afferent impulses from the carotid body are transmitted as follows: inferior ganglion --> nucleus tractus solitarius and paramedian nucleus --> nucleus ambiguus and vagus nerve.

FURITHER READING

Guyton AC, Hall JE. *Textbook of Medical Physiology.* 10th ed. Philadelphia, PA: W.B. Saunders; 2000:188–189.

2. C. The vertebral arteries enter via C6-C1 transverse foramina, prior to exiting the transverse foramina of the atlas (C1). The vertebral arteries are not enclosed in the vertebral body below the cervical level.

FURTHER READING

Katsuta T. The jugular foramen: microsurgical anatomy and operative approaches. *Neurosurgery.* 1997;41(1):149–201.

3. A. The coronal plane. By comparison, the lumbar articular facets are typically found in the sagittal plane.

FURTHER READING

Epstein NE. Lumbar synovial cysts: a review of diagnosis, surgical management, and outcome assessment. *J Spinal Disord Tech.* 2004;17(4):321–325. Review.

4. C.The supratentorial compartment.

FURTHER READING

MacFarlane MR, McAllister VL. Posterior circulation aneurysms: results of direct operations. *Surg Neurol.* 1983;20(5):399–413.

5. B. The anatomy of the Circle of Willis is described in Figure 22.6, but is it important to recall that the circle begins to form from the basilar artery at the level of the upper pons and upon the entry of the internal carotid artery after entering the skull base.

6. D. At birth the dura mater ends at the level of the third or fourth sacral vertebra and the cord (conus medullaris) at the L3 or L4 level. It is only at the end of the first year of life that adult level is attained, namely, L1 for the conus medullaris and S2 for the dural sac.

FURTHER READING

Miller RD, Eriksson LI, Fleisher LA, Wiener-Kronish JP, Young WL, eds. *Miller's Anesthesia* 7th ed. Philadelphia, PA: Elsevier Churchill Livingstone; 2009.

7. E. The oculocardiac reflex can be triggered by stimulating any of the orbital contents, though it is most commonly associated with traction on the medial rectus muscle.

FURTHER READING

Miller RD, Eriksson LI, Fleisher LA, Wiener-Kronish JP, Young WL, eds. *Miller's Anesthesia* 7th ed. Philadelphia, PA: Elsevier Churchill Livingstone; 2009.

8. A. In the neck there are three special paired sympathetic ganglia. These are the superior cervical, middle cervical, and cervicothoracic ganglia. The last is known as the stellate ganglion and is formed by the fusion of the inferior cervical and first thoracic SNS ganglia. The superior and middle cervical ganglia are discrete entities.

FURTHER READING

Barash PG, Cullen BF, Stoelting RK, Stock MC, Ortega R. *Clinical Anesthesia.* 7th ed. Philadelphia, PA: Wolters Kluwer/Lippincott Williams & Wilkins; 2013.

23.

RESPIRATORY PHYSIOLOGY

Marie-Francoise Doursout, Shruti Deshpande, and George W. Williams

LUNG FUNCTIONS

The primary and most basic function of the lungs is respiration, that is, uptake of oxygen and exchange of CO_2. Other than respiratory gas exchange, lungs also perform many nonrespiratory functions, such as storage and filtering of blood for systemic circulation and metabolism of vasoactive substances like PGE1, E2, and F2α. The lung also synthesizes and secretes chemical substances, which are locally used, such as pulmonary surfactant, mucus, other tracheobronchial secretions, surface enzymes, proteins and other factors, and immunologically active substances. Histologically, the lung contains two types of pneumocytes: I and II. Type I pneumocytes constitute the alveolus. Pulmonary surfactant is mainly produced by type II pneumocytes and in some amounts by Clara cells; this surfactant is released into the alveoli to decrease surface tension. Type II pneumocytes may also spontaneously convert to type I pneumocytes in order to preserve the alveolus.

Additionally, the lung produces and releases substances into the bloodstream such as bradykinin, histamine, serotonin, heparin, prostaglandins E2 and F2α, and the endoperoxides (prostaglandins G2 and H2). These are also stored by cells in the lung and may be released into the general circulation under various circumstances.

LUNG VOLUMES AND CAPACITIES

Lung volume is an important measurable parameter that can provide insight for comparison between normal and abnormal measurements. Normal lung volumes vary according to size, weight, gender, and most importantly height. Lung *capacities* can be calculated by adding two or more lung *volumes*. (See Figure 23.1.)

Lung volumes can be discussed from two perspectives:

1. Static lung volumes: Lung volumes that are not affected by the rate of respiration are termed *static lung volumes.*
2. Dynamic lung volume: Lung volumes that change according the rate of gas moving in and out.

Most lung volumes (except for the residual volume, functional residual capacity, and total lung capacity) can be measured with spirometry, which is a common pulmonary function test. These are difficult to measure and require sophisticated techniques like nitrogen washout, closed circuit helium dilution, and body plethysmography.

STATIC VOLUMES

1. Tidal volume (TV): The volume of air that moves in and out of the lungs during quiet breathing is called the tidal volume. It measures around 500–700 mL or 6–8 mL/kg. It is when a normal individual take a relaxed breath in and out without any efforts.
2. Inspiratory reserve volume: The maximum volume of air that could be inhaled above the tidal volume with maximum inspiratory effort. It is approximately 2–3 L.
3. Expiratory reserve volume (ERV): The maximum volume of air that can be exhaled with an active expiratory effort below tidal volume. It does not have diagnostic value and measures around 1–1.2 L.
4. Residual volume (RV): It is the volume of air remaining in the lung after forced expiration and amounts to 2 to 2.5 L. This volume of lung cannot be expelled out by any maneuver, hence difficult to measure by direct spirometry.
5. Total lung capacity (TLC): It is the maximum volume to which lung can be inflated. It is the sum of all volumes

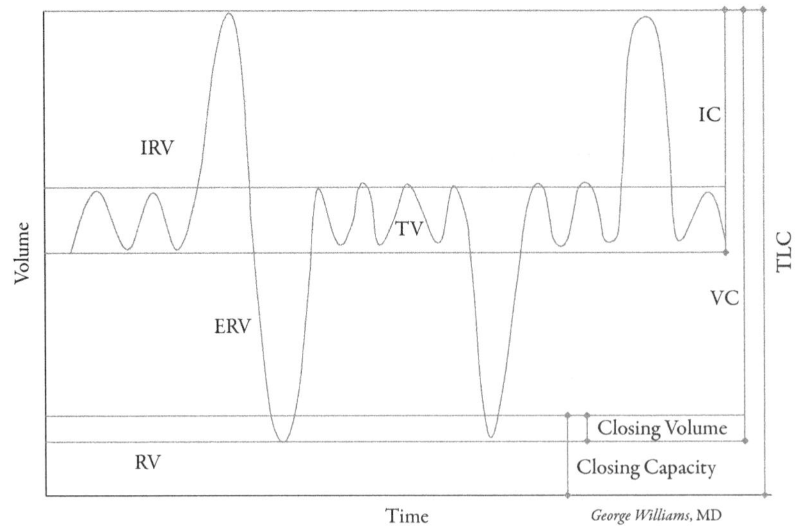

Figure 23.1 Lung volumes and capacities diagrammatically displayed.

described above. Therefore TLC = TV + IRV + ERV + RV, and is typically 6 to 8 L.

6. Functional Residual Volume (FRC): It is the volume of air that remains in the lung after normal expiration (ERV + RV). It is around 3–4 L or 30–35 mL/kg. There is equal balance between inward elastic recoil of the lung and outward force of the chest wall at FRC. Elastic fibers of the lung, contractile forces of the airway, and surface tension determine the inward elastic recoil of the lungs, whereas outward force of the thorax is determined by the force exerted by the ribs, muscles, and joints. FRC prevents lung collapse at end expiration. Thus it eliminates the resistance offered by collapsed alveoli with a liquid-gas interface to reopen. It has been proved that less resistance is encountered to inflate alveoli in an open lung with liquid-gas interface units than in a collapsed lung with a liquid-gas interface unit. This volume has clinical significance, as it determines the oxygen reserve of humans when apnea occurs or is induced by anesthesia. Thus FRC improves the ventilation–perfusion relationship in the lungs because blood gets oxygenated even though respiration is stopped for some time as in apnea. In essence, FRC is an oxygen reserve tank, and when a patient is apneic, the more FRC available, the longer they can sustain an oxygen saturation (hence, obese patients desaturate more quickly, even when preoxygenated).

Functional residual capacity is dependent on factors that have an influence on both the chest and the lung recoil forces.

- Body habitus: FRC decreases with obesity. With increase in body weight the outward chest recoil force decreases, and increased weight also affects the diaphragmatic movement negatively, decreasing the FRC. The opposite is true of the lean body. Height has no effect on the FRC.
- Sex: FRC is lower by 10% in females compared with males because of the smaller size of the lung.
- Posture: FRC increases in the upright and sitting positions. It decreases in the supine and prone positions because of the decrease in the movement of the diaphragm in these positions (hence, in the postanesthesia care unit [PACU] or intensive care unit [ICU], sitting patients up helps them wean off of oxygen faster).
- During exercise: With rapid respiration, FRC decreases as tidal volume increases with increased inspiration and expiration.
- Lung diseases: FRC decreases in restrictive lung disease as the compliance of the lung goes down. In contrast, FRC increases in COPD patients because of less elastic recoil and excessively compliant lungs. A phenomenon of "gas trapping" is seen in these patients at the end of expiration.

Functional residual capacity, TLC, and residual volume are difficult-to-measure lung volumes and require special techniques to be assessed. They can be measured with different techniques like closed-circuit helium dilution, closed-circuit nitrogen washout, and body plethysmography. The most commonly used methods are helium dilution (closed circuit) and nitrogen washout (modern open circuit) methods. These techniques are able to measure the FRC communicating with the airways; when a bleb or pocket of gas is trapped it will not be measured using these techniques. Additionally, the nitrogen washout technique is more commonly used in small or sick infants because the circuit resistance is lower. The data acquired from these studies and the subsequent calculations are easily programmable for determination by personal computer.

Body Plethysmography

Body plethysmography measures the compressible air content in the thorax and the very small amount of air in the abdomen irrespective of whether it is freely communicating or trapped. This method requires the patient to sit in a sealed box with a known volume of gas. The patient is connected to a mouthpiece through which he pants gently at a frequency of 1 breath per second against a closed shutter at FRC (the patient is asked to use both hands to collapse both cheeks). The compression and decompression of air in the chest forms a pressure volume curve, which is used to calculate the total air in the thorax. It is based on Boyle's law (i.e., at a constant temperature, the product of gas volume and pressure is a constant). The technique makes it possible to determine the absolute volume of FRC regardless of whether there are parts of FRC not communicating to the conducting airways.

Nitrogen Washout

After breathing room air, the patient is asked to breathe 100% oxygen in and out normally in a special instrument with continuous collection and monitoring of the exhaled nitrogen gas. The test proceeds until the alveolar nitrogen concentration is reduced to <7%, usually requiring 7 to 10 minutes. The RV, FRC, and TLC are calculated based on the assumption that the mass of displaced nitrogen is equal to the mass of nitrogen in the lungs at the beginning of the test and that the initial concentration of nitrogen in the lungs was ~75% in the mixture of air (see Figure 23.2).

Helium Dilution Method

This test is based on the assumption of the mass balance approach. The known concentration and volume of an inert gas like helium (He) is inhaled by the subject. Determining the exhaled concentration of the inert gas allows the calculation of the volume present in the patient's lungs at the moment tracer gas breathing began, as we already know the concentration and volume that is inhaled at the beginning. The circuit required for this technique has higher resistance than the nitrogen washout method.

Both nitrogen washout and helium dilution techniques may underestimate FRC, because they measure only the lung volume that communicates with the airways. In patients with severe airflow limitation, a considerable volume of trapped gas may communicate very poorly or not at all.

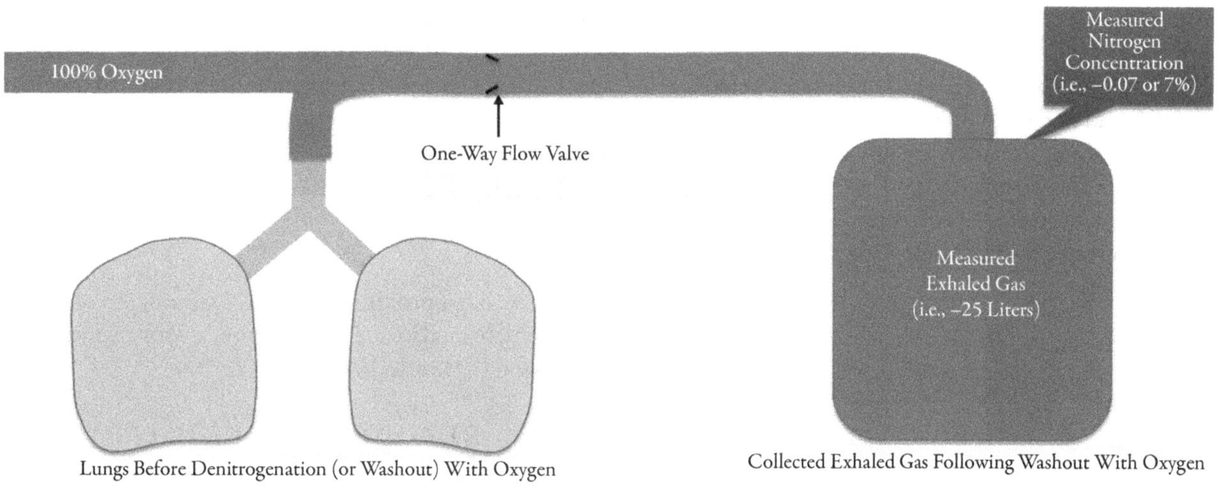

$$C_1V_1 = C_2V_2 \quad \rightarrow \quad V_1 = \frac{C_2V_2}{C_1}$$

Where...

C_1 = Concentration of nitrogen (N_2) (known, usually 0.75 or 75%) = $C_{alv}N_2$

V_1 = Volume of FRC (unknown) = V_{FRC}

C_2 = Postwashout concentration of N_2 (i.e., ~0.07 or 7%) = $C_{washout}\,N_2$

V_2 = Measured volume of collect gas following set time/exhaled volume (i.e., ~25 liters) = $V_{totalgas}$

So that...

$$V_{FRC} = \frac{C_{washout}N_2 * V_{totalgas}}{C_{alv}N_2} \quad \rightarrow \quad V_{FRC} = \frac{(0.07) * 25 \text{ liters}}{0.75} = 2.33 \text{ liters}$$

Figure 23.2 Nitrogen washout method. The patient is connected to a circuit that collects all exhaled gas. Nitrogen concentration at room air is known, then the patient is administered 100% oxygen in order to calculate the FRC. Sample calculations as shown.

7. Inspiratory capacity (IC): The maximum volume that can be inspired from end expiratory level or resting respiratory level. It is about 2.5–3.5 L. It is the sum of IRV and TV. Measurement of IC can be a simple test to determine the extrathoracic obstruction.
8. Vital capacity (VC): It is the maximum volume of gas expired from the maximal inspiratory level or fully inflated lungs. It is obtained by summing IRV, TV, and ERV and measures around 4 to 6 L or 60–70 mL/kg in a healthy subject. Changes in inspiratory capacity have a similar effect on VC. Vital capacity depends on the body habitus, respiratory muscle strength, and lung compliance. It can be correlated clinically with maximal deep inspiration and effective coughing. Various pathological conditions like restrictive lung diseases including pulmonary edema, atelectasis, pleural effusion, and pneumothorax and physiological conditions such as pregnancy decrease the vital capacity (VC).
9. Closing volume (CV): The volume of lung at which small airways unsupported by cartilage and more dependent parts of lung begin to close during expiration. Closing volume is normally less than FRC and more than RV. It is clinically demonstrated by expiration to residual volume, which is inevitably followed by a sigh to reexpand the collapsed lung.
10. Closing capacity (CC): This is the sum of closing volume and residual volume. It increases by age. At 44 years of age, CC equals FRC in the supine position, and at 66 years of age, CC is greater than FRC in the upright position. This increase of CC is due to the decrease in FRC with age. As age increases, FRC goes below the CC and the alveoli collapse at the resting state. This creates a shunt called the "intrapulmonary shunt," causing hypoxemia.

DYNAMIC LUNG VOLUMES

1. Forced vital capacity (FVC): It is measured as the volume of air that can be expired forcefully and rapidly after maximal inspiration. It is an important component of pulmonary function testing. When exhalation is occurring rapidly and forcefully, it increases the intrapleural pressure significantly without an effect on airway pressures. Thus this causes more bronchiolar collapse and air trapping in patients with obstructive lung diseases, leading to low FVC even though VC appears within normal limits. The FVC is also lower in the restrictive lung diseases. Forced vital capacity is important to determine the airway resistance and gives useful information about the strength of the respiratory muscles and other aspects of pulmonary function. Normal FVC is ~4L or 50–60 mL/kg in normal 70-kg adults. Measurement of FVC depends on the patient's efforts.
2. Forced expiratory volume: The volume of air exhaled forcefully over a given time interval during the FVC maneuver. Around 75% volume of FVC is expired during the first second (FEV1), which is the most significant clinical value. The FEV1/FVC ratio clinically correlates with the degree of airway obstruction. The FEV1/FVC is normal in restrictive pathology, as the total lung volume is uniformly decreased. But patients with obstructive lung pathology show reduced FEV1/FVC, as FEV1 is reduced significantly as compared with FVC. Normal FEV1/FVC is greater than 0.75, or 75% of FVC.

VENTILATION

During normal respiration, oxygen in the fresh air enters the lung and CO_2 is exhaled. *Minute ventilation* is TV times the respiratory frequency, which is usually 7–8 L/min (may be approximated as 0.1 L/kg). It is important to note that all the fresh air from the tidal breath does not reach the alveoli. Some air remains in the conducting airways and does not actually participate in gas exchange. This is called *dead space ventilation* (VD), which is about 100–150 mL (0.1–0.2 mL/kg). Alveolar ventilation is the part of ventilation that reaches alveoli and participates in gas exchange.

$$\text{As such: Alveolar ventilation } (\dot{V}A) = \text{respiratory rate} \times (TV - VD)$$

The VA is approximately 5 L, similar to cardiac output, which is also 5 L. Therefore, overall ventilation ($\dot{V}$) Perfusion ($\dot{Q}$) ratio $\dot{V}/\dot{Q} \sim 1$.

DEAD SPACE VENTILATION

There are three types of dead space ventilation: anatomical, alveolar, and physiological.

Anatomical Dead Space

The part of inspired volume that is expired without taking part in the alveolar gas exchange (unchanged gas) is called dead space. Most of the dead space belongs to this category (anatomical dead space) in a normal individual and constitutes about 2 mL/kg of body weight. For example, the trachea would fall into this category. An endotracheal tube in effect extends anatomical dead space up unto the point where the Y-connector is located (effectively, where the lips or nose would equivalently be located).

Alveolar Dead Space

The air in unperfused alveoli constitutes alveolar dead space. The cause is inadequate perfusion of the alveoli, as seen in a pulmonary embolus, with normal gas distribution. Alveoli with no perfusion → $\dot{V}/\dot{Q} = \infty$

Physiological Dead Space

The sum of more than two dead spaces is called physiological dead space. These three types of dead space are explained in Figure 23.3. As we have already discussed, TV in an average adult is 450 mL, and VD/TV is about 33%. This ratio can be derived by the Bohr equation:

$$\frac{VD}{VT} = \frac{P_{ACO_2} - P_{ECO_2}}{P_{ACO_2}},$$

where $PACO_2$ is alveolar CO_2 tension and $PECO_2$ is mixed expired oxygen tension. This equation is based on the concept that all the CO_2 expired is from the alveolar gas. The Bohr equation is important because in classical respiratory physiologic teaching, the dead space fraction should be ≤ 0.60 (60%) in order for a patient to meet extubation criteria.

Factors Affecting Dead Space

1. Factors that increase dead space
   - Upright posture
   - Neck extension
   - Age
   - Positive pressure ventilation
   - Anticholinergic causing bronchodilation
   - Pulmonary emboli, hypotension
   - Lung diseases like COPD
2. Factors that decrease dead space
   - Supine posture
   - Neck flexion
   - Artificial airway like endotracheal tube

Total dead space can be calculated from partial pressure of CO_2 in the alveolus ($P_{Alv}CO_2$), the PCO_2 of arterial blood ($PaCO_2$), the PCO_2 of inspired air ($PICO_2$), and the TV Bohr equation. It is important to note that end-tidal CO_2 as acquired on the average anesthesia machine is not an accurate reflection of alveolar CO_2; this would have to be attained using a Douglas bag.

$$P_{Alv}CO_2 \times VT = PaCO_2 \times (V_T - V_D) + P_ICO_2 \times V_D$$

LUNG MECHANICS

The movement of the lung is passive and occurs secondary to external forces produced by ventilator muscles. These forces are divided into *elastic resistance* and *nonelastic resistance.*

ELASTIC RESISTANCE

Elastic resistance is exerted by (1) the elastic resistance of the tissue and (2) the gas-liquid interface.

Elastic Resistance of the Tissue (Lung and Chest)

Elastic resistance of the tissue plays a significant role in the mechanism of normal breathing. When exposed to

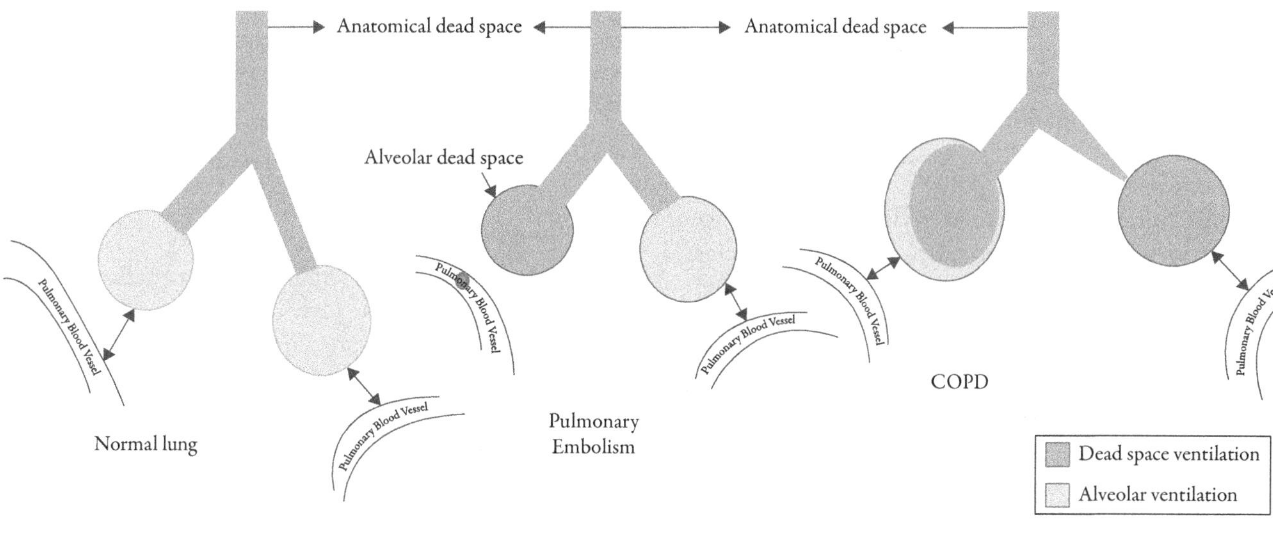

Figure 23.3 Dead space ventilation physiologically described. Adapted from Hedenstierna G. Respiratory physiology. In: Miller R, ed. *Miller's Anesthesia*. 7th ed. Philadelphia, PA: Elsevier; 2010. Figure 15–1.

the atmosphere, the lung has tendency to expand outward. The normal tendency of lung is to collapse due to its composition of elastic fibers, resulting in resting passive expiration. The elastic behavior of the lung can be measured in terms of *compliance.* Compliance of any tissue is its tendency to return back to its original size and shape after the deforming pressure is withdrawn.

Measurements of compliance for the lung, chest wall, or both combined can be obtained under static or dynamic conditions:

1. **Static compliance**—measures the elastic resistance to airflow when the airflow rate is 0.
2. **Dynamic compliance**—measures elastic as well as nonelastic resistance to airflow.

Static Compliance

Static compliance is called effective compliance. Compliance of the lung (C_L) is defined as the amount of pressure required to change per unit volume of lung.

$$C_L = \frac{\text{Change in unit lung volume}}{\text{Change in Transpulmonary pressure}} = \frac{\Delta V}{\Delta P}$$

Normal lung compliance is 0.2–0.3 L/cmH_2O. The pressure needed to keep the lung inflated at a certain volume is the *transpulmonary pressure*, which is defined as the difference between the intrapleural pressure and the alveolar pressure. Compliance has a critical relationship with lung volume. Compliance is high at low lung volumes and low at high lung volumes. Compliance also differs with the different phases of breathing. It increases slightly during deflation and decreases during inflation. To calculate static compliance in mechanically ventilated and paralyzed patients, the plateau pressure is used, which is measured during an inspiratory pause on the ventilator.

Factors influencing lung compliance are lung volume, pulmonary blood volume, extravascular lung fluid, and pathological process (inflammation and fibrosis).

Dynamic Compliance

Dynamic compliance is measured during actual movement of air in the airway. Normally, at low or moderate flow, static and dynamic compliance are approximately same. But dynamic compliance decreases at high frequency due the difference in time constants. This is because the time to fill the alveoli depends on product of airway resistance (R_{aw}) and compliance. Due to the difference in compliance in different parts of the lung, some alveoli in reduced-compliance zones distend slowly as compared with those in very compliant zones. To calculate dynamic compliance, peak airway pressure is used when patient is on ventilator.

Surface Tension Forces (Gas-liquid interface)

The alveoli are lined with a gas-fluid interface, causing them behave like bubbles. This creates surface tension forces, which favor alveolar collapse. According to Laplace's law, pressure within the alveoli can be measure as:

$$\text{Pressure} = \frac{2 \times \text{surface tension}}{\text{radius}}$$

Therefore, alveolar collapse is directly proportional to surface tension. To nullify the effect of surface tension, the alveolar lining produces surfactant. This helps in reducing alveolar surface tension. The ability to decrease surface tension depends on the concentration of surfactant. The smaller the alveoli, the more concentrated the surfactant and the less collapse of alveoli. Larger alveoli have decreased concentration and increased surface tension. This prevents smaller alveoli from collapsing and larger alveoli from overdistention.

Hysteresis

Surface tension in alveoli increases up to 40 mN/m during inspiration and decreases to 15 mN/m during expiration. The pressure within larger alveoli increases due to the decreased concentration of surfactant, and vice versa. Thus gas flow develops from larger to smaller alveoli. The difference in surface tension during inspiration and expiration creates hysteresis of alveoli, forming two pressure volume curves. These two curves form a hysteresis loop that becomes wider with an increase in tidal volume. Hysteresis plays an important role in maintaining normal lung compliance. See Figure 23.4.

NONELASTIC RESISTANCE

Nonelastic resistance is composed of (1) airway resistance to gas flow (R_{aw}) and (2) tissue resistance.

Airway Resistance

Pressure is required to overcome the resistance offered by the airway to the airflow. Airway resistance (R_{aw}) can be calculated as:

$$R_{aw} = \frac{\text{Driving pressure}}{\text{Gas flow}}$$

During inspiration, the driving pressure equals the atmospheric pressure minus the alveolar pressure. During expiration, the driving pressure equals the transpulmonary pressure minus the pleural pressure. The gas flow pattern plays a major role in determining airway resistance. Gas flow is a combination of laminar and turbulent flows.

Laminar Flow

Laminar flow is a streamlined flow composed of concentric cylinders having variable velocities that are greater

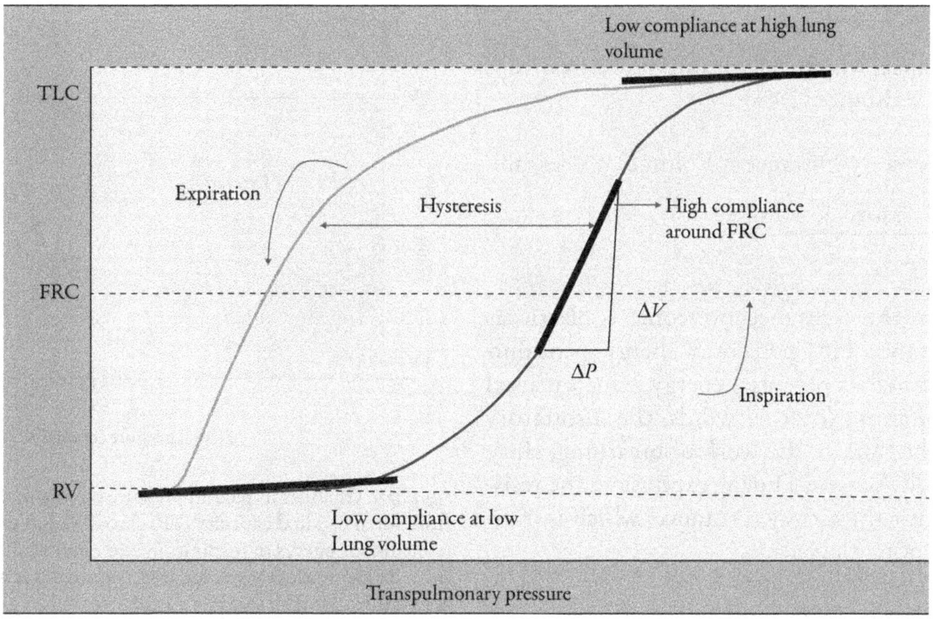

Figure 23.4 Pressure volume curve showing lung volumes related to compliance.

Adapted from: http://www.biomedsearch.com/attachments/00/16/91/91/16919173/1471-2466-6-21-7.jpg

at the center and lesser at the walls of airway (imagine soldiers marching in an organized formation, they would move efficiently though a conduit or stricture). Molecularly, this forms a cone-shaped flow.

R_{aw} during laminar flow is calculated with Poiseuille's equation (easily testable concept):

$$R_{aw} = \frac{8 \times \text{length} \times \text{gas viscosity}}{\pi \times \text{radius}^4}$$

Resistance to laminar flow is directly related to the length of the airway and the viscosity of the gas. And it is inversely related to the fourth power of the radius of the airway. Thus, as the radius of smaller airway decreases due to bronchospasm, the airway resistance increases by the fourth power. And as the length of the tube and viscosity of air increase, the resistance also increases.

Turbulent Flow

Turbulent flow takes place when the airway diameter, density of gas, and velocity are greater. The probability of turbulent flow is decided by the Reynolds number:

$$\text{Reynolds number} = \frac{\text{linear velocity} \times \text{diameter} \times \text{gas density}}{\text{Gas viscosity}}$$

A low Reynolds number (<1000) yields laminar flow, whereas a high Reynolds number (>1500) yields turbulent flow. Turbulent flow is mathematically described as:

$$\text{Pressure gradient} \approx \text{Flow}^2 \times \frac{\text{Gas density}}{\text{Radius}^5}$$

Therefore resistance is directly proportional to density and inversely proportionate to the fifth power of the radius. Density is the most relevant physical property in turbulent flow.

Normal airway resistance is approximately 0.5–1.5 $cmH_2O/L/s$, calculated by body plethysmography with a 0.5-L/s flow rate (quiet breathing).

Tissue Resistance

Tissue resistance is resistance offered by viscoelastic tissue to airflow. It offers around 20% of total nonelastic resistance. This type of resistance is less clinically significant than airflow resistance.

TIME CONSTANT

There are regional differences in ventilation due to differences in compliance and resistance, as discussed previously. Lung alveoli in different parts require variable time to inflate to maximum capacity. The time constant is the time required to inflate alveoli to 60% of filling capacity if the filling pressure is constant. An increase in resistance and/or decrease in compliance increases the time constant. A normal time constant is 0.5 seconds; this concept is usually applied when managing patients with acute respiratory distress syndrome (ARDS) or COPD.

WORK OF BREATHING

The act of breathing is performed by respiratory muscles, which require mechanical work as well as metabolic work reflected by oxygen consumption. The work of breathing (WOB) is performed to overcome two major factors:

- Elastic recoil (65% WOB)
- Nonelastic resistance, which includes airway resistance (80%) and tissue resistance (20%)

$$\text{Work} = \text{Force} \times \text{Distance} = \text{Volume} \times \text{Pressure}$$

$$\text{Elastic work} = \frac{\text{Pressure} \times \text{volume}}{2}$$

During inspiration, the resistance overcome is elastic as well as airway resistance. Fifty percent of energy spent during inspiration is stored as potential energy, which is used during passive expiration; in other words, the inspiratory process performs the bulk of the work of breathing, since expiration is primarily passive. During expiration, the resistance overcome is just the airway resistance, which is overcome by the stored potential energy.

Work of Breathing During Different Ventilator Patterns:

As respiratory rate increases, flow rate increases, which in turn increases the airway resistance.

As tidal volume (TV) increases, elastic work increases.

To decrease the work of breathing, patients with decreased lung compliance increase respiratory frequency, and patients with obstructive lung disease with increased airflow resistance have slow and deep breaths. Figure 23.5 explains the work of breathing.

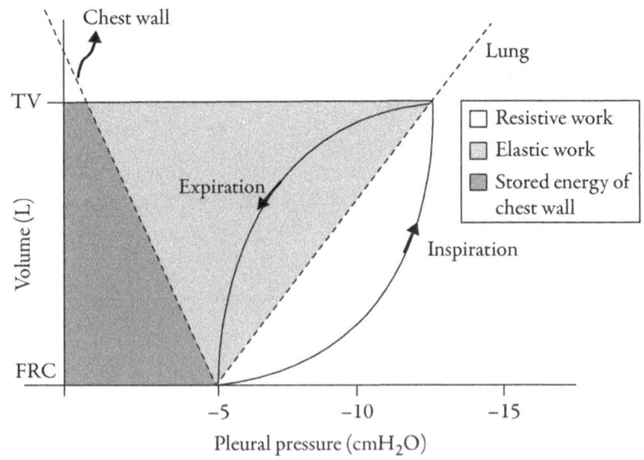

Figure 23.5 Changes in pleural pressure during inspiration from functional residual capacity (FRC) to TV, and the following expiration (continuous curves of inspiration and expiration). The dashed lines indicate the static P-V curves of lungs and chest wall (which are not seen clinically). The total inspiratory work is represented by the whole area at the left of the inspiration P-V curve. A portion of it (gray-dotted area diagonal lines) is contributed by the expanding action of the chest wall.

FLOW-VOLUME LOOP

The flow-volume loop depicts flow generated by breathing deeply to total lung capacity and then forcibly and rapidly breathing out to residual volume, which is plotted on the Y-axis, against the volume of air expired, which is plotted on the X-axis. It is graphically recorded using a spirometer. The normal flow-volume loop is shown in Figure 23.6.

Changes in the flow-volume loop contour help in diagnosis of large airway and extrathoracic airway obstruction in addition to providing the values of FEV1 and FVC. This is a part of pulmonary function testing and is highly dependent on the patient's efforts. Due to the availability of high-resolution imaging techniques, the flow-volume loop plays a less prominent role in the diagnosis of obstructive lung disease.

REGULATION OF AIRWAY CALIBER

Airway caliber is controlled by various factors like neural, humoral, and physical properties of inspired air and locally released molecules, for example, inflammatory mediators (Figure 23.7).

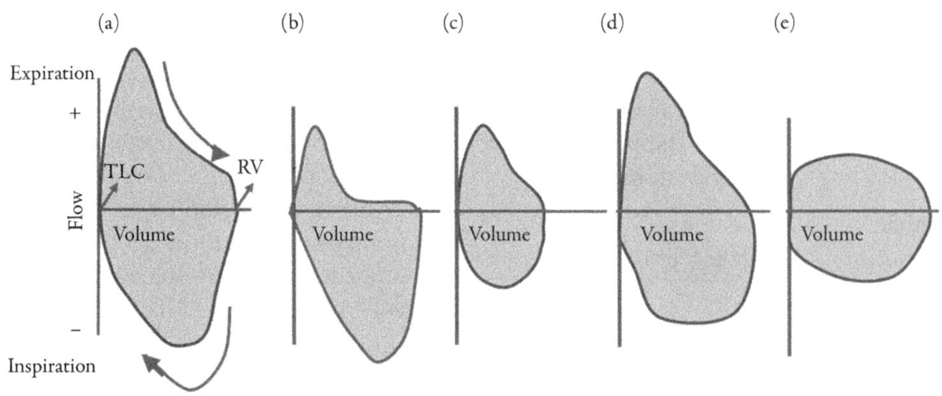

Figure 23.6 Normal flow-volume loops with variations resulting from disease processes. a: Normal. b: Intrathoracic obstruction. c: Restriction. d: Variable extrathoracic obstruction. e: Fixed airway obstruction.

Adapted from: Anatomy, development, and physiology of the lungs, Figure 5—Flow-volume loops. Nature.com. http://www.nature.com/gimo/contents/pt1/fig_tab/gimo73_F5.html#figure-title. Accessed April 2, 2015.

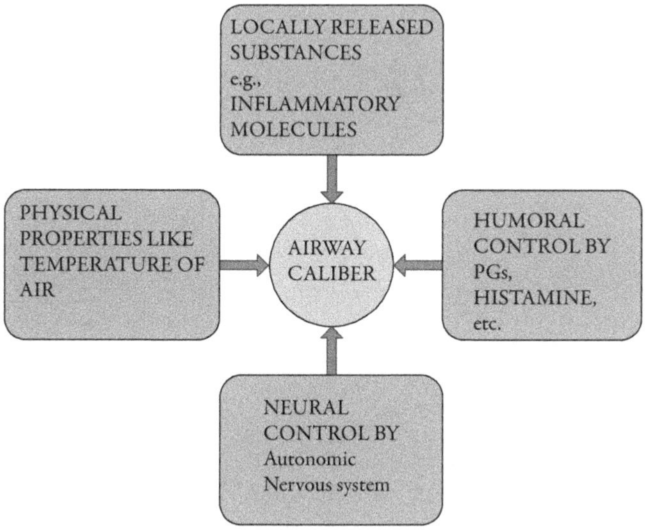

Figure 23.7 Physiologic factors regulating airway caliber.

AUTONOMIC NERVOUS SYSTEM

Cholinergic muscarinic receptors are stimulated by the vagus nerve and cause bronchoconstriction. Additionally, adrenalin can stimulate the adrenergic β_2 receptors, which causes bronchodilation.

DISTRIBUTION OF VENTILATION AND PERFUSION

The primary function of the lung is oxygenation of the blood and removal of CO_2, which occurs at the alveolar-capillary membrane level. To achieve that, alveolar ventilation and pulmonary capillary perfusion matching is most important.

DISTRIBUTION OF PULMONARY BLOOD FLOW

The distribution of pulmonary blood flow in the lungs is not uniform. Because of the nonrigid composition of the alveolar-capillary beds, the pressure of the surrounding tissues, such as alveolar pressure and pulmonary venous pressure, has an effect on the resistance to the blood flow in the capillaries. Also pulmonary blood flow is gravity dependent, therefore pulmonary artery pressure increases by 1 cmH2O/cm distance down the lung (as blood density ~ 1). According to the different relationship between alveolar, pulmonary artery, and venous pressures, West et al. described three *physiologic* zones of the lung (Figure 23.8). It is important to note that these zones describe physiology and not necessarily anatomic position.

Zone I

Alveolar pressure (PA) is uniform throughout the lung, and pulmonary artery pressure (Pa) is approximately 0 at the apex in the upright position. Pulmonary venous pressure (Pv) is always lower than pulmonary arterial pressure in normal physiological conditions. The relation between the three pressures is PA > Pa > Pv. So the blood flow depends on the alveolar arterial pressure difference. This is called the collapse zone or alveolar dead space, which does not exist normally. It occurs with hypovolemia and

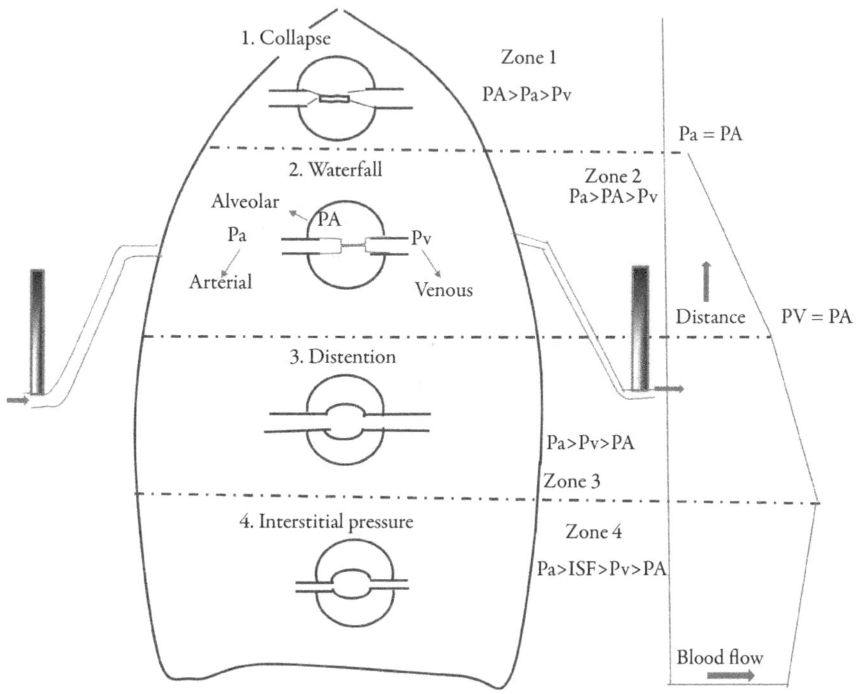

Figure 23.8 West zones diagrammatically described.

increased alveolar pressures. In effect, it is all gas and no blood in the lung.

Zone II

As we go down the lung (physiologically) Pa increases above PA. Therefore Pa > PA > Pv. This is described as a waterfall zone. The perfusion pressure is determined by the difference between the arterial and alveolar pressures. The capillary blood flow is intermittent and varies with respiration.

Zone III

Farther down the lung (physiologically) arterial as well as venous pressures exceed that of alveolar pressure. Pa > Pv > PA. Capillary perfusion is continuous and depends on the arterial and venous pressure gradients. This becomes clinically relevant with situations such as pulmonary artery catheter (PAC or Swan-Ganz) placement; if the catheter is intended to measure the pressure in the left atrium, there needs to be a continuous fluid column between the catheter and the atrium. If the Swan is pointing upward, toward Zone 1, then theoretically the pressures measured do not reflect the left atrium because there is no continuous fluid column.

Recently, **Zone IV** has been added, in which the interstitial pressure causes compression of the vessel wall, interrupting the flow.

DISTRIBUTION OF VENTILATION

Although alveolar pressure is constant throughout the lung, alveolar ventilation is unevenly distributed. The right lung, the base of the lung, and dorsal portions of lung in upright and supine postures, respectively, are better-ventilated parts of the lung. Different parts of the lungs are placed on different points of the compliance curve, and as such, dependent parts are better ventilated due to the effect of gravity. It increases the intrapleural pressure (less negative) and decreases the transpulmonary pressures as one samples further caudally in the lung (Figure 23.9). Pleural pressure becomes less negative by 1 cmH_2O per 3-cm decrease in height of the lung (specific density of fluid filled and perfused lung ~ 0.3). Compliance of the lung increases as the transpulmonary pressure decreases. As a result, during inspiration, the alveoli in the dependent parts, with smaller resting volumes and lower transpulmonary pressures, expand more easily than the alveoli at the apex, which are fully inflated.

VENTILATION ($\dot{V}_A$) AND PERFUSION ($\dot{Q}$) RELATIONSHIP

As we discussed previously, the gravity-dependent parts of lung receive more perfusion as well as ventilation compared with the apical region. Also, ventilation and perfusion are not perfectly matched, as perfusion increases more rapidly

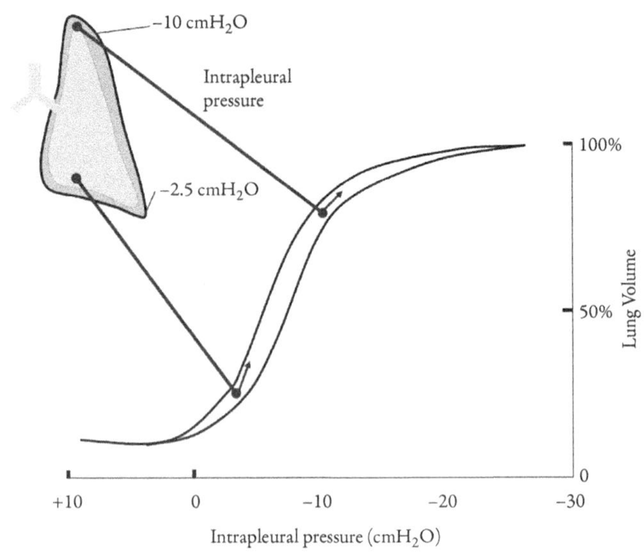

Figure 23.9 Intrapleural pressure and its relationship to lung volume.

than ventilation down the lung. This creates $\dot{V}_A/\dot{Q}$ ratios throughout the lung. The ideal $\dot{V}_A/\dot{Q}$ is 1 and it occurs somewhere in midportion of the lung. Above this portion, the $\dot{V}_A/\dot{Q}$ is greater than 1 (trending more toward dead space), and below this more perfusion is reflected by a $\dot{V}_A/\dot{Q}$ that is less than 1 (trending more toward shunt).

Hypoxic Pulmonary Vasoconstriction

Hypoxic pulmonary vasoconstriction (HPV) is a physiological mechanism by which the $\dot{V}_A/\dot{Q}$ ratio is maintained near normal. When bronchiolar constriction/obstruction occurs, hypoxia develops due to underventilation of that part of lung. Hypoxia directly acts on vascular smooth muscles, producing vasoconstriction shunting the blood away from the hypoxic area; this process is called hypoxic pulmonary vasoconstriction. Also, CO_2 accumulation leads to acidic pH in that area, which results in vasoconstriction of pulmonary vessels. This regional decrease in pulmonary blood flow reduces alveolar PCO_2, which leads to bronchiolar constriction shifting ventilation to better-perfused parts.

Shunt is described as a process whereby desaturated mixed venous blood from the right heart returns to the left heart without being resaturated with oxygen in the lungs. Intrapulmonary shunts occur when unventilated alveoli get perfused, causing dilution of arterial oxygen content.

Intrapulmonary shunts are of two types:

1. Absolute shunts are anatomic shunts where $\dot{V}/\dot{Q}$ is 0, which cannot be corrected.
2. Relative shunts are areas of the lung with low $\dot{V}/\dot{Q}$, which can be partially corrected by increasing the inspired oxygen concentration.

3. Atelectactic shunts are those where blood passes through the collapsed alveoli.

Venous admixture (Qs) mainly results in an increase in the difference between PAO_2 and PaO_2 across the alveolar-capillary membrane. It is the amount of mixed venous blood that would have to be mixed with the pulmonary end-capillary blood to account for the difference in oxygen tension between arterial and pulmonary end-capillary blood.

Venous admixture in a physiological shunt is typically less than 5% and can be used to calculate the virtual shunt fraction. The virtual shunt fraction is a calculation that reflects the degree of shunting occurring. The equation is:

$$\textbf{Virtual shunt fraction} = Qs / Q_t = (CcO_2 - CaO_2)/(CcO_2 - CvO_2)$$

CcO_2—oxygen content of the end-capillary blood in mL/100mL blood.

CaO_2—oxygen content of the arterial blood in mL/100mL blood

CvO_2—oxygen content of mixed venous blood in mL/100mL blood

Qs—Venous admixture

Q_t—Total cardiac output

DIFFUSION CAPACITY

The rate at which the gas molecules transfer through a membrane is diffusion capacity.

According to Fick's principle, diffusion capacity is proportionate:

- Directly to the area for transfer (A)
- Directly to gas tension difference across the membrane (P_1–P_2)
- Inversely to the thickness of the membrane (T)

Diffusion of gas:

$$\dot{V}\text{ gas} = \frac{A \times D}{T} \times (P_1 - P_2)$$

where D is diffusion constant.

Gas diffusion is determined by the following factors:

1. **Surface area available for diffusion**: has a linear relation with the diffusion capacity, but the surface area of the lung should be well perfused for better diffusion of oxygen.
2. **Thickness of the membrane**: has an inverse relation with diffusion capacity of gas. As thickness increases, solubility decreases. This is also true with fibrosis of the membrane.
3. **Difference in partial pressure (gas tension) across the membrane:** the greater the gradient across the alveolar-capillary membrane, the greater the diffusion of gas. Normal alveolar oxygen tension or partial pressure (PAO_2) is 100 mmHg, and partial pressure of oxygen in mixed venous blood (PvO_2) is 40 mmHg. This creates a gradient of 60 mmHg, which drives gases from alveoli to capillaries.
4. **Molecular weight of the gas:** diffusion capacity is inversely proportional to the molecular weight of the gas.
5. **Solubility of gas**: This can be explained by *Henry's law*, which states the amount of gas that dissolves in a unit volume of liquid at a given temperature is directly proportional to the partial pressure of the gas in the equilibrium phase. The more solubility, the more the partial pressure increases diffusion.

Diffusion of gases can be limited by flow or perfusion. Traditionally, the diagnostic gas to measure diffusion capacity is carbon monoxide, due to its high solubility; the resulting measure is termed the diffusion capacity of carbon monoxide (DLCO).

Factors influencing DLCO are:

1. Hemoglobin: carbon monoxide gets chemically bound to hemoglobin after it is diffused in the blood from alveoli. This causes a decrease in the partial pressure of carbon monoxide in the plasma. This creates a gradient between the alveolar and arterial partial pressure of carbon monoxide and increases further diffusion. Hence, a decrease in in Hb% decreases the DLCO.
2. Posture: Supine posture increases DLCO due to changes in the pulmonary circulation in supine posture.
3. Blood volume: Increased pulmonary capillary blood volume increases the DLCO.
4. Body size: Increased body size increases the surface area of diffusion.

OXYGEN UPTAKE AND CONTENT

Oxygen uptake depends on the function of ventilation and circulatory system. To know the oxygen uptake we need to know about the arterial oxygen content and oxygen flux. Oxygen content is the addition of hemoglobin (Hb)-bound oxygen and the physically dissolved oxygen in the plasma.

$$O_2Content = [SaO_2 \times Hb \times 1.38\ ml / dL\ blood] + [0.003ml\ O_2 / dl\ blood / mmHg \times PaO_2]$$

The solubility coefficient of oxygen is 0.003 mL/dL/mmHg. When Hemoglobin is 15 gm/dL, oxygen saturation of hemoglobin (SaO_2) is 98%, and PaO_2 is 100 mmHg, arterial oxygen content (CaO_2) and venous oxygen content (CvO_2) can be calculated. Total oxygen delivery to the tissues is synonymous with oxygen flux (DO_2), which is defined as cardiac output (Q_t) × CaO_2.

According to Fick's equation, the oxygen consumption or uptake ($\dot{V}O_2$) can be calculated as:

$$\dot{V}O_2 = Q_t \times (CaO_2 - CvO_2)$$

From this equation the normal extraction fraction for oxygen is (CaO_2 – CvO_2)/CaO_2, and body consumption of oxygen can be calculated.

ALVEOLAR GAS EQUATION

It is difficult to sample the air in the alveoli for measuring the partial pressure of oxygen. The alveolar gas equation calculates the partial pressure of oxygen in the alveoli (PAO_2). It is required to know how much inspired oxygen is finally available at the pulmonary capillary level or arterial level, and also calculates the alveolar-arterial oxygen difference. It is given as:

$$PAO_2 = PIO_2 - Pa_{CO2} / RQ$$

Where PIO_2 is partial pressure of oxygen in the inspired air, which is 21% in room air; Pa_{CO2} is partial pressure of CO_2 in arterial blood, and RQ is oxygen consumption over carbon dioxide production (must be measured). The PIO_2 can be calculated as: $PIO_2 = FIO_2 \times (P_B - P_{H2O})$. The FIO_2 is the fraction of oxygen in inspired air, P_B and P_{H2O} are barometric pressure (~760 mmHg) and water vapor pressure (47 mmHg), respectively, as the air gets humidified in the upper airway.

Carbon Dioxide Transport

Carbon dioxide is carried in the blood in three forms: dissolved in plasma, in the form of HCO_3, and chemically combined with proteins to form carbamino compounds. These three forms combine to give the total CO_2 content in the blood.

Dissolved CO_2 is more soluble in blood than oxygen. The solubility coefficient is 0.067 mL/dL/mmHg. In presence of enzyme carbonic anhydrase, erythrocytes and endothelial cells can combine CO_2 and H_2O to form carbonic acid and bicarbonate. The reaction is given as:

$$CO_2 + H_2O \leftrightarrow H_2CO_3 \leftrightarrow H^+ + HCO3^-.$$

Bicarbonate is the largest fraction of CO_2 in the blood. The CO_2 is transported to and fro from alveoli to pulmonary capillaries, which can be explained by the *Hamburger shift*. According to this effect, the CO_2 on the venous side enters red blood cells and is converted to HCO_3, as shown in the above reaction. The HCO_3 diffuses out of red blood cells into the plasma, and to maintain electrical neutrality, chloride ions move into red blood cells from the plasma. In the pulmonary capillaries reverse reactions happen. The HCO_3 reenters red blood cells in exchange with chloride ions and changes to CO_2, to be exhaled after diffusing in to the alveoli.

Apneic Oxygenation

Apneic oxygenation is an important process when performing a rapid-sequence intubation. In apneic patients, oxygen and CO_2 continue to diffuse from alveoli into the blood stream. Around 250 mL of oxygen and 8–10 mL of CO_2 moves from alveoli to capillary blood per minute. This causes a pressure drop in alveoli to become subatmospheric, generating a mass flow of air form pharynx to alveoli. Apneic oxygenation can help extend the safe apnea period that can be achieved with preoxygenation. Thus oxygenation can be maintained, but the individual can become hypercapneic and develop significant acidosis subsequently due to lack of ventilation.

DIFFUSION HYPOXIA

Diffusion hypoxia is also known as the Fink effect and the third gas effect. This is seen in patients who receive N_2O during anesthesia. When soluble gases like nitrous oxide are inhaled in large quantities, they are dissolved in body fluids rapidly. This results in a temporary increase in the concentration of oxygen and CO_2 in the alveolus, leading to an increase in their respective partial pressures. During recovery from N_2O anesthesia, large quantities of gas diffuse from pulmonary capillaries to the alveoli down their concentration gradient. Thus, for that period the oxygen and CO_2 concentrations in alveoli decrease, reducing their respective partial pressures. The decrease in the partial pressure of oxygen causes hypoxia temporarily, which is known as diffusion hypoxia. The decrease in CO_2 concentration can depress ventilation, which can lead to hypoxemia.

Diffusion hypoxia last only for few minutes and can be avoided by increasing the inspired oxygen concentration during recovery from anesthesia. This was first explained by Bernard Fink, and hence is named after him.

Anemia Blood

Physically dissolved in plasma (2%). Compared with CO_2, oxygen is relatively insoluble in plasma. 100 mL blood contains 0.3 mL of oxygen at PO_2 = 100 mmHg.

- Chemically bound to the hemoglobin molecule (Hb) in the red blood cells (98%). Hemoglobin can combine rapidly and reversibly with oxygen. The reversibility of this reaction allows oxygen to be released to the tissues. $Hb + O_2 = HbO_2$ (oxyhemoglobin).

Each gram of Hemoglobin can combine with 1.34 mL of oxygen. Normally, blood contains about 15 g Hemoglobin per 100 mL of blood [or 150 g/L]. Hence, the oxygen-carrying capacity of Hemoglobin is 15 × 1.34 = 20 mL oxygen/100 mL blood. The amount of oxygen in the blood (sum of both forms, dissolved and bound to Hemoglobin) is called the oxygen content of blood and is described in mL oxygen per 100 mL blood (or volume %). The oxygen content of arterial blood (CaO_2) is about 20 vol%; the oxygen content of venous blood (CvO_2) about 15 vol%. Therefore, each time blood circulates through the circulation, 5 vol % of oxygen is taken up by the tissues. The proportion of Hemoglobin that is bound to oxygen is called percent saturation and is written as % Hb saturation or, often clinically for arterial blood, as S_aO_2.

It is important to note that both oxygen-carrying capacity and oxygen content depend on the amount of Hemoglobin in an individual's blood and are expressed as volume of oxygen per unit volume of blood. The S_aO_2 and oxygen content are not interchangeable. For example, two patients may have the same S_aO_2, but if one has a low blood Hemoglobin concentration because of anemia, that patient will have lower oxygen content. Combining these concepts, one can more easily recall the formula describing oxygen content:

$$\mathbf{CaO_2\,(oxygen\ content)} = 1.34 \times Hb \times SaO_2 + PaO_2 \times 0.0034$$

FACTORS THAT AFFECT OXYGEN TRANSPORT IN THE BLOOD

- *Anemia*: The association of oxygen and hemoglobin expressed as % Hb saturation is not affected, but the association of oxygen and hemoglobin expressed as arterial content of blood is reduced because the decreased amount of hemoglobin per 100 mL blood decreases the oxygen-carrying capacity of the blood.
- *Carbon monoxide (CO):* The affinity of hemoglobin for carbon monoxide is 240 times that for oxygen. Carbon monoxide competitively blocks the combination of oxygen with hemoglobin. Carbon monoxide-bound hemoglobin is called carboxyhemoglobin (COHb). Carbon monoxide also shifts the oxyhemoglobin dissociation curve to the left. Together these characteristics of CO can lead to severe tissue hypoxia. A patient breathing CO can slowly reach life-threatening levels of COHb. Carbon monoxide is colorless, odorless, and tasteless, and does not elicit reflexes such as coughing or sneezing. It does not increase ventilation or result in a sensation of shortness of breath (dyspnea). Small amounts of COHb are present in normal individuals due to urban pollution or smoking. A nonsmoker living in a rural area may have only 1% COHb in the blood; whereas a heavy smoker living in urban area can have 5%–8% COHb in the blood.

THE OXYHEMOGLOBIN DISSOCIATION CURVE

Functions of Hemoglobin

Hemoglobin is a conjugated protein consisting of heme and globin, which is found in red blood cells (erythrocytes). Hemoglobin is responsible for giving red color to our blood. It is a great source of energy metabolism and also plays a pivotal role in respiration. It interacts with nitric oxide in order to regulate the blood pressure. Hemoglobin also acts as an antioxidant and regulates metabolism of iron in macrophages and alveolar and mesangial cells in the kidney. Importantly, hemoglobin carries CO_2 from tissues to the lungs and oxygen from the lungs to the tissues (see Figure 23.10).

The oxyhemoglobin dissociation curve describes the nonlinear tendency for oxygen to bind to hemoglobin. The oxyhemoglobin dissociation curve is an important tool for understanding how our blood carries and releases oxygen. Specifically, the oxyhemoglobin dissociation curve relates oxygen saturation (SO_2) and partial pressure of oxygen in the blood (PO_2), and is determined by what is called "hemoglobin's affinity for oxygen," that is, how readily hemoglobin acquires and releases oxygen molecules from its surrounding tissue. The lack of linearity of the curve makes interpretation of the oxygen content of blood difficult.

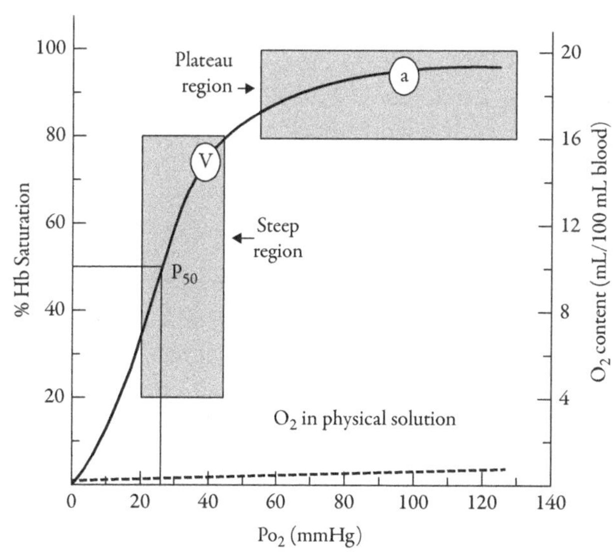

Figure 23.10 Oxyhemoglobin dissociation curve comparing arterial and venous oxygen content.

Understanding the Dissociation Curve

In its basic form, the oxyhemoglobin dissociation curve describes the relation between the partial pressure of oxygen (X-axis) and the oxygen saturation (Y-axis). Hemoglobin's affinity for oxygen increases as successive molecules of oxygen bind. More molecules bind as the oxygen partial pressure increases, until the maximum amount that can be bound is reached. As this limit is approached, very little additional binding occurs, and the curve levels out as the hemoglobin becomes saturated with oxygen. Hence, the curve has a sigmoidal or S shape. At oxygen partial pressures above about 60 mmHg, the standard dissociation curve is relatively flat, which means that the oxygen content of the blood does not change significantly even with large increases in the oxygen partial pressure (see formula for oxygen content). To get more oxygen to the tissue would require blood transfusions to increase the hemoglobin count (and hence the oxygen-carrying capacity), or supplemental oxygen that would increase the oxygen dissolved in plasma.

2,3-DIPHOSPHOGLYCERATE

2,3-Bisphosphoglycerate (2,3-BPG) is formed from 1,3-BPG by the enzyme BPG mutase. It can then be broken down by 2,3-BPG phosphatase to form 3-phosphoglycerate (Figure 23.11). Its synthesis and breakdown are, therefore, a way around a step of glycolysis, with the net expense of one ATP per molecule of 2,3-BPG generated as the high-energy carboxylic acid-phosphate mixed anhydride bond is cleaved by bisphosphoglycerate mutase.

As such, 2,3-bisphosphoglycerate is an organophosphate, which is created in erythrocytes during glycolysis. The production of 2,3-DPG is likely an important adaptive mechanism, because the production increases for several conditions in the presence of diminished peripheral tissue oxygen availability, such as hypoxemia, chronic lung disease, anemia, and congestive heart failure, among others. High levels of 2,3-DPG shift the curve to the right (as in childhood), while low levels of 2,3-DPG cause a leftward shift, seen in states such as septic shock, and hypophosphataemia.[1] In the absence of 2,3-DPG, hemoglobin's affinity for oxygen increases. 2,3 DPG as a heteroallosteric effector of hemoglobin, lowers hemoglobin's affinity for oxygen by binding preferentially to deoxyhemoglobin. An increased concentration of DPG in red blood cells favors formation of the T, low-affinity state of hemoglobin and so the oxygen-binding curve will shift to the right (Figure 23.12).

RESPIRATORY ENZYMES

Respiratory enzymes and mitochondrial membranes are normally synthesized in a coordinated fashion, the proportions of the various components being characteristic for a given cell.[2] Regulation of the amounts of enzyme in mammalian cells depends on environmental conditions; for example, on oxygen tension[3–6] and on hormonal levels but not on glucose levels.[4–7] **P50** is the oxygen tension at half saturation (50%) of blood and is calculated from the measured oxygen tension and oxygen saturation by extrapolation along the oxygen dissociation curve to 50% saturation.

Some Important Terms

Factors that increase hemoglobin-oxygen affinity will shift the curve to the left and decrease p50, and factors decreasing hemoglobin-oxygen affinity will shift the curve to the right and increase p50. These shifts are a result of changes in the molecular configuration of hemoglobin (allosteric effects), which influence the avidity of hemoglobin-oxygen binding. For example, when 2,3-DPG binds to the beta chain of reduced hemoglobin, it causes the molecular configuration to change from the relaxed to the tense form. The tense molecular form has a smaller central cavity to bind oxygen, and hemoglobin-oxygen affinity is decreased. Factors increasing p50 include acidemia, hypercapnia (which has an additional right-shifting influence independent of its effect on pH), high levels of erythrocytic organic phosphates (of which 2,3-DPG is the most important in humans), and fever. Conversely, p50 is decreased by alkalemia, hypocapnia, low 2,3-DPG levels, and hypothermia.

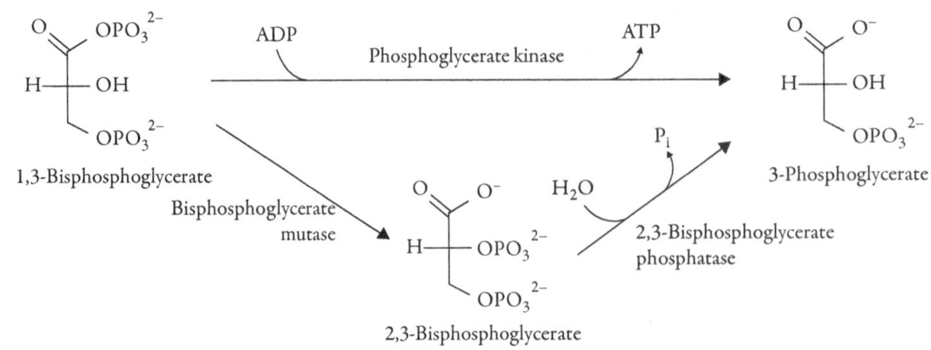

Figure 23.11 Pathway of generation of 2,3-bisphosphoglycerate http://en.wikipedia.org/wiki/File:Pathway_of_generation_of_2,3-bisphosphoglycerate.png

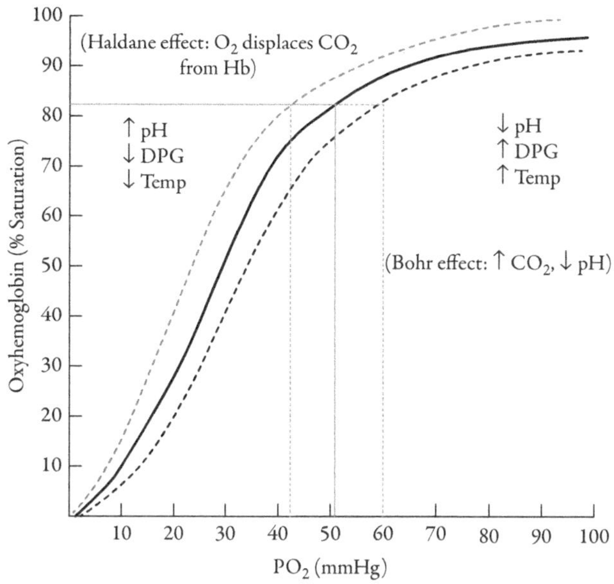

Figure 23.12 Oxyhemoglobin dissociation curve. Dotted red line corresponds with shift to the right caused by Bohr Effect. http://en.wikipedia.org/wiki/Oxygen–haemoglobin_dissociation_curve#mediaviewer/File:Oxyhaemoglobin_dissociation_curve.png

How to Calculate p50

Highly accurate determination of p50 requires construction of the hemoglobin-oxygen dissociation curve, or at least a Hill plot, both of which are laboratory procedures. In the intensive care unit or the operating room, measurement of blood gases and hemoglobin-oxygen saturation with a blood gas analyzer and a co-oximeter allows calculation of p50 using the Siggaard-Andersen oxygen status algorithm, provided the hemoglobin-oxygen saturation is less than 97%.[8] If this value is exceeded, venous blood can be used. These single-point calculations of p50 are sufficiently accurate for clinical purposes unless there are severe perturbations of acid-base balance or 2,3-DPG concentrations, which change the shape of the hemoglobin-oxygen dissociation curve.[9]

CARBON DIOXIDE TRANSPORT AND CONTENT

Carbon dioxide is transported in blood more readily than oxygen because CO_2 is *20 times more soluble than oxygen* in plasma (this is a key fact). The amount of CO_2 in the blood (CO_2 content) is described as mL CO_2 per 100 mL blood (or volume %). The CO_2 content of arterial blood ($CaCO_2$) is 48 vol%; the CO_2 content of venous blood ($CvCO_2$) is 52 vol%. Therefore, each time blood circulates through the body, 4 vol% of CO_2 is removed from the tissues and delivered to the lungs to be exhaled. Carbon dioxide is transported in three forms in the blood (Figure 23.13):

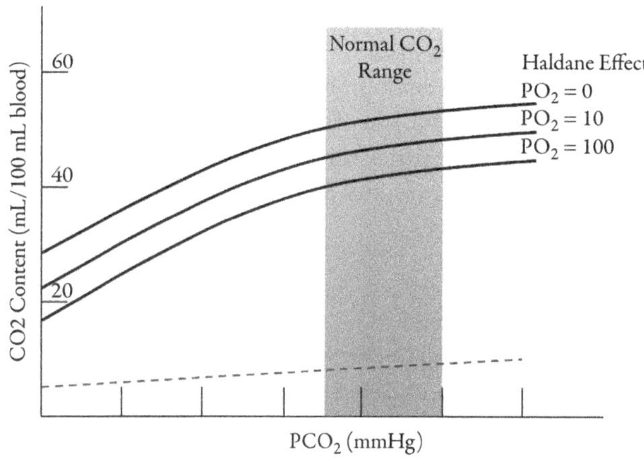

Figure 23.13 CO_2 content in blood as described by the Haldane effect. Image courtesy of George Williams, MD.

- physically dissolved (5%)
- physically dissolved as bicarbonate ion (90%)
- combined with hemoglobin as carbamino-compound (5%)

THE CARBON DIOXIDE DISSOCIATION CURVE

The relationship between the PCO_2 and the whole blood CO_2 content (in all three forms mentioned above) is known as the CO_2 dissociation curve. Within the range of normal blood PCO_2, the curve is nearly a straight line. Transport of CO_2 is dependent on oxygen release. The CO_2 dissociation curve is influenced by the state of oxygenation of the hemoglobin (Haldane effect). The *Haldane effect* is a property of hemoglobin first described by John Scott Haldane.[10,11] Deoxygenation of the blood increases its ability to carry CO_2; this property is the Haldane effect. Conversely, oxygenated blood has a reduced capacity for CO_2. The Haldane effect describes how oxygen concentrations determine hemoglobin's affinity for CO_2. For example, high oxygen concentrations enhance the unloading of CO_2. The converse is also true: low oxygen concentrations promote loading of CO_2 onto hemoglobin. In both situations, it is oxygen that causes the change in CO_2 levels.

The *Bohr effect* is a physiological phenomenon first described in 1904 by the Danish physiologist Christian Bohr, stating that hemoglobin's oxygen-binding affinity is inversely related both to acidity and to the concentration of CO_2.[12] In other words, it is an effect by which an increase of CO_2 in the blood and a decrease in pH results in a reduction of the affinity of hemoglobin for oxygen.

The simplest way to differentiate the two effects is to identify which molecule is the cause of the change. To further illustrate the difference, it might help to look at specific examples. In the lungs, when hemoglobin loaded with CO_2 is exposed to high oxygen levels, hemoglobin's affinity for CO_2 decreases. *This is an example of the Haldane effect.*

In active muscles, CO_2 and H^+ levels are high. Oxygenated blood that flows past is affected by these conditions, and the affinity of hemoglobin for oxygen is decreased, allowing oxygen to be transferred to the tissues. Because we are looking at the situation from the perspective of CO_2 changing oxygen affinity, *this is an example of the Bohr effect.*

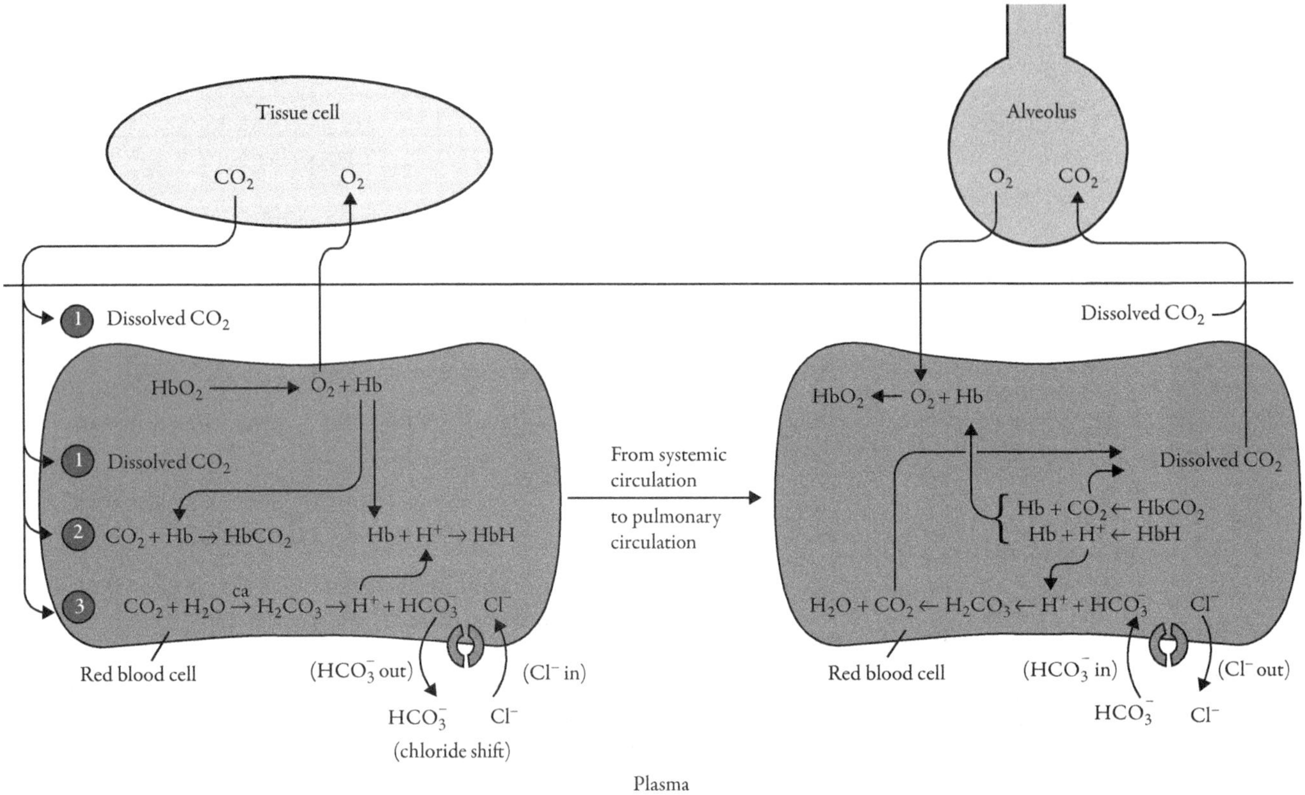

Gas Exchange at the Tissues

As CO_2 leaves the tissue cells and enters the red blood cells, it causes more oxygen to dissociate from hemoglobin (Bohr shift); thus more CO_2 combines with hemoglobin and more HCO_3^- is produced.

Gas Exchange at the Lungs

As oxygen passes from the alveoli into the red blood cells, hemoglobin becomes saturated with oxygen and becomes a stronger acid. The more acidic hemoglobin releases more H^+ that binds to more HCO_3^- to form carbonic acid. The carbonic acid dissociates into CO_2 and water. The CO_2 diffuses from the blood into the alveoli.

SYSTEMIC EFFECTS OF HYPERCARBIA AND HYPOCARBIA

In intensive care, acute hypercapnia is mainly encountered in acute respiratory failure, in cardiorespiratory arrest, and during mechanical ventilation. In the latter circumstance, it can be nonintentional (ventilator malfunction, extreme derangement of lung mechanics) or intentional (permissive hypercapnia).[13] Permissive hypercapnia (acceptance of raised concentrations of CO_2 in mechanically ventilated patients) may be associated with increased survival as a result of less ventilator-associated lung injury. Conversely, hypocapnia is associated with many acute illnesses (e.g., asthma, systemic inflammatory response syndrome, pulmonary edema), and is thought to reflect underlying hyperventilation. Accumulating clinical and basic scientific evidence points to an active role for CO_2 in organ injury, in which raised concentrations of CO_2 are protective and low concentrations are injurious. Foëx et al. hypothesize that therapeutic hypercapnia might be tested in severely ill patients to see whether supplemental CO_2 could reduce the adverse effects of hypocapnia and promote the beneficial effects of hypercapnia.[14] Such an approach could also expand our understanding of the pathogenesis of disorders in which hypocapnia is a constitutive element.[15]

The possibility that systemic CO_2 tension may have a role in protection against organ injury has not been considered in the clinical context. Although hypercapnic acidosis may indicate tissue dysoxia and predict adverse outcome, it is not necessarily harmful per se. In fact, it may be beneficial. There is increasing evidence that respiratory (and metabolic) acidosis can exert protective effects on tissue injury and, furthermore, that hypocapnia may be deleterious. Laffey et al. discussed current insights into the effects of CO_2 on organ injury, and proposed an integrated concept of the mechanism of action of CO_2 in acute disease processes. The authors draw on this evidence to propose the concept of "therapeutic hypercapnia"—that is, the prevention of hypocapnia, and the induction of hypercapnia—whereby increased partial pressure of CO_2 in arterial blood ($PaCO_2$) might be a goal of therapy in critical illness, rather than something to be avoided.[15]

Hypercapnia in Disease

One of the most important concepts in the care of critically ill patients is the recognition that mechanical ventilation—the supportive therapy commonly used in respiratory failure—can worsen, or even cause, lung injury, by repetitive overstretching of lung tissue.[16] If hypoventilation is allowed in an effort to limit lung stretch, CO_2 tension increases. Such "permissive hypercapnia" may be associated with increased survival in acute respiratory distress syndrome (ARDS).[17] This association is supported by outcome data from a 10-year study.[18] Although explanations for this apparent decline in mortality remain speculative, recognition of the potential impact of ventilator-induced lung injury has led to the suggestion that the adoption of "protective" ventilatory strategies may have been a factor. However, attribution of any improvements solely to the emergence of new ventilatory strategies may be premature. Death in ARDS results largely from multisystem organ failure, not hypoxia.[19] Furthermore, improved survival may be attributable to nonventilatory issues, such as improvements in resuscitation, fluid management, sepsis diagnosis or treatment, supportive measures for organ dysfunction, nutritional support, staff training, or other unidentifiable clinical factors. Nevertheless, permissive hypercapnia resulting from protective ventilatory strategies[20] has been identified as an important technique in the management of patients with ARDS. Such an approach assumes that the hypercapnic acidosis generated reflects the underlying protective hypoventilatory strategy rather than having any direct therapeutic role. The possibility that hypercapnic acidosis may exert clinically important organ protection has received little attention.

Hypocapnia in Disease

Acute injury can be caused by hyperventilation; hyperventilation causes hypocapnic alkalosis; and hyperventilation and hypocapnic alkalosis frequently coexist in lung (or other organ) injury. Although separation of these entities is difficult, the association of hyperventilation, hypocapnia, and worsened lung injury is well documented.[21] In fact, hypocapnia and hyperventilation may be independent causes of bronchopulmonary dysplasia.[21] Possible mechanistic insights into the direct effect of hypocapnia are provided by studies showing that hypocapnia increases microvascular permeability in tracheal mucosa,[22] decreases lung compliance,[23] and increases dysfunctional surfactant production.[24] In nonpulmonary organs, the differentiation between the effect of altered ventilation and that of altered $PaCO_2$ is more clear-cut. For example, prophylactic hyperventilation to produce hypocapnia in acute head injury (a traditional and only briefly applied therapy) is associated with a worsened neurological outcome.[25] Hypocapnia is also a pathogenetic factor in pontosubicular necrosis,[26] a pattern of acute brain injury seen in infants with perinatal anoxia.

HYPEROXIA AND HYPOXEMIA

Both hypoxia and hyperoxia have major effects on cardiovascular function. However, both states affect ventilation, and many previous studies have not controlled CO_2 tension. Variations in oxygen tension beyond the physiological range have complex effects on cardiovascular function. Hypoxia and hyperoxia have been studied extensively and shown to alter heart rate, cardiac output, and vascular resistance.[(27–32)] A variety of mechanisms contribute to these cardiovascular responses after changes in oxygen tension. Vascular smooth muscle cell tone is directly affected by altered conduction through L-type Ca^{2+} channels[33] and ATP-sensitive[34] and voltage-dependent K^+ channels.[35] In addition, oxygen tension may affect release of angiotensin II, with ensuing changes in endothelin-1 levels.[36] A number of other vasoactive substances are also produced by the endothelium in an oxygen-sensitive manner, including prostaglandins,[37] adenosine,[38] and nitric oxide (NO).[39] Both hyperoxic[40] and hypoxic[41] conditions can increase formation of reactive oxygen species (ROS) that may subsequently alter cell function by reacting with various cellular components, including cell membranes, enzymes, and ion channels. Reactive oxygen species created in this way may also play fundamental roles in intracellular signaling. Hyperoxia also reduces the bioavailability of NO, via production of superoxide anions.[42] Finally, changes in autonomic balance have been implicated in some of the cardiovascular responses, with hypoxia leading to sympathetic activation, whereas hyperoxia reduces sympathetic and possibly increases parasympathetic tone.[32,43] Many of the previous studies of changes in oxygenation in intact organisms, particularly those investigating hyperoxia, are hard to interpret because CO_2 levels were not controlled. This is important because CO_2 has profound effects on cardiovascular function through local vascular, chemoreceptor-mediated, and central effects.[44] Both hyperoxia and hypoxia stimulate ventilation and reduce arterial CO_2 tension.[45,46] It is therefore possible that some of the changes attributed to alterations in oxygen tension may in fact be caused by these secondary changes in ventilation. This potential confounding effect was addressed in part in some previous studies of hypoxia under stable CO_2 conditions.[47,48] These studies suggested that short periods of isocapnic hypoxia had smaller but similar effects on cardiovascular function than hypoxia when CO_2 is not controlled.

CONTROL OF VENTILATION

The respiratory center (RC) is located in the medulla oblongata, which is the lower part of the brain stem. The RC receives controlling signals of neural, chemical, and hormonal nature and controls the rate and depth of respiratory movements of the diaphragm and other respiratory muscles. Injury to this center may lead to central respiratory failure, which necessitates mechanical ventilation; usually the prognosis is grave. In healthy individuals, the presence of elevated CO_2 levels in the blood is the stimulant that the RC responds to in order to signal the respiratory muscles to breathe. Chemoreceptors found in carotid bodies and aortic bodies are responsible for detecting decrease in blood pH by this CO_2.

RECEPTORS, MUSCLES, AND REFLEXES

The respiratory chemoreceptor control system is composed of central and peripheral respiratory chemoreceptors that operate in a classic feedback loop to control breathing. The central chemoreceptors detect brain tissue CO_2, and the peripheral chemoreceptors detect blood oxygen and CO_2 levels. Using different time scales, inputs from central and peripheral chemoreceptors are integrated in the central nervous system to precisely match pulmonary ventilation to metabolic demands and maintain blood gases within narrow limits during wakefulness and sleep.

Central chemoreceptors of the central nervous system, located on the ventrolateral medullary surface in the vicinity of the exit of the 9th and 10th cranial nerves, are sensitive to the pH of their environment. These receptors act to detect the changes in pH of nearby cerebrospinal fluid (CSF) that are indicative of altered oxygen or CO_2 concentrations available to brain tissues. An increase in CO_2 tension of the arteries, often resulting from increased CO_2 intake (hypercapnia), indirectly causes the blood to become more acidic; the CSF pH is closely comparable to plasma, as CO_2 easily diffuses across the blood-brain barrier. However, a change in plasma pH alone will not stimulate central chemoreceptors, as H^+ are not able to diffuse across the blood-brain barrier (BBB) into the CSF. Only CO_2 levels affect this as it can diffuse across the blood-brain barrier, reacting with H_2O to form carbonic acid and thus decrease pH. Central chemoreception remains, in this way, distinct from peripheral chemoreceptors. The central chemoreception system has also been shown experimentally to respond to hypercapnic hypoxia (elevated CO_2, decreased oxygen).

Peripheral chemoreceptors (carotid and aortic bodies) and central chemoreceptors (medullary neurons) primarily function to regulate respiratory activity. This is an important mechanism for maintaining arterial blood pO_2, pCO_2, and pH within appropriate physiological ranges. For example, a fall in arterial pO_2 (hypoxemia) or an increase in arterial pCO_2 (hypercapnia) leads to an increase in the rate and depth of respiration through activation of the chemoreceptor reflex. Chemoreceptor activity, however, also affects cardiovascular function either directly (by interacting with medullary vasomotor centers) or indirectly (via altered pulmonary stretch receptor activity).

Proprioceptors are specialized sensory receptors on nerve endings found in muscles, tendons, joints, and the inner ear. These receptors relay information about motion or position and make us aware of our own body position and movement in space. Proprioceptors detect subtle changes in movement, position, tension, and force within the body.

Given the importance of the ventilatory "pump" muscles, it would not be surprising if they were endowed with both sensory and motor specializations. The present paragraph focuses on some unexpected properties of the respiratory muscle system in human subjects. (1) Although changes in blood gas tension were long held not to influence sensation directly, studies in subjects who are completely paralyzed show that increases in arterial CO_2 levels elicit strong sensations of respiratory discomfort. (2) Stretch reflexes in human limb muscles contain a monosynaptic spinal excitation and a long-latency excitation. However, inspiratory muscles show an initial inhibition when tested with brief airway occlusions during inspiration. This inhibition does not depend critically on input from pulmonary or upper airway receptors. (3) Human inspiratory muscles (including the diaphragm) have been considered to fatigue during inspiratory resistive loading. However, recent studies using phrenic nerve stimulation to test the force produced by the diaphragm show that CO_2 retention (hypoventilation) and voluntary cessation of loading occur before the muscles become overtly fatigued.[49]

CARBON DIOXIDE AND OXYGEN RESPONSE CURVES

The chemical control of breathing is based on a negative feedback loop and chemoreflex. Thus, when the central and peripheral chemoreceptors sense an increase in $[H^+]$, breathing is stimulated by a chemoreflex that includes the central nervous system, respiratory muscles, and changes in alveolar ventilation resulting in correction of the [H+], hence the negative feedback designation of the system. However, in addition to chemical stimuli, non-chemical drives to breathe also contribute to the level of ventilation, independently of the chemoreflexes. These drives include the central nervous system "state" of the subject, which is referred to as the "waking neural drive," because it is withdrawn during sleep. Inspiration of CO_2 in healthy, awake subjects increases minute ventilation by approximately 3 L/min per 1 mm Hg of arterial CO_2 tension. All inhaled anesthetics depress the ventilatory response to hypercarbia in a dose-dependent fashion. High concentrations of volatile anesthetics may almost entirely eliminate hypercarbia-induced increases in ventilatory drive. The slope of the minute ventilation-arterial CO_2 tension relation returns toward normal after 6 hours of halothane anesthesia, but ventilatory responsiveness to CO_2 remains profoundly depressed despite this observation. The effects of small doses of inhaled anesthetics on ventilatory responses to hypercarbia remain somewhat controversial despite intense investigation. Several studies have demonstrated that subanesthetic concentrations (e.g., 0.1 MAC) of inhaled anesthetics (with the exception of desflurane and nitrous oxide) depress the peripheral chemoreflex loop by approximately 30% to inhibit the ventilatory response to hypercarbia. The response was also attenuated during administration of desflurane when a level of sedation comparable with sleep was achieved. At higher concentrations of volatile agents, other sites, including the central chemoreceptors, may also be affected[50,51].

CARBON DIOXIDE RESPONSE CURVE

- **Volatile Anesthetics**: decrease the response (slope and right-shift) to CO_2 (although low doses ~ 0.1 MAC controversial)
- **Opioids**: right-shift the ventilatory response curves (slope may change at high doses)
- **Benzodiazepines**: decrease the slope of the ventilatory response curves
- **Propofol**: decrease the slope of the ventilatory response curves (58% reduction at 100 ucg/kg/min)
- **Hypoxemia**: at less than 65 mm Hg paO2, the CO2 response curve is left-shifted

NONRESPIRATORY FUNCTIONS OF LUNGS

The primary function of the lungs is gas exchange. However, the lungs perform several important nonrespiratory functions that are vital for normal physiology.

- The lung, with its unique ability to distend and recruit pulmonary vasculature, acts as a reservoir of blood, fine-tuning preload to the left heart to optimize cardiac output.
- The lung acts as a filter against endogenous and exogenous emboli, preventing them from accessing systemic circulation.
- Pulmonary epithelium forms the first line of defense against inhaled particles.
- Pulmonary endothelial cells are responsible for uptake, metabolism, and biotransformation of several exogenous and endogenous substances.
- Pulmonary metabolic capacity is easily saturated, but pulmonary endothelial binding of some drugs alters their pharmacokinetics.

VOLUME RESERVE

The volume of the blood passing through the pulmonary vessels is equal to the right ventricular output, of which 70–100 mL is within the pulmonary capillaries,[52] and takes part in gas exchange. The remaining blood volume is held within the pulmonary vasculature.

RECRUITMENT AND DISTENTION

The lung has an extremely distensible vasculature, which enables it to cope with large variations in venous return, especially during postural changes, exercise, and increased intravascular volume. The two mechanisms involved are recruitment and distention of the pulmonary vasculature.[53] At resting cardiac output, the pulmonary vascular bed is not fully perfused. In the face of an increased cardiac output, underperfused areas of the pulmonary vasculature are "recruited" to accommodate an increase in blood flow and to prevent an increase in pulmonary arterial pressures. The walls of the pulmonary vasculature are thin and contain relatively little smooth muscle, which make it compliant to increased blood volume. The pressure in the pulmonary circulation is approximately six times less than that of the systemic circulation, and both arteries and veins increase in caliber with lung expansion. This "distention" along with "recruitment" helps in altering the lung blood volume by 500–1000 mL.

POSTURAL AND VENTILATORY CHANGES

A change in posture from supine to erect in normal individuals results in ~400 mL of pulmonary blood volume being redistributed to the systemic circulation. During forced expiration against a closed glottis (e.g., valsalva maneuver), the pulmonary blood volume decreases by 50%. On the other hand, the pulmonary blood volume doubles with forced inspiration. Changes in pulmonary vascular volume are also influenced by the activity of the sympathetic nervous system.[52]

FILTER FOR BLOOD-BORNE SUBSTANCES

The lung is ideally positioned to filter out particulate matter such as clots, fibrin clumps, and other endogenous and exogenous materials from entering the systemic circulation. This plays an important role in preventing ischemia or even infarction to vital organs.

CHEMICAL FILTRATION

Pulmonary capillaries also produce substances that break down blood clots. Pulmonary endothelium is a rich source of fibrinolysin activator, which converts plasminogen present in plasma to fibrinolysin, which subsequently breaks down fibrin-to-fibrin degradation products. Thus, the lung has an efficient fibrinolytic system, which lyses clots in the pulmonary circulation.[53] In addition, the lung is the richest source of heparin (which inhibits coagulation) and thromboplastin (which by converting prothrombin to thrombin, promotes coagulation). Hence the lung may play a role in the overall coagulability of blood to promote or delay coagulation and fibrinolysis.

DEFENSE AGAINST INHALED SUBSTANCES

Every day, about 10,000 liters of air comes in to contact with 50–100 m^2 of alveolar epithelium. There are various mechanisms along the respiratory tract that are involved in providing protection against inhaled physical and chemical substances.

DEFENSE AGAINST INHALED PARTICLES

A pseudostratified ciliated epithelium lines the upper airway from the posterior two-thirds of the nose to the respiratory bronchioles. This is covered with a "mucous blanket" that is composed of a highly viscous mucopolysaccharide gel secreted by goblet cells in the epithelium and mucous cells of the submucosal glands, floating on a low-viscosity serous fluid layer secreted by the bronchial glands. This "mucous blanket" forms the first line of defense against inhaled physical substances.

IMMUNE FUNCTION

Optimal lung defenses require coordinated action of multiple cell types. Immune function within the lung is mediated by pulmonary alveolar macrophages (PAMs) and a variety of immune mediators.

Amoeboid PAMs engulf the particles that reach the alveoli and deposit them on the mucociliary escalator or remove them via blood or lymph. The macrophages are particularly effective against bacteria and ensure that the alveolar region of the lung is effectively sterile.[52] The PAMs also have a role in antigen presentation, T-cell activation, and immunomodulation. When PAMs ingest large amounts of inhaled particles, especially cigarette smoke, silica, and asbestos, they release lysosomal products into the extracellular space causing inflammation and eventually fibrosis. Neutrophil activation within the lung also leads to the release of proteases such as trypsin and elastase. These chemicals, while very effective at destroying pathogens, can also damage normal lung tissue. This is prevented by the proteases being swept away by the mucus coating the respiratory tree, and by conjugation with alpha$_1$-antitrypsin, which renders them inactive.[54] Hence, in alpha$_1$-antitrypsin deficiency, surplus trypsin and elastase leads to tissue destruction that in turn leads to pulmonary emphysema.

IMMUNE MEDIATORS

The airway epithelial cells secrete a variety of substances such as mucins, defensins, lysozyme, lactoferrin, and nitric oxide, which nonspecifically shield the lung from microbial attack.[55] They also produce a number of mediators of inflammation such as reactive oxygen species, cytokines (tumor necrosis factor [TNFα], interleukins [IL-1β], granulocyte/macrophage colony stimulating factor [GM-CSF]), and platelet activating factor to recruit inflammatory cells to the site of inflammation. Immunoglobulins, mainly IgA, present in the bronchial secretions resist infections and help maintain the integrity of the respiratory mucosa.[56]

In conclusion, the lung is responsible for several important nonrespiratory functions, vital for maintenance of normal physiology. Evolving research has not only contributed to improved understanding of these roles but also opened new diagnostic and therapeutic avenues for a variety of medical conditions.

REFERENCES

1. Jacquez J. *Respiratory Physiology*. Oxfordshire, England: Taylor & Francis; 1979:156–175.
2. Novikoff A. Cells and their component parts. In: Brachet J, Mirsky AE. *In the Cell*. Vol. 2. New York: Academic Press; 1961.
3. Adebonojo F, Bensch, K, King D. The effect of nitrogen on the enzymatic pattern of strain L-cells. *Cancer Res*. 1961;21:252–256.
4. Hakami N, Pious D. Regulation of cytochrome oxidase in human cells in culture. *Nature*. 1967;216(5120):1087–1090.
5. King M, King D. Effect of oxygen deficiency on cytochrome c, heme a, and iron protoporphyrin of L-cells. *Arch Biochem Biophys*. 1968;127(1):302–309.
6. King M, King D. Respiratory enzyme activity and mitochondrial morphology of L-cells under prolonged oxygen deprivation. *Lab Invest*. 1971;25(5):374–379.
7. Ernster L. Control of cell metabolism at the mitochondrial level. *Fed Proc*. 1965;24(5):1222–1236.
8. Siggaard-Andersen O, Siggaard-Andersen M. The oxygen status algorithm: a computer program for calculating and displaying pH and blood gas data. *Scand J Clin Lab Invest Suppl*. 1990;203:29–45.
9. Morgan T, Endre Z, Kanowski D, Worthley L, Jones R. Siggaard-Andersen algorithm-derived p50 parameters: perturbation

by abnormal hemoglobin-oxygen affinity and acid-base disturbances. *J Lab Clin Med.* 1995;126(4):365–372.
10. Miller R, ed. *Miller's Anesthesia.* 7th ed. Philadelphia, PA: Elsevier; 2010:ch. 49.
11. Klocke R. Mechanism and kinetics of the Haldane effect in human erythrocytes. *J Appl Physiol.* 1973;35(5):673–681.
12. Bohr C, Hasselbalch K, Krogh A. Concerning a biologically important relationship: the influence of the carbon dioxide content of blood on its oxygen binding. Trans. Ulf Marquardt. *Skand Arch Physiol.* 1997;401–412.
13. Servillo G, De Robertis E, Coppola M, Tufano R. Local and systemic effects of hypercapnia. In: Gullo A, ed. *Anaesthesia, Pain, Intensive Care, and Emergency Medicine —A.P.I.C.E.* Milan, Italy: Springer; 2001:189–194.
14. Foëx P, Ryder W. Effect of CO2 on the systemic and coronary circulations and on coronary sinus blood gas tensions. *Bull Eur Physiopathol Respir.* 1976;15(4):625–638.
15. Laffey J, Kavanagh B. Carbon dioxide and the critically ill: too little of a good thing? *Lancet.* 1999;354(9186):1283–1286.
16. Slutsky A. Mechanical ventilation. *Chest.* 1993;104(6):1833–1859.
17. Hickling K, Walsh J, Henderson S, Jackson R. Low mortality rate in adult respiratory distress syndrome using low-volume, pressure-limited ventilation with permissive hypercapnia: a prospective study. *Crit Care Med.* 1994;22(10):1568–1579.
18. Milberg J, Davis D, Steinberg K, Hudson L. Improved survival of patients with acute respiratory distress syndrome (ARDS): 1983–1993. *JAMA.* 1995;273(4):306–309.
19. Montgomery A, Stager M, Carrico C, Hudson L. Causes of mortality in patients with the adult respiratory distress syndrome. *Am Rev Respir Dis.* 1985;132(3):485–489.
20. Amato MB, Barbas CS, Medeiros DM, et al. Effect of a protective-ventilation strategy on mortality in the acute respiratory distress syndrome. *N Engl J Med.* 1998;338(6):347–354.
21. Garland J, Buck R, Allred E, Leviton A. Hypocarbia before surfactant therapy appears to increase bronchopulmonary dysplasia risk in infants with respiratory distress syndrome. *Arch Pediatr Adolesc Med.* 1995;149(6):617–622.
22. Reynolds A, Zadow S, Scicchitano R, McEvoy, R. Airway hypocapnia increases microvascular leakage in the guinea pig trachea. *Am Rev Respir Dis.* 1992;145(1):80–84.
23. Cutillo A, Omboni E, Perondi R, Tana F. Effects of hypocapnia on pulmonary mechanics in normal subjects and in patients with chronic obstructive lung disease. *Am Rev Respir Dis.* 1974;110(1):25–33.
24. Oyarzún M, Donoso P, Quijada D. Role of hypocapnia in the alveolar surfactant increase induced by free fatty acid intravenous infusion in the rabbit. *Respiration.* 1986;49(3):187–194.
25. Muizelaar J, Marmarou A, Ward J, et al. Adverse effects of prolonged hyperventilation in patients with severe head injury: a randomized trial. *J Neurosurg.* 1991;75(5):731–739.
26. Hashimoto K, Takewuchi Y, Takashina S. Hypocarbia as a pathogenic factor in pontosubicular necrosis. *Brain Dev.* 1991;13(3):155–157.
27. Asmussen E, Nielsen M. The cardiac output in rest and work at low and high oxygen pressures. *Acta Physiol Scand.* 1955;35(1):73–83.
28. Daly W, Bondurant S. Effects of oxygen breathing on the heart rate, blood pressure, and cardiac index of normal men: resting, with reactive hyperemia, and after atropine. *J Clin Invest.* 1962;41:126–132.
29. Haque W, Boehmer J, Clemson B, Leuenberger U, Silber D, Sinoway L. Hemodynamic effects of supplemental oxygen administration in congestive heart failure. *J Am Coll Cardiol.* 1996;27(2):353–357.
30. Keys A, Stapp J, Violante A. Responses in size, output, and efficiency of the human heart to acute alteration in the composition of inspired air. *Am J Physiol.* 1943;138:763–771.
31. Mak S, Azevedo E, Liu P, Newton G. Effect of hyperoxia on left ventricular function and filling pressures in patients with and without congestive heart failure. *Chest.* 2001;120(2):467–473.
32. Waring W, Thomson A, Adwani S, Rosseel A, Potter J, Webb D, Maxwell S. Cardiovascular effects of acute oxygen administration in healthy adults. *J Cardiovasc Pharmacol.* 2003;42(2):245–250.
33. Welsh D, Jackson W, Segal S. Oxygen induces electromechanical coupling in arteriolar smooth muscle cells: a role for L-type Ca2+ channels. *Am J Physiol.* 1998;274(6 Pt2):H2018–2024.
34. Daut J, Maierrudolph W, Vonbeckerath N, Mehrke G, Gunther K, Goedelmeinen L. Hypoxic dilation of coronary arteries is mediated by ATP-sensitive potassium channels. *Science.* 1990;247(4948):1341–1344.
35. Coppock E, Martens J, Tamkun M. Molecular basis of hypoxia-induced pulmonary vasoconstriction: role of voltage-gated K+ channels. *Am J Physiol Lung Cell Mol Physiol.* 2001;281(1):L1–L12.
36. Winegrad S, Henrion D, Rappaport L, Samuel J. Self-protection by cardiac myocytes against hypoxia and hyperoxia. *Circ Res.* 1999;85(8):690–698.
37. Messina E, Sun D, Koller A, Wolin M, Kaley G. Role of endothelium-derived prostaglandins in hypoxia-elicited arteriolar dilation in rat skeletal muscle. *Circ Res.* 1992;71(4):790–796.
38. Leuenberger U, Gray K, Herr M. Adenosine contributes to hypoxia-induced forearm vasodilation in humans. *J Appl Physiol* (1985). 1999;87(6):2218–2224.
39. Pohl U, Busse R. Hypoxia stimulates release of endothelium-derived relaxant factor. *Am J Physiol.* 1989;256(6 Pt 2):H1595–H1600.
40. Jamieson D, Chance B, Cadenas E, Boveris A. The relation of free-radical production to hyperoxia. *Annu Rev Physiol.* 1986;48:703–719.
41. Liu J, Sham J, Shimoda L, Kuppusamy P, Sylvester J. Hypoxic constriction and reactive oxygen species in porcine distal pulmonary arteries. *Am J Physiol Lung Cell Mol Physiol.* 2003;285(2):L322–L333.
42. Rubanyi G, Vanhoutte P. Superoxide anions and hyperoxia inactivate endothelium-derived relaxing factor. *Am J Physiol.* 1986;250(5 Pt 2):H822–H827.
43. Lund V, Kentala E, Scheinin H, et al. Heart rate variability in healthy volunteers during normobaric and hyperbaric hyperoxia. *Acta Physiol Scand.* 1999;167(1):29–35.
44. Price H. Effects of carbon dioxide on the cardiovascular system. *Anesthesiology.* 1960;21:652–663.
45. Easton P, Slykerman L, Anthonisen N. Ventilatory response to sustained hypoxia in normal adults. *J Appl Physiol* (1985). 1986;61(13):906–911.
46. Keys A, Stapp J, Violante A. Responses in size, output, and efficiency of the human heart to acute alteration in the composition of inspired air. *Am J Physiol.* 1943;138:763–771.
47. Richardson D, Kontos H, Shapiro W, Patterson J. Role of hypocapnia in the circulatory responses to acute hypoxia in man. *J Appl Physiol.* 1966;21(1):22–26.
48. Slutsky A, Rebuck A. Heart rate response to isocapnic hypoxia in conscious man. *Am J Physiol.* 1978;234(2):H129–H132.
49. Gandevia S, Allen G, Butler J, Gorman R, McKenzie D. Human respiratory muscles: sensations, reflexes, and fatiguability. *Clin Exp Pharmacol Physiol.* 1998;25(10):757–763.
50. Miller R, ed. *Miller's Anesthesia.* 7th ed. Philadelphia, PA: Elsevier; 2010:ch. 22, 26.
51. Barash P, Cullen B, Stoelting R, Cahalan M, Stock M. *Clinical Anesthesia.* 6th ed. Philadelphia, PA: Lippincott Williams & Wilkins; 2009:242.
52. Davies A, Moores C. *The Respiratory System: Basic Science and Clinical Conditions.* Oxford, England: Churchill Livingstone; 2003.
53. Ganong W. Pulmonary function. In: *Review of Medical Physiology.* 22nd ed. San Francisco, CA: McGraw-Hill; 2005:664–665.
54. Levitzky M. *Pulmonary Physiology.* 6th ed. New York, NY: McGraw-Hill; 2003.
55. Moldoveanu B, Otmishi P, Jani P. Inflammatory mechanisms in the lung. *J Inflamm Res.* 2009;2:1–11.
56. Bartlett J, Fischer A, McCray P. Innate immune functions of the airway epithelium. *Contrib Microbiol.* 2008;15:147–163.

FURTHER READING

Miller R, ed. *Miller's Anesthesia*. 7th ed. Philadelphia, PA: Elsevier; 2010: ch. 15.

QUESTIONS

1. Lung compliance:
   A. Can be expressed as change in pressure per unit volume
   B. Is greater when measured during inflation than deflation
   C. Increases with lung fibrosis
   D. Decreases in emphysema
   E. Increases in pulmonary congestion

2. Which of the following statements BEST describes pulmonary surfactant?
   A. Produced by type I pneumocytes
   B. Promotes alveolar collapse
   C. Enhances the effect of surface tension
   D. Reduces microbial growth
   E. Loses effect with alveolar distention

3. Physiologic dead space is:
   A. Decreased by a pulmonary embolus
   B. Increased by a snorkel
   C. Underventilated alveoli
   D. Transitional respiratory zones
   E. About 250 mL in a healthy adult

4. According to Fick's law of diffusion, capacity of gas exchange varies:
   A. Proportionally to the area of gas exchange
   B. Inversely to the thickness of gas exchange surface
   C. Proportionally to the pressure difference across the membrane
   D. All of the above
   E. None of the above

5. Which of the following techniques could be used to reduce airflow resistance in an intubated patient?
   A. Withdrawing the endotracheal tube to the carina
   B. Heating the ventilated air
   C. Cutting 2 cm from the tip of the endotracheal tube
   D. Administering systemic beta blockade

ANSWERS

1. A. Lung compliance is change in pressure to change in a unit of volume in the lung, so more compliant lungs result in more of a change in volume associated with less of a change in pressure. In effect, patients with pulmonary edema, congestions, or fibrosis require higher pressures in order to achieve the same ventilation. Patients with emphysema have destruction of the lung parenchyma and highly (overly) compliant lungs. Lung compliance increases during deflation and decreases during inflation. It should be noted that static lung compliance should be measured during the plateau phase.
2. D. Surfactant is produced by type II pneumocytes and Clara cells. Its primary function is to reduce tension and prevent collapse of the alveoli. Surfactant retains its effect with alveolar distention. Surfactant may play a role in opsonizing pathogens (bacteria and viruses) and to facilitating phagocytosis by macrophages and monocytes.
3. B. Pulmonary embolism is the pathopneumonic lesion describing dead space; when you hear PE, think dead space. A snorkel effectively makes the trachea longer, so its use would result in an increase in dead space. Underventilated alveoli would result in shunt, whereas *underperfused* alveoli would result in dead space. Dead space in a normal adult is approximately 100–150 mL (1–2 mL/kg). The sum of anatomic and alveolar dead space is physiologic dead space.
4. D. According to Fick's principle, diffusion capacity is directly to the area for transfer, gas tension difference across the membrane (P1-P2) and inversely to the thickness of the membrane. This observation is described by the formula: Diffusion of gas (V gas) = (A.D)/T×(P1-P2), where D is diffusion constant.
5. C. Withdrawing the endotracheal tube will increase resistance, as it will increase anatomic dead space (space beyond the lips). Based on the kinetic theory of gas, increases in gas temperature increase the gas's viscosity, which increases resistance (μ in the Poiseuille equation); this is the opposite of what is seen in liquids. Administration of systemic beta blockers will promote bronchoconstriction and lead to increased resistance. Cutting two centimeters from the tip of the tube will reduce the length of the circuit and thereby reduce resistance.

24.

RESPIRATORY FUNCTIONAL ANATOMY AND PHARMACOLOGY

Omonele Ohen Nwokolo and Tolutope Coker

NASAL ANATOMY

The nose is an organ of respiration, olfaction, humidification, and filtration. Through the nose lies the nasal cavity, which consists of two main chambers separated by a midline nasal septum. The septum is made up of cartilage joined to the vomer and ethmoid bone. The roof of the nasal cavity is made up of the nasal and frontal bones, the cribriform plate of the ethmoid, and the body of the sphenoid. The floor of the nasal cavity is made up of the maxilla and palatine bones.

The lateral wall of the nose has three shelf-like projections known as the superior, middle, and inferior conchae. Inferior to every concha is the meatus. The conchae are covered with fibrovascular tissue to form turbinates. This covering allows for filtration and humidification of the air. The superior turbinate is located just below the cribriform plate and receives drainage of the sphenoidal air cells. The middle turbinate forms the medial wall of the ethmoid sinus and receives the drainage of the maxillary and frontal sinus. The inferior turbinate is the largest turbinate and receives the termination of the lacrimal duct (see Figure 24.1).

Sensation is supplied is via the ophthalmic and maxillary branches of the trigeminal verve. The olfactory fibers supply the respiratory epithelium in the upper part of the nose. The sympathetic and parasympathetic innervations are from the pterygopalatine ganglion, which is derived from the maxillary nerve.

The blood supply of the nose derives from the anterior and posterior and ethmoidal artery the branches of the ophthalmic, sphenopalatine, greater palatine, maxillary, and superior labial artery. The four arteries anastomose in Kiesselbasch's plexus, which is located in Little's area, defined as the region located in the anteroinferior part of the nasal septum. This is the most common site for epistaxis (see Figure 24.2).

DIVISIONS OF THE PHARNYX

The pharynx is a fibromuscular tube that extends from the base of the skull to the level of the sixth vertebra. It links the oral and nasal cavities to the larynx and esophagus. Furthermore, it serves as a conduit for oral intake as well as respiratory gases. It is divided into the nasopharynx, oropharynx, and laryngopharynx. The nasopharynx extends from the base of the skull to the soft palate. It contains the pharyngeal tonsils and the openings of the auditory tubes. The nasopharyngeal tonsil lies on the roof on the posterior wall of the nasopharynx (see Figure 24.3). Sensory supply to the nasopharynx is derived from the second division of the trigeminal nerve.

The oropharynx is bordered by the tonsillar pillars anteriorly; the oropharynx extends from the soft palate to the tip of the epiglottis. It houses the palatine tonsils in its lateral walls. Sensory innervation to the oropharynx is supplied by the glossopharyngeal nerve. The laryngopharynx (or hypopharynx) extends from the tip of the epiglottis to the lower border of the cricoid cartilage. The sensory innervation to the laryngopharynx is supplied by the glossopharyngeal and vagus nerves (so when these are directly blocked, an intubation can be performed without an IV induction). The motor supply of the pharynx is supplied by the pharyngeal branch of the vagus. Exceptions to this include (1) the stylopharyngeus muscle, which is supplied by the glossopharyngeal nerve, and (2) the tensor palatine, which is supplied by cranial nerve III (oculomotor).

THE LARYNX

Understanding the larynx and its anatomy is a component of mastering the airway (see Figure 24.4). The larynx is the gateway to the pharyngeal inlet, which is commonly viewed and familiar anatomy for the anesthesiologist. Apart from

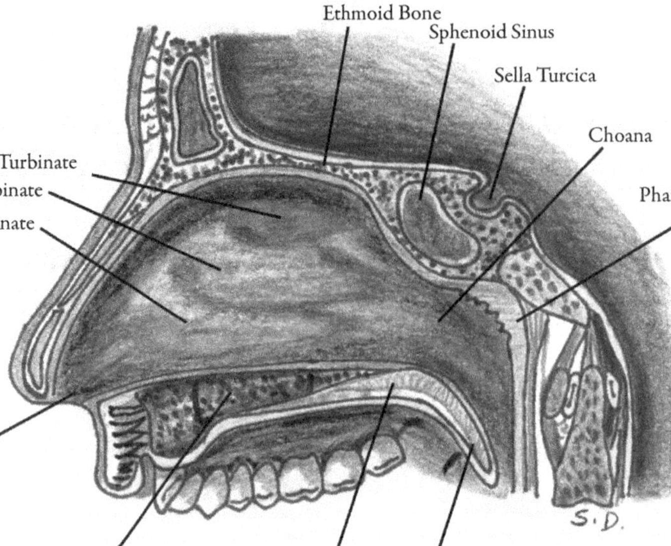

Figure 24.1 Nasal anatomy. Image courtesy of Shilpa Dabhade, MD. Adapted from *Nasal Cavity*. Edoctoronline.com website. http://www.edoctoronline.com/medical-atlas.asp?c=4&id=21657&m=2. Accessed April 6, 2015.

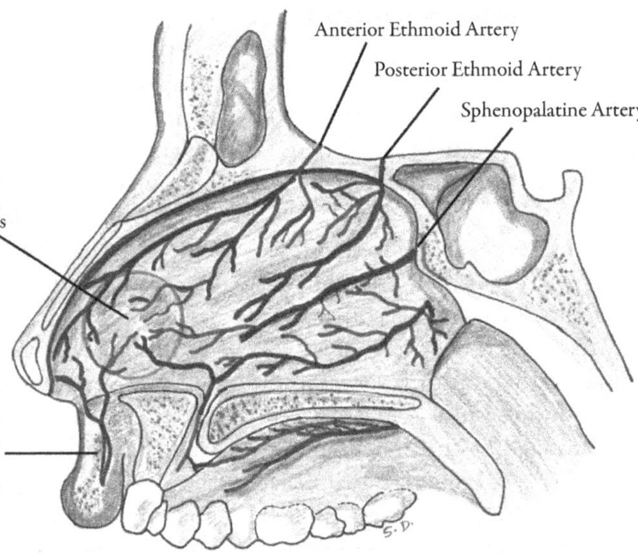

Figure 24.2 Nasal vascular anatomy. Image courtesy of Shilpa Dabhade, MD. Adapted from *Management of Epistaxis*. American Academy of Family Physicians website. http://f.pepst.com/c/d/B652D1/406342-8266/ssc3/home/013/medicalpictures/albums/blood_supply.jpg. Accessed April 6, 2015.

its function as a respiratory conduit, the larynx also serves in phonation and airway protection. The larynx is located midline from C-3 to C-6. It is suspended from the hyoid bone (C-3 level) by the thyrohyoid membrane. The hyoid bone is a unique bone in that it does not articulate with any other bone. This section reviews the cartilages, ligaments, and muscles that enable the larynx perform its functions.

CARTILAGES

The larynx is made up of three unpaired cartilages (epiglottis, thyroid, cricoid) and three smaller contributing paired cartilages (arytenoids, corniculate, cuneiform) (Figure 24.5).

Epiglottis cartilage: The epiglottis guards the pharyngeal inlet; it prevents food from entering the trachea by covering the tracheal inlet during swallowing. It is leaf shaped with the stem of the leaf connected to the posterior surface of the thyroid cartilage by the thyroepiglottic ligament. Additionally, hypoepiglottic ligaments connect the epiglottis to the hyoid bone. The superior component is free and facilitates coverage of the laryngeal inlet during swallowing.

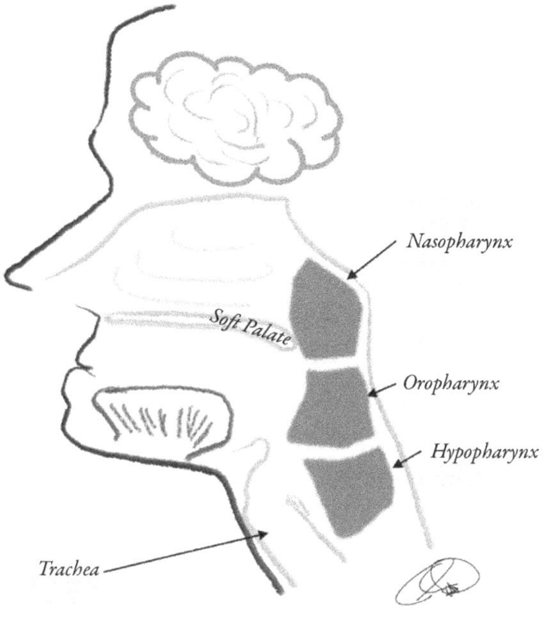

Figure 24.3 Pharyngeal anatomy. Image courtesy of George Williams, MD.

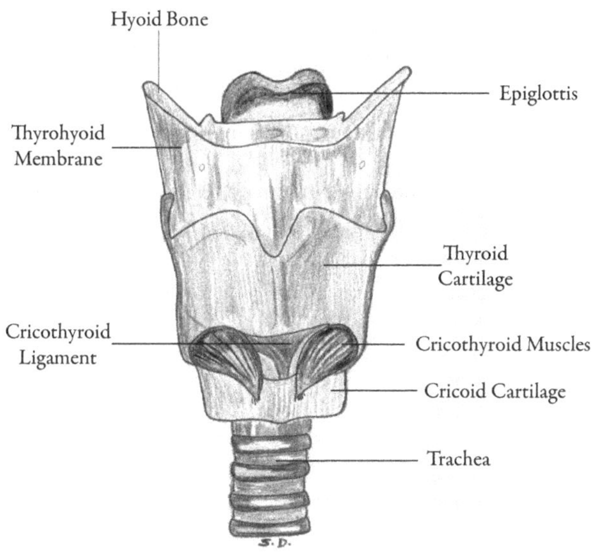

Figure 24.4 The larynx. Image courtesy of Shilpa Dabhade, MD.

Adapted from: *Laryngeal Anatomy*. Airway Education Web Resource website. http://airwayeducation.homestead.com/Larynxfrontsm.jpg. Accessed April 6, 2015.

Thyroid cartilage: The largest of the unpaired cartilages, the thyroid cartilage consists of two lamina that fuse anteriorly and diverge posteriorly. Its anterior portions join at different angles in males and females. In the male the angle is about 90 degrees, which causes a greater laryngeal prominence in males called the "Adams apple."

Cricoid cartilage: The cricoid cartilage is a complete ring of cartilage located inferior to the thyroid cartilage at the level of C6. Its anterior portion is called the arch and is palpable. The posterior portion forms the back wall of the larynx. The circular structure of the cricoid cartilage comes into play during Sellick's maneuver (cricoid pressure) during a rapid-sequence intubation; compression of the cricoid cartilage will compress the esophagus behind and prevent aspiration. Sellick's maneuver is commonly applied incorrectly (on the thyroid cartilage) when this anatomical fact is not taken into consideration.

Arytenoid cartilages: The arytenoids are paired pyramidal cartilages located posteriorly on top of the cricoid lamina; the bases of the arytenoid cartilages are l-shaped. Intrinsic muscles attach to the lateral process called the muscular process. The medial process is called the vocal process, which is where the vocal cords attach. The arytenoid cartilages articulate with the cricoid cartilage, forming the cricoarytenoid joints. This joint allows rotation, abduction, and adduction of the vocal cords. During intubation, the endotracheal tube can cause the arytenoids to dislocate or subluxate. If the normal position of the arytenoids is affected, it can interrupt the normal movement of the vocal cords.

Corniculates: These rod-shaped cartilages are located on the apex of the arytenoid cartilages.

THE LIGAMENTS OF THE LARYNX

The ligaments of the larynx connect the cartilages of the larynx together. They are divided into intrinsic or extrinsic ligaments.

Extrinsic Ligaments

The thyrohyoid membrane connects the thyroid cartilage to the hyoid bone. It is thickened anteriorly to form the median thyrohoid ligament and laterally to form the thyrohyoid ligament. The membrane is pierced by the superior laryngeal vessels. The cricothyroid membrane connects the thyroid cartilage to the cricoid cartilage. The cricotracheal ligament connects the cricoid cartilage to the first tracheal ring, and the hypoepiglottic ligament connects the thyroid cartilage to the epiglottis.

Intrinsic Ligaments

Intrinsic ligaments connect the laryngeal cartilages with *each other*. The thyroepiglottic ligaments attach the epiglottis to the thyroid cartilage. The conus elasticus connects the cricoid cartilage (Figure 24.6) with the thyroid and arytenoid cartilage. It is made up of the medial cricothyroid ligament and the lateral cricothyroid membrane.

The lateral cricothyroid membrane attaches to the vocal process of the arytenoid cartilages posteriorly and anteriorly to the inside of the median part of the thyroid cartilage. Its free borders form the vocal ligaments.

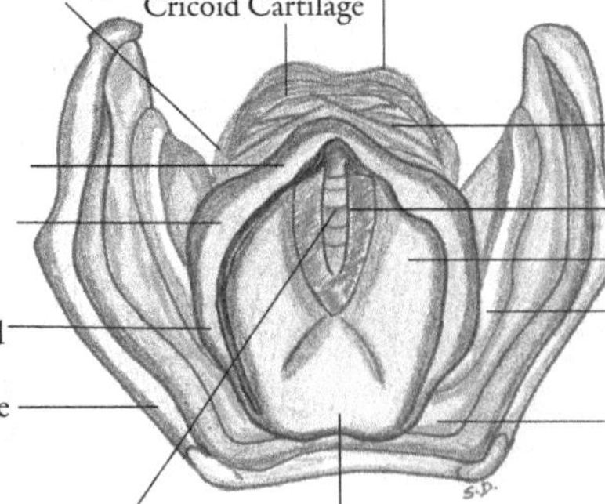

Figure 24.5 Larynx cartilages. Image courtesy of Shilpa Dabhade, MD. Adapted from: *Laryngeal Anatomy.* Airway Education Web Resource website. http://airwayeducation.homestead.com/Larynxtop.jpg. Accessed April 6, 2015.

The medial cricothyroid ligament connects the anterior part of the arch of the cricoid cartilage to the inferior border of the thyroid membrane. The quadranqular membrane is the upper part of a fibrous sheet that connects the arytenoids to the thyroid cartilages. The free inferior borders of the quadrangular membrane form the ventricular ligaments, or false focal cords and the superior margins form the aryepiglottic folds.

INNERVATION OF THE LARYNX

The larynx is innervated by two branches of the vagus nerve: the superior laryngeal nerve and the recurrent laryngeal nerve (Figure 24.6). The vagus exits the skull via the jugular foramen and descends in the carotid sheath. It gives off three branches, a pharyngeal branch, the recurrent laryngeal nerve, and the superior laryngeal nerve.

The superior laryngeal nerve (SLN) arises from the middle sympathetic ganglion. It receives a branch from the superior sympathetic cervical ganglion and descends behind the internal carotid. It then branches into the internal and external branches at the level of the cornu of the hyoid. The internal branch of the superior laryngeal nerve originates from the superior laryngeal nerve, lateral to the greater cornu of the hyoid bone. This branch enters the larynx by piercing the posterior part of the hyothyroid membrane above the superior laryngeal vessels. As such, it provides sensory innervation above the cords, to the base of the tongue, posterior surface of the epiglottis, aryepiglottic fold, and arytenoids. The external branch provides motor innervation to the cricothyroid muscle.

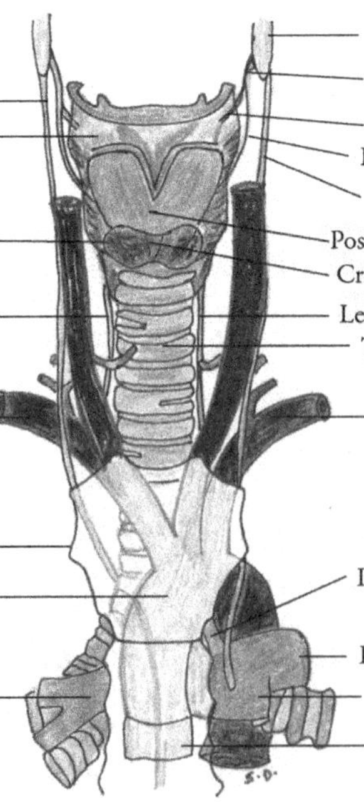

Figure 24.6 Laryngeal anatomy. Image courtesy of Shilpa Dabhade, MD.

The recurrent laryngeal nerve in its course loops under the subclavian artery on the right and under the aortic arch on the right and then travels back into the neck in the tracheo-esophageal groove. It enters the pharynx posteriorly, adjacent to the cricothyroid joint. The recurrent laryngeal nerve provides sensory innervation below the cords and motor innervation to all intrinsic muscles of the larynx except the cricothyroid muscle (this is innervated by the external branch of the superior laryngeal nerve, as mentioned in the previous paragraph).

THE VOCAL CORDS

Loss of the cricothyroid muscle affects tensing of the vocal cords, the voice will be weak and easily fatigued, and the pitch of the patient's voice will be lower. Sensation to the supraglottic area will be affected via injury to the internal division of the superior laryngeal nerve. Patients will complain of frequent throat clearing and a feeling of foreign body sensation in throat. Injury to the external branch of the superior laryngeal nerve will affect the cricothyroid muscle. The cricothyroid muscle is the tensor of the vocal cord. Injury to this branch of the nerve will cause hoarseness.

Recurrent Laryngeal Nerve

The left laryngeal nerve takes different courses on the left and on the right. On the left the recurrent laryngeal nerve circles the arch of the aorta. This longer course makes it more prone to injury. In unilateral recurrent laryngeal nerve paralysis the affected vocal cord assumes a median or paramedian position and does not move on inspiration (Figure 24.7). The patient will present with hoarseness.

In bilateral recurrent laryngeal nerve paralysis, both cords lie in median or paramedian position due to unopposed cricothyroid muscles. The patient will present with stridor and dyspnea.

MUSCLES OF THE LARYNX

The extrinsic muscles of the larynx position and support the larynx. They can be divided into the suprahyoid, infrahyoid, and pharyngeal muscles as follows:

- The suprahyoid muscle moves the hyoid bone upward and forward.
- The infrahyoid bone depresses the larynx.
- The pharyngeal constrictor assists in swallowing.

The suprahyoid muscles include the stylohyoid, thyrohyoid, diagastric, mylohyoid, and geniohyoid. The infrahyoid muscle group includes the omohyoid, sternohyoid, thyrohyoid, and sternothyroid muscles.

The intrinsic muscles of the larynx have their attachments within the larynx. They are responsible for closing the laryngeal inlet, adjusting the tension of the vocal ligaments, and regulating the space between the vocal cords. They include the aryepiglottic, thyroepiglottic, thyroarytenoid, vocalis, oblique and transverse arytenoid, lateral and posterior cricoarytenoid, and cricothyroid muscles. To facilitate memory, a good way to remember the intrinsic muscles is to group them by action.

A**b**duction: Posterior cricoarytenoid.

A**d**duction: Lateral cricoarytenoid and transverse arytenoid.

Closing of the laryngeal inlet: Aryepiglottic and oblique arytenoid.

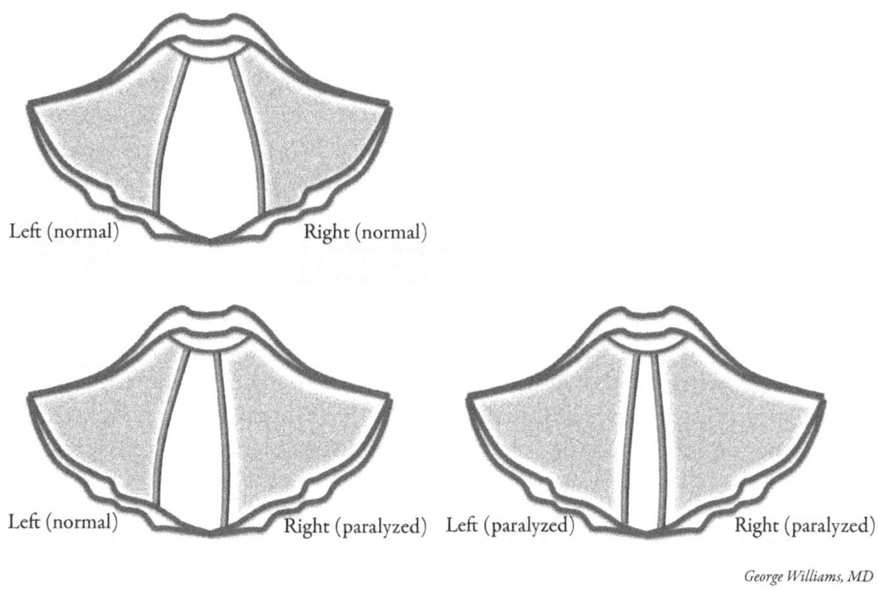

Figure 24.7 Demonstration of differing degree of vocal cord paralysis. Notice that the paralyzed cord has greater length (yielding longer wavelengths/lower tones) and more adduction providing greater potential for airway obstruction.

Relaxation of vocal cords: Vocalis and thyroarytenoid.

Tension of vocal cords: Cricothyroid.

BLOOD SUPPLY

The larynx receives blood supply from the superior laryngeal artery (branch of the superior thyroid artery) and the inferior laryngeal artery (branch of the inferior thyroid artery).

The external branch of the superior laryngeal artery travels with the superior thyroid artery. The superior laryngeal artery branches off the external carotid artery from the external carotid and gives off an infrahyoid branch. It then bifurcates at the tip of the superior cornu of the thyroid cartilage to give off the superior laryngeal artery that travels with the internal branch of the superior laryngeal nerve to pierce the thyrohyoid membrane and supply the interior of the larynx. It continues as the superior thyroid artery on the lateral surface of the middle and inferior constrictor muscle.

The inferior laryngeal artery is a branch of the inferior thyroid artery from the subclavian artery. It runs with the recurrent laryngeal nerve into the larynx. It enters the larynx and anastomoses with the superior laryngeal artery.

PEDIATRIC VERSUS ADULT AIRWAY

There are anatomical differences between the adult and the pediatric patient that must be noted for proper anesthetic management. The pediatric patient has a larger head, a larger tongue, and a more prominent occiput. For airway management purposes, this means any further extension of the neck during intubations or bag masking will produce airway obstruction. Also, a larger tongue in relation to the oral cavity will easily obstruct the airway.

The pediatric epiglottis is long and stiffer than the adult epiglottis, which makes it difficult to lift with a laryngoscope. In the pediatric patient, the larynx is more cephalad, located at the C3-C4 level versus C5-C6 in the adult. The vocal fold in the pediatric patient has a lower attachment, therefore it has an anterior angle when compared with the adult. This leads to increased likelihood of mistakenly placing the endotracheal tube in the anterior commissure rather than into the trachea during nasal intubations.

In the pediatric patient the airway is funnel shaped and narrowest at the cricoid cartilage, while in the adult the narrowest component of the airway is the laryngeal inlet. These facts can be expected to be commonly tested.

TRACHEAL STRUCTURE

The trachea is composed of 18–22 C-shaped cartilaginous rings; the trachea begins at the lower border of the cricoid cartilage at the C6 vertebra and ends at T4-T5 the level of the sternum. It travels anterior to the esophagus into the superior mediastinum and divides into the left and the right bronchi at the T4-T5 vertebral level. Anterior to the trachea in the neck lies the isthmus of the thyroid gland, cervical fascia, and inferior thyroid veins.

Posteriorly the trachea is covered by the trachealis muscle, which allows for expansion of the esophagus during swallowing.

Laterally, in the neck the trachea is surrounded by the common carotid sheath, right and left lobes of the thyroid gland, and the recurrent laryngeal nerves. In the chest on the right side the trachea lies near the root of the neck of the innominate artery, while on the left it lies next to the aortic arch, left common carotid artery, and subclavian artery.

MUSCLES OF RESPIRATION

Respiration is a process that requires contraction of skeletal muscles. There are several muscles in the chest and upper torso that assist in the mechanism of respiration and work of breathing. The muscles that aid in inspiration are those with the ability to contract and expand the thoracic cavity, while those compressing the thoracic cavity help induce exhalation. There are principal muscles of respiration as well as the accessory muscles of respiration. These muscles can be affected by several different factors including poor nutrition, fatigue, inadequate ventilation, and increased work in conditions like COPD. These muscle groups can be categorized as the muscles of inspiration and muscles of expiration based on their function on the thoracic cavity.

INSPIRATION MUSCLES

The diaphragm is the principal muscle of inspiration. This is a dome-shaped muscle that separates the thoracic cavity from the abdominal cavity. Its insertion point is a mobile, central tendon that originates from fibers attached to the xiphoid process, lower six ribs, and lumbar vertebral bodies. About half of its muscle fibers are made up of slow-twitch, high-oxidative-capacity (hence fatigue-resistant) fibers. It accomplishes about 75% of inspiration effort. The contraction of the diaphragm causes the dome to flatten, moving down into the abdominal cavity, raising intra-abdominal pressure. It also causes the lower ribs to move upward and forward. These movements function to increase the volume of the thoracic cavity by an increase in the transverse diameter and create a negative pressure proportional to the force of contraction. The diaphragm moves about 1 cm during normal tidal breathing but can move up to 10 cm during forced inspiration.

The external intercostal muscles are located between the ribs on the outer layer of the thoracic cage alongside the expiratory muscle fibers; they slope downward and forward.

Table 24.1 MUSCLES INVOLVED IN RESPIRATION

MUSCLES OF INSPIRATION	MUSCLES OF EXPIRATION
Diaphragm	Diaphragm
External Intercostal Muscles	Internal Intercostal Muscles
Accessory Muscles of Inspiration • Scalene Muscles • Sternocleidomastoid • Serratus Anterior • Serratus Posterior Superior and Inferior • Pectoralis Major and Minor • Upper Trapezius • Latissimus Dorsi • Levator Scapulae • Rhomboids • Levatores Costarum • Alae Nasi • Cervical Strap Muscles	Abdominal Muscles • Rectus Abdominus • Internal Obliques • External Obliques • Transverse Abdominus

The contraction of these muscles pulls the ribs upward and outward as well as stabilizing the ribcage. The stabilization of the ribcage helps oppose the tendency of the thoracic cage to collapse that comes from the negative pressure from diaphragmatic contraction. These muscles provide about 25% of the work of inspiration. Due to the efficiency of the diaphragm during respiration, paralysis of the intercostal muscles does not significantly impair breathing.

The accessory muscles of inspiration include mainly the scalene muscles, which elevate the first two ribs, and the sternocleidomastoids, which in turn elevates the sternum. These muscles rarely function during normal tidal breathing but come into play during increased work of breathing (i.e., exercise and disease states). There are several other muscles listed in Table 24.1 that play minor roles in achieving forced inspiration.

EXPIRATION MUSCLES

Expiration is a passive process during normal tidal breathing. This occurs from the relaxation of the diaphragm and therefore the recoil of the lungs and ribcage. However during forced expiration such as during exercise, coughing, or hyperventilation, some muscles actively contract to assist in expiration.

Abdominal muscles contribute by depressing the ribs, pushing the diaphragm up, and increasing intra-abdominal pressure in order to enable forced exhalation. The internal intercostal muscles pull the ribs downward and inward in the opposite direction of the external intercostal muscles. This action effectively decreases the thoracic volume.

RESPIRATORY PHARMACOLOGY

The smooth muscles in the airway system can transiently become irritated, causing an increase in tone and, therefore, increased airway resistance. This can occur in normal individuals undergoing general anesthesia without previous lung pathology, but is more common in patients with a history of asthma and or chronic obstructive pulmonary disease (COPD). The treatment of these patients is based on bronchodilators and anti-inflammatory therapy. The most commonly used bronchodilators are β2-adrenergic agonists and anticholinergics. These medications can be short acting and used in the acute phase of bronchospasm from any source or long acting and used in the maintenance phase.

β2-ADRENERGIC AGONISTS

These are sympathomimetic agents that bind to the Gs-protein-coupled beta adrenoreceptors. This action activates adenylyl cyclase, which in turn catalyzes the production of cyclic adenosine monophosphate (cAMP) from ATP. Cyclic adenosine monophosphate inactivates myosin light chain kinase, which is what phosphorylates smooth muscle myosin (facilitating muscle relaxation and thereby bronchodilation). Cyclic adenosine monophosphate also causes a decrease in the intracellular calcium concentration.

A combination of these results in an intracellular increase in cAMP and, therefore, smooth muscle relaxation in the lungs. Selective β2-adrenergic agonists have an equivalent bronchodilating effect with less cardiac stimulation than the nonselective agonists. A commonly used selective β2-adrenergic agonist is levalbuterol.

The short-acting β2-adrenergic agonists' onset of action is typically 3–5 minutes and lasts 4–6 hours. Albuterol is the most commonly prescribed short-acting β2-adrenergic agonist. The long-acting β2-adrenergic agonists' onset of action is within 30–45 minutes and can lasts up to 12 hours (Table 24.2). The prototypical agent is salmeterol. Most of these medications are available through an inhaled route, which has the highest therapeutic ratio, and have the added benefit of improved mucociliary clearance. These properties make them useful in treatment of asthma and COPD.

Epinephrine, while not a specific β2-adrenergic agonist, can be used for bronchodilation in extremis. When severe bronchoconstriction occurs particularly during anaphylaxis, small doses of epinephrine can be life saving. However, a longer-acting medication will need to be instituted due to the short half-life. Initiating a low-dose infusion is an example of how to achieve prolonged action with epinephrine.

ANTICHOLINERGIC DRUGS

Anticholinergic drugs are agents that bind reversibly with cholinergic (muscarinic and nicotinic) receptors in the central and peripheral nervous system, inhibiting parasympathetic impulses. This site binding blocks acetylcholine's access to these sites, inhibiting release of intracellular cAMP. This overall cascade prevents the bronchoconstriction caused by a release of acetylcholine.

Table 24.2 EXAMPLES OF BETA-2 ADRENERGIC AGONISTS

SHORT-ACTING β2-ADRENERGIC AGONISTS	LONG-ACTING β2-ADRENERGIC AGONISTS
Albuterol 1–2 puffs q 4–6 hours	Salmetarol 1–2 puffs q 12 hours
Levalbuterol • Liquid Nebs 0.63–1.25 mg q 6–8 hours • MDI 1–2 puffs q 4 hours	
Terbutaline 1–2 puffs q 6–8 hours	Formoterol 1–2 puffs q 12 hours
Pirbuterol 1–2 puffs q 4–6 hours	
Tornalate 1–2 puffs q 8 hours	

In the lungs, the subset of muscarinic receptors responsible for bronchial smooth muscle contraction are the M3 receptors and are predominantly in the medium- to large-size bronchioles. Medications that have the most affinity to blocking the M3 receptors, therefore, have the most bronchodilating properties. Similar to the β2-adrenergic receptor agonists, the anticholinergic medications can be divided into short acting and long acting (Table 24.3). The short-acting medications take 15 minutes for onset of action and last 6–8 hours. They have a longer time to onset and thus are not preferred as the rescue treatment for acute asthma or COPD exacerbation. The long-acting medications take about 20 for onset of action and lasts 24 hours. This is more commonly used for maintenance therapy.

The β2-adrenergic agonists are regarded as first line in the treatment of an acute bronchospasm; however, anticholinergics have been used extensively in as an adjuvant therapy. The anticholinergics are also less absorbed systemically than the β2-adrenergic agonists, and therefore have decreased systemic side effects in comparison to the former.

Table 24.3 EXAMPLES OF ANTICHOLINERGICS

SHORT-ACTING ANTICHOLINERGIC	LONG-ACTING ANTICHOLINERGIC
Ipratropium Bromide • MDI 2–4 puffs 3–4 times daily • DPI 40–80 μg 4 times daily	Tiotropium • DPI inhale contents if 1 capsule daily
Oxitropium Bromide • MDI 2 puffs 2–3 times daily • DPI 200 μg twice daily	
MDI: Metered dose inhaler DPI: Dry power inhaler μ: micro	

ANTI-INFLAMMATORY MEDICATIONS

Inflammation is a release of chemical mediators from tissues and cells. This can be a normal defense mechanism again pathogens. The most common of these chemicals are leukotrienes, histamine, bradykinin, prostaglandins, platelet-activating factor, and interleukin-1. When triggered, an excessive release of these mediators can result in significant airway inflammation, edema, and mucus plugging with resulting difficulty in breathing. There are a wide variety of medications to aid in preventing or stopping the cascade of inflammation in order to decrease the morbidity and mortality.

Corticosteroids are four-ringed steroid hormones produced by the adrenal cortex from the biochemical precursor cholesterol. There are two major groups: the glucocorticoids and the mineralocorticoids. However, the term *corticosteroids* became colloquially used to refer to glucocorticoids. The mineralocorticoids primary act on sodium balance through aldosterone with little or no role in anti-inflammatory processes. The glucocorticoids, on the other hand, possess the properties to help reduce the inflammatory response by various mechanisms, some not fully understood. One method is by binding to the glucocorticoid receptors and therefore up-regulating the expression of anti-inflammatory proteins in the nucleus. They also bind and inhibit the activation of inflammatory cells such as cytokines, arachidonic acid metabolites. Corticosteroids are also associated with a reduction of mast cells in in the bronchus. Furthermore, corticosteroids alter the vascular inflammatory response to bronchial injury as well as decreasing microvascular leakage, mucus formation, and mediator production. The use of systemic corticosteroids in patients with acute asthma attack refractory to bronchodilators is essential (Figure 24.8). They should be given as quickly as possible whenever inflammation is suspected, however, significant clinical effect can be

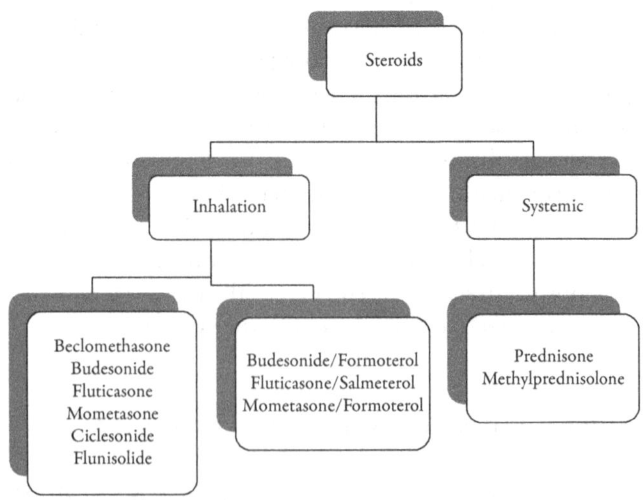

Figure 24.8 Corticosteroids.

delayed up to 6 hours after administration. They can also be used typically via inhalation route for chronic control of airway inflammation. They can also be used in combination with anticholinergic medication for symptoms relief.

The side effect profile of the inhaled steroid is favorable at the usual doses; however, the long-term use of systemic steroids can include adrenal suppression, oral candidiasis, hypertension, and hyperglycemia.

LEUKOTRIENE MODIFIER DRUGS

Leukotrienes are fatty compounds that are produced by the immune system, causing inflammation and bronchoconstriction. Leukotriene modifiers are the first classification of drugs that are mediator-specific therapy for asthma. They can be used in place of inhaled steroids or as an adjuvant therapy. There are two classifications of these drugs. One class, the receptor antagonists, blocks the actions of cysteinyl leukotrienes at the level of the CycLT1 receptors. The second class blocks 5-lipocygenase and inhibits the synthetic pathway of leukotriene (Figure 24.9).

While these may not be as efficacious as the other treatments for asthma and bronchospasm, they are well tolerated with few side effects, the most serious being elevated liver enzymes—the mechanism is unknown but may be due to altered metabolism. They are metabolized by the cytochrome P450 system (CYP3A4 and CYP2C9), and hepatotoxicity may be caused by formation of toxic intermediates. This was discovered in the clinical trials of these medications and therefore necessitated monitoring liver function while taking them.

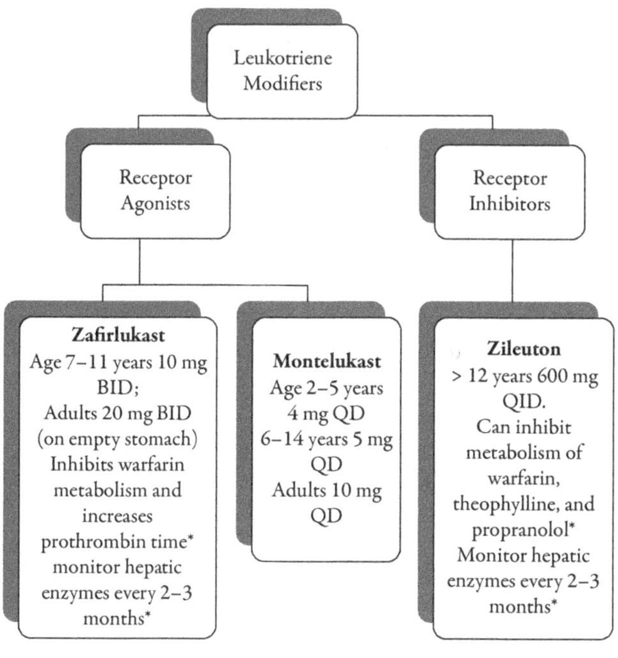

Figure 24.9 Leukotrienes.

MAST CELL STABILIZERS

Mast cells play a significant role in allergic reactions and inflammation. These are granulocytes that contain histamine. When these cells are activated, they release their histamine-filled granules causing a histamine-mediated inflammatory response. The mast cell stabilizers work by blocking IgE-regulated calcium channels. This prevents the influx of the intracellular calcium needed for degranulation and histamine release. These are not effective for moderate to severe asthma, but can be useful in mild asthma and prior to exposure to an asthma-triggering substance. Cromolyn sodium is an example of this drug type that may be prescribed for mastocytosis and food allergy (200 mg po QID 30 minutes before meals, or inhaled 20 mg via nebulizer QID). Mast cell stabilizers have a very low bioavailability with minimal systemic effects.

IMMUNOGLOBULIN E BLOCKERS

Immunoglobulin E (IgE) blockers are a newer agent in the treatment of asthma. This subset of drugs can be used in moderate to severe allergic asthma or other allergic conditions that do not respond to high doses of corticosteroids. The IgE are a class of immunoglobulins. They have low plasma levels as well as a short half-life. When allergic individuals are exposed to a triggering agent, IgE molecules bind to the high-affinity IgE receptor (FcεRI) on the surface of mast cells and basophils, triggering immediate-hypersensitivity reactions and late-phase responses. They also augment humoral and cellular immune responses to allergens.

The prototypical drug in this class is omalizumab (Xolair). This is a recombinant DNA–derived monoclonal antibody that binds to free IgE in the blood as well as to membrane-bound IgE on the surface of the lymphocytes. This binding reduces the surface-bound IgE, thereby limiting the release of mediators, decreasing the allergic response. This medication is different from most other asthma and inflammation medication because of the delivery mode (Tables 24.4 and 24.5). It is not available orally or via inhalation. It administered in doses of 150 to 375 mg by subcutaneous (SC) injection every 2 or 4 weeks. It is approved for patients age 12 years of age and above. Patients should have serum total IgE level (IU/mL), measured before the start

Table 24.4 XOLAIR DOSING—EVERY 4 WEEKS

PRETREATMENT SERUM IGE (IU/ML)	BODY WEIGHT (KG)			
	30–60	61–70	71–90	91–150
30–100	150 mg	150 mg	150 mg	300 mg
101–200	300 mg	300 mg	300 mg	
201–300	300 mg			
>300	See Table 24.5			

Table 24.5 XOLAIR DOSING—EVERY 2 WEEKS

PRETREATMENT SERUM IGE (IU/ML)	BODY WEIGHT (KG) 30–60	61–70	71–90	91–150
30–100	See Table 24.4			
101–200				225 mg
201–300		225 mg	225 mg	300 mg
301–400	225 mg	225 mg	300 mg	
401–500	300 mg	300 mg	375 mg	
501–600	300 mg	375 mg	Do not Dose	
601–700	375 mg			

of treatment, and body weight (kg). Serum IgE can remain elevated for up to 1 year after discontinuation of treatment. Hence retesting serum IgE during treatment cannot be used as a guide.

REFERENCES

1. Agur A, Dalley A. *Grant's Atlas of Anatomy*. 12th ed. Philadelphia, PA: Lippincott Williams & Wilkins; 2008.
2. Bateman E, Kornmann O, Schmidt P, et al. Tiotropium is non-inferior to salmeterol in maintaining improved lung function in B16-Arg/Arg patients with asthma. *J Allergy Clin Immunol*. 2011;128:315–322.
3. Butterworth I, Mackey D, Wasnick J. *Clinical Anesthesiology*. 5th ed. Philadelphia, PA: McGraw-Hill; 2013.
4. Celli B. Respiratory muscle function. *Clin Chest Med*. 1986;7:567.
5. Chabner B, Knollman B. *Goodman and Gilman's The Pharmacological Basis of Therapeutics*. 12th ed. New York, NY: McGraw-Hill; 2011:277–333.
6. Diamant Z, Mantzouranis E, Bjermer L. Montelukast in the treatment of asthma and beyond. *Expert Rev Clin Immunology*. 2009;5(6):639–658.
7. Diong B, Rajagiri A, Goldman M, Nazeran H. The augmented RIC model of the human respiratory system. *Med Biol Eng Comput*. 2009;47(4):395–404.
8. Drake RL, Vogl A, Mitchell A. *Gray's Anatomy for Students*. 2nd ed. Philadelphia, PA: Churchill Livingstone; 2009.
9. Gosens R, Zaagsma J, Meurs H, Halayko A. Muscarinic receptor signaling in the pathophysiology of asthma and COPD. *Resp Res*. 2006;7:73.
10. Jarvis B, Markham A. Montelukast: a review of its therapeutic potential in persistent asthma. *Drugs*. 2000;59(4):891–928.
11. Kaiser H, Parasuraman B, Boggs R, Miller C, Leidy N, O'Dowd L. Onset of effect of budesonide and formoterol administered via one pressurized metered-dose inhaler in patients with asthma previously treated with inhaled corticosteroids. *Ann Allergy Asthma Immunol*. 2008;101(3):295–303.
12. Lewis J. Nonsteroidal anti-inflammatory drugs and leukotriene receptor antagonists. In: Kaplowitz N, DeLeve L. *Drug-Induced Liver Disease*. 3rd ed. Amsterdam, Netherlands: Elsevier; 2013:389–390.
13. Masoli M, Williams M, Weatherall M, Beasley R. The 24 h duration of bronchodilator action of the budesonide/formoterol combination inhaler. *Respir Med*. 2006;100(1):20–25.
14. Matera M, Cazzola M. Ultra-long-acting beta2-adrenoceptor agonists: an emerging therapeutic option for asthma and COPD? *Drugs*. 2007;67:503–515.
15. Maurer M, Rosén K, Hsieh H, et al. Omalizumab for the treatment of chronic idiopathic or spontaneous urticaria. *N Engl J Med*. 2013;368:924–935.
16. McKenna S. Respiratory physiology. In: Vacanti C, Sikka P, Urman R, Dershwitz M, Segal B. *Essential Clinical Anesthesia*. Cambridge, England: Cambridge University Press; 2011.
17. Palmqvist M, Arvidsson P, Beckman O, Peterson S, Lötvall J. Onset of bronchodilation of budesonide/formoterol vs salmeterol/fluticasone in single inhalers. *Pulm Pharmacol Ther*. 2001;14(1):29–34.
18. Rochester D. The diaphragm: contractile properties and fatigue. *J Clin Invest*. 1985;75:1397.
19. Roussos C, Macklem P. The respiratory muscles. *N Engl J Med*. 1982;307:786.
20. Tashkin D, Celli B, Senn S, et al. A 4-year trial of tiotropium in chronic obstructive pulmonary disease. *N Engl J Med*. 2008;359:1543–1554.
21. van der Wiel E, ten Hacken N, Postma D, van den Berge M. Small-airways dysfunction associates with respiratory symptoms and clinical features of asthma: a systematic review. *J Allergy Clin Immunol*. 2013;131(3):646–657.
22. West J. *Respiratory Physiology: The Essentials*. 8th ed. Philadelphia, PA: Lippincott Williams & Wilkins; 2007.
23. Zimmerman H. Respiratory supportive drugs. In: Zimmerman H. *Hepatotoxicity: The Adverse Effects of Drugs and Other Chemicals on the Liver*. 2nd ed. Philadelphia, PA: Lippincott; 1999:717.
24. Xolair Product information. Genentech website. http://gene.com/download/pdf/xolair_prescribing.pdf. Accessed April 6, 2015.

FURTHER READING

Barash P, Cullen B, Stoelting R, Cahalan M, Stock M. *Clinical Anesthesia*. 7th ed. Philadelphia, PA: Lippincott Williams & Wilkins; 2013.

Cheeseman K, Burdett E. Anatomy of the nose and pharynx. *Ann Intensive Care*. 2011;12(7):283–286. doi: 10.1016/j.mpaic.2011.04.013.

Ellis H, Lawson A. Part 1: The respiratory pathway, lungs, thoracic wall, and diaphragm. In Ellis H, Lawson A. *Anatomy for Anaesthetists*. 9th ed. Hoboken, NJ: Wiley; 2013:3–42.

Rajagopal, P. Anatomy and physiology of airway and breathing. *Indian J Anaesth*. 2005;49(4):251–256.

QUESTIONS

1. Which turbinate receives the termination of the lacrimal duct?
   - A. Inferior turbinate
   - B. Superior turbinate
   - C. Middle turbinate
   - D. Frontal sinus
   - E. Maxillary turbinate

2. Vocal cord abduction is achieved with which of the following muscles?
   - A. Cricothyroid
   - B. Posterior cricoarytenoid
   - C. Vocalis
   - D. Thyroarytenoid
   - E. Lateral cricoarytenoid

3. In the pediatric patient, which anatomic structure is the narrowest part of the airway?
   A. Laryngeal inlet
   B. Cricoid cartilage
   C. False vocal cords
   D. Tracheal rings
   E. Thyroid cartilage

4. Through what ligament is an incision made to create an emergency airway?
   A. Thyroid cartilage
   B. Cricothyroid membrane
   C. Cricotracheal ligament
   D. Tracheal ligament
   E. Thyrohyoid ligament

5. Which of the following statements regarding the diaphragm is FALSE?
   A. It is made up of fast-twitch, high-oxidative-capacity, and fatigue-resistant fibers, making it an ideal principal muscle of inspiration.
   B. Its insertion point is a mobile, central tendon that originates from fibers and is attached to the xiphoid process, lower six ribs, and lumbar vertebral bodies.
   C. Relaxation of the diaphragm and elastic recoil of the lungs constitute the mechanism for passive exhalation.
   D. The diaphragm can move up to 10 cm during forced inspiration.
   E. It accomplishes 75% of inspiratory effort.

6. What subset of muscarinic receptors is responsible for bronchial smooth muscle contraction?
   A. M1
   B. M2
   C. M3
   D. M4
   E. M5

7. Which of the following statement about IgE blocker omalizumab (Xolair) is FALSE?
   A. It is only available via subcutaneous injection route.
   B. It is a recombinant DNA–derived monoclonal antibody.
   C. It is imperative to monitor serum IgE before and during the treatment.
   D. It approved for patients 12 years and older.
   E. It is approved for moderate to severe asthma unresponsive to high-dose steroids.

8. Which of the following drugs is an example of a mediator-specific therapy for the treatment of asthma?
   A. Budesonide
   B. Montelukast
   C. Terbutaline
   D. Cromolyn
   E. Tiotropium

9. What is the mechanism of anticholinergic drugs in the treatment of asthma and bronchospasm?
   A. They block IgE-regulated calcium channels.
   B. They block 5-lipocygenase and inhibit the synthetic pathway of leukotriene.
   C. They bind to receptors blocking acetylcholine's access to these sites, therefore inhibiting release of intracellular cAMP.
   D. They stabilize mast cells.
   E. They directly inhibit histamine.

10. Which of the following medications is available only via an injection route?
   A. Omalizumab
   B. Cromolyn sodium
   C. Zileuton
   D. Mometasone
   E. Methylprednisolone

ANSWERS

1. A. The inferior turbinate is the largest turbinate and receives the termination of the lacrimal duct. The other answers are distractors.
2. B. The posterior cricoarytenoid. The posterior cricoarytenoid originates from the posterior aspect of the cricoid cartilage and inserts into the muscular process of the arytenoid cartilage. It laterally abducts the arytenoid cartilage, which opens the laryngeal inlet. It is the only abductor of the vocal cords.
3. B. In the pediatric patient the airway is funnel shaped and narrowest at the cricoid cartilage, while in the adult the laryngeal inlet is the narrowest component. The other responses are not narrowed in the pediatric patient.
4. B. Cricothyrotomy is an emergency procedure that accesses the airway by making a midline cut through the cricothyroid membrane.
5. A. The diaphragm has muscle fibers that are made up of slow- (not fast-) twitch, high-oxidative-capacity, hence fatigue-resistant fibers. This makes it an effective and efficient muscle for respiration. All other answers are correct.

FURTHER RE1ADING

ButterworthJF, MackeyDC, WasnickJD. *Morgan and Mikhail's Clinical Anesthesiology*. 5th ed. New York, NY: McGraw-Hill;2013:ch. 23.

West JB. *Respiratory Physiology: The Essentials*. 8th ed. Philadelphia, PA: Lippincott Williams & Wilkins; 2007:ch. 7.

6. C. In the lungs, the subset of muscarinic receptors responsible for bronchial smooth muscle contraction are the M3 receptors, which are predominantly found in the medium- to large-size bronchioles. Medications that have the most affinity to blocking the M3s therefore

have the most bronchodilating properties. There are five subtypes of muscarinic receptors; M1s, which are common in exocrine glands, increase secretions from salivary glands and acid secretions in stomach. M2s are mostly located in the heart, where they can act to slow down heart rate to normal sinus by slowing the speed of depolarization and decreasing contractile forces of the atrial cardiac muscle. M4s and M5s are mostly in the CNS, and also decrease calcium conduction.

FURTHER READING

Gosens R, Zaagsma J, Meurs H, Halayko A. Muscarinic receptor signaling in the pathophysiology of asthma and COPD. *Resp Res.* 2006;7:73.

7. C. Serum IgE is elevated during treatment with omalizumab and can remain elevated up to 1 year after stopping treatment. Therefore, it is imperative to draw IgE prior to starting treatment, but not during treatment. It cannot be used to guide treatment once it has started. All other choices are correct.

FURTHER READING

Maurer M, Rosén K, Hsieh H, et al. Omalizumab for the treatment of chronic idiopathic or spontaneous urticaria. *N Engl J Med.* 2013;368:924–935. http://gene.com/download/pdf/xolair_prescribing.pdf.

8. B. Leukotrienes are fatty compounds that are produced by the immune system, causing inflammation and bronchoconstriction. Leukotriene modifiers are the first classification of drugs that are mediator-specific therapy for asthma. Montelukast is a receptor agonist. Budesonide is a glucocorticoid; terbutaline is a β2-adrenergic receptor agonist; cromolyn is a mast cell stabilizer; and tiotropium is an anticholinergic bronchodilator; none of these is a mediator-specific therapy for treatment of asthma.

FURTHER READING

Diamant Z, Mantzouranis E, Bjermer L. Montelukast in the treatment of asthma and beyond. *Expert Rev Clin Immunology.* 2009;5(6):639–658.
Jarvis B, Markham A. Montelukast: a review of its therapeutic potential in persistent asthma. *Drugs.* 2000;59(4):891–928.

9. C. These are agents that bind reversibly with cholinergic (muscarinic and nicotinic) receptors in the central and peripheral nervous system, inhibiting parasympathetic impulses. This site binding blocks acetylcholine's access to these sites, inhibiting release of intracellular cAMP. This overall cascade prevents the bronchoconstriction caused by a release of acetylcholine. The other listed mechanisms have their specific agents for that mechanism of action including IgE blockers, leukotriene inhibitors, mast cell stabilizers, and antihistamines.

FURTHER READING

Butterworth JF, Mackey DC, Wasnick JD. *Morgan and Mikhail's Clinical Anesthesiology.* 5th ed. New York, NY: McGraw-Hill; 2013:ch. 24.

10. A. Omalizumab is the only medication in this group that is available neither via inhalation nor oral route but via subcutaneous injection only. Cromolyn sodium is available via oral concentrate of nebulized solution. Zileuton is a leukotriene receptor inhibitor that is available via oral route. Mometasone is a steroid available as a nasal spray or a dry power inhaler. Methylprednisolone can be oral or IV formulation. See text and package insert.

25.

CARDIOVASCULAR SYSTEM

Erin A. Gottlieb and Timothy Pawelek

CONTROL OF HEART RATE

The heart rate is controlled by the firing of the sinoatrial node. Its rate of firing is influenced by neural and humoral factors. Parasympathetic vagal cell bodies are located in the dorsal vagal nucleus and the nucleus ambiguus in the medulla. The fibers make up the vagus nerve. They primarily innervate the sinoatrial (SA) and atrioventricular (AV) nodes, and the released neurotransmitter acetylcholine binds M_2 muscarinic receptors. Increased vagal stimulation has a negative chronotropic (decrease in heart rate) and negative dromotropic effect (slower AV conduction).

The neurons of the sympathetic system originate in the rostral ventrolateral medulla. The preganglionic fibers synapse in the stellate, middle cervical, and thoracolumbar sympathetic paravertebral ganglia. Postganglionic fibers innervate the SA and AV nodes, the conduction system, and cardiac myocytes. Stimulation of primarily β_1 receptors by the sympathetic neurotransmitter norepinephrine results in a positive chronotropic effect (increase in heart rate) and a positive dromotropic effect (faster AV conduction).

Stimulation of the right vagus and right sympathetic nerves mostly affects the sinoatrial node, while stimulation of the left vagus and left sympathetic nerves mostly affects the atrioventricular node.

Parasympathetic or sympathetic system dominance varies with age. For example, the parasympathetic system predominates in neonates; neonates often become bradycardic during laryngoscopy due to vagal stimulation. Certain parasympathetic or sympathetically mediated changes in heart rate are due to reflexes. A number of them are described in Table 25.1.

There is also humoral control of the cardiovascular system via circulating catecholamines and the renin-angiotensin-aldosterone system. Catecholamines are secreted by the adrenal medulla into the bloodstream. The adrenal medulla secretes about 80% epinephrine and 20% norepinephrine. The other endogenous source of circulating norepinephrine is sympathetic nerves innervating the blood vessels. These catecholamines bind to β_1 receptors, causing an increase in heart rate. The other humoral substance that affects heart rate is angiotensin II. Angiotensin II increases the release of norepinephrine from sympathetic nerve endings, inhibits its reuptake, and increases sympathetic efferent activity in the rostral ventrolateral medulla.[1]

SYNCHRONICITY OF PRESSURE, FLOW, ELECTROCARDIOGRAPHY, SOUNDS, VALVE ACTION

There is a timing correspondence between the ECG, aortic blood flow, filling, aortic pressure, jugular venous pressure, heart sounds, and valve action during the cardiac cycle. It is necessary to understand the phases and timing of the cardiac cycle.[2,3]

The jugular venous pressure waveform has three waves and two descents. The *a wave* corresponds to atrial contraction. The *c wave* is caused by the bulging of the tricuspid valve into the atrium and occurs at the time of ventricular contraction. The *v wave* is caused by the buildup of blood in the venous system prior to the opening of the tricuspid valve. The *x descent* is the decrease in pressure between the c and v waves and is caused by a downward distortion of the atrium during ventricular contraction. The *y descent* after the v wave corresponds to the decrease in central venous pressure following the opening of the tricuspid valve and beginning of rapid ventricular filling.[4]

IMPULSE PROPAGATION

As blood is ejected into the aorta with each ventricular systole, the arterial tree is filled with blood and the aorta

Table 25.1 CARDIOVASCULAR REFLEXES AFFECTING HEART RATE

Carotid Sinus Reflex	**Afferent impulses travel to nucleus tractus solitarius via Hering's nerve, which connects with the glossopharyngeal nerve; results in a decrease in heart rate from increased parasympathetic outflow via the efferent pathway, the vagus nerve**
Valsalva Maneuver	**Forced expiration against a closed glottis increases intrapleural pressure, compresses vessels in thorax, and transiently increases aortic pressure. Aortic baroreceptors trigger an afferent signal via the vagus nerve to the nucleus tractus solitarius; results in a transient decrease in heart rate due to an increase in parasympathetic outflow via vagal efferents**
Bezold-Jarisch Reflex	**Afferent signals from the left ventricular wall from increased intraventricular pressure, mechanical distortion, or ischemia cause a decrease in heart rate and hypotension from an increase in parasympathetic activity; vagus nerve carries both afferent and efferent signals**
Bainbridge Atrial Reflex	**Stretch receptors at the venoatrial junction are stimulated when there is an increase in venous return; afferent signal carried by vagus nerve, results in increase in sympathetic outflow and heart rate**
Chemoreceptor Reflex	**Activation of specialized cells in carotid and aortic bodies detects hypoxemia, hypercarbia, and acidemia. Efferent signals from carotid bodies are carried by Hering's nerve and the glossopharyngeal nerve; efferent signals from aortic bodies are carried by the vagus nerve; results in increased vasomotor center activity and an increase in sympathetic outflow and heart rate**

Adapted from: Klabunde RE. Neurohumoral control of the heart and circulation. In: *Cardiovascular Physiology Concepts.* 2nd ed. Philadelphia, PA: Lippincott Williams & Wilkins; 2012:124–147; Barth CD, Ebert TJ. Autonomic nervous system. In: Hemmings HC Jr, Hopkins PM, eds. *Foundations of Anesthesia: Basic Sciences for Clinical Practice.* 2nd ed. Philadelphia, PA: Mosby Elsevier; 2006:403–420.

distends. In diastole, the aorta recoils so that there is continuous flow in the arterial system during all phases of the cardiac cycle. Various arterial waveforms are shown in Figure 25.1. The highest point is the systolic pressure, the lowest point is the diastolic pressure, and the difference between systolic and diastolic blood pressure is the pulse pressure. The notch in the training is called the incisura and corresponds to the closing of the aortic valve.[5]

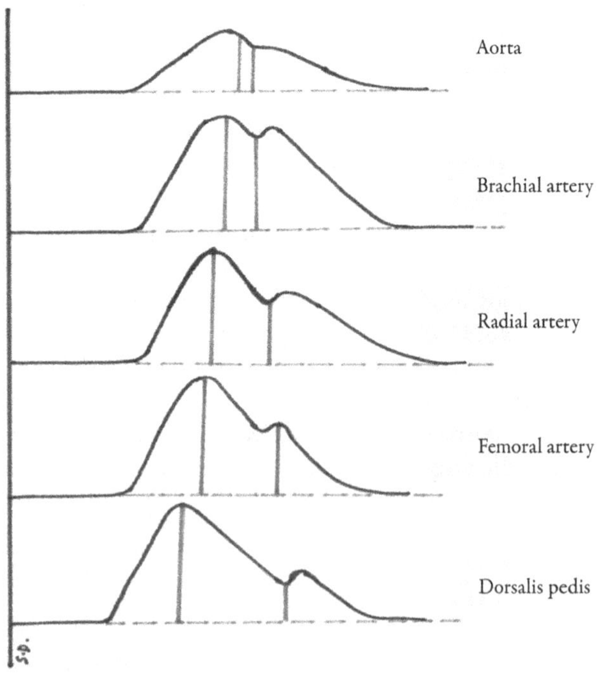

Figure 25.1 Arterial waveforms adjusted for sample site. Image courtesy of Shilpa Dabhade, MD.

The pulse pressure and contour are affected by disease states. In atherosclerotic aortic disease, the aorta is noncompliant. The systolic pressure is very high due to the stiff aorta that does not distend. In valvar aortic stenosis, the systolic peak is lower due to the obstruction at the valve and to the decrease in blood flow across it. In aortic regurgitation and in patent ductus arteriosus, the pulse pressure is large. This is due to the diastolic runoff back through the regurgitant valve and through the ductus arteriosus, respectively. The low diastolic pressure in these disease states can lead to coronary ischemia.[5]

The pulse waveform changes as the site of measurement moves from central to peripheral locations. In general, distal pressure waveforms have greater amplitude, a more pronounced diastolic wave, and a lower mean and diastolic pressure (Figure 25.2). This change in waveform is due to forward propagation of the pressure wave and wave reflection from higher resistance vessels, mainly the arteriole.[6]

NORMAL ELECTROCARDIOGRAM

The ECG is an average of all action potentials in the heart. The ECG is important for the recognition and diagnosis of arrhythmias, ischemia, and electrolyte disturbances. The components of an ECG tracing are summarized in Table 25.2.[7]

ELECTROPHYSIOLOGY, ION CHANNELS, CURRENTS

There are two kinds of action potentials in cardiac cells, those in atrial and ventricular myocytes and Purkinje fibers and those in sinoatrial and atrioventricular (AV) nodal cells (Figure 25.3). The action potential in atrial

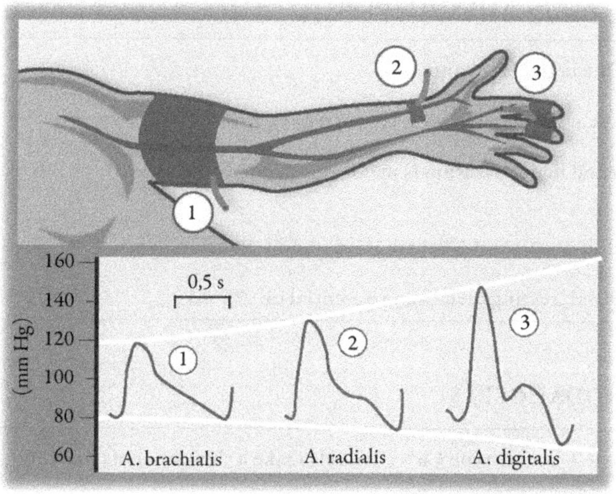

Figure 25.2 Arterial pressure waveform. From PhysiologyWeb. http://upload.wikimedia.org/wikipedia/commons/f/f5/Arterial_Pathway.jpg Accessed: April 8, 2015.

and ventricular myocytes and Purkinje fibers has five phases (Table 25.3). The action potential in nodal cells has three phases (Table 25.4).[7,8]

VENTRICULAR FUNCTION

Cardiac output is influenced by a number of factors including preload, afterload, inotropic state, heart rate, and right and left ventricular function.

FRANK-STARLING LAW, PRELOAD AND AFTERLOAD, INTRACARDIAC PRESSURES

Preload represents the volume and stretch of myocytes prior to contraction. An indirect measure of preload is the end diastolic volume or pressure (EDV or EDP). Preload is very dependent on diastolic function. Diastolic

Table 25.2 ECG COMPONENTS

P wave	Atrial depolarization, normally 0.08–0.1 seconds
QRS complex	Ventricular depolarization, normally 0.06–0.1 seconds; if prolonged, ventricular conduction defect exists
T wave	Ventricular repolarization
U wave	Small upward deflection following the T wave; prominent with marked hypokalemia or bradycardia
PR interval	Time between the start of atrial depolarization to the beginning of the QRS complex; if > 0.2 seconds, a conduction defect exists most likely in the AV node
ST segment	Isoelectric period following the QRS complex when the ventricle is depolarized; it is important in the diagnosis of myocardial ischemia
QT interval	Ventricular depolarization and repolarization, the duration of the action potential, normally 0.2-0.4 seconds; longer QT interval can indicate susceptibility to arrhythmias
QTc interval	The QT interval divided by the square root of the RR interval (the interval between ventricular depolarizations); allows assessment of the QT interval independent of heart rate

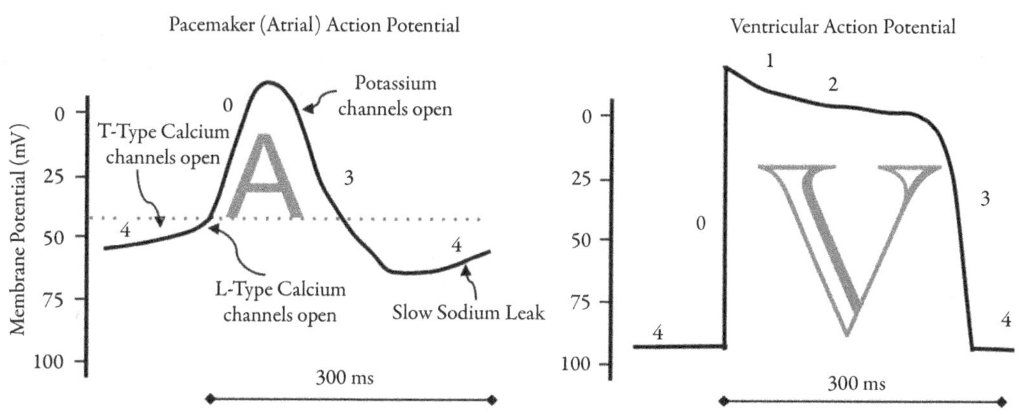

Figure 25.3 Atrial (pacemaker) and ventricular membrane potentials. Notice how the ventricular membrane potential is sharper (more like the edges of a V) than the pacemaker. Adapted from *Cardiac Action Potentials: Figure 2*. Natalie's Casebook Website. http://www.nataliescasebook.com/img/Case-7/Cardiac_APs.png Accessed April 8, 2015.

Table 25.3 PHASES OF ACTION POTENTIAL IN MYOCYTES AND PURKINJE FIBERS

Phase 0	Initial depolarization	Inward Na^+ current (I_{Na}) through Na^+ channels
Phase 1	Early repolarization	Transient outward K^+ current (I_{TO}) and inward Cl^- current (I_{Cl})
Phase 2	Plateau	Repolarization is delayed and depolarization is maintained mostly by inward Ca^{2+} current (I_{Ca})
Phase 3	Repolarization	Termination by rapid and slow outward K^+ currents (I_{Kr} and I_{Ks})
Phase 4	Resting potential	Cell is maximally repolarized; resting membrane potential of −90 mV

Table 25.4 PHASES OF ACTION POTENTIAL IN AV AND SA NODAL CELLS

Phase 0	Initial depolarization	Inward Ca^{2+} current through T- and L-type Ca^{2+} channels make a slower depolarization upstroke
Phase 3	Repolarization	Inactivation of slow inward Ca^{2+} channels and increased outward movement of K^+
Phase 4	Resting potential	Pacemaker ("funny") current (I_f) predisposes to spontaneous depolarization; some inward movement of Na^+ and Ca^{2+}; Resting membrane potential of these nodal cells is −50 to −70 mV

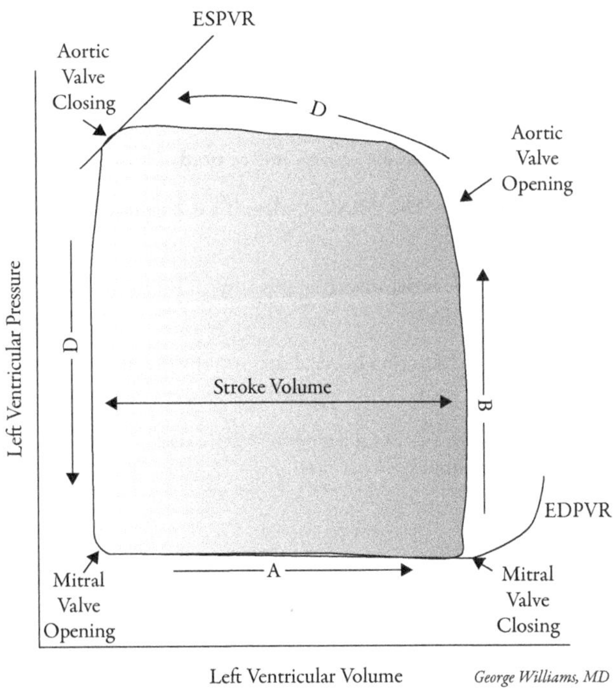

Figure 25.4 Pressure volume loop of the cardiac cycle. Image courtesy of George Williams, MD.

dysfunction results in reduced ventricular compliance and reduced preload.

Changes in preload (ventricular filling) change the ability of the myocyte to generate force. As preload increases and myocyte length increases, active tension increases; this is known as the *length-tension relationship*. There is a limit to this increase.

Frank-Starling curves show the relationship between left ventricular end diastolic pressure (LVEDP) and stroke volume (SV). The *Frank-Starling mechanism* describes the effect of increasing venous return to the heart. An increase in venous return results in an increase in ventricular filling, an increase in preload. The increase in preload results in an increase in the force generated by the ventricle. This increase in force results in an increase in stroke volume. If preload gets too high, then the curve changes to reflect a reduction in cardiac output due to fluid overload. Preload is affected by venous pressure, ventricular compliance, heart rate, atrial contraction, resistance to inflow, resistance to outflow, and inotropy.

Afterload is the pressure that the heart must overcome in order to eject. The afterload for the left ventricle is the aortic pressure, and the afterload for the right ventricle is the pulmonary artery pressure. The *force-velocity relationship* describes the effect of a change in afterload on the velocity of shortening. An increase in afterload results in a decrease in the velocity of shortening, and a decrease in afterload results in an increase in the velocity of shortening.

A change in afterload affects Frank-Starling curves as well. An increase in afterload shifts the Frank-Starling curve downward (reduced cardiac output), and a decrease in afterload shifts the Frank-Starling curve upward (increased cardiac output).[3]

MYOCARDIAL CONTRACTILITY, MEASUREMENT LIMITATIONS

Myocardial contractility or *inotropy* is the ability of cardiac muscle to generate tension in the face of a specific load. Changes in the inotropic state of the heart lead to changes in stroke volume.

Therefore, inotropy has a large effect on cardiac output. At a given preload, an increase in inotropy leads to an increase in stroke volume, and the Frank-Starling curve is moved upward. A decrease in inotropy leads to a decrease in stroke volume, and the Frank-Starling curve is moved downward.

Sympathetic stimulation and increases in circulating catecholamines have a positive inotropic effect due to β_1 adrenergic stimulation. An increase in afterload can also lead to an increased inotropic state (Anrep effect). The increase in inotropic state due to an increase in heart rate is called the Bowditch or Treppe effect.[3]

Contractility is difficult to quantify in vivo as it is dependent on loading conditions. There are a number of different indices of contractility that are useful in experimental preparations, but that are not easily applied in clinical situations.

Left ventricular pressure monitoring during the phase of isovolumic contraction phase can also provide useful information regarding contractility. During this phase, pressure is developed in the left ventricle until it is greater than the pressure in the aorta, and the aortic valve opens. The first derivative of the developed pressure, dP/dt_{max}, is an index of contractility. It is relatively independent of afterload, but it is affected by preload, valvular pathology, and wall properties. It also requires special monitoring.

Information about contractility can be derived from pressure-volume loops. The end-systolic pressure volume relationship (ESPVR) is the point at the upper left hand corner of the pressure volume loop (see Figure 25.4). Elastance is defined as delta P/Delta V. The maximal elastance is at end-systole, and it provides an index of contractility that is independent of load.

Preload recruitable stroke work describes the amount of stroke work that the left ventricle can perform for a given preload. The slope of this line changes with changes in contractility; as contractility increases, the ventricle can perform more work for a given preload. The opposite is also true.[9]

The most commonly used index of ventricular contractility is the ejection fraction (EF). It is defined as the stroke volume divided by end-diastolic volume. The normal EF for the left ventricle is 60%–70%. The normal ejection fraction for the right ventricle is 45%–50%. The EF can be determined using various imaging techniques including echocardiography, angiography, and MRI. It can also be measured using indicator dilution techniques. The ejection fraction is useful for describing systolic function only, and it is influenced substantially by changes in afterload.[3]

In clinical practice, pulmonary artery catheters can be used to assess right ventricular contractility, but they do not have access to the left side of the heart. Right ventricular preload recruitable stroke work can be calculated by measuring right ventricular end-systolic and end-diastolic volumes using thermodilution. Another reported approach uses Doppler flow and pulmonary artery pressure measurements to index RV power generation.[9]

Echocardiography is often used for assessment of contractility. Motion mode (M-mode) imaging, two-dimensional imaging, and Doppler techniques can all be used to quantify systolic function. In M-mode, the change in LV short axis diameter during systole can be calculated as a percentage called fractional shortening (FS). Fractional shortening is a good assessment of global systolic function in the absence of segmental wall motion abnormalities (SWMAs). The formula for FS is below where the LVEDD is the left ventricular end-diastolic dimension and the LVESD is the left ventricular end-systolic dimension.

$$FS = (LVEDD - LVESD / LVEDD) \times 100$$

Mitral annular descent can also be examined using M-mode imaging. The magnitude of mitral annular descent in systole provides an index of global LV function. It can characterize function as normal, mildly depressed, and moderately to severely depressed; that is, it cannot differentiate between moderately and severely depressed LV function.

Two-dimensional imaging can be used to quantify systolic function by determining the fractional area change (FAC) and the ejection fraction (EF). The FAC examines the proportional change in LV area during systole and expresses it as a percentage. Images are obtained in the transgastric mid-short-axis view. The FAC is influenced by loading conditions and SWMAs. The EF is the calculated from the proportional change in LV volume during systole. It is also highly dependent on loading, influenced by diastolic function and RV function. It can also be unpredictable if SWMAs exist. The equations for FAC and EF are below. The LVEDA is the left ventricular end-diastolic area, and the LVESA is the left ventricular end-systolic dimension. The LVEDV is the left ventricular end-diastolic volume and the LVESV is the left ventricular end-systolic volume.

$$FAC = \left[(LVEDA - LVESA) / LVEDA\right] \times 100$$

$$EF = \left[\left(LVEDV - LVESV\right) / LVEDV)\right] \times 100$$

Doppler techniques can also be used to quantify left ventricular function, including examination of the rate of rise of LV pressure, the peak mitral jet velocity, myocardial performance index, and tissue Doppler imaging.[10]

CARDIAC OUTPUT: DETERMINANTS AND REGULATION

The cardiac output (CO) is the volume of blood ejected from the left ventricle into the aorta during systole multiplied by the number of systoles in one minute.

$$CO = SV \times HR$$

The CO is therefore determined by the stroke volume and the heart rate, and changes in these parameters result in changes in the CO. The CO is expressed in liters per minute. The cardiac index is the CO divided by the body surface area of the subject and is expressed in liters per minute per square meter. The normal cardiac index is 2.6–4.2 L/min/m^2.

Changes in heart rate are generally modulated by the autonomic nervous system, with increases in heart rate due to a preponderance of sympathetic activity compared with parasympathetic activity at the sinoatrial node. Increases in heart rate increase the CO up to a point where the rapid heart rate does not allow for adequate ventricular filling and where stroke volume is impaired.

During times of increased metabolic need such as exercise, stroke volume can also be increased due to increased sympathetic stimulation. Sympathetic stimulation augments preload by decreasing venous compliance and by improving ventricular filling. Ventricular filling is also enhanced by an increase in atrial inotropy leading to an improved atrial systole and enhanced ventricular relaxation (lusitropy). An increase in ventricular inotropy leads to a decreased end-systolic volume, as well.[3,11]

MYOCARDIAL OXYGEN UTILIZATION

The heart requires oxygen in order to replenish ATP, which is required for contraction and relaxation of cardiac muscle. Any factor that increases myocardial demand increases myocardial oxygen utilization. These factors include increases in heart rate, contractility, afterload, and preload. Myocardial oxygen consumption (mVO_2) is the product of coronary blood flow (CBF) and the oxygen extraction of the myocardium, the difference in oxygen content between arterial and venous blood.

$$mVO_2 = CBF\left(CaO_2 - CvO_2\right)$$

The mVO_2 at rest is approximately 8 mL O_2/min/100 g of myocardium. It can increase to more than 70 mL O_2/min/100 g during exertion, and the mVO_2 of an arrested heart is 2 mL O_2/min/100 g, for cellular maintenance alone. It is difficult to directly measure myocardial oxygen consumption. The pressure-rate product (double product) is the product of the heart rate (HR) and systolic blood pressure (SBP) and correlates with myocardial oxygen consumption.

$$\text{Pressure-Rate Product} = HR \times SBP$$

Although myocardial oxygen consumption is increased with an increase in heart rate and with an increase in contractility, preload, and afterload, it is important to recognize that the increase in mVO_2 associated with an increase in preload is much smaller than the increase due to increases in the other variables.[3]

SYSTOLIC AND DIASTOLIC FUNCTION

Left ventricular systolic function is the ability of the ventricular to eject blood into the aorta. It is determined by preload, afterload, contractility, and ventricular configuration. On a cellular level, it is an energy-dependent process, and calcium handling is important. Inotropy can be increased by increasing the influx of calcium into the myocyte, increasing the affinity of troponin-C for calcium, increasing the uptake of calcium by the sarcoplasmic reticulum and inhibiting calcium efflux from the myocyte.

Diastolic function is defined by the adequacy of ventricular filling during diastole. Myocardial relaxation is required for effective and efficient filling. The four phases of diastole are isovolumic relaxation, rapid ventricular filling, slow ventricular filling, and atrial systole. Inadequate relaxation reduces the amount of filling during the rapid and slow filling phases and increases the importance of filling due to the atrial systole. Relaxation is also active and requires energy. At a cellular level, relaxation requires the removal of calcium from troponin-C binding sites so that actin and myosin dissociate. It requires ATP for the removal of cytosolic calcium by reuptake into the sarcoplasmic reticulum and exchange of calcium for sodium across the cell membrane. Diastolic function can be compromised by ineffective calcium removal from insufficient time (tachycardia), insufficient ATP (ischemia), or enhanced calcium binding to Troponin-C.

β-adrenergic activation enhances both systolic and diastolic function by affecting calcium handling. For example, sympathetic activation leads to the phosphorylation of phospholamban and troponin-I. The phosphorylation of phospholamban allows calcium to be picked up faster by the sarcoplasmic reticulum, and the phosphorylation of troponin-I reduces the affinity of calcium for troponin-C so that unbinding is faster.[12]

VENOUS RETURN

VASCULAR COMPLIANCE AND CAPACITANCE

Venous return can be augmented by several factors: an increase in the volume of blood, an increase in the tone of large vessels leading to increased peripheral venous pressure, and a dilation of arterioles leading to a decrease in peripheral vascular resistance and resulting in a rapid transit of blood from the arterial to the venous side.[13] Vascular tone is regulated via substances that act on the endothelial cells. The production of endothelium-derived relaxing factors is diminished if the endothelium is damaged, such as in atherosclerosis, leading to constriction of blood vessels. In intact vessels, acetylcholine causes vasodilation via release of NO.[14] Most of the peripheral vasculature is controlled by the thoracolumbar sympathetic chain with increases in sympathetic stimulation resulting in increased vascular tone. This increased tone forces the blood out of venous capacitance vessels, resulting in increased preload. At the same time, sympathetic output causes a reduction in splanchnic and lower extremity perfusion via vasoconstriction as well.[15]

POSITIONING AND MUSCLE ACTION

Venous return is augmented by negative intrathoracic pressure generated by inspiration, and so preload is higher during the inspiration phase of the respiratory cycle. Positive pressure ventilation abolishes this increase.[16] Venous return can also be increased by isometric muscle contraction, such as squatting or bilateral hand grip, and by changing position: lowering the head or raising or crossing legs.[17] This principle is applied to patients with preload-dependent cardiac lesions, such as tetralogy of Fallot ("Tet spells"), where the patient squats in order to relieve the spell.

BLOOD VOLUME AND DISTRIBUTION

Blood volume varies with age and can be estimated at 100 mL/kg for a premature infant, 90 mL/kg for a term infant, 80 mL/kg for a 3- to 12-month-old, and 70 mL/kg for an over-1-year-old (recall this fact; blood volume calculations are an easily tested concept for anesthesiology residents).[18] Various organ systems serve as capacitance vessels for blood that can be redistributed to the central circulation in case of a hemorrhage. The release of epinephrine leads to arterial vasoconstriction in tissue beds and shifts the blood into central compartments.[19] The venous system serves as a reservoir for blood that can increase preload when needed (like a strategic blood reserve); however, with age the venous system becomes less compliant and the ability to augment the preload by venoconstriction is diminished.[20]

BLOOD PRESSURE

SYSTOLIC, DIASTOLIC, MEAN, AND PERFUSION PRESSURES

The classic formula for mean arterial pressure is the sum of the systolic pressure and two times the diastolic pressure divided by 3. This means that about 67% of the mean arterial pressure is determined by diastolic pressure (a double-weighted average favoring the diastolic pressure). This is based on the fact that during normal heart rates a greater portion of the cardiac cycle is spent in diastole. At very high heart rates less time is spent in diastole, and the mean arterial pressure then is closer to the average of systolic and diastolic pressure.[21] Arterial pulsation dampens as blood travels from the bigger arteries to the arterioles and capillaries. This is caused by the compliance of the vessels and the resistance to blood movement in the vessels.[22] Short-term control of blood pressure is achieved by the nervous system effect on peripheral vascular resistance and capacitance and cardiac output. Long-term effects on blood pressure are exerted by the renal control of volume status.[23]

THORACIC CIRCULATION FACTS

Normal intracardiac pressures are as follows in mmHg. Right atrium 0–6, right ventricle pressure of 15–30/0–6, pulmonary artery 15–30/5–12 with a mean PAP of 9–18, and pulmonary artery occlusion pressure 5–12, which is also the left atrial pressure. On the systemic side, the left ventricular pressure of 120/0–5 and the aortic pressure of 120/80. The pulmonary veins contribute 40% of total resistance of the pulmonary circulation and can have an even higher resistance in states of hypoxemia, acute respiratory distress syndrome (ARDS), or sepsis due to pulmonary venous vasoconstriction.

VASCULAR RESISTANCE

The drop in mean pressure from systemic artery to arteriole is more pronounced across the systemic vessels versus the pulmonary vessels. Sympathetic innervation in the pulmonary vessels is important for the optimization of V/Q caused by gravity and position.[24] The pulmonary circulation vasoconstricts due to a drop in oxygen tension so that the V/Q relationship is optimized.

BARORECEPTOR FUNCTION

Arterial baroreceptors are found in the aortic arch and at the bifurcation of the carotids and respond to increased stretch from increased blood pressure by sending a signal to the carotid sinus nerve. The stimulus is then transmitted via the glossopharyngeal nerve to the postsynaptic nucleus ambiguus and vagal motor nucleus, causing a decrease in heart rate.[25]

THE MICROCIRCULATION

Pressure/Starling's Law

The capillaries vary in the sizes of their clefts between the endothelial cells by tissue depending on the function of the involved organ. For example, brain capillaries have tight junctions that allow passage of only small molecules such as water, oxygen, and carbon dioxide (CO_2). The liver has wide clefts to accommodate plasma proteins, and the glomerular capillaries have fenestrae through the cells that allow filtration of small molecules and ions without the need to pass through clefts between endothelial cells.[26] Starling noted that under normal conditions a near-equilibrium exists in most capillaries. This means that the volume of fluid filtered out from the arterial side of the capillary approximates the volume of fluid reabsorbed to the circulatory system with the small amount of fluid missing returning via the lymphatic system at a rate of about 2 mL/min in a healthy adult.[27] Osmotic pressure is created by sodium, glucose, urea, and the oncotic pressure by plasma proteins.

$$Q = kA\left[(Pc - Pi) + \sigma(\pi_i - \pi_c)\right]$$

Q = fluid filtration, k = capillary filtration coefficient (conductivity of water), A = the area of the capillary membrane, P_c = capillary hydrostatic pressure, P_i = interstitial hydrostatic pressure, σ = reflection coefficient for albumin, π_i = interstitial colloid osmotic pressure, and π_c = capillary colloid osmotic pressure.

Capillary Sphincter Control

Arterioles have an internal diameter of 10–15 micrometers and are highly muscular. The terminal arterioles are intermittently covered by smooth muscle cells and at the transition point to a true capillary, a smooth muscle fiber encircles the capillary, creating a precapillary sphincter that can open and close. The local conditions of the tissue cause direct effect on the precapillary sphincters, controlling local blood flow.[28]

Viscosity/Rheology

Poiseuille's law states that blood flow in inversely proportional to the viscosity of the fluid. Whole blood is about three times more viscous then water, and when the hematocrit approaches 60%–70% the viscosity rises to about 10 times that of water. The concentration and type of plasma proteins play a minor role in viscosity as opposed to hematocrit.[29] Remember that chronic hypoxia such as from intracardiac shunt or living at altitude (or sleeping in a hypoxic chamber like elite cyclists) will also result in an increase of hematocrit. From a viscosity standpoint only, the optimal hematocrit for oxygen delivery is actually 30%.

REGIONAL BLOOD FLOW AND ITS REGULATION

CEREBRAL AND SPINAL CORD

In healthy adults, cerebral blood flow is autoregulated between mean arterial pressures of 50 and 150 mmHg. The autoregulation is impaired by high volatile anesthetic concentration and/or hypercarbia, and is shifted toward higher pressures (curve shifts to the right) in patients with chronic hypertension. Arterial CO_2 is a major factor in effecting cerebral blood flow. Cerebral blood flow increases 1–2 mL/100 g/min for every 1-mmHg rise in CO_2. This is relevant in the short term, as over a longer period the pH of the CSF normalizes. Oxygen tension also affects cerebral blood flow, most notably at PaO_2 below 60, leading to a dramatic increase in cerebral blood flow. Neural control plays a minor role in cerebral blood flow. Areas with regional cerebral ischemia (strokes) do no autoregulate cerebral blood flow, and it becomes pressure dependent.[30] Spinal cord perfusion pressure is a function of MAP minus the CSF pressure, and draining CSF can improve spinal cord perfusion during high-risk surgery such as a TAAA.

CARDIOPULMONARY PERFUSION

Coronary perfusion of the right ventricle occurs during systole and diastole, while the left ventricular subendocardium relies on perfusion during diastole. Coronary perfusion pressure is the difference between aortic diastolic pressure and the pressure in the left ventricle at end diastole. Pulmonary wedge pressure can be used as an estimate of the left ventricular diastolic pressure. As diastolic time decreases with increasing heart rate, so does the time for left ventricular coronary flow. Tachycardia is the most important trigger of intraoperative and perioperative ischemia. Coronary arteries autoregulate flow and at maximal vasodilation will receive 3–5 times the flow at baseline.

The pulmonary circulation is unique in its response to hypoxia, which leads to pulmonary vasoconstriction. This serves to optimize the V/Q match to provide blood flow to the areas of the lung that are ventilated. The mechanism of hypoxic pulmonary vasoconstriction (HPV) is thought to be via an oxygen sensor. Hypoxic pulmonary vasoconstriction is thought to be mediated by a calcium-calmodulin and phosphorylation of myosin light chains.[31]

RENAL

Renal blood flow is about 20% of cardiac output and is autoregulated in healthy adults at mean arterial pressures between 75 and 170 mmHg. The greatest resistance is provided by the efferent arterioles providing a pressure of 10–20 mmHg, which allows net reabsorption to occur (recall *A*fferent is on the *A*rterial side of the Glomerulus, and *E*fferent is on the v*E*nous side). Most of the renal blood flow goes to the renal cortex with the medulla and papillae receiving about 10% of flow. The kidney regulates its flow by either the afferent arteriole responding to the stretch of increased flow by vasoconstriction or by the tubular-glomerular mechanism. The macula densa at the juxtoglomerular apparatus senses changes in the flow of filtrate and signals the afferent arterioles to modulate renal blood flow. At low blood pressures, sympathetic input results in compensatory water retention and an increase in plasma volume by inducing renal vasoconstriction, lowering GFR and reducing renal capillary hydrostatic pressure.[32]

SPLANCHNIC/HEPATIC

Splanchnic circulation has only a small degree of autoregulation and is primarily controlled by metabolic factors. Feeding releases cholecystekinin and gastrin, and the absorption of glucose and other nutrients causes an increase in splanchnic blood flow. Sympathetic activity causes arterial and venous constriction via alpha receptors and diverts blood from the large capacitance of the splanchnic circulation to the central circulation. Hepatic blood flow is about 25% of cardiac output, and 75% of hepatic blood flow is from the portal vein. The hepatic artery provides the remaining 25% and delivers oxygen to the liver. The liver is a blood capacitance organ and has about 15% of blood volume. The liver received 50% of its oxygen supply from the hepatic artery and the other 50% from the hepatic vein. Sympathetic stimulation causes constriction of perisinusoidal resistance vessels and diverts blood from the liver back into central circulation.[33]

MUSCLE AND SKIN

The percent of cardiac output to the muscles is 15% at rest and 6% to the skin in cool weather. The blood flow to the inactive muscles is very low at only 750 mL/min considering that they can constitute up to 40% of total body mass. With exercise and the increase in metabolic activity, blood flow can increase by up to 20 times the resting value.[34] The skin blood flow is linked to the temperature regulation of the body and is controlled by the sympathetic nervous system. With skin warming, blood flow to the skin can be as high as 7-8 L/min. The blood flow necessary for the metabolic demand of skin is very low and sufficient with even severe vasoconstriction.[35]

UTERINE AND PLACENTAL

The blood flow to the uterus increases significantly as the pregnancy progresses due to low vascular resistance of the uterus and a 15%–25% increase in heart rate. The increased cardiac output, which is at 50% of baseline is increased during labor (up to 12–14 L/min) and postpartum, when blood volume is augmented from the contracting uterus. The decrease in vascular resistance is due to estrogens, progesterone, and prostacyclin. Placental blood flow can be decreased by aortocaval compression, hypotension, hemorrhage/hypovolemia, and uterine contraction.[36]

HEMODYNAMIC REGULATION

CENTRAL

The vasomotor center is located in the medulla and pons and sends parasympathetic impulses via the vagus nerve to the heart and via sympathetics to the spinal cord and vasculature. The vasomotor center can be activated by the reticular system, the hypothalamus, and several parts of the cerebral cortex.[37] Any increase in serum osmolality stimulates the release of antidiuretic hormone (ADH) via stimulation of osmoreceptors in the hypothalamus and atrial stretch receptors. Positive pressure ventilation, stress, and beta stimulation can also cause release of ADH. The posterior pituitary secretes ADH in the supraoptic and paraventricular nuclei. Antidiuretic hormone increases the permeability of membranes to water in the renal collecting tubules and increases reabsorption of water. This causes an increase in blood volume and a decrease in serum osmolality. Antidiuretic hormone also causes vasoconstriction of vascular smooth muscle, increasing blood pressure. This effect is most potent on the splanchnic, renal, and coronary vasculature. As such, vasopressin may be used to treat gastrointestinal bleeding.[38,39] Antidiuretic hormone also increases the levels of circulating von Willebrand factor and factor VIII. An analogue of ADH, DDAVP, is used for this effect to treat intraoperative bleeding.[40]

PERIPHERAL

Arterial baroreceptor reflexes and the cardiopulmonary reflexes respond to decreases in blood pressure and blood volume (as discussed earlier in the chapter). They are located in the high-pressure regions of the aortic arch and the carotid sinus as baroreceptors and in the cardiac atria in the low-pressure system as stretch receptors. The afferent stimuli travel via the vagus and glossopharyngeal nerves and synapse in the nucleus solitarius. From there, the signals are conducted to the hypothalamus and trigger ADH control and secretion. The Bainbridge reflex is caused by atrial stretch via the vagus nerve to the medulla, and the efferent effect via the vagus and sympathetic nerves is to increase the heart rate and contractility. This is thought to improve blood flow through the atria and pulmonary circulation.[41]

HORMONAL CONTROL

Blood volume and extracellular fluid volume are interdependent. Even a small change in blood volume causes a significant effect on cardiac output, this in turn affects blood pressure, and blood pressure affects urine output. The interplay of these factors results in a stable blood volume despite widely varying fluid intake. Hormonal control is primarily a more long-term mechanism as opposed to the almost instantaneous control of the circulation based on the tone of various vascular systems. When low pressure is sensed in the pulmonary circulation, a reflex activation of the sympathetic nervous system occurs. This increased activity causes constriction of the renal arterioles, resulting in a decreased GFR and increased tubular reabsorption of sodium and water. It also causes release of renin and formation of angiotensin and aldosterone, which also increases tubular reabsorption. If the blood pressure is still low, the stretch receptors become activated, as discussed in the previous section.[42]

MIXED VENOUS OXYGEN TENSION AND SATURATION

Mixed venous oxygen is measured in the proximal pulmonary artery as it captures the blood returning from all areas that receive perfusion, including the coronary sinus. This means that one cannot use a triple lumen or other nonpulmonary arterial catheter to obtain a true mixed venous gas. The mixed venous saturation is an indicator of global extraction of oxygen and is dependent on cardiac output, hemoglobin, and oxygen saturation on the arterial side. Mixed venous oxygen below 65% is indicative of an imbalance between supply and demand of oxygen at the tissue level. When the mixed venous saturation rises above 80% it may indicate a maldistribution of peripheral blood flow, which can occur in a state of high cardiac output such as sepsis, liver disease, inflammation, or pregnancy.

ANATOMY OF THE NORMAL HEART AND SYSTEMIC VASCULATURE

The heart is typically found in the middle mediastinum near ribs 5–8 to the left of the sternum and rests above the diaphragm. It consists of four chambers operating as two circuits in a series with the atria as receiving chambers and the ventricles as discharging chambers and with valves at the exit of each chamber to prevent reverse flow. The right side of the heart receives deoxygenated blood form the venous system (via the superior vena cava and inferior vena cava primarily) and pumps it through the pulmonary system for oxygenation and ventilation. The left side of the heart receives the oxygenated ventilated blood and pumps it systemically through the body. The atria are composed of two thin muscle layers oriented perpendicular to each other and are constructed similarly to each other. They function as reservoirs during systole and passively empty during ventricular diastole, with a contraction immediately prior to subsequent ventricular systole to aid in ventricular filling. The atria and ventricles are separated by the atrioventricular valves (the tricuspid and mitral). The two ventricles are constructed differently from each other due to the different pressure systems they pump against. The right ventricle is more anterior in the chest and pumps against a low-pressure system. It can deliver a large volume of blood with less contraction, as the wall shortens toward the tricuspid valve and toward the septum. This configuration will suffer if the pulmonary resistance rises rapidly. Conversely, the left ventricle has three layers of muscle fibers (longitudinal, lateral, and oblique) and functions in "wringing" fashion to generate higher cavitary pressures to pump against the higher resistance of the systemic vasculature. The ventricles also have valves at their outflow to the arteries to prevent regurgitant flow. The right ventricle pumps into the main pulmonary artery, which divides into a right and left PA to further divide into smaller divisions into the lung parenchyma. The parenchymal capillaries empty into the pulmonary venous system, which will confluence into four pulmonary veins that empty into the left atrium. The left ventricle ejects into the aorta, which leads to the rest of the systemic vasculature. The aorta has sinuses surrounding each cusp of the trileaflet aortic valve (right coronary, left coronary, noncoronary), which function to direct blood flow down the coronary arteries.

SYSTEMIC ARTERIAL SYSTEM

The aorta subdivides into major arteries that will either empty directly into the "vessel rich" organs or into arterioles for the rest of the body. The vessel rich vasculature primarily includes the brain, heart, kidney, hepatic, and splanchnic circulation. The cerebral vasculature is fed by a combination of the two carotids and by the vertebral circulation via the basilar artery. The brain receives 15%–20% of the cardiac output and regional cerebral flow is closely related to the metabolic rate of the region perfused. Thus the more active gray matter in the cerebral cortex receives significantly more blood flow and has a higher metabolic rate than the subcortical white matter. This coupling is tightly regulated by local metabolites in the cortex, CO_2 partial pressures and O_2 partial pressures.

The pulmonary circulation has a lower mean pressure than the systemic circulation and facilitates gas exchange due to the proximity of the alveoli to the capillaries. The alveoli and bronchial smooth muscle are regulated by the autonomic system. The pulmonary vasculature typically has approximately one-fifth of the blood volume in it at any given time and can function as a reservoir during traumatic hemorrhage. These shifts are regulated by the sympathetic system as well as regulators such as the renin-angiotensin-aldosterone system, prostaglandins, and endogenous nitric oxide. Low oxygen tension also regulates the vasculature by hypoxic pulmonary vasoconstriction, which shifts blood flow away from poorly ventilated areas by contraction of the arterial smooth muscle. This reflex also leads to the development of refractory pulmonary hypertension under chronically low oxygenation.

The hepatic circulation is a combination of the arterial system and venous system. The liver receives approximately 20%–25% of the cardiac output, with about 75% of the blood flow from the portal vein and the remainder from the hepatic artery. Most of the hepatic oxygen is supplied by the artery and is autoregulated by the sympathetic system in response to decreased oxygen tension (abolished by volatile anesthetics). The portal venous system does not autoregulate like the arterial system but is sensitive to downstream increases in pressure from right ventricular failure or cirrhosis and can lead to dilation of the surrounding veins (esophageal varices) or transudation of fluid (ascites).

The splanchnic circulation supplies the gastrointestinal tract, spleen, pancreas, and a portion of the hepatic circulation. It is weakly autoregulated and primarily responds to decreases in circulating blood volume by arterial and venous vasoconstriction. It exhibits some local metabolically driven autoregulation and hormonal response to food ingestion as well.

HEART CONDUCTION INNERVATION

The sinoatrial node (SAN) is a spindle-shaped structure located lateral to the junction of the superior vena cava and the right atrium. Evidence suggests that the SAN consists of three distinct regions, each responsive to a separate group of neural and circulatory stimuli. The interrelationship of these three regions appears to determine the ultimate rate of output of the SAN. Although the SAN is the primary site of impulse formation, numerous other subsidiary sites are present in both atria and can generate impulses as well. The SAN transmits electrical impulses through atrial muscle bundles to the AVN rather than discrete conduction pathways. These muscle bundles are anatomically separated by the orifices of the vena cavae, coronary sinus, and fossa ovalis. The atrioventricular (AV) node within the medial right atrium (RA) gives rise to the bundle of His, which enters the membranous septum at the distal left ventricular outflow tract (LVOT). The right bundle branch (RBB) travels along the septal aspect of the right ventricle (RV). The left bundle branch (LBB) travels superficially along the septal aspect of the left ventricle (LV) to branch into the left anterior fascicle (LAF) and left posterior fascicle (LPF). Purkinje fibers then become the distal extent of the conduction system.

The heart is richly supplied with sympathetic and parasympathetic innervation. The sympathetic nerves originate from the superior and middle cervical sympathetic ganglia, as well as the stellate ganglion (a major source of cardiac sympathetic innervation). Sympathetic activation results in increases in heart rate, contractility, and blood pressure, which lead to a marked, metabolically mediated increase in coronary blood flow. The vagus nerves deliver parasympathetic efferent cholinergic endings, which result in bradycardia, decreased contractility, and lower blood pressure. A decline in oxygen delivery causes a metabolically mediated coronary vasoconstriction. However, if myocardial oxygen needs are constant, cholinergic coronary dilation is observed in response to vagal stimulation, and reflex activation through baroreceptors, chemoreceptors, and ventricular receptors.

DIGOXIN

The most commonly used digitalis glycoside that will be encountered by anesthesiologists is digoxin. Digoxin is a helpful adjuvant in the treatment of symptomatic CHF and LV dysfunction by reducing the incidence of CHF exacerbations in those under optimal therapy and is the only positive inotropic agent approved for use in chronic heart failure. It indirectly increases inotropy by increasing intracellular Na + through inhibition of the myocardial sarcolemmal Na^+/K^+-ATPase. The increase in Na+ prompts the Na^+/Ca^+ exchanger to extrude Na^+ from the cell, increasing intracellular concentration of Ca+, allowing more interaction between contractile proteins and Ca+. It provides some sympatholysis by direct action on the carotid sinus baroreceptor resulting in decreased sympathetic efferent nerve activity to the heart and circulation. It slows conduction velocity through the AV node and conduction system and results in a decrease in ventricular response to atrial fibrillation while allowing more heart rate variability than beta blockade. It also reduces Na+ absorption in the renal tubules by inhibition of the Na^+/K^+-ATPase. Unfortunately, it has a narrow therapeutic range, resulting in toxic effects in the presence of hypokalemia, hypercalcemia, hypomagnesemia, or renal insufficiency. Treatment of digoxin toxicity is accomplished by administration of digoxin-specific antibodies.

INOTROPES

Inotropes increase the contractility of myocardium by increasing the amount of calcium available to contractile elements. Beta-1 agonists increase intracellular cAMP, resulting in increased concentrations of intracellular calcium, phophodiesterase inhibitors inhibit the breakdown of cAMP (independent of the beta receptor), and calcium sensitizers (levosimendan) increase the sensitivity of the cardiomyocyte contractile proteins to calcium. Beta-1 agonists used as inotropes include epinephrine, dobutamine, isoproterenol, and dopamine. These drugs have varying effects in addition to β1 agonism. It is also should be noted that β-receptor activation causes dilation of both large and small coronary vessels even in the absence of changes in blood flow. Both subtypes are present in the coronary circulation, however β1 predominate in the conductance vessels and β2 in the resistance vessels.

Isoproterenol is the most potent β1 agonist, and its inotropic effect is accompanied by an increase in HR and a decrease in coronary perfusion pressure due to its equally potent β2 activity in the peripheral circulation. This β2 effect will allow blood to preferentially go to the cutaneous and muscular beds at the expense of coronary blood flow. It will extend ischemic areas due to a dysrhythmogenic effect in addition to the decreased coronary blood flow with increased cardiac demand. It will result in a net increase in CO and contractility and decreased SVR. It is very useful as a chemical pacemaker until artificial pacing can be instituted and has some utility in managing asthma and elevated pulmonary pressures.

Epinephrine has potent β1 and β2 activity, but adds alpha activity as well. Its beta effects predominate at lower doses, and because of the alpha stimulation, epinephrine allows an adequate perfusion pressure in conjunction to positive inotropy. At higher doses tachycardia will manifest and prolonged infusions will elicit hyperglycemia and increased lactate due to the metabolic effects from β2 stimulation.

Dobutamine is structurally derived from isoproterenol and retains the β1 agonism with a less potent β2 activity. It allows an increase in coronary blood flow due to coronary vasodilation and mildly dilates the pulmonary vasculature resulting in a net increase in CO, decreased LV filling pressures, and a decrease in SVR with less chronotropic activity at lower doses. It does possess a weak α1 activity, but it is significantly less than that of epinephrine.

Dopamine has activity at all the catecholamine receptors and, historically, was administered at varying doses to take advantage of these effects. As an inotropic agent, it can increase CO by increasing chronotropism and contractility in conjunction with some increase in preload through venoconstriction and by reducing SVR for afterload reduction. At higher doses the α-agonist properties of dopamine can cause increases in pulmonary artery pressure, PVR, and LV filling pressure. The "low/medium/high" (renal dose, etc.) dosing to take advantage of varying effects on different receptors has been unfounded and is also widely varying in individual patient responses.

PHOSPHODIESTERASE III INHIBITORS

The phosphodiesterase (PDE) III inhibitors (milrinone, amrinone, and enoximone) have positive inotropic effects independent of the β1-adrenergic receptor and unique vasodilatory actions independent of endothelial function or nitrovasodilators. Milrinone is most commonly used and increases intracellular cAMP by inhibition of its breakdown by PDE III. These agents also cause vasodilation in the arterial and capacitance beds. Phosphodiesterase inhibitors increase CO, decrease SVR and PVR, and decrease pulmonary wedge pressure.

ANTIARRHYTHMICS

Antiarrythmics are classified based on where they interact with the cardiac conduction cycle. The different classes have a large amount of overlap and affect the rate of depolarization, the duration of the cardiac action potential, and the duration of the refractory period (Table 25.5). Class I drugs have the common effect of decreasing sodium entry through the fast Na+ entry channels, resulting in a decrease in the rate of depolarization. They have been further subdivided into classes IA, IB, and IC based on the other effects they exhibit on the conduction system. Class II drugs are beta antagonists, which decrease the rate of depolarization, the duration of the action potential, and the length of the refractory periods. Class III drugs prolong repolarization by altering potassium, sodium, and calcium channels. Class IV antiarrythmics decrease slow channel calcium conductance, thus slowing the rate of depolarization.

Amiodarone is a first-line agent for treating arrhythmia in CPR and effectively treats SVT, ventricular arrhythmias, ventricular tachycardia, ventricular fibrillation, and a number of other preexcitation arrhythmias. It decreases the rate of depolarization and prolongs the rate of repolarization in the SA node. It also prolongs the refractory period and rate of repolarization in the myocardium, AV

Table 25.5 ANTIARRYTHMICS

CLASS	ELECTROPHYSIOLOGIC EFFECT	PHARMACOLOGIC EFFECT	COMMONLY SEEN EXAMPLES
IA	1. Decrease conduction 2. Prolong depolarization 3. Increased ERP, APD, QRS	Fast inward sodium blockade	Quinidine, Procainamide, Disopyramide
IB	1. Minimal effect on conduction, depolarization, ERP, QRS 2. Decreased APD	Fast inward sodium blockade	Lidocaine, Mexiletine
IC	1. Minimal effect on ADP, conduction 2. Slight increase in ERP 3. Significant increase of QRS duration	Fast inward sodium blockade	Flecainide
II	1. Decreased MaxV 2. Increased APD, ERP	Beta antagonist	Metoprolol, Atenolol, Esmolol, Sotalol
III	1. Increased APD, ERP	Repolarization prolonged	Amiodarone, Sotalol
IV	1. Decreased APD 2. Decreased slow channel depolarization	Calcium channel blockade	Verapamil, Diltiazem
Other	1. Will vary depending on the agent	See text for individual agents	Digoxin, Adenosine, Potassium, Magnesium

node, and in the remainder of the conduction system. Amiodarone also has some effects on sodium channels, calcium channels, and alpha and beta antagonism in addition to its effects on potassium channels. The side effects of amiodarone are numerous and affect multiple organ systems. Pulmonary effects include dyspnea, decreased lung capacity, and hypoxia from decreased diffusion capability and may lead to the formation of infiltrates or inflammation. It can lead to severe hypotension if infused too rapidly and affects the myocardial response to endogenous T3.

Lidocaine (oral formulation is mexiletine) is an antiarrhythmic that affects phase 4 depolarization in the Purkinje system, increases the threshold for ventricular fibrillation, and also affects potassium transmission through its effects on sodium channels. Changes in the APD vary in the different tissues of the myocardium, and this is the likely source of its antiarrhythmic effects. Its major side effects are related to changes in the ion flows in the CNS. It will present as drowsiness or hallucinatory symptoms and progress to agitation, muscle twitching, and eventual seizure (despite being an anticonvulsant). Treatment at this point is supportive, and seldom are there long-term sequelae.

Sotalol is available in a mixture of d- and l-isomers and has both class II activity resulting in decreased heart rate and increased refractory period and class III activity blocking the delayed rectifier potassium current, leading to an additional increase in the refractory period. It is often prescribed for SVT and ventricular tachyarrhythmias and is associated with increased risk of torsades de pointes and prolongation of the QT interval.

Vasodilators treat vascular hypertension and are employed perioperatively to decrease LV depression, decrease oxygen consumption, decrease suture line stress, and prevent CVA or MI.

Nitroprusside is a very potent vasodilator that acts on the venous and arterial systems, lowering preload and afterload. It has been hypothesized that ischemia can be worsened by shifting blood away from ischemic myocardium in the presence of occlusive coronary artery disease. Nitroprusside has a rapid onset and short duration of action (minutes for both) and functions by reduction to nitric oxide. Due to its structure, this reduction also releases cyanide molecules, which are typically further reduced to thiocyanate in the liver. Thiocyanate can accumulate in renal failure. Cyanide toxicity is also a side effect marked by tachyphylaxis, metabolic acidosis, and increasing mixed venous PaO_2 secondary to interference of the electron transport chain at the cytochrome level. Cyanide toxicity can be treated by amyl nitrite (inhaled or in the circuit), injected sodium nitrite, or injected thiosulfate.

Nitroglycerin is a potent venodilator and is a coronary artery dilator, making it one of the first drugs of choice in acute coronary syndromes and angina. It dilates stenotic coronary arteries as well as the collateral vessels, however, at higher doses it will also dilate the systemic arterial system. Dosing should be reduced in those with hepatic or renal disease, and it can lead to methemoglobinemia in patients deficient in methemoglobin reductase.

Hydralazine is a direct-acting arteriodilator by activating ATP-sensitive potassium channels and does not affect the cholinergic or adrenergic systems. It has minimal effect on the venous system, decreasing instances of orthostatic hypotension, however it does promote the formation of peripheral edema and reflex sympathetic manifestations such as flushing, tachycardia, and headache. It can cause pancytopenia, peripheral neuropathy, rash, and fever. It can also lead to a lupus-like syndrome and is consequently typically used on patients who are refractory to other classes of antihypertensives. Its vasodilatory effects appear to be very effective in the cerebral vasculature, renal vasculature, splanchnic vasculature, and coronary vessels; the decrease in afterload, while beneficial to the myocardium, can be associated with a tachycardia that is excessive to the point of negating these benefits, and it often must be given concurrently with a beta agonist or calcium channel blocker for rate control.

Nesiritide is a recombinant version of brain natriuretic peptide, which is secreted by the ventricles in response to volume overload and increased wall tension. It acts on cGMP (similar to nitric oxide) to promote vasodilation and decreases the synthesis of norepinephrine, angiotensin II, and endothelin. It functions as a diuretic and natriuretic, and endogenous levels increase with worsening heart function. Therapeutically, it is used in acute dyspnea and severe acute heart failure, but it has been associated with diminished renal function. When compared with nitroglycerin, it is more effective at lowering right atrial pressure, pulmonary capillary wedge pressure, and systemic vascular resistance without tolerance development, but it was associated with increased mortality at 30 days and at 6 months.

Calcium channel blockers are a diverse group with a range of effects. Calcium is a universal messenger in various enzymatic processes such as muscle contraction, coagulation, nervous transmission, bone metabolism, and cellular membrane electrical processes. In the myocardium, it aids initiation of automaticity and contractility and plays a role in various components of the action potential. Calcium transport controls the contraction of smooth muscle in locations such as the bronchi and in the arterial system to varying degrees. Calcium's influence in the vascular muscle contraction and its role in myocardial conduction and contractility have led to the development of a number of agents designed to antagonize the channels responsible for calcium transport. Pharmaceutical agents consequently have been developed with varying degrees of specificity for these tissues.

Verapamil is highly specific for the myocardial conduction system and is a first-line therapy for SVT involving the AV or SA node. It slows nodal conduction to provide a block against reentrant conduction. It affects the calcium channels responsible for automaticity of the pacemaker cells and slows conduction velocity and increases refractoriness of the AV node and decreases the rate of SA node discharge, leading to increase in the PR interval without changes in the QRS or QT (as compared with the IA antiarrhythmics). Consequently it should not be used in those with sick sinus syndrome, AV block, or in those with CHF. If the SVT is extranodal in origin or uses accessory pathways (WPW), then verapamil may lead to accelerated heart rate, due to the unopposed conduction through the accessory pathway. It can also lead to cardiovascular collapse from bradycardia. Administration concurrent with digoxin, benzodiazepines, and hypoglycemics may increase the toxicity of these substances and should be monitored appropriately.

Diltiazem, like verapamil, will slow the conduction through the cardiac conduction system, however it will also dilate the coronary arteries and (poorly) dilate the systemic vasculature. It is effective in SVT such as A-fib, A-flutter, and paroxysmal atrial tachycardia, and it slows AV nodal conduction.

Nifedipine is a very potent vasodilator and has use as a coronary arterial dilator. It is useful in coronary vasospasm and in treating angina (superior to nitroglycerin). It is hypothesized that the decrease in afterload and left ventricular volume is the basis for the relief in angina despite a reflex tachycardia that often develops.

Nicardipine is a titratable intravenous antihypertensive that is specific for the arterial system with minimal effect on the myocardium. It is quick acting with a short duration of action and does not demonstrate the reflex tachycardia seen in nifedipine.

ANGIOTENSIN-CONVERTING ENZYME INHIBITORS AND ARBS

Angiotensin-converting enzyme (ACE) inhibitors prevent the conversion of angiotensin I to the active angiotensin II, allowing a decrease in peripheral vascular resistance by interrupting the renin-angiotensin-aldosterone system (RAAS). They also inhibit degradation of bradykinin, a potent vasodilator. They are used extensively in the treatment of hypertension as well as CHF. Effects of treatment include reductions in angiotensin, aldosterone, NE, and plasma antidiuretic hormone and increased plasma potassium levels. Preoperative administration of ACE inhibitors is associated with severe hypotension when volatile anesthetic agents are used and should be avoided when feasible. Additionally, ACE inhibitors may cause life-threatening angioedema, which can be treated with fresh frozen plasma administration.

ELECTROLYTES

Potassium is a cation found in the intracellular fluid in high concentrations and in the extracellular fluid in low concentrations and is maintained in an inverse equilibrium with sodium concentrations by the sodium-potassium pump (ATPase). Numerous actions in the body are dependent on this concentration gradient, and the myocardial conduction and impulse generation are extremely influenced by it. Hypokalemia and hyperkalemia both exhibit cardiac sequelae, and both are often seen in perioperative patients. The cardiac conduction action potential is dependent on the extracellular level of potassium.

Hypokalemia will consequently decrease the rate of repolarization due to a decrease in the permeability of the myocardial membrane to potassium. The increased length of repolarization can allow a slowing of overall conduction and increases the amount of time the membrane is susceptible to excitability in the refractory period. Hypokalemia can be seen in the ECG as a U-wave or in an increased amplitude of the P-wave and the most common arrhythmias seen are SVT, atrial tachycardia, and premature atrial contractions. Treatment is with potassium (possibly concurrent with magnesium) and avoidance of rapid changes in pH.

Hyperkalemia, as opposed to hypokalemia, increases the membrane permeability to potassium and will increase the rate of repolarization, thus decreasing the action potential duration. This will decrease the chance of arrhythmias, however the increased concentration gradient will slow the spontaneous depolarization of the SA node leading to bradycardia and eventual asystole. Electrocardiogram tracings will show peaked T-waves, decreases in the QRS amplitude, increased QRS duration, and increased PR interval. Treatment of hyperkalemia is dependent on the clinical picture, as rapid correction may be necessary to prevent demise. Calcium will directly antagonize potassium at the level of the cellular membrane. Sodium bicarbonate will alkalize the extracellular environment, encouraging the transport of protons extracellularly and, to maintain electroneutrality, driving potassium intracellularly, and thus decrease the concentration gradient. A less rapid correction can be achieved with glucose/insulin, β2 agonists, and loop diuretics.

Magnesium is another cation found in large quantities in the extracellular space. It is used in many enzymatic processes in the body and is often deficient in ill or older patients. It is vital in the sodium-potassium ATPase and necessary to maintain normal potassium concentrations. The ECG will be consistent with hypokalemia. Magnesium functions as a myocardial membrane stabilizer much like calcium and may aid in preventing some arrhythmias. Torsades de pointes is a particular arrhythmia that is related to magnesium depletion (and can be elicited by some antidysrhythmic agents) and often is refractory to other therapies.

Calcium is a key electrolyte responsible for not only muscle contraction but also cardiac conduction fluid transport and virtually every cellular function. Calcium exists (1) bound to protein, (2) chelated with phosphate, sulfate, and so forth, or (3) in the free ionized (biologically active) form. As such, it is important to know the ionized calcium or calculate the corrected calcium level in the blood in the setting of hypoalbuminemia.

$$\text{Corrected Calcium} = [0.8 \times (\text{Normal Albumin} - \text{Patient's Albumin})] + \text{Serum Ca}$$

VASOPRESSIN AND DESMOPRESSIN

Vasopressin and desmopressin are exogenous synthetic analogues of ADH. Vasopressin targets renal collecting ducts, vascular smooth muscle, and cardiac myocytes, resulting in increased water reabsorption, vasoconstriction, and inotropism. Vasopressin demonstrates large increases in SVR, cerebral perfusion pressure, and coronary perfusion pressure, is an effective vasoconstrictor in the presence of tissue hypoxia and acidosis, and does not increase myocardial oxygen consumption or lactate production. Acidosis and lactate increase cellular nitric oxide generation, which activates potassium channels, leading to hyperpolarization inhibiting calcium entry to the contractile elements, and consequently is refractory to norepinephrine and angiotensin II. It is important to note that vasopressin selectively causes splanchnic vasoconstriction (in fact it was originally used in much higher doses for gastrointestinal bleeding) and can, in some cases, compromise bowel perfusion in settings of prolonged administration.

REFERENCES

1. Klabunde E. *Cardiovascular Physiology Concepts*. 2nd ed. Philadelphia, PA: Lippincott Williams & Wilkins; 2012:124–147.
2. Hall J. *Guyton and Hall: Textbook of Medical Physiology*. 12th ed. Philadelphia, PA: Saunders Elsevier; 2011:101–113.
3. Klabunde E. *Cardiovascular Physiology Concepts*. 2nd ed. Philadelphia, PA: Lippincott Williams & Wilkins; 2012:60–92.
4. Reich D, Mittnacht A, London M, Kaplan J. Monitoring of the heart and vascular system. In: Kaplan J, Reich D, Lake C, Konstadt S, eds. *Kaplan's Cardiac Anesthesia*. 5th ed. Philadelphia, PA: Saunders Elsevier; 2006:385–436.
5. Hall J. *Guyton and Hall: Textbook of Medical Physiology*. 12th ed. Philadelphia, PA: Saunders Elsevier; 2011:167–176.
6. Teplick R. Basic principles and limitations of hemodynamic monitoring. In: Hemmings H, Hopkins P, eds. *Foundations of Anesthesia: Basic Sciences for Clinical Practice*. 2nd ed. Philadelphia, PA: Mosby Elsevier; 2006:173–188.
7. Klabunde E. *Cardiovascular Physiology Concepts*. 2nd ed. Philadelphia, PA: Lippincott Williams & Wilkins; 2012:9–40.
8. Balser J, Thompson A. Cardiac electrophysiology. In: Hemmings H, Hopkins P, eds. *Foundations of Anesthesia: Basic Sciences for Clinical Practice*. 2nd ed. Philadelphia, PA: Mosby Elsevier; 2006:485–497.
9. Heerdt PM, Dickstein ML. Regulation and assessment of cardiac function. In: Hemmings H, Hopkins P, eds. *Foundations of Anesthesia: Basic Sciences for Clinical Practice*. 2nd ed. Philadelphia, PA: Mosby Elsevier; 2006:511–523.
10. Kruger C, Sidebotham D. Systolic left ventricular function. In: Sidebotham D, Merry A, Legget M, Edwards M, eds. *Practical Perioperative Transesophageal Echocardiography with Critical Care Echocardiography*. 2nd ed. Philadelphia, PA: Saunders Elsevier; 2011:101–123.
11. Klabunde E. *Cardiovascular Physiology Concepts*. 2nd ed. Philadelphia, PA: Lippincott Williams & Wilkins; 2012:198–234.
12. Nyhan D, Blanck T. Cardiac physiology. In: Hemmings H, Hopkins P, eds. *Foundations of Anesthesia: Basic Sciences for Clinical Practice*. 2nd ed. Philadelphia, PA: Mosby Elsevier; 2006:473–484.
13. Hall J. *Guyton and Hall Textbook of Medical Physiology*. 12th ed. Philadelphia, PA: Saunders, Elsevier; 2010:172.
14. Miller R, ed. *Miller's Anesthesia*. 7th ed. Philadelphia, PA: Elsevier; 2010.
15. Barash P, Cullen B, Stoelting R, Cahalan M, Stock M. *Clinical Anesthesia*. 6th ed. Philadelphia, PA: Lippincott Williams & Wilkins; 2009:221.
16. Barash P, Cullen B, Stoelting R, Cahalan M, Stock M. *Clinical Anesthesia*. 6th ed. Philadelphia, PA: Lippincott Williams & Wilkins; 2009:429.
17. Rowland L, Pedley T. *Merritt's Neurology*. 12th ed. Philadelphia, PA: Lippincott Williams & Wilkins; 2009:19.
18. Barash P, Cullen B, Stoelting R, Cahalan M, Stock M. *Clinical Anesthesia*. 6th ed. Philadelphia, PA: Lippincott Williams & Wilkins; 2009:1215.
19. Barash P, Cullen B, Stoelting R, Cahalan M, Stock M. *Clinical Anesthesia*. 6th ed. Philadelphia, PA: Lippincott Williams & Wilkins; 2009:227.
20. Barash P, Cullen B, Stoelting R, Cahalan M, Stock M. *Clinical Anesthesia*. 6th ed. Philadelphia, PA: Lippincott Williams & Wilkins; 2009:882.
21. Hall J. *Guyton and Hall Textbook of Medical Physiology*. 12th ed. Philadelphia, PA: Saunders, Elsevier; 2010:171.
22. Hall J. *Guyton and Hall Textbook of Medical Physiology*. 12th ed. Philadelphia, PA: Saunders, Elsevier; 2010:213.
23. Barash P, Cullen B, Stoelting R, Cahalan M, Stock M. *Clinical Anesthesia*. 6th ed. Philadelphia, PA: Lippincott Williams & Wilkins; 2009:227.
24. Barash P, Cullen B, Stoelting R, Cahalan M, Stock M. *Clinical Anesthesia*. 6th ed. Philadelphia, PA: Lippincott Williams & Wilkins; 2009:221.
25. Hall J. *Guyton and Hall Textbook of Medical Physiology*. 12th ed. Philadelphia, PA: Saunders, Elsevier; 2010:178.
26. Hall J. *Guyton and Hall Textbook of Medical Physiology*. 12th ed. Philadelphia, PA: Saunders, Elsevier; 2010:185.
27. Hall J. *Guyton and Hall Textbook of Medical Physiology*. 12th ed. Philadelphia, PA: Saunders, Elsevier; 2010:177.
28. Hall J. *Guyton and Hall Textbook of Medical Physiology*. 12th ed. Philadelphia, PA: Saunders, Elsevier; 2010:164–165.
29. Barash P, Cullen B, Stoelting R, Cahalan M, Stock M. *Clinical Anesthesia*. 6th ed. Philadelphia, PA: Lippincott Williams & Wilkins; 2009:229.
30. Barash P, Cullen B, Stoelting R, Cahalan M, Stock M. *Clinical Anesthesia*. 6th ed. Philadelphia, PA: Lippincott Williams & Wilkins; 2009:228.
31. Barash P, Cullen B, Stoelting R, Cahalan M, Stock M. *Clinical Anesthesia*. 6th ed. Philadelphia, PA: Lippincott Williams & Wilkins; 2009:230.
32. Barash P, Cullen B, Stoelting R, Cahalan M, Stock M. *Clinical Anesthesia*. 6th ed. Philadelphia, PA: Lippincott Williams & Wilkins; 2009:230–231.
33. Hall J. *Guyton and Hall Textbook of Medical Physiology*. 12th ed. Philadelphia, PA: Saunders, Elsevier; 2010:191–200.
34. Hall J. *Guyton and Hall Textbook of Medical Physiology*. 12th ed. Philadelphia, PA: Saunders, Elsevier; 2010:195.

35. Barash P, Cullen B, Stoelting R, Cahalan M, Stock M. *Clinical Anesthesia*. 6th ed. Philadelphia, PA: Lippincott Williams & Wilkins; 2009:1141–1142.
36. Hall J. *Guyton and Hall Textbook of Medical Physiology*. 12th ed. Philadelphia, PA: Saunders, Elsevier; 2010:202.
37. Walker T, Salazar G, Waltman A. Angiographic evaluation and management of acute gastrointestinal hemorrhage. *World J Gastroenterol*. 2012;18(11):1191–1201.
38. Law A, Gales M. Octreotide or vasopressin for bleeding esophageal varices. *Ann Pharmacother*. 1997;31(2):237–238.
39. Barash P, Cullen B, Stoelting R, Cahalan M, Stock M. *Clinical Anesthesia*. 6th ed. Philadelphia, PA: Lippincott Williams & Wilkins; 2009:1301.
40. Hall J. *Guyton and Hall Textbook of Medical Physiology*. 12th ed. Philadelphia, PA: Saunders, Elsevier; 2010:208.
41. Hall J. *Guyton and Hall Textbook of Medical Physiology*. 12th ed. Philadelphia, PA: Saunders, Elsevier; 2010:371, 373.
42. Irwin R, Lilly C, Rippe J. *Irwin and Rippe's Manual of Intensive Care Medicine*. 6th ed. Philadelphia, PA: Lippincott Williams & Wilkins; 2013.

QUESTIONS

1. All of the following increase myocardial oxygen consumption except:
   A. A decrease in heart rate
   B. An increase in contractility
   C. An increase in afterload
   D. An increase in preload
   E. An increase in ventricular wall stress

2. The reflex that originates from stretch or mechanical distortion of the left ventricle and results in an increase in parasympathetic outflow and a decrease in heart rate is known as the:
   A. Carotid Sinus Reflex
   B. Bainbridge Reflex
   C. Valsalva Reflex
   D. Bezold-Jarisch Reflex
   E. Oculocardiac Reflex

3. The v wave on the central venous pressure waveform corresponds to:
   A. Atrial contraction
   B. Ventricular contraction
   C. The bulging of the tricuspid valve into the right atrium
   D. Buildup of blood in the venous system before the opening of the tricuspid valve
   E. The closing of the pulmonary valve

4. All of the following can result in an increase in stroke volume during exercise except:
   A. Increase in inotropy
   B. Increase in ventricular filling
   C. Increase in sympathetic stimulation
   D. Decrease in lusitropy
   E. Decrease in venous compliance

5. The left ventricular ejection fraction is all of the following except:
   A. Normally greater than 55%
   B. The stroke volume divided by the end-diastolic volume
   C. The most frequently used clinical index of contractility
   D. Easily calculated using a pulmonary artery catheter
   E. Estimated using transesophageal echocardiography

6. The property of the ventricle that is important for diastolic function and relaxation is:
   A. Dromotropy
   B. Inotropy
   C. Lusitropy
   D. Bathmotropy
   E. Chronotropy

7. Which of the following is NOT a part of the baroreceptor control system?
   A. Carotid sinus nerve
   B. Nucleus ambiguous
   C. Sympathetic chain
   D. Glossopharyngeal nerve
   E. Vagal motor nucleus

8. Placental perfusion is improved by all of the following, EXCEPT
   A. Prostacyclin
   B. Increased in cardiac output
   C. Left uterine displacement
   D. Fluid bolus
   E. Uterine contraction

Which of following factors serves to increase circulating blood volume:
   A. Renal vasodilation
   B. Reduction in renal capillary hydrostatic pressure
   C. Increase in GFR
   D. Decreased ADH release
   E. Decreased tubular permeability to free water

9. Which of the following circulating systems do NOT rely significantly on autoregulation in maintaining their blood flow?
   A. Renal
   B. Cerebral
   C. Uterine
   D. Splanchnic
   E. Coronary

10. All of the following are true statements about the effect of ADH, EXCEPT:
   A. Increases synthesis of von Willebrand factor
   B. Vasoconstricts vascular smooth muscle
   C. Increases reabsorption of free water
   D. Increases circulating factor VIII
   E. It is secreted from the posterior pituitary

11. Preload is increased by all of the following EXCEPT
    A. An increase in blood volume
    B. A decrease in peripheral vascular resistance
    C. An increase in peripheral venous pressure
    D. An increase in peripheral vascular resistance
    E. An increase in the vascular tone in the splanchnic circulation

12. All of the following actions will increase the spinal cord perfusion pressure EXCEPT?
    A. Increasing MAP
    B. Draining CSF via lumbar drain
    C. Increasing pCO2 from 30 to 40mmHg
    D. Increasing pO2 from 90 to 150mmHg
    E. Draining an epidural hematoma

ANSWERS

1. A. Myocardial oxygen consumption is increased by anything that increases myocardial work. An increase in heart rate increases myocardial work, but a decrease in heart rate decreases myocardial work.[1p86]
2. D. The Bezold-Jarisch reflex is a baroreceptor reflex that results from rapid increases in pressure, mechanical distortion, and ischemia of the left ventricle, resulting in bradycardia and hypotension.[2p406]
3. D. The v wave is caused by right atrial filling before the tricuspid valve opens at the beginning of diastole.[44p393]
4. D. A decrease in ventricular relaxation during diastole, lusitropy, results in decreased ventricular filling and a resulting decrease in stroke volume.[1p199]
5. D. It is possible to calculate some indices of right ventricular contractility including right ventricular power generation and preload recruitable stroke work, but the left ventricular ejection fraction is most easily estimated using echocardiography.[10p519]
6. C. Lusitropy is the relaxation of the ventricular myocardium. Effective relaxation during diastole results in enhanced ventricular filling when the atrioventricular valve opens.[13p477]
7. C. Sympathetic chain. Arterial baroreceptors are found in the aortic arch and at the bifurcation of the carotids and respond to increased stretch from increased blood pressure by sending a signal to the carotid sinus nerve. The stimulus is then transmitted via the glossopharyngeal nerve to the postsynaptic nucleus ambiguus and vagal motor nucleus, causing a decrease in heart rate.[16p221]
8. E. Uterine contractions cause an increase in the resistance of the uterine blood vessels, which leads to decreased uterine blood flow and oxygen delivery.[16pp1141–1142]
9. B. A reduction in renal capillary hydrostatic pressure leads to increased reabsorption of water and increases circulating blood volume.[16p230]
10. D. Splanchnic. Splanchnic circulation has only a small degree of autoregulation and is primarily controlled by metabolic factors. Feeding releases cholecystekinin, gastrin and the absorption of glucose and other nutrients cause an increase in splanchnic blood flow. Sympathetic activity causes arterial and venous constriction via alpha receptors and diverts blood from the large capacitance of the splanchnic circulation to the central circulation.[16pp230–231]
11. A. Increase in synthesis of von Willebrand factor. While ADH does increase the level of circulating von Willebrand factor, it does so by increasing the release of bound vWF and not by increasing the synthesis of the factor.[16p1301]
12. D. An increase in peripheral vascular resistance. The following factors cause an increase in preload: an increase in the volume of blood, an increase in the tone of large vessels leading to increased peripheral venous pressure, and a dilation of arterioles leading to a decrease in peripheral vascular resistance and resulting a rapid transit of blood from the arterial to the venous side.[14p172] Vasoconstriction of the splanchnic circulation causes a shift of that blood volume to the central circulation leading to an increase in preload.

26.

GASTROINTESTINAL AND HEPATIC SYSTEMS

Olakunle Idowu and Sarah Guzman-Reyes

LIVER PHYSIOLOGY

The liver is one of the largest organs in the body, and demands 25% of cardiac output, using a dual vascular supply consisting of the hepatic artery and portal vein.[1] Hepatic blood flow is roughly 1500 mL/min, of which 75% passes through the portal vein and 25% percent passes through the hepatic artery[2] (Figure 26.1). Despite this discrepancy, the portal vein is responsible for providing 50%–55% of the liver's oxygen requirements and the hepatic artery is responsible for providing the balance.[2] In effect, both the hepatic artery and vein equally support the metabolic demand of the liver. Portal vein oxygen saturation normally approximates 85%, and portal vein pressure is 7–10 mmHg.[2] The low resistance caricature of the portal vein allows it to be a large reservoir for blood. Blood supply in the portal vein stems from the superior mesenteric vein and splanchnic veins, which drain venous blood from the stomach, spleen, pancreas, small intestine, and colon. This is in contrast to the hepatic artery, which approximates aortic pressure and is supplied by the common hepatic artery.

There are several regulatory mechanisms that autoregulate hepatic blood flow, which can be intrinsic, extrinsic, or extrahepatic. The liver prioritizes its oxygen delivery, preserving the oxygen and substrates needed to carry out essential functions.[3] The liver autoregulates blood flow, however, there are still regions of the liver that are more susceptible to ischemia.

INTRINSIC PERFUSION CONTROL

The hepatic artery serves as a large buffer for portal vein blood flow, because the liver cannot directly control portal vein blood flow.[1] For example, when portal vein blood flow is low, the hepatic artery increases blood flow reciprocally to compensate. The mechanism of this response is closely regulated by adenosine. With low portal venous blood flow, adenosine accumulates in periportal regions, causing arterial vasodilation and a subsequent increase in hepatic artery blood flow. The contrary is also true for elevated portal vein blood flow. Hence, high portal vein flows will decrease periportal adenosine, causing arterial vasoconstriction and a decrease in hepatic artery blood flow.[1]

The postprandial state, decreases in pH, decreases in oxygen content, or increases in $PaCO_2$ can modulate the liver's blood flow. After a meal, both hepatic and portal vein blood flow increase in response to the hyperosmolarity of the food bolus. This increase does not apply to the fasting state. Decreases in pH, decreases in oxygen content, or increases in $PaCO_2$ increase hepatic blood flow to improve oxygen delivery.

Liver blood flow is also controlled by myogenic responses. Myogenic responses are arterial in origin and protect against significantly elevated or decreased transmural pressures. Stretching of arterial smooth muscle causes vasoconstriction to avoid uncontrolled spikes in liver blood flow. In contrast, during acute drops in transmural pressure, a loss of myogenic response causes vasodilation, which increases blood flow for organ protection.[1] Myogenic responses are not existent in the portal vein, which is a major limitation of this reflex. Hence, systemic hypotension can lead to proportional decreases in portal vein blood flow.

EXTRINSIC PERFUSION CONTROL

The liver receives neural input from the vagus and splanchnic nerves. Vagal stimulation redistributes hepatic blood flow without increasing it. In contrast, sympathetic stimulation causes vasoconstriction of the splanchnic vasculature, increasing hepatic blood flow. Sympathetic responses are critical because the splanchnic vasculature serves as a large reservoir for blood.[1] Another important consideration is that modulation of splanchnic tone can be mediated by adrenal stimulation.

Humoral regulators such as epinephrine, norepinephrine, dopamine, glucagon, angiotensin II, and vasopressin act on various receptors to alter splanchnic and hepatic blood flow.[3] The hepatic artery has alpha 1, beta 2, and

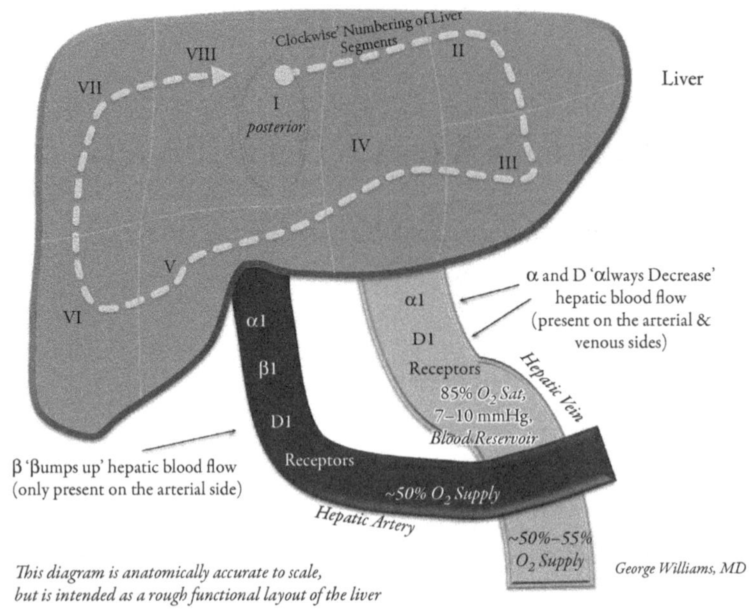

Figure 26.1 Hepatic blood flow and structure.

dopamine 1 receptors, whereas the portal vein has alpha 1 and dopamine 1 receptors.[2] Liver blood flow decreases with stimulation of dopamine 1 and alpha 1 receptors and increases with stimulation of beta 2 receptors.[1] Epinephrine and norepinephrine have significantly more vasoactive activity than dopamine on the hepatic adrenergic receptors. Glucagon causes dilation of hepatic arterioles and antagonizes sympathetic mediated vasoconstriction. Angiotensin II causes vasoconstriction of the hepatic artery and portal vein, leading to decreased hepatic blood flow. Lastly, vasopressin causes vasoconstriction of the splanchnic vasculature, also leading to a decrease in hepatic blood flow.

METABOLIC ACTIVITY

The liver plays a vital role in the production and metabolism of proteins.[8] Almost all plasma proteins (i.e., albumin) are produced in the liver, with the exception being immunoglobulins. Hepatocytes deaminate proteins and are responsible for forming proteins, which serve as hormones, cytokines, transport proteins, and procoagulants. Most of the liver's protein production, roughly 15%, is due to the synthesis of albumin.[2] Albumin is the body's most abundant protein, and it is largely responsible for maintaining plasma oncotic gradients in the body and serving a transporter of free fatty acids, hormones, and unconjugated bilirubin, to name a few. Alpha fetoprotein genetically and functionally resembles albumin in neonates and infants up to 1 year of life. Hence, it can be a marker for liver injury or hepatocellular carcinoma.

Hepatocytes are responsible for the mobilization of amino acids to keto acids, glutamine, and ammonia, which are broken down into byproducts that are used for other metabolic needs or removed from the body.[1] Ammonia is sent to the urea cycle to be combined with carbon dioxide to produce urea that is excreted in the urine and keto acids that can be used as substrates in the Krebs cycle. Hepatocytes also transaminate nonessential amino acids, which may become vital with nutritional deficiency.

The liver is largely responsible for carbohydrate metabolism and the control of blood glucose. Net blood glucose levels are the result of the balance between gluconeogenesis, glycogen breakdown, and glycogen storage. Insulin is a neuroendocrine factor that is anabolic and helps to stimulate glycogen storage, whereas glucagon and catecholamines are catabolic factors that cause glycogen breakdown and gluconeogenesis. Other factors that play a key role in the liver's regulation of blood glucose are the fasting and fed state. In the fasting state the body breaks down glycogen for the body's use, and in the fed state the body has the opposite effect.[1] Gluconeogenesis is facilitated by using lactate, glycerol, and amino acids, which are metabolic byproducts to produce glucose.

Excess carbohydrates and proteins are converted to fat that is stored in the liver or adipose tissue. Free fatty acids can be mobilized for fuel after carbohydrate stores have been depleted. This occurs as fatty acids are oxidized to acetyl Coenzyme A (acetyl CoA), which is used in the citric acid cycle for the generation of ATP. Overproduction of acetyl CoA from the breakdown of free fatty acids leads to the formation of ketone bodies, which serve as a reservoir for acetyl CoA. Insulin inhibits the breakdown of free fatty acids whereas glucagon and catecholamines facilitate the catabolic state.[2]

Factor VIII and Von Willibrand factor are the *only* coagulation factors not produced by the liver. Hepatocytes are responsible for the production of all other coagulation factors along with the synthesis of antithrombin III (important in mechanism of action of heparin), plasminogen activating factor, protein C, and protein S, which are regulators of coagulation and fibrinolytic pathways. Hepatocytes are essential for the carboxylation of vitamin K dependent factors, which facilitate their procoagulant activity. The liver is also responsible for the production of heme and the metabolism of bilirubin.[2]

SECRETORY FUNCTION OF THE GASTROINTESTINAL SYSTEM

The gastrointestinal (GI) tract has multiple secretory glands. Their main function is to produce enzymes for food breakdown and mucus to lubricate and protect the GI epithelium. The enzyme-producing glands are located from the mouth to the distal end of the ilium, and the mucus-producing glands are found from the mouth to the anus. The amount and type of secretion produced depends on the type of food ingested and the segment of the GI tract where the ingested food is located or passing through. The GI tract secretes approximately 7 L of fluid per day.

Anatomically, the secretory glandular cells are classified as mucus gland or goblet cells, crypts of Lieberkuhn, tubular glands, and complex glands. These represent specialized secretory glands like the pancreas, liver, and the salivary glands. The principal glands of salivation include the parotid, submandibular, and sublingual glands. Daily secretion of saliva is approximately 1500 mL. It contains ptyalin, which initiates digestion of starches, and mucin for lubrication and protection. The parotid gland secretes ptyalin exclusively. The submandibular and sublingual glands secrete both. The pH of saliva is approximately 6–7, which promotes the digestive action of ptyalin.

Innervation is provided primarily by the parasympathetic nervous system. Salivation also occurs in response to reflexes originating from the stomach and the intestines. Decreased blood supply to the glands proportionally affects its secretory function.[5]

GASTRIC SECRETION

In addition to the mucus-secreting glands, the stomach mucosa has two important types of tubular glands:

1. Oxyntic gastric glands—composed of three different types of cells: (1) mucous neck cells, which secrete mucus and some pepsinogen; (2) peptic (or chief cells), which secrete a large amount of pepsinogen; and (3) parietal cells, which secrete hydrochloric acid and intrinsic factor (essential for absorption of B12 in the ilium).
2. Pyloric glands—are similar to the oxyntic glands but with fewer peptic cells, and almost no parietal cells. They secrete gastrin, mucus, and a small amount of pepsinogen.

The parietal cells secrete an acid solution, which contains 160 mmol/L of hydrochloric acid, with a pH of 0.8. This H+ concentration is 3 million times greater than that of the arterial blood gas, and it requires 1500 calories of energy per liter to be produced. Hydrochloric acid is necessary for the proteolytic activity of pepsin, which is almost inactive at a pH greater than 5.[5]

Gastric secretion processes are regulated by nervous system and hormonal mechanisms. The secretion of H+ by parietal cells is directly stimulated by acetylcholine (M3), histamine (H2), and gastrin (CCK2). The receptors are found on the basolateral membrane of the parietal cells in the body and fundus of the stomach.[6]

The H2 receptor is a GPCR that activates the Gs-adenyl cyclase-cAMP-PKA-pathway. Acetylcholine and gastrin signal through GPCRs that couple via the Gq – PLK – IP3 – Ca2+ pathway in parietal cells. The cAMP and Ca2+ dependent pathway, activates a H+, K+ ATPase pump, which exchanges hydrogen and potassium ions across the parietal cell membrane. This mechanism is inhibited by proton pump inhibitors (i.e., pantoprazole, lansoprazole, and other "azoles").[6]

The CNS modulates the activity of the enteric nervous system via acetylcholine, stimulating gastric secretion in response to smell, taste, or anticipation of food. This is known as the cephalic phase of acid secretion. Acetylcholine also affects parietal cells by increasing histamine release from the ECL (enterochromatin-like) cells and gastrin from G cells. Histamine acts as paracrine mediator, diffusing from its site of release to nearby area total cells, where it activates H2 receptors, the place of action for H2 antagonists.[7]

Somatostatin (SST) is produced by antral D cells and inhibits gastric secretions. This hormone is secreted when gastric pH is less than 3, and it suppresses gastrin secretions, facilitating a negative feedback loop. It is found to be decreased in patients with *H. pylori* infection. This phenomenon may contribute to excess gastrin production in these patients.

Pepsinogen is the precursor of pepsin, necessary for protein digestion. Its secretion rate is dependent on the amount present in the stomach.

GHRELIN

Ghrelin is a recently identified brain-gut peptide with properties resulting in release of growth hormone and induction of appetite. It has been isolated from human and rat stomach and was first reported in the late 1990s. Originally, ghrelin was discovered as an endogenous ligand for the growth hormone (GH) secretagogue receptor, and as such ghrelin strongly and dose-dependently stimulates GH secretion. Ghrelin stimulates more GH than GH-releasing hormone (GHRH). Subsequent reports showed that it increases food intake and body weight as well. Wren et al. found out that both intracerebroventricular and intraperitoneal administration of ghrelin in freely feeding rats stimulated food intake and increased the plasma growth hormone level.[15]

Ghrelin is produced mainly by the stomach, but is also synthesized in the hypothalamus. Within the stomach, ghrelin is produced most abundantly in the gastric fundus by the enteroendocrine cells in the oxyntic mucosa that were previously dubbed "X/A-like cells."[19]

Regulation of Appetite by Ghrelin

Plasma ghrelin levels increase before meals and decrease strongly postprandially, indicating that ghrelin plays a role in meal initiation.[16]

Central action: Ghrelin stimulates appetite by acting on the hypothalamic arcuate nucleus, a region known to control food intake.[16]

Peripheral action: It also has a peripheral modulatory effect on satiety by affecting the mechanosensitivity of gastric vagal afferents, making them less sensitive to distention, resulting in overeating.[16]

Regulation of Energy Homeostasis by Ghrelin

Chronic administration of ghrelin increases body weight by stimulating food intake, decreasing energy expenditure, decreasing utilization of fat, and increasing utilization of carbohydrates.[17]

The increase in the plasma ghrelin level with diet-induced weight loss is consistent with the hypothesis that ghrelin has a role in the long-term regulation of body weight. Gastric bypass is associated with markedly suppressed ghrelin levels, possibly contributing to the weight-reducing effect of the procedure.[18]

HORMONAL CONTROL OF DIGESTION

Physiologic control of gastrointestinal motility is provided by GI hormones. One of the most important is gastrin. Gastrin is produced by G cells and stimulates gastric acid secretion and mucosal growth, stimulated by presence of protein and gastric distention as well as neural stimulation. Gastrin is the most potent inducer of acid secretion of all the GI hormones.

Another important hormone in the endocrinology of digestion is cholecystokinin. Cholecystokinin is secreted by I cells in presence of protein, fat, and acid. It controls the enzyme secretion by the pancreas (pancreatic enzymes and bicarbonate), relaxation of the sphincter of Oddi, and gallbladder contraction. It inhibits gastric emptying and appetite.[9] A third hormone, secretin, is produced by the as cells of the small intestine and stimulated when acid stomach content (pH less 5) enters the duodenum (and in a lesser way by fatty acids). It stimulates the secretion of pepsin, pancreatic bicarbonate, and liver ductal secretion.[9]

The fourth GI hormone is gastric inhibitory peptide, which is produced by K cells of the duodenum and the jejunum. It is produced in response to the presence of protein, fat, and carbohydrate in the gut. Its release inhibits acid secretion and gastric motility. Finally, the fifth GI hormone is motilin, which is produced by M cells of duodenum and jejunum. Motilin stimulates gastric and intestinal motility.[9]

An important take-home point of the endocrinology of digestion is that gastric volume is controlled not only by the amount of per os (PO) intake but also by the content of that intake and its ramifications on gastric pH, volume, and motility.

PANCREATIC SECRETION

The enzymes secreted by the pancreas are important in the digestion of protein carbohydrates and fats (Table 26.1). The pancreas also secretes copious amount of bicarbonate, which helps neutralize the acid chyme as it passes from the stomach into the duodenum. The most important proteolytic enzymes are trypsin, chymotrypsin, and carboxypolypeptidase. Other pancreatic digestive enzymes include amylase (hydrolyzes starches), lipase (hydrolyzes fats), and phospholipase (splits fatty acids from phospholipids). The pancreas also secretes trypsin inhibitor to prevent autodigestion of the pancreas. All proteolytic enzymes are secreted inactive into the duodenum, where they become activated.

Pancreatic secretion is regulated by acetylcholine, cholecystokinin, and secretin (Table 26.2). The first two stimulate production of digestive enzymes, and control the enzyme secretion of the pancreas. Secretin stimulates the secretion of sodium bicarbonate.[11]

SECRETION OF BILE BY THE LIVER

One of the liver's many functions is secretion of bile (600–1200 mL/day). Bile is important in fat digestion and absorption and it also serves to excrete waste products from the blood, especially bilirubin. Bile is secreted by hepatocytes into the bile canaliculi. From there, it flows to the terminal bile duct to progressively larger ducts until it reaches the hepatic duct, and common bile duct, from which it empties into the duodenum or is diverted to the cystic duct into the gallbladder. The bile ducts serve as a conduit for the bile without modifying its composition other than adding mucus from peribiliary glands, protecting the epithelium and avoiding bacterial invasion of the biliary tract. It is important to mention that the cystic duct has a spiral lumen, which increases the level of turbulence in the ductal flow, decreasing the risk of bile precipitation and stone formation.[11]

Table 26.1 PANCREATIC SECRETIONS (EXOCRINE)

ENZYMES		TYPE	REACTION CATALYZED
	Proteases	Trypsin	Proteins → Peptides
		Chymotrypsin	Proteins → Peptides
		Carboxypeptidase	Peptides → Amino Acids
	Polysaccharidase	Amylase	Starch & Glycogen → Maltose/Limit Dextrins
	Lipases	Phospholipases A & B	Phospholipids → Phosphate/FA/Glycerol
		Esterases	CHOL. ESTERS → FREE CHOL./FA
		Triacylglycerol lipases	TGL → FA/MGL
	Nucleases	Ribonuclease	RNA → Ribonucleotide
		Deoxyribonuclease	DNA → Deoxyribonucleotide
Bicarbonate			

FA—fatty acids; TGL—triglycerides; MGL—monoglycerides; CHOL—cholesterol

Table 26.2 HORMONAL CONTROL OF SECRETIONS FROM EXOCRINE PANCREAS

HORMONE INVOLVED	RELEASED FROM	IN RESPONSE TO	ACTION ON PANCREAS
Cholecystokinin (CCK)	Duodenum	Acid in stomach	Release of pancreatic enzymes
Secretin	Duodenum	Partially digested foods in stomach	Release of bicarbonate

DRUG METABOLISM

Drug metabolism is primarily a hepatic event. It influences the plasma concentration and systemic availability of most orally and parenterally administered drugs. Plasma proteins produced in the liver (particularly albumin and alpha-1-acid glycoprotein) act as sinks to decrease free drug concentration.[12]

In hepatic drug metabolism, hepatocytes change the drug into an inactive water-soluble substance (biotransformation) to be eliminated or excreted via bile or urine. Most drugs contain a lipophilic functional group to facilitate passage through the membrane barrier to improve its gastrointestinal absorption. This same characteristic inhibits their secretion. The liver detoxifies these drugs and terminates their pharmacological activity. This process has been classified as the following:

Phase 1 reactions—oxidation, reduction, and N-alkylation modify the drug, making it more polar. This requires the participation of the cytochrome P450 isoenzymes from the hepatic microsomes.

Phase 2 reactions—catalyzed by transferases. The chemical group generated from phase 1 are used as receptors for conjugation. The enzymes that carry out these reactions are glucoronyl-, acetyl-, sulfo-, and methyltransferase.

The resulting water-soluble glucuronide conjugates are unlikely to be reabsorbed into the systemic circulation and are excreted in the bile and the urine. Occasionally, liver metabolism of specific drugs can lead to the production of toxic intermediates, especially if an overdose is ingested, overwhelming the normal pathway of safe metabolism. This scenario accounts for the liver injury that can occur if patients ingest an overdose of acetaminophen.[13]

CYTOCHROME P450

The enzymes responsible for the oxydative drug metabolism are called mixed-function oxidases or monooxygenases. The activity of these enzymes requires a reducing agent (NADPH) and molecular oxygen. In this oxidation-reduction process, two microsomal enzymes play a key role. These are: (1) NADPH-cytochrome P450 oxidoreductase and (2) cytochrome P450 (CYP or P450). The relative abundance of P450s, compared with that of the reductase in the liver, contributes to making P450 heme reduction a rate-limiting step in hepatic drug oxidations. Approximately 14 genetically different isoforms of P450 have been identified; they are responsible for the metabolism of most of hepatic drug metabolism.[10]

The most studied of these enzymes is CYP2D6. Its polymorphism has been found to affect a large number of lipophilic-based drugs like antidepressants, antipsychotics, antiarrhythmics, beta blockers, and opioids (the latter three commonly used in anesthetic practice). The clinical consequence of this could be an altered drug response or a severe drug reaction. For example, genetically caused inactivity of CYP2D6 causes increased levels of codeine the prodrug and decreased, or no, formation of morphine. On the other hand, highly active CYPD26 leads to rapid metabolism of codeine to morphine and potential opioid drug toxicity. Drugs that inhibit CYP2D6 include quinidine and SSRIs. Therefore, codeine, oxycodone, and hydrocodone are poor analgesic choices for patients receiving SSRIs.[14,15]

The importance of discussing the polymorphism of these isoenzymes relates to the possibility in the future of incorporating pharmacogenetics into clinical practice.

REFERENCES

1. Miller R, ed. *Miller's Anesthesia.* 7th ed. Philadelphia, PA: Elsevier; 2010.
2. Butterworth I, Mackey D, Wasnick J. *Clinical Anesthesiology.* 5th ed. Philadelphia, PA: McGraw-Hill; 2013.
3. Barash P, Cullen B, Stoelting R, Cahalan M, Stock M. *Clinical Anesthesia.* 6th ed. Philadelphia, PA: Lippincott Williams & Wilkins; 2009.
4. Murray M, Rose S, Wedel D, Wass C, Harrison B, Mueller J. *Anesthesiology Review.* 4th ed. Philadelphia, PA: Saunders; 2014.
5. Guyton A, Hall J. *Guyton and Hall Textbook of Medical Physiology.* 1st ed. Philadelphia, PA: Saunders, Elsevier; 1996: 798, 818–828.
6. Wallace JL, Sharkey KA. Pharmacotherapy of gastric acidity, peptic ulcers, and gastroesophageal reflux disease. In Goodman LS, Brunton LL, Chabner BA; Knollmann BC, eds. *Goodman and Gilman's The Pharmacological Basis of Therapeutics.* 12th ed. New York, NY: McGraw-Hill; 2011: ch. 45.
7. Steadman R, Braunfeld M, Park H. Liver and gastrointestinal physiology. In: Hemmings H. *Pharmacology and Physiology for Anesthesia.* New York, NY: Elsevier; 2013:475–486.
8. Barash P, Cullen B, Stoelting R. *Clinical Anesthesia.* 5th ed. Philadelphia, PA: Lippincott Williams & Wilkins; 2006:1079.
9. Correia M. Drug biotransformation In: Katzung B, Masters S, Trevor AJ, eds. *Basic and Clinical Pharmacology.* 12th ed. Philadelphia, PA: McGraw-Hill; 2012.
10. Zhou S. Polimorphism of human P450 2D6 and its clinical significance. *Clin Pharmakokinet.* 2009;48(11):689–723.
11. Vuilleumier P, Stamer U, Landau R. Pharmacogenomic considerations in opioid analgesia. *Pharmagenomics Pers Med.* 2012;5:73–87.
12. Korbonits M, Goldstone A, Gueorguiev M, Grossman A. Ghrelin: a hormone with multiple functions. *Front Neuroendocrinol.* 2004;25:27–68.
13. Date Y, Kojima M, Hosoda H, Sawaguchi A, et al. Ghrelin, a novel growth hormone-releasing acylated peptide, is synthesized in a distinct endocrine cell type in the gastrointestinal tracts of rats and humans. *Endocrinology.* 2000;141(11):4255–4261.
14. Lengyel A. From growth hormone-releasing peptides to ghrelin: discovery of new modulators of GH secretion *Arq Bras Endocrinol Metabol.* 2006;50:17–24.
15. Wren A, Small Y, Ward H, et al. The novel hypothalamic peptide ghrelin stimulates food intake and growth hormone secretion *Endocrinology.* 2000;141:4325–4328.
16. De Vriese C. Ghrelin: a new peptide regulating growth hormone release and food intake. *Int J Biochem Cell B.* 2008;40:1420–1424.
17. Klok M, Jakobsdottir S, Drent M. The role of leptin and ghrelin in the regulation of food intake and body weight in humans: a review. *Obes Rev.* 2007;8:21–34.
18. Cummings D, Weigle D, Frayo R, et al. Plasma ghrelin levels after diet-induced weight loss or gastric bypass surgery. *N Engl J Med.* 2002;346:1623–1630.

FURTHER READING

Kieth J, Moore E. Hepatic and biliary trauma. In: Harken A, Moore E. *Abernathy's Surgical Secrets.* 6th ed. Philadelphia, PA: Mosby; 2009.

Malhotra V, Pamnani A. Renal, liver, and biliary tract disease. In: Miller R, Pardo M. *Basics of Anesthesia.* 6th ed. Philadelphia, PA: Elsevier; 2011.

QUESTIONS

1. Dual blood supply to the liver consists of:
   A. The hepatic artery and hepatic vein
   B. The hepatic vein and portal vein
   C. The hepatic artery and portal vein
   D. The portal vein and inferior vena cava
   E. The inferior vena cava and hepatic artery

2. What receptors are responsible for the humoral response of the portal vein and hepatic artery?
   A. The portal vein has alpha 1 adrenergic, beta 2 adrenergic, and dopaminergic 1 receptors. The hepatic artery has beta 2 adrenergic receptors only.
   B. The hepatic artery has alpha 1 adrenergic, beta 2 adrenergic, and dopaminergic 1 receptors. The portal vein has alpha 1 adrenergic and dopaminergic 1 receptors.
   C. The portal vein has alpha 1 adrenergic, beta 2 adrenergic, and dopaminergic 1 receptors. The hepatic artery has beta 2 adrenergic and dopaminergic 1 receptors.
   D. The portal vein only has alpha 1 adrenergic receptors. The hepatic artery only has beta 2 adrenergic receptors.
   E. The portal vein has alpha 1 adrenergic, beta 2 adrenergic, and dopaminergic 1 receptors. The hepatic artery has cholinergic receptors only.

3. Which of the following BEST describes the action of insulin?
   A. Stimulates gluconeogenesis, inhibits glycogen storage, promotes protein catabolism
   B. Stimulates glycogenolysis, inhibits oxidation of free fatty acids, inhibits gluconeogenesis
   C. Stimulates glycogenolysis, protein catabolism, and gluconeogenesis
   D. Inhibits lipolysis, protein catabolism, and glycogenolysis
   E. Inhibits lipolysis, protein catabolism, and glycogenolysis

4. Which coagulation factors are not produced in the liver?
   A. Factors III, IV, VII
   B. Factors II, IX, X
   C. Factor VIII, Von Willibrand Factor
   D. Factors II, VII, IX, X
   E. Factors III, VII, VIII, X

5. A 36-year-old male received an axillary block using lidocaine 2% for carpal tunnel release. He has history of taking propanolol to treat his tremors. How does beta blockade affect hepatic biotransformation (clearance) of lidocaine, and how should the dose of lidocaine be adjusted?
   A. Clearance of lidocaine is increased; thus increase the dose
   B. Clearance of lidocaine is decreased; thus decrease the dose
   C. There is no effect on the clearance of lidocaine
   D. The clearance of lidocaine is increased; thus decrease the dose

6. Which of the following drugs will have the highest blood concentration after one pass through the liver?
   A. Warfarin
   B. Lidocaine
   C. Morphine
   D. Metoprolol
   E. Ranitidine

7. A 46-year-old Hispanic female with history of depression, on bupropion and Zoloft, undergoes an urgent laparoscopic cholecystectomy. Which of the following regimens is most appropriate for her postop pain management?
   A. Acetaminophen and codeine PO Q8H
   B. Norco (hydrocodone/acetaminophen) 7.5/325 one tablet PO Q6H PRN
   C. Morphine 4 mg IV Q6H PRN
   D. Acetaminophen 500mg PO Q12H

8. A 70-year-old female presents to the OR with a diagnosis of small bowel obstruction. She has been symptomatic for 2 days. Her HR is 121, B/P is 96/49, and temperature is 96.9. Understanding the daily secretion of fluid produced in the gastrointestinal tract, and not including vomiting, approximately how many liters of fluid might be accumulated above the obstruction?
   A. 9 L
   B. 15.5 L
   C. 25 L
   D. 6 L

ANSWERS

1. B. The liver is one of the largest organs in the body and demands 25% of cardiac output, using a dual vascular supply consisting of the hepatic artery and portal vein.

FURTHER READING

Miller R, ed. *Miller's Anesthesia*. 7th ed. Philadelphia, PA: Elsevier; 2010:417.

2. B. The hepatic artery has alpha 1, beta 2, and dopamine 1 receptors, whereas the portal vein has alpha 1 and dopamine 1 receptors.

FURTHER READING

Butterworth I, Mackey D, Wasnick J. *Clinical Anesthesiology*. 5th ed. Philadelphia, PA: McGraw-Hill; 2013:693.

3. E. Insulin is a neuroendocrine factor that is anabolic and helps to stimulate glycogen storage, whereas glucagon and catecholamines are catabolic factors that cause glycogen breakdown and gluconeogenesis.

FURTHER READING

Miller R, ed. *Miller's Anesthesia*. 7th ed. Philadelphia, PA: Elsevier; 2010:420.

4. C. Hepatocytes produce all coagulation factors except factor VIII and Von Willibrand Factor.

FURTHER READING

Butterworth I, Mackey D, Wasnick J. *Clinical Anesthesiology*. 5th ed. Philadelphia, PA: McGraw-Hill; 2013:696.

5. B. Drug removal from the blood is a function of hepatic blood flow and intrinsic clearance (extraction ratio ER). The ER is the amount or percentage of drug that is metabolized after just one pass through the liver. Lidocaine is a high extraction drug with approximately 70%–80% of the drug being cleared after one pass through the liver. Thus hepatic blood flow (HBF) is the determiner of clearance, and anything that lessens HBF will decrease the clearance of the drug and thus increase the risk of toxicity. The dose of lidocaine should be decreased.

FURTHER READING

Rosow C, Levine W. Drug interaction. In: Barash P, Cullen B, Stoelting R, Cahalan M, Stock M, eds. *Clinical Anesthesia*. 6th ed. Philadelphia, PA: Lippincott Williams; 2009:554–555.

6. A. Warfarin is a poorly extracted drug, while the other drugs are all efficiently extracted drugs. With high extraction drugs the liver is able to eliminate the drug easily, whereas with low extraction drugs the hepatic elimination rate is limited by the availability for protein binding. The elimination of high extraction drugs is affected by blood flow, not changes in protein binding or the activity of drug-metabolizing enzymes.

FURTHER READING

Miller R, ed. *Miller's Anesthesia*. 7th ed. Philadelphia, PA: Elsevier; 2010:424.

7. C. The enzyme CYPD26 converts codeine into morphine. Quinidine, fluoxetine, and paroxetine can inhibit such conversion. Therefore codeine, oxycodone, or hydrocodone would not be best in a patient on SSRIs.

FURTHER READING

Miller R, ed. *Miller's Anesthesia*. 7th ed. Philadelphia, PA: Elsevier; 2010:511.

8. A. The salivary glands secrete approximately 1500 mL of fluid per day and the stomach secretes approximately 7000 mL per day.

FURTHER READING

Guyton A, Hall J. *Guyton and Hall Textbook of Medical Physiology*. Philadelphia, PA: Saunders, Elsevier; 1996:798, 818–828.

27.

RENAL AND URINARY SYSTEMS

Katya H. Chiong

PHYSIOLOGY

BLOOD FLOW

Although the kidneys represent a very small volume of total body weight, the amount of blood flow they receive is significant, approximately 20%–25% of cardiac output. Most of this blood flow is distributed to the renal cortex. Autoregulation maintains relatively constant renal blood flow (RBF) and glomerular filtration rate (GFR) through a range of mean arterial blood pressures (60–160 mmHg). Autoregulation is thought to be achieved by the adjustment of afferent arteriolar tone (myogenic response), altering the resistance to blood flow in response to increases and decreases in mean arterial blood pressure. Tubularglomerular feedback via the juxtaglomerular apparatus is thought to also play a role. Autoregulation is impaired by calcium channel blockade and is reset in chronic hypertension. It may be lost in the diabetic kidney as well as acute renal failure through the excessive release of nitric oxide caused in endothelial dysfunction by renal ischemia-reperfusion injury.[1]

Urinary flow rate is not subject to autoregulation and is affected by changes in blood pressure. It is tubular water reabsorption, closely related to the hydrostatic pressure in the peritubular capillaries, that determines the urinary flow rate.[1]

GLOMERULAR FILTRATION

Glomerular filtration directly reflects glomerular function. Approximately 90% of fluid filtered at the glomeruli is resorbed and returned to the circulation. The glomerular filtration rate (GFR) is dependent on glomerular filtration pressure (GFP) and is approximately 125 mL/min. The GFP is a function of renal arterial pressure, both afferent and efferent tone, and glomerular oncotic pressure. The GFR is reduced by significant decreases in mean arterial pressures and renal blood flow as well as by increases in afferent tone. On the other hand, afferent dilation and mild increase in efferent tone increase GFP and GFR.[2]

TUBULAR REABSORPTION AND SECRETION

The tubule is composed of four major segments: the proximal tubule, the loop of Henle, the distal tubule, and the connecting segment. It has a large capacity for reabsorption of both water and sodium, almost 99%. Many other filtered substances are completely absorbed, but some, such as glucose, have a maximum rate of absorption (tubular maximum, 375 mg/dL). Once plasma glucose exceeds the tubular maximum, glucose is no longer reabsorbed and glycosuria results. Thus, the amount of glucose excreted in the urine is directly proportional to the filtered load.[1]

There are a number of active transport systems within the tubule system; the most important one is the sodium-potassium adenosine triphosphatase (Na^+-K^+-ATPase) system. It pumps sodium of the tubular cell into the interstitial fluid against a concentration and electrical gradient in exchange for potassium inside the tubular cell. The subsequent decrease in sodium concentration inside the cell facilitates passive reabsorption of sodium from the tubular lumen into the cell. The transport of virtually all solutes is coupled to this active transport of sodium.[1]

Many endogenous and exogenous solutes are secreted into the tubular lumen from the capillary blood. The most metabolically active components of the tubules are the proximal tubule, the thick ascending loop of Henle, and the first part of the distal tubule. Structure and function of these segments go hand in hand and typically have invaginations with varying characteristics with anywhere from few to a rich amount of mitochondria.[1]

RENAL FUNCTION TESTS

Renal function tests can be measured preoperatively but must be interpreted carefully, as significant renal disease may exist before affecting lab values. In fact, a 50% decrease in renal function may exist while laboratory values remain normal.[2] Trends are more useful for evaluating renal function than one isolated lab value. Complicating the picture even more, reported lab values may not be adjusted for age.

TESTS OF GLOMERULAR FILTRATION

Blood Urea Nitrogen (BUN): a byproduct of protein metabolism with a normal range of 8–20 mg/dL. The BUN values may increase independently of renal function as a result of dehydration, increase in protein intake, degradation of blood (hematoma) or bleeding (GI tract), or increased metabolic state (trauma, sepsis, burns). Dehydration is suspected in patients with a BUN:CR ratio greater than 20:1.[3] Although BUN concentration is susceptible to many extraneous factors, values greater than 50 mg/dL inevitably reflect a decreased GFR.[2]

Serum Creatinine (Cr): an end product of skeletal muscle breakdown, excreted primarily by the kidneys and often used as a marker of GFR. Normal lab values range from 0.5 to 1.2 mg/dL. It can be influenced by age, skeletal muscle mass, and catabolism. Considering that elderly patients typically have decreased muscle mass, and that creatinine production is proportional to skeletal muscle mass, elderly patients may show normal Cr despite substantial reductions in renal function. Thus even mild increases in Cr in the elderly can suggest significant renal disease. Likewise, in patients with chronic renal disease, Cr may not accurately reflect GFR due to various ongoing factors such as decreases in Cr production, decreases in muscle mass, and any nonrenal excretion of Cr, such as in the GI tract.[2]

Creatinine Clearance (CrCL): measures glomerular ability to filter creatinine, and because it is only affected by accurate urine volume measurements, it is considered a more reliable measurement of GFR than both BUN and Cr. Creatinine clearance provides a simple alternative in calculating GFR via the use of the following equation: CrCl = [(Urine Cr) (urinary flow rate *mL/min*)/(plasma Cr). Normal range for CrCL is 110–150 mL/min. Additionally, the Cockcroft-Gault equation may be used to estimate creatinine clearance when urine studies cannot be conducted. The Cockcroft-Gault equation is estimated $Cr_{Clearance}$ = {[(140 - Age)(mass in kg)] / [(Serum Creatinine × 72)]} × (*0.85 if female*).

Cystatin C: a cysteine-protease inhibitor that is released into the circulation by nucleated cells. It is completely filtered by the glomerulus; therefore serum levels bear a close relationship to serum creatinine levels (and GFR). Serum cystatin C shows promise as, unlike creatinine, is not affected by muscle mass, age, and gender. In certain clinical situations, it even appears to be a more accurate predictor of low GFR than serum creatinine. However, there is evidence that factors such as cigarette smoking, inflammation (elevated c-reactive protein), and immunosuppressive therapy affect cystatin c levels independently of GFR and thus it remains an investigational marker at this time.[1]

TESTS OF TUBULAR FUNCTION

Results of urine specific gravity (1.003–1.030), urine osmolality (350–500 mOsm), and urine sodium (20–40 mEq/L) tests reflect the kidney's ability to perform its homeostatic functions. Urine sodium (UNa), for example, is useful in assessing volume status. A value below 20 mEq/L suggests intravascular volume depletion, whereas a value over 40 mEq/L suggests a decreased ability to resorb sodium by the renal tubules such as occurs in acute tubular necrosis (ATN). Calculating the fractional excretion of sodium (FENa) can be helpful in differentiating between prerenal and renal tubular causes of azotemia. A FENa above 1% indicates tubular damage and would be consistent with ATN. A FENa below 1% may be seen in normal or hypovolemic patients. While this formula may be expressed in many ways, the authors suggest FENa = $(Urine_{Na}/Plasma_{Na}) / (Urine_{Cr}/Plasma_{Cr}) \times$ 100%.[3] Written/memorized in this fashion, the fractional excretion of sodium (which means that sodium is in the numerator) can be expressed as $(U/P_{Sodium})/(U/P_{Creatinine})$ ... or, "if you pee, you pee" (think about it a couple of times and it makes sense).

HORMONAL REGULATION OF EXTRACELLULAR FLUID AND OSMOLALITY

Two mutually dependent and opposing neurohormonal systems maintain blood pressure, intravascular volume, as well as salt and water hemostasis. The vasoconstrictor system group consists of the sympathoadrenal system, the renin-angiotensin system, aldosterone, and antidiuretic hormone (ADH), which all work to *decrease* RBF, GFR, urine flow, and excretion of sodium. The vasodilation system group, on the other hand, consists of prostraglandins, kinins, and atrial natriuretic peptide (ANP), which work to *increase* RBF, GFR, urine flow, and sodium excretion.

REGULATION OF ACID-BASE BALANCE

Hydrogen ion concentration can be described in terms of volatile and metabolic acids. The body has evolved various intra- and extracellular weak acid buffering systems to prevent rapid changes in the extracellular electrochemical balance that may interfere with transcellular ion pumps.[4]

The lungs are the main eliminators of CO_2, the major source of acid in the body. Volatile acids are principally buffered by hemoglobin. When respiratory failure occurs, the principle CO_2-buffering system, hemoglobin, becomes overwhelmed, which leads to acidosis. The kidney responds by excreting an increased chloride load using NH_4^+, a weak cation, maintaining electrochemical balance, referred to as metabolic compensation.

The bicarbonate buffering system is probably the most important extracellular buffer. It manages the numerous acid-base imbalances that can be produced by normal as well as abnormal physiology, including the handling of CO_2 waste produced in cellular respiration.

DRUG EXCRETION

Excretion of drugs and their metabolites depends on glomerular filtration as well as the *active* secretion and *passive* absorption by the renal tubules. The glomerular filtration of anesthetic drugs and other small drugs depends on the GFR and the fractional plasma protein binding. Drugs that are highly protein bound will not be efficiently filtered at the glomerular site. Protein binding influences the elimination of drugs, because it is the unbound portion that is available for metabolism and clearance by the kidney (or liver). Nonionized compounds undergo passive tubular reabsorption; because nonionized compounds are reabsorbed, this group is more available and subject to metabolism and elimination. Drugs can also be conjugated to water-soluble metabolites that can then be eliminated in the urine by the kidney. Ionized compounds, on the other hand, are more likely trapped within renal tubules accounting for an increased renal elimination by either urine alkalization or acidification.[2]

WATER BALANCE, DISTRIBUTION, AND ELECTROLYTES

Total body water (TBW) is 60% of total body weight. The TBW is divided into two compartments: two-thirds intracellular (or TBW = 40% total body weight) and one-third extracellular (or TBW = 20% total body weight). The extracellular compartment is further divided into two compartments: three-fourths interstitial (or TBW = 15% total body weight) and one-fourth intravascular (or TBW = 5% total body weight). It is the extracellular compartment to which crystalloids such as Lactated Ringer's and normal saline distribute.

Sodium is the most abundant positive ion in the extracellular compartment. Normal sodium serum levels are 135–145 mEq/L. Serum osmolality is tightly regulated in the body primarily through ADH and ranges from 275–290 mOsm/kg. Serum osmolality is estimated by using the following equation:

$$\text{Serum Osmolality} = [(2 \times \text{Na}) + (\text{glucose}/18) + (\text{urea}/2.8)]$$

Hyponatremia, typically defined as a sodium concentration of less than 135 mEq/L results from excessive loss of sodium in the body (e.g., sweat, vomiting, diarrhea, burns, iatrogenic from diuretics). Most commonly it results from an excess of TBW and not a deficiency of sodium itself. Rapid correction of hyponatremia can lead to *central pontine myelolysis*. Management of hyponatremia should include eliminating the underlying cause and should guide overall therapy. Severe hyponatremia may lead to an altered level of consciousness, seizures, weakness, and coma. At levels at or below 123 mEq/mL, brain edema occurs. At 100 mEq/L, severe cardiac effects include ventricular fibrillation and cardiac arrest. The most likely cause of postoperative hyponatremia is SIADH. The optimal rate of correction seems to be 0.6–1 mmol/L/h until the sodium concentration is 125 mEq/L and then the rate is slowed down further.[5] Half of the deficit can be replaced over the first 8 hours, and the next over the next few days if symptoms remit. Appropriate treatment for patients with neurologic deficits remains controversial. Hypernatremia is an increased extracellular sodium concentration. The major causes of hypernatremia include an excess loss of water, inadequate water intake, ADH deficiency, or excessive intake of sodium including iatrogenic causes with treatment that includes hypertonic saline and other drugs. The most common objective sign of hypernatremia is lethargy or mental status changes, which can proceed to seizures and a state of coma.[5] With acute and severe hypernatremia, the rapid osmotic shift of water from the brain cells can lead to brain shrinkage with tearing of the meninges and subsequent intracranial hemorrhage. Treatment involves restoration of normal serum osmolality and volume using diuretics and hypotonic fluids. Rapid correction may cause harmful or lethal brain edema and should be avoided.

Chloride is the predominate anion in the extracellular compartment. Excessive chloride intake or inadequate elimination secondary to renal dysfunction can cause hyperchloremic metabolic acidosis. Excess loss of chloride, either by gastric secretion or loss in urine for example, results in hypochloremic alkalosis. Depletion of chloride affects the ability of the kidney to excrete bicarbonate. The reabsorption of sodium bicarbonate is augmented because total body chloride depletion results in both extracellular volume contraction (which stimulates HCO_3 reabsorption) and decreased quantities of filtered chloride available for reabsorption with sodium. Metabolic alkalosis also increases potassium excretion, which may lead to hypokalemia. Sodium or potassium chloride should be administered in the setting of intravascular depletion or hypokalemia.[5]

Potassium is the most abundant positive ion in the intracellular fluid compartment. In fact, nearly all (nearly 98%) of the potassium in the body is intracellular. Normal serum potassium concentrations range from 3.5 to 5.5 mEq/L. In the short term (within minutes), all of the following can influence potassium balance: insulin, pH, β-adrenergic agonists, and bicarbonate concentrations. Long-term regulation and balance of potassium primarily involve the kidney and aldosterone. Increases in potassium intake increase its excretion in the kidney through various cellular mechanisms. Multiple factors regulate the normal transmembrane potassium gradient, most importantly involving the Na^+K^+-ATPase. In response to an increase in extracellular potassium concentration, aldosterone is secreted from the zona glomerulosa of the adrenal gland to increase potassium secretion into the renal tubules and increase potassium excretion. Hypokalemia (<3.5 mEq/L) can occur due to a deficiency or redistribution into the intracellular space. The most common causes of hypokalemia are reduced intake, increased GI losses, excess renal loss (e.g., mineral corticosteroids, diuretics), and a shift of concentration from the extracellular fluid compartment to the intracellular compartment (insulin, acute alkalosis, stress, or increased catecholamine activity). Severe hypokalemia in the range of 2–2.5 mEq/L is likely to cause muscular weakness, arrhythmias, and EKG changes (sagging of the ST segment, t-wave depression, u-wave elevation). Cardiac dysrhythmias are more predictable with severity of hypokalemia and most frequently involve atrial fibrillation and ventricular asystoles. [5] The rate of potassium repletion is typically limited to 0.5 mEq/kg/h. Hyperkalemia (>5.5 mEq/L) can be caused by drugs that decrease potassium excretion, or after sudden shifts of potassium from the intracellular fluid compartment to the extracellular compartment. Some examples of drugs that may cause hyperkalemia include amiloride, angiotensin II antagonists, ACE-I, mannitol, succinylcholine, spironolactone, and triamterene.[5] Reperfusion after long periods of ischemia (>4 hours) results in significant acidosis, and subsequent outflow of intracellular potassium can result in fatal hyperkalemia. Conditions or drugs that decrease adrenal function or decrease levels of aldosterone can also cause hyperkalemia via retention of potassium. Other potential causes of hyperkalemia include lysis of blood cells and renal failure. Hyperkalemia can cause muscle weakness and paralysis. Mild elevations (6–7 mEq/L) may cause peaked t-wave on EKG. Levels approaching 10–12 mEq/L may manifest as prolonged P-R interval, widened QRS complex, ventricular fibrillation, or asystole.[5] Therapy centers around the cause as well as stabilization of cardiac effects of hyperkalemia. Treatment consists of physiologic antagonists (calcium), agents to shift potassium into cells (insulin, hyperventilation, bicarbonate, β-adrenergic agonists), and drugs or interventions to eliminate potassium from the body (diuretics, dialysis, kayexalate).[5]

PHARMACOLOGY

DIURETICS: COMPARISON OF DRUGS

Acetazolamide (Carbonic Anhydrase Inhibitor)[6]

Mechanism of Action (MOA): Reversible inhibition of the enzyme carbonic anhydrase resulting in reduction of hydrogen ion secretion at renal tubule and an increased renal excretion of sodium, potassium, bicarbonate, and water. Uses: treatment for glaucoma, acute mountain sickness, and significant metabolic alkalosis, and to induce an alkaline urine in drug overdoses (salicylates).

Effect on Electrolytes and Acid-Base Balance: Hyperchloremia, hypokalcemia, metabolic acidosis.

Adverse Effects: Flushing, CNS effects (ataxia, depression, dizziness, paresthesias), hyper-/hypoglycemia, electrolyte and metabolic disturbances, dermatologic (TEN, skin photosensitivity) and hematologic effects (aplastic anemia, agranulocytosis, thrombocytopenia), sulfa allergy cross-reactivity.

Furosemide, Bumetanide, Ethacrynic Acid, Torsemide (Loop Diuretics)[6]

MOA: Inhibits reabsorption of sodium and chloride in the ascending loop of Henle and distal renal tubule, interfering with the chloride-binding cotransport system, causing increased excretion of water, sodium, chloride, magnesium, and calcium.

Effect on Electrolytes and Acid-Base Balance: Can produce electrolyte imbalances: hypokalemia, hypomagnesemia, hypocalcemia. May result in metabolic (contraction) alkalosis.

Adverse Effects: Ototoxicity, nephrotoxicity, sulfa allergy cross-reactivity (except ethacrynic acid), hyperuricemia, renal and hepatic dysfunction, can lead to profound diuresis resulting in fluid and electrolyte depletion.

Mannitol (Osmotic Diuretic)[6]

MOA: Increases the osmotic pressure of the glomerular filtrate, reducing the efficiency of sodium (and water) reabsorption, causing significant diuresis. Decreases ICP within 30 minutes with max effect at 1–2 hours, duration of action for approximately 6 hours. Additionally, used to decrease IOP and to promote urinary excretion (e.g., toxic substances).

Effect on Electrolytes and Acid-Base Balance: Can produce electrolyte imbalances (Na, K, Mg). May result in hyponatremic, hyperkalemic metabolic acidosis.

Adverse Effects: Can lead to volume depletion and electrolyte abnormalities, serum osmolality > 320 mOsm/kg may increase the risk of acute renal tubular damage. If very high doses of hypertonic mannitol are infused, or if the drug is given to patients with renal failure, mannitol is retained in the circulation, which results in the osmotic movement of water and potassium out of cells leading to extracellular fluid volume expansion (and possibly pulmonary edema), hyponatremia, metabolic acidosis (by dilution), and hyperkalemia.

Spironolactone (Potassium-Sparing Diuretic)[6]

MOA: Spironolactone is an aldosterone antagonist—it competes with aldosterone for receptor sites in the distal renal tubules, increasing sodium chloride and water excretion while conserving potassium and hydrogen ions. It is used in the management of edema associated with excessive aldosterone, CHF refractory to other therapy, primary hyperaldosteronism, cirrhosis of liver, ascites, and hypokalemia.

Effect on Electrolytes and Acid-Base Balance: Results in electrolyte imbalance (hyperkalemia) and may result in hyperchloremic metabolic acidosis.

Adverse Effects: Hepatoxicity, gynocomastia, hyperkalemia, agranulocytosis, dermatologic manifestations, and nausea/vomiting.

Triamterene, Amiloride (Potassium-Sparing Diuretics)[6]

MOA: Diuretics in this subcategory have no effect on aldosterone but have the same effect on the nephron by blocking sodium channels and inhibiting sodium reabsorption.

Effect on Electrolytes and Acid-Base Balance: The reduction in intracellular sodium decreases the function of Na+/K+ ATPase, leading to potassium retention and decreased calcium, magnesium, and hydrogen excretion. May result in metabolic acidosis.

Adverse Effects: Hematologic abnormalities, dizziness, fatigue, headache, weakness, nausea/vomiting, jaundice, and cough.

Hydrochlorothiazide (Thiazide Diuretics)[6]

MOA: Primarily inhibits sodium transport in the distal tubule, the connecting segment at the end of the distal tubule, and possibly the cortical collecting tubule. Commonly used to treat primary hypertension.

Effect on Electrolytes and Acid-Base Balance: Can produce electrolyte imbalances (Na, K, Mg, Ca), may result in metabolic (hypochloremic) alkalosis.

Adverse Effects: Hypotension, hypokalemia, hypercalcemia, hyperuricemia, hyponatremia, and can also increase glucose and cholesterol concentration in the blood. Other adverse effects: hypersensitivity reactions, photosensitivity, gout, ocular effects, sulfa allergy cross-reactivity.

DOPAMINERGIC DRUGS

Dopaminergic agonists selectively increase renal blood flow and may oppose renal vasoconstriction. Dobutamine, dopexamine, and fenoldopam are all pharmacologic analogs of dopamine. Dobutamine, however, is devoid of dopaminergic activity and has predominately β1- and β2-adrenergic activity, causing a marked increase in both cardiac output and therefore RBF. Fenolopam is a pure, selective $dopamine_1$-receptor agonist, whereas dopexamine is a mixed $dopamine_1$- and $dopamine_2$-receptor agonist.[1] Fenoldopam increases renal blood flow and GFR and may have beneficial effects in the treatment of acute renal injury, however its exact role in therapy of renal failure is unclear at this time. It is presently approved for short-term parenteral treatment of severe hypertension.[2] Dopamine works at numerous receptors: $dopamine_1$- and $dopamine_2$-receptors (at lower concentrations), and β1-, β2-, and α1-receptors (at higher concentrations).

REFERENCES

1. Sladen R. renal physiology. In: Miller R, ed. *Miller's Anesthesia*. 7th ed. Philadelphia, PA: Elsevier; 2010:441–476.
2. Malhotra V, Pamnani A. Renal, liver, and biliary tract disease. In: Miller R, Pardo M. *Basics of Anesthesia*. 6th ed. Philadelphia, PA: Elsevier; 2011:448–455.
3. Wass C. Renal function tests. In: Faust R, Cucchiara R, Rose S, Spackman T, Wedel D, Wass C. *Anesthesiology Review*. 3rd ed. Philadelphia, PA: Churchill Livingstone; 2002:85–86.
4. Neligan PJ, Deutschman CS. Perioperative acid-base balance. In: Miller R, ed. *Miller's Anesthesia*. 7th ed. Philadelphia, PA: Elsevier; 2010:1557–1572.
5. Kaye A, Riopelle J. Intravascular fluid and electrolyte physiology. In: Miller R, ed. *Miller's Anesthesia*. 7th ed. Philadelphia, PA: Elsevier; 2010:1705–1737.
6. Drug Information. UpToDate® website. http://www.uptodate.com/contents/acetazolamide-drug-information?source=search_result&search=acetazolamide&selectedTitle=1~95. Accessed April 8, 2015.

FURTHER READING

Malhotra V, Pamnani A. Renal, liver, and biliary tract disease. In: Miller R, Pardo M. *Basics of Anesthesia*. 6th ed. Philadelphia, PA: Elsevier; 2011.

QUESTIONS

1. Which of the following renal function tests best correlate with glomerular filtration?
   A. Cystatin C
   B. Creatinine clearance
   C. Serum creatinine
   D. Blood urea nitrogen
   E. Urine osmolality

2. You have been called to the bedside to evaluate a patient with oliguria on POD 1 s/p hysterectomy. Which of the following findings is MOST consistent with an intrarenal etiology for oliguria?
   A. Urine sodium > 40 mEq/L
   B. FENa <1%
   C. Urine specific gravity > 1.030
   D. Urine osmolality > 1200 mOsm/kg
   E. Absence of casts on urinalysis

3. Which of the following electrolytes is MOST likely to increase with chronic furosemide therapy?
   A. Potassium
   B. Magnesium
   C. Chloride
   D. Calcium
   E. Bicarbonate

4. A 65-year-old male is admitted to the ICU on POD 3 s/p femur fracture repair for new-onset hypotension and decreased urine output, no gross hematuria.

Vitals: Temperature—36.9°C, pulse—87, blood pressure—113/65, respiratory rate—18, oxygen saturation—98% on room air. Lab findings include:

Blood urea nitrogen 63 mg/dL
Creatinine 1.6 mg/dL
Urine Sodium 10 mEq/L
FENA <1%
Urinalysis: few cells, no casts, no proteinuria

Based on the above findings, which of the following is the MOST likely cause of his acute kidney injury?
   A. Acute tubular necrosis (ATN)
   B. Dehydration
   C. Sepsis associated ATN
   D. Methyl methacrylate
   E. Obstructive uropathy

5. All of the following drugs may cause hyperkalemia EXCEPT:
   A. Succinylcholine
   B. Mannitol
   C. Amiloride
   D. Furosemide
   E. ACE inhibitors

6. Which of the following drugs is MOST likely to result in metabolic alkalosis if given chronically and in excess?
   A. Triamterene
   B. Spironolactone
   C. Hydrochlorothiazide
   D. Mannitol
   E. Acetazolamide

7. Which of the following values represents the interstitial volume of a 90-kg male?
   A. 54 L
   B. 36 L
   C. 18 L
   D. 13.5 L
   E. 4.5 L

ANSWERS

1. B. Creatinine clearance measures glomerular ability to filter creatinine, and because it is only affected by accurate urine volume measurements, it is considered a more reliable measurement of GFR than both BUN and Cr. Cysplastin C currently remains only an investigational marker, as many factors still interfere with levels.
2. A. The other options are most consistent with prerenal causes of oliguria rather than intrarenal etiologies. Recall that urine sodium retention is a function that the kidney uses to retain water, and that elevations in urine sodium reflect dysfunction of this process (in oliguria) or appropriate function of this process (as in cerebral salt wasting, or polyuria).
3. E. Chronic loop diuretics can cause many electrolyte imbalances (K+, Mg+, Ca+, Cl-) and lead to contraction alkalosis. Specifically, the depletion of chloride affects the kidney's ability to excrete bicarbonate.
4. B. Noted findings reflect a prerenal cause of oliguria, not intrarenal etiologies. Methyl methacrylate can cause systemic hypotension and embolic events intraoperatively and are less likely to cause findings as described.
5. D. One of the side effects of furosemide is hypokalemia, which may require potassium supplementation. All other drugs listed may contribute to hyperkalemia.
6. C. Hydrochlorothiazide may result in metabolic (hypochloremic) alkalosis. All others listed may result in metabolic acidosis.
7. D. 13.5 L represents the interstitial compartment (or 15% total body weight). Calculation: $90 \times .15 = 13.5$ L).

28.

HEMATOLOGIC SYSTEMS

Sam Gumbert

RED BLOOD CELLS

The administration of packed red blood cells (pRBCs) is indicated for the treatment of anemia and the associated complications of inadequate oxygen delivery. One unit of RBCs has a volume of 250–300 mL with an average hematocrit of 70%–80%. Transfusion of one RBC unit in a 70-kg adult will increase the hemoglobin by 1.0 g/dL and hematocrit by 3%, improve oxygen-carrying capacity, and increase intravascular volume.

Red blood cells are typically reconstituted with 100–150 mL of normal saline. Hypotonic glucose solutions pose a potential risk of hemolysis, while a theoretical risk of reconstituting RBCs with Lactated Ringer's solution is that it may cause calcium to bind with the citrate in the blood preservative, raising the risk of micro emboli.

Previously published guidelines for the use of RBC transfusions, including those from the American Society of Anesthesiologists task force, the British Committee for Standards in Haematology, the Australian and New Zealand Society of Blood Transfusion, and the American Association of Blood Banks (AABB) Practice Guidelines recommend that RBC transfusions should not be dictated solely by a single hemoglobin "trigger" but instead should be based on the patient's risks of developing complications associated with inadequate oxygenation.

The decision to transfuse should be based on clinical considerations such as a patient's medical history, anticipated bleeding, actual rate of blood loss, and the patient's ability to compensate with a low hemoglobin level. Red blood cell transfusion is rarely indicated in the stable patient with a hemoglobin concentration greater than 10 g/dL with evidence supportive of a restrictive transfusion strategy in the stable patient to a hemoglobin level of 6 to 7 g/dL. A recent Cochrane Review of current published evidence suggests that a restrictive transfusion trigger does not adversely affect mortality, cardiac morbidity, function, or length of hospital stay. A restrictive transfusion trigger should be used with caution in patients from high-risk groups such as acute coronary syndrome, as future randomized controlled trials are needed to guide treatment. For intermediate hemoglobin concentrations (6–10 g/dL), RBC transfusion should be based on the patient's risk for complications of inadequate oxygenation.

PLATELETS

The administration of platelets is indicated in the perioperative and peripartum setting when a quantitative or qualitative platelet defect is suspected as a source of bleeding. Prospective randomized trials recommend withholding platelet transfusion until platelet counts drop below 10×10^9/L with a higher threshold of 20×10^9/L in patients with additional bleeding risks. The determination of therapy for patients with intermediate platelet counts of 50×10^9/L to 100×10^9/L should be based on the risk of significant bleeding, type of surgery, and site of operation, for example, a closed space like the brain or eye. Additionally, platelet transfusion may be indicated despite an apparently adequate platelet count if there is known platelet dysfunction or the presence of microvascular bleeding.

In thrombocytopenic patients requiring invasive procedures or surgery, some general guidelines should be used in the prophylactic transfusion of platelets. A platelet count of greater than 100×10^9/L should be maintained in those operative cases with significant risk of major bleeding, neurosurgical or eye procedures, and in patients with intracranial trauma. In operative procedures with a risk of intraoperative bleeding and invasive procedures like epidural anesthesia, platelets should be maintained above 50×10^9/L. For minimally invasive procedures such as endoscopy or procedures associated with lower risk of blood loss, a platelet count of $20–50 \times 10^9$/L is sufficient.

Platelets are derived from three primary methods, the platelet rich plasma (PRP) method, the buffy coat method, and apheresis. The PRP method separates platelets from a unit of whole blood and suspends them in the plasma of the same donor. One platelet unit typically contains 55×10^9 platelets and is pooled in the blood bank with five other units to form an average adult dose. In contrast, the buffy coat method pools platelets from four donors and suspends them in the plasma of a single donor. This prepooled unit constitutes one dose and typically contains 240×10^9 platelets. In contrast to PRP, the buffy coat method limits the recipient's exposure to multiple donors, requires less plasma in preparation, and allows for quicker release because of the prepooled production method. An apheresis procedure removes only platelets from the donor's circulation and contains approximately 250×10^9 platelets in an adult unit. In patients who are likely to be transfused multiple times, apheresis platelets reduce the risk of alloimmunization to platelet and WBC antigens by limiting the number of donors to which the recipient is exposed.

Patients with low platelet counts or documented platelet function abnormalities are likely to benefit from platelet transfusions. However, prophylactic platelet transfusion is ineffective and rarely indicated in the presence of the immunologic destruction of platelets (e.g., idiopathic thrombocytopenic purpura or heparin-induced thrombocytopenia).

FRESH FROZEN PLASMA

Approximately 2,000,000 units of fresh frozen plasma (FFP) are transfused each year in the United States. FFP contains all the coagulation factors with the exception of platelets, and is primarily used for the treatment of hemorrhage from coagulation factor deficiencies.

Fresh frozen plasma is prepared by separating plasma from whole blood by centrifugation and then freezing (200–250 mL) plasma within 8 hours of collection, although in the United States plasma units are often frozen within 24 hours after phlebotomy (FP24). Fresh frozen plasma and FP24 can be transfused interchangeably. The primary difference between the products is that cryoprecipitate can be manufactured from FFP but not FP24. The centrifugation and freezing process maintains the activity of labile coagulation factors, specifically factors V and VIII. Once frozen, FFP may be stored for up to 1 year and requires a period to thaw prior to transfusion. Fresh frozen plasma should then be transfused within 24 hours to obtain adequate coagulation levels of Factors V and VIII, which diminish after 6 hours.

Transfusion of FFP is generally indicated during the perioperative period when the prothrombin time (PT) or partial thromboplastin time (PTT), are 1.5 times longer than normal. Fresh frozen plasma is indicated in patients with coagulation factor deficiencies secondary to liver disease, dilution coagulopathy, disseminated intravascular coagulation (DIC), and the rapid reversal of warfarin in neurosurgical patients.

Fresh frozen plasma is no longer the treatment of choice for coagulopathies such as factor VIII (hemophilia A) or factor IX (hemophilia B) deficiency, where virally inactivated or recombinant blood products exist. Plasma is ineffective in replacing individual clotting factors secondary to volume requirement and associated transfusion risks.

Fresh frozen plasma should be administered in a directed manner (10–15 mL/kg) to achieve a minimum of 30% of plasma factor concentration. Risk factors of FFP transfusion include transfusion-related acute lung injury, transfusion-associated circulatory overload, allergic/anaphylactic reaction, blood-borne illness, RBC alloimmunization, and hemolytic transfusion reaction.

CRYOPRECIPITATE

Cryoprecipitate is the fraction of plasma that precipitates when FFP is thawed, and contains factor VIII, von Willebrand factor (vWF), fibrinogen, fibronectin, and factor XIII. It is a critical component in the formation of clots, providing substrate for fibrin formation and clot stability. It is indicated for fibrinogen deficiency in the setting of bleeding, invasive procedures, trauma, or DIC. Crossmatching and ABO compatibility testing are not required before infusion of cryoprecipitate.

A single unit of cryoprecipitate is prepared from a single unit of thawed FFP after harvesting the cryosupernatant plasma following centrifugation. Each unit typically contains 80 IU factor VIII and 150 mg fibrinogen in approximately 5–20 mL of plasma. Five single units of cryoprecipitate are typically pooled into one bag with a fibrinogen concentration of approximately 7.5 g/L. A standard two-pooled adult dose of cryoprecipitate (or 10 single units) will increases the plasma fibrinogen level by 1–2 g/L.

Cryoprecipitate has associated transfusion risks that include allergic reaction, hemolytic transfusion reaction, transfusion-related acute lung injury, and blood-borne infection. With the effectiveness of concentrates and factor therapy, guidelines no longer recommend using cryoprecipitate in the treatment of hemophilia, von Willebrand disease, or fibronectin deficiency.

BLOOD COMPATIBILITY TESTING—GROUPING AND TYPING

BLOOD GROUP

The blood group is determined by the presence or absence of the A, B, and D antigens on the surface of the RBC membrane. If the A antigen or B antigen is present, a patient has Type A blood or Type B blood, respectively. When both A and B antigens are present, the patient has Type AB blood.

When neither antigen A nor B is present, the blood type is group O. The presence of the Rhesus group antigen D on the surface of the red cell is designated by a (+) or (-) sign. Approximately 85% of the population is Rh positive.

Acute hemolytic transfusion reactions (AHTRs) are most often caused by the recipient's plasma antibody against A, B, or D antigens on donor RBC. The antibody-antigen interaction activates the complement, resulting in hemolysis. Patients whose blood type is Type A have anti-B antibodies in their plasma; those whose blood type is Type B have anti-A antibodies in their plasma. Patients with AB blood types have neither A nor B antibodies in their plasma, whereas patients with group O blood type have both anti-A and anti-B antibodies in the plasma. In contrast to the A and B antigens, the anti-D antibodies are not present in the serum of the Rh-negative patient. However, 60%–70% of Rh-negative patients exposed to Rh-positive blood will develop anti-D antibodies with the possibility of AHTR with future exposure. Thus, a universal recipient is AB positive (AB+), lacks the A, B, and D antibodies in their plasma, and may receive all types of blood (i.e., A-, B-, AB-, A+, B+, AB+, O+ or O- blood). In contrast, the universal blood donor is O-negative, which has the fewest number of antigens on the cells and may be administered to all blood types.

BLOOD TYPING

Blood typing classifies blood into four groups designated A, B, AB, and O. Donor and recipient blood groups are identified by forward (i.e., cell) and reverse (i.e., serum) blood typing tests. The "forward type" determines which antigens in the ABO blood group system are on the patient's red blood cells. This is determined by mixing anti-A and anti-B reagent antibodies with the patient's RBC. To confirm the blood type, a "reverse type" identifies the isohemagglutinin in the patient's serum and should correlate to red blood cell antigen. Determination of the ABO group and Rh type takes approximately 5 minutes to process.

ANTIBODY SCREENING AND ANTIBODY IDENTIFICATION

The Antibody Screen

Antibody screening is a test used to detect atypical antibodies in the serum that may have been formed as a result of previous transfusion or pregnancy. The antibody screen is an indirect Coombs test used to identify the recipient's serum antibodies to possible RBC antigens. A patient's serum is mixed with commercially available RBCs with 25 to 30 clinically significant hemolytic antigens. Only 4 in 1,000 potential recipients demonstrate unexpected antibodies, and the likelihood that a screen will miss a potentially dangerous antibody is less than 1 in 10,000. If a positive plasma screen occurs, then the antibody must be identified to allow for the selection of compatible units. The performance of an ABO/Rh type and antibody screen testing is 30–45 minutes (when antibody negative) and should be repeated every 3 days in patients that require ongoing transfusion.

The Crossmatching

Crossmatching is performed to determine the compatibility between a specific donor's blood and a recipient's blood. A type and cross is typically requested when blood will likely be transfused, has a known history of antibodies, or is at high risk of alloimmunization. Crossmatch procedures vary, but at a minimum entail incubation of the recipient plasma with the donor RBCs at 37°C for 10–15 minutes followed by an indirect antiglobulin test and examination for agglutination. A full crossmatch takes 45 minutes to complete. Once compatibility testing is complete, crossmatched blood is removed from blood bank inventory and is typically reserved for the patient for 24-48 hours.

Uncrossmatched Blood

Uncrossmatched blood that is ABO and Rh compatible can be administered with greater than 99.8% assurance of safety to patients with negative antibody screens. In patients with a previous history of transfusion or pregnancy, a cumulative 1 per 200 exposures exists of developing an anti-RBC antibody. The addition of a 30–45 minute antibody screen further increases the likelihood of compatibility to greater than 99.9%. The administration, in emergency situations, of type-specific, uncrossmatched blood in patients with no history of prior transfusion or pregnancy is safe.

AUTOLOGOUS

Autologous blood transfusion is the collection of blood from a single patient and retransfusion back to the same patient when required. Autologous blood donation has been used as an alternative or adjunct to allogeneic blood administration in the form of predonation, isovolemic hemodilution, or operative field blood salvage. The decision to use autologous blood donation is predicated on the type of surgery, the patient's hematocrit, and the predicted erythropoietic response to donation.

TRANSFUSION REACTIONS

ACUTE HEMOLYTIC TRANSFUSION REACTION

About 20 people die yearly in the United States as a result of AHTR. The most common cause of AHTR is ABO incompatibility, with recipient plasma antibodies reacting to donor RBC antigens. Other antibodies such as Kell, Kidd, Duffy, Rhesus, and Ss antigens can also cause AHTR. When incompatible blood is administered, antibodies and complements in the recipient plasma attack the corresponding RBC surface antigen, causing intravascular RBC hemolysis and to a lesser extent extravascular hemolysis. The signs and symptoms of AHTR include the acute onset of fever, chills, nausea, rigors, diarrhea, dyspnea, and tachycardia. During an AHTR, patients will often complain of back and chest pain and appear restless. Hemoglobinuria will occur if plasma Hb rises above the renal threshold (25 mg/dL). Jaundice may follow acute hemolysis. Acute hemolytic transfusion reaction is life threating with profound hypotension, shock, acute renal failure, and potential development of DIC. The severity of AHTR depends on the degree of incompatibility, the amount of blood given, the rate of administration, and the integrity of the kidneys, liver, and heart.

Clerical errors of the recipient's pretransfusion sample at collection or misidentification of the recipient with the blood product immediately prior to transfusion are the two primary causes of AHTR. If a reaction is suspected, stop the transfusion, verify the identity of the patient, and immediately notify the blood bank. Suspected AHTR should be monitored and treated to maintain systemic blood pressure, mitigate the onset of DIC, and preserve renal function. Confirmation occurs with direct antiglobulin (Coombs) test and visual examination for hemoglobinemia. If positive, a repeat ABO/Rh type, antibody screen, and crossmatch must be performed.

DELAYED HEMOLYTIC TRANSFUSION REACTIONS

The cause of delayed hemolytic transfusion reactions (DHTRs) is an IgG-mediated antibody from red cell exposure associated with pregnancy or prior transfusion. In DHTRs, patients have an undetectable antibody level on pretransfusion screen but after exposure to the RBC antigen an anamnestic response occurs, with eventual lysis of the foreign RBCs in the spleen or sequestered extravascularly in the reticuloendothelial system. In contrast to acute hemolytic reactions, DHTR symptoms typically appear after 1–2 weeks and are typically less severe secondary to the extravascular nature of the RBC lysis. Symptoms include low-grade fever, mild increased indirect bilirubin, and a small reduction in hemoglobin. The diagnosis is made with direct antiglobulin test (Coombs test) and is associated with Kell, Kidd, and Rhesus antigens. Treatment of DHTRs is supportive, with monitoring of hemoglobin levels.

TRANSFUSION RELATED ALLERGIC REACTIONS—TYPES AND TREATMENT

Minor Allergic Reactions

Allergic reactions vary from minor uticaria to fulminant anaphylactic shock. Allergic reactions are caused by reactions to allergens in donor plasma and occur most frequently with the transfusion of FFP and platelets. In the classic type I hypersensitivity response, IgE antibodies react with plasma proteins and activate mast cells to release histamine, proteases, and chemotactic factors. Clinically, mild allergic reactions present in the immediate transfusion period with symptoms of fever, uticaria, edema, dizziness, and headache. Mild allergic symptoms may be treated prophylactically with antihistamine and steroids.

Anaphylactic Reaction

Anaphylaxis, though less common, may result in a life-threatening clinical presentation that includes dyspnea, bronchospasm, angioedema, and hypotension. Classically, anaphylaxis occurs in patients with hereditary IgA-deficient recipients with a prior exposure of foreign IgA immunoglobulin from previous transfusions or pregnancy. Patients with severe IgA deficiency require transfusion of washed RBCs, washed platelets, and plasma from an IgA-deficient donor. Severe reactions may require pretransfusion treatment with steroids, close monitoring, and epinephrine.

Febrile Reactions

White blood cell–related transfusion reaction, or febrile reactions, are caused by patient antibodies directed against human leukocyte antigens (HLA) present on transfused lymphocytes or granulocytes. This cause is most common in patients with a significant transfusion history or multiparous patients. Cytokines released from WBCs during storage, particularly in platelet concentrates, are a second possible cause. A white blood cell transfusion reaction occurs in up to 2% of platelet, FFP, and RBC transfusions. Febrile reactions should be distinguished from AHTRs with a direct Coombs test.

Clinically, febrile reactions consist of a temperature increase of ≥ 1°C within 4 hours of transfusion and are associated with myalgia, chills, respiratory distress, headache, and back pain. White cell related transfusion reactions are treated with acetaminophen and can be minimized through the administration of leukoreduced blood products.

INFECTION COMPLICATIONS AND RISKS

Bacterial Contamination

Bacterial contamination of packed RBCs rarely occurs secondary to refrigeration and aseptic techniques in collection and administration. All RBC units are inspected before issue for bacterial growth. The most common organism found to contaminate RBCs is *Pseudomonas fluorescens*, the bacterial source for mupirocin (which is given nasally to patients found positive for MRSA). Because platelet concentrates are stored at room temperature, they have greater potential for bacterial growth and endotoxin production.

Storage of platelets is subsequently limited to 5 days, and platelets are rigorously evaluated for bacteria prior to administration. The risk of bacterial growth is further reduced with the administration of apheresis platelets.

An immediate septic reaction is observed with the transfusion of a bacterial contaminated blood product with symptoms of fever, chills, tachycardia, dyspnea, shock, acute renal failure, and disseminated intravascular coagulation. If contaminated blood is suspected, blood cultures should be sent and supportive measures should be undertaken.

Hepatitis

Hepatitis may occur after the transfusion of any blood product and necessitates the screening of all donated blood products. The risk has been reduced by viral inactivation through heat treatment of serum albumin and plasma proteins and by the use of recombinant factor concentrates. The estimated risk of hepatitis B is 1:500,000; of hepatitis C, 1:2.6 million. Transmission of hepatitis A virus is very rare. Because of its relatively transient viremic phase (1-2 weeks) and concomitant clinical illness, blood banks are able to successfully preclude blood donation by patient history and antibody seroconversion.

Human Immunodeficiency Virus

Currently the risk of human immunodeficiency virus (HIV) transmission from a unit of blood is exceedingly remote. Human immunodeficiency virus, a retrovirus, is propagated via the translation of RNA to DNA. Infection in the United States is almost entirely HIV-1, although HIV-2 is a viable concern. Through the evaluation of at-risk behaviors in blood donors and the screening of blood products for HIV-1 and HIV-2 strains, the risk of HIV transmission due to transfusion is estimated to be 1:2.6 million.

Cytomegalovirus

Cytomegalovirus (CMV) constitutes a serious and potentially fatal complication in the immunocompromised patient (e.g., premature neonates, pregnant females, and severe immune depression such as organ transplant recipients and cancer patients). Cytomegalovirus is transferred via leukocytes in the blood. The onset of infection is usually asymptomatic and occurs 4 to 12 weeks after exposure to blood products. The risk of infection appears to increase with the number of blood products and the number of seropositive blood donors. To minimize risk of CMV transmission, at-risk patients receive leukoreduced blood from CMV seronegative donors.

Parasitic and Prion Diseases

Transmission of blood-borne parasitic diseases such as malaria or Chagas's disease have been reported but are exceeding rare in the United States. Creutzfeldt-Jakob disease, a prion, has never been reported to be transmitted by transfusion. Current practice precludes donation from a person who has received human-derived growth hormone or a dura mater transplant or who has a family member with Creutzfeldt-Jakob disease.

Citrate Intoxication

The rapid transfusion of a large quantity of stored blood results in the risk of citrate toxicity. Citrate, an anticoagulant used in the blood-collection process, is a preservative that binds ionized calcium and is present in PRBCs, FFP, and platelets. Citrate is normally metabolized by the liver, however liver impairment or rapid transfusion rates associated with massive transfusion (i.e., exceeding 1 mL/kg per minute) may exceed the liver's ability to process citrate and causes hypocalcemia. Signs of citrate toxicity associated with hypocalcemia include decreased cardiac contractility, hypotension, arrhythmias, muscle tremors, nausea, and narrow pulse pressure. Hypocalcemia should be treated with calcium chloride.

ELECTROLYTE

Hyperkalemia

During the storage of RBC, the Na+/K+ ATP function deteriorates, allowing intracellular potassium to leak into the plasma from RBCs to maintain electrochemical neutrality as hydrogen ions redistribute across the impaired RBC membrane. The magnitude of potassium redistribution directly correlates to the duration of red cell storage and may exceed 30 mEq/L after 21 days. Because the volume of plasma is relatively small, 20 to 60 mL per unit of PRBC, standard transfusion rates rarely result in hyperkalemia. Hyperkalemia may manifest with rapid infusion devices with transfusion rates exceeding 500 mL/min or in infants and small children.

Patients at risk of experiencing hyperkalemia benefit from either fresh RBCs (<8 days old), plasma reduced, or RBCs washed in saline if rapid transfusion is expected.

ACID BASE CHANGES

Acid base alterations occur from the blood collection and preservation process. Citrate phosphate dextrose (CPD) solution is added to freshly drawn blood and decreases the pH to 7.0–7.1. Over the course of 21 days of storage, a further reduction in pH to 6.84 occurs as glucose is metabolized to lactate and an increase in partial pressure of carbon dioxide is present. Following transfusion, the lactic acid and carbon dioxide are rapidly cleared and the RBC buffering capacity is restored.

ALTERED OXYGEN AFFINITY

A progressive decrease in RBC 2,3-diphosphoglycerate (DPG) occurs with the storage of blood until it is significantly reduced at 7 days and then absent after 10 days. This reduction in 2,3-DPG produces a left-shift of the oxygen dissociation curve, resulting in an increased affinity for oxygen and slower release of oxygen into the tissue. The 2,3-DPG levels return to normal with efficient oxygen delivery similar to native Hb after 12 to 24 hours.

MASSIVE BLOOD LOSS AND MASSIVE TRANSFUSION

Massive blood loss is the total loss of a blood volume within 24 hours or an acute 50% reduction of the total blood volume within minutes of injury. Massive transfusion is generally accepted to be a transfusion of greater than 10 units of PRBCs or an equivalent patient's blood volume in a 6- to 2-hour period. Massive transfusion is a lifesaving treatment of hemorrhagic shock with associated complications that include hypothermia, coagulopathy, citrate toxicity, electrolyte abnormalities, and metabolic derangements.

COAGULOPATHIES

In massive transfusion, coagulopathy occurs as a consequence of the dilution of coagulation factors and platelets, platelet consumption at the injury site, and impaired platelet function secondary to hypothermia.

Dilution Coagulopathy

Administration of large volumes of fluids deficient in clotting factors and platelets produces a coagulopathy secondary to clotting factor dilution. With isovolemic dilution, clinically significant reduction of fibrinogen, platelets, and factors II, V, and VII are evidenced. Platelet counts can decrease to less than 50,000 cells/mm^3 in adult patients who receive 10 to 15 units of packed RBCs. With the exception of trauma resuscitation, the decision to transfuse FFP, platelets, or cryoprecipitate should be directed by clinical and laboratory evidence of coagulopathy.

HYPOTHERMIA

Hypothermia associated with massive transfusion has been shown to be an independent predictor of mortality and morbidity in the trauma patient. Evidence suggests that mortality rates approach 100% if a patient's core temperature falls below 32°C regardless of the injury severity score. The administration of a unit of RBC at 4°C will reduce the core temperature of a 70-kg patient an estimated 0.25°C. Hypothermia results in a left shift of the oxygen-hemoglobin dissociation curve and exacerbates coagulopathy, acidosis, infection, and organ failure. Hypothermia is avoided by using active warming devices and fluid warmers.

SUBSTANTIAL BLEEDING PROTOCOLS

Substantial bleeding protocols (SBPs) were developed to preemptively mitigate the lethal triad of acidosis, hypothermia, and coagulopathy in the massive transfusion patient. The purpose of an SBP is to establish an institutional system that efficiently and continuously delivers blood products from the blood bank to the point of care, reducing the risk of coagulopathy, blood loss, and morbidity. In the massive transfusion a SBP reduces provider variability, facilitates staff communication and compliance, and simplifies the administration of predefined ratios of blood components.

PULMONARY

TRANSFUSION-RELATED ACUTE LUNG INJURY

Transfusion-related acute lung injury (TRALI) is a noncardiogenic form of pulmonary edema that occurs after the administration of blood products. It is now the leading cause of transfusion-related mortality. Acute respiratory symptoms of dyspnea, tachypnea, hypoxia, tachycardia, and bilateral radiographic pulmonary infiltrates occur within 6 hours of transfusion. It has been associated with all plasma-containing blood components; platelets and FFP are most commonly associated with TRALI.

In most instances, TRALI occurs when donor antileukocyte or anti-HLA antibodies recognize recipient leukocytes or recipient HLA cell surface markers and activate an inflammatory response. These activated leukocytes are sequestered in the lung, causing granulocyte enzymes to be released, damaging the pulmonary epithelium and increasing capillary permeability and pulmonary edema. Treatment for TRALI is largely supportive, with no evidence supporting the use of diuretics or steroids. Most cases improve within 2 days.

Blood donors with prior transfusion history or multiparous females are more likely to have antibodies that cause TRALI. For this reason, efforts are now being made to use male donor plasma for FFP transfusion.

TRANSFUSION-ASSOCIATED CIRCULATORY OVERLOAD

Transfusion-associated circulatory overload (TACO) occurs when the transfused volume exceeds a patient's cardiopulmonary capacity, inducing congestive heart failure. Transfusion-associated circulatory overload manifests as dyspnea, severe headache, and peripheral edema, with symptomatic congestive heart failure following a transfusion. Susceptible patients commonly have a history of diminished cardiac and pulmonary function and are unable to compensate for rapid intravascular volume expansion. Treatment of TACO includes supportive therapy and diuretics. The goal of transfusing patients susceptible for TACO is the slow administration of blood product and, when possible, the limitation of total volume.

GRAFT VERSUS HOST DISEASE

Red blood cells and platelets contain a significant number of donor lymphocytes. Graft versus host disease (GVHD) occurs when transfused donor lymphocytes from cellular blood components engraft and proliferate in an immunocompromised patient (e.g., organ transplant patients, bone marrow transplant recipients, or patients with hematologic cancers). The newly engrafted lymphocytes attack the host, causing symptoms of rash, bloody diarrhea, lymphadenopathy, pancytopenia, and often death. Graft versus host disease occurs 4 to 30 days after transfusion and is diagnosed based on clinical suspicion and skin and bone marrow biopsies. Cellular components should be irradiated to inactivate donor lymphocytes in patients at risk for GVHD.

TRANSFUSION-RELATED IMMUNOMODULATION

In transfusion-related immunomodulation (TRIM), red cell transfusions modulate the immune responsiveness. The mechanism of immunosuppression are still not fully known, however the transfusion of mononuclear white cells is thought to play a principal role. A dose-related relationship of adverse affects such as increased mortality, accelerated recurrence of malignancy, and increased hospital infection rates have been reported. This same dose-related relationship is not observed in autologous blood. In fact, prior to the availability of modern antirejection drugs, renal transplant recipients were commonly admitted to the hospital the night before surgery in order to receive a transfusion of two units of packed red cells in order to reduce the rate of transplant rejection. Keeping this fact in mind, it is no surprise that each unit of blood is associated with greater risk of infection.

COAGULATION

The coagulation cascade is a flow diagram that describes the enzymatic components of coagulation in their logical order and should be memorized (Figure 28.1). The two limbs of the coagulation cascade are the intrinsic and extrinsic components. The intrinsic cascade gets its name from the fact that when these factors were first being discovered, there was something "intrinsic" to the blood that allowed it to clot, meaning that nothing had to be introduced in order for the process to initiate. Conversely, the extrinsic cascade is activated by tissue factor; this is the "extrinsic" element that needs to be added to the blood in order to activate coagulation. Thus, enzymatic coagulation is designed to activate regardless of the source.

ANTICOAGULATION

Anticoagulants target specific parts of the coagulation cascade in order to exert their effects (see Figure 28.1). Warfarin effects factors II, VII, IX, and X. Unfractionated heparin

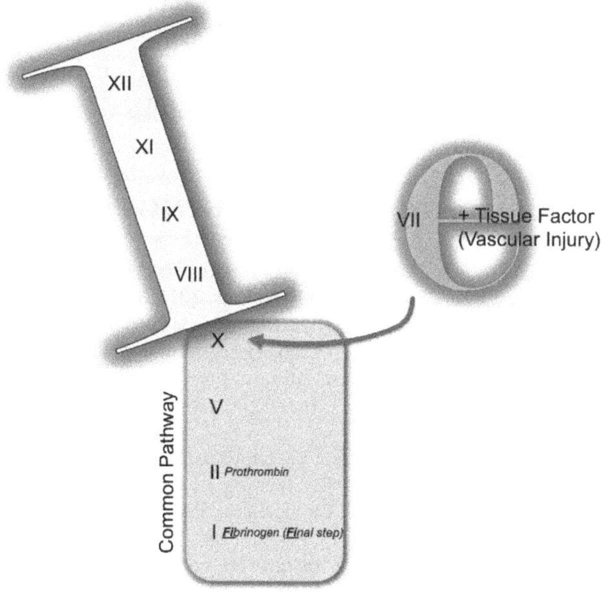

Figure 28.1 An overall perspective of the coagulation cascade (cofactors and inactive vs. active enzyme forms omitted for brevity). The intrinsic cascade describes clotting factors that are "instrinsic" to the blood, meaning that no other factors are needed in order for clotting to take place. The extrinsic cascade requires something "extra," meaning that vascular injury (or something that releases tissue factor) needs to take place in order to activate this portion of the cascade. The activation of any part of the cascade leads to the common pathway, ending in fibrinogen, the final factor (factor I). Image courtesy of George Williams, MD.

exerts its effect by potentiating antithrombin III (ATIII), thus heparin is not a direct anticoagulant but enhances an existing physiologic anticoagulant. If a patient does not have enough ATIII, heparin would not work, effectively leading to no change in coagulation status; this could paradoxically lead to needing FFP administration in order to facilitate anticoagulation from heparin. Heparin can be reversed by administering protamine (another anticoagulant); protamine neutralizes heparin via an acid-base reaction, but can lead to lethal anaphylactic reactions, so care must be taken. Protamine is derived from the spermatozoa of salmon. Recall that spermatozoa are immunologically isolated from the circulation, so potential allergic reactions can be deduced, though protamine allergic reactions are not universally seen.

Low molecular weight heparin (LMWH) also activates ATIII, but the resulting complex has an increased affinity for factor X specifically. Low molecular weight heparin also has more limited binding to plasma proteins, leading to a more predictable level and clinical effect (dose needs to be reduced in renal insufficiency).

New oral anticoagulants are available that bypass the "middle man" of ATIII, so to speak, by directly inhibiting factor X or factor II (thrombin). Direct thrombin inhibitors were originally isolated from leech saliva, leading to the hirudins (lepirudin and desirudin). Bivalrudin was synthetically generated and is easily metabolized, allowing for reduced bleeding risk and more rapid loss of activity. Dabigatran is an orally absorbed direct thrombin inhibitor. As of now, there is no reversal of these agents.

FURTHER READING

Allman K, Wilson I, Baker B, et al. *Oxford Handbook of Anesthesia*. 3rd ed. Oxford, UK: Oxford University Press; 2011.

American Association of Blood Banks. Standards for blood bank transfusion services. http://www.aabb.org/sa/standards/Pages/sigchngstds29.aspx. Accessed April 9, 2015.

Atlee J. *Complications in Anesthesia*. 2nd ed. Philadelphia, PA: Saunders; 2006.

Drummond J, Petrovitch C, Lane T. Hemostasis and transfusion medicine. In: Barash P, Cullen B, Stoelting R, Cahalan M, Stock M. *Clinical Anesthesia*. 7th ed. Philadelphia, PA: Lippincott Williams & Wilkins; 2013.

Blaney K, Howard P. *Basic and Applied Concepts of Blood Banking and Transfusion Practices*. 3rd ed. Philadelphia, PA: Elsevier Health Sciences; 2013.

Carson J, Carless P, Hebert P. Transfusion thresholds and other strategies for guiding allogeneic red blood cell transfusion. *Cochrane Database Syst Rev*. 2012;4:CD002042.

Carson J, Grossman B, Kleinman S, et al. Red blood cell transfusion: a clinical practice guideline from the AABB. *Ann Intern Med*. 2012;157:49–58.

Carless P, Henry D, Carson J, Hebert P, McClelland B, Ker K. Transfusion thresholds and other strategies for guiding allogeneic red blood cell transfusion. *Cochrane Database Syst Rev*. 2010;CD002042.

Dreger V, Tremback T. Blood and blood product use in perioperative patient care. *AORN J*. 1998;67(1):154–156, 158, 160, passim; quiz 193–196.

Hillyer C, Silberstein L, Ness P, Anderson K, Roback J. *Blood Banking and Transfusion Medicine: Basic Principles and Practice*. 2nd ed. Philadelphia, PA: Churchill Livingstone; 2007.

Miller R, Eriksson L, Fleisher L, Wiener-Kronish J, Cohen N, Young W, eds. *Miller's Anesthesia*. 8th ed. Philadelphia, PA: Elsevier; 2015.

Practice guidelines for blood component therapy: a report by the American Society of Anesthesiologists Task Force on Blood Component Therapy. *Anesthesiology*. 1996;84:732–747.

Prout J, Jones T, Martin D. *Advanced Training in Anaesthesia*. Oxford, UK: Oxford University Press; 2014.

Porter R, Kaplan J. The Merck Manual: Professional Edition v1.0 website. http://www.merckmanuals.com/Professional. Retrieved October 3, 2014.

The 2009 national blood collection and utilization survey report. US Department of Health and Human Services website. https://wayback.archive-it.org/3919/20140402175927/http:/www.hhs.gov/ash/bloodsafety/2009nbcus.pdf. Accessed April 9, 2015.

Vacanti C, Segal S, Sikka P, Urman R. *Essential Clinical Anesthesia*. Cambridge, UK: Cambridge University Press; 2011.

QUESTIONS

1. Which of the following blood components requires the highest number of donor units to achieve one normal adult aliquot for transfusion?
   A. PRBCs
   B. Platelets
   C. FFP
   D. Cryoprecipitate

2. Which of the following complications is NOT associated with massive blood transfusion?
   A. Acute lung injury
   B. Hypercalcemia
   C. Hypotension
   D. Circulatory overload
   E. Bacterial infection

3. Which of the following is FALSE when it come to describing one unit of packed red blood cells (pRBCs)?
   A. Packed RBCs are given to treat anemia and the associated complications of inadequate oxygen delivery.
   B. A unit of pRBCs has a volume of approximately 250–300 mL with an average hematocrit of 50%.
   C. Transfusion of one unit of pRBCs in a 70-kg adult increases the hemoglobin by 1.0 g/dL.
   D. Transfusion of one unit of pRBCs in a 70-kg adult increases the hematocrit by 3%.
   E. When pRBCs are administered, oxygen-carrying capacity is improved.

4. Which of the following is FALSE regarding thrombin formation in coagulation cascade?
   A. Prothrombin, also known as factor II, is the active precursor of thrombin.
   B. Thrombin serves to cleave fibrinogen, which forms fibrin monomers for clot formation.
   C. Thrombin formation is the key enzymatic step that regulates hemostasis.
   D. Thrombin activates formation of active conformations of factors V and VIII.
   E. Thrombin activates platelets.

5. Which statement best describes the action of a direct thrombin inhibitor?
   A. Direct thrombin inhibitors work by blocking formation of factors IX to IXa.
   B. Direct thrombin inhibitors function in the extrinsic pathway.
   C. Direct thrombin inhibitors inactivate circulating thrombin and thrombin bound to clot.
   D. Direct thrombin inhibitors work by inactivating factor IIIa.
   E. Direct thrombin inhibitors inactivate factor XIIa.

ANSWERS

1. B. Platelets, while generally resulting in an increase of serum platelet count by ~50,000, requires five to six donors to make the characteristic "5" or "6" pack normally used in transfusion practice. In essence, the recipient is being exposed to five donors in order to receive the

pack of platelets. By contrast, PRBCs, FFP and cryoprecipitate each come from one donor per unit transfused.

2. B. Acute lung injury (TRALI) occurs in 1:5,000 units of transfused RBCs and is a well-known complication of RBC transfusion. Hypercalcemia is not seen with blood product administration, but hypocalcemia may result from citrate toxicity, resulting in hypotension (answer C). This may be treated by administering calcium chloride. Circulatory overload (TACO) may occur with transfusion, especially in patients with limited cardiac function. Bacterial infection, while uncommon, may occur from transfusion of contaminated blood products.
3. B. Packed RBCs have the same amount of hemoglobin as whole blood, but the hematocrit is higher at 70% compared with 40% for whole blood. Patients who are stable and are not actively bleeding should have hemoglobin increased by 1g/dL and by 3% for hematocrit. Oxygen delivery to the tissues is dependent on the following: cardiac output (CO), regional blood flow, and oxygen-carrying capacity, also known as the oxygen content of blood (CaO_2), thus by transfusing pRBCs the hemoglobin is increased, which will thereby increase the oxygen-carrying capacity. This ultimately serves to avoid tissue hypoxia when blood cells are functioning appropriately.

FURTHER READING

Carabini L, Ramsey G. Hemostasis and transfusion medicine. In: Barash P et al. *Clinical Anesthesia*. 7th ed. Philadelphia, PA: Lippincott Williams & Wilkins; 2013:419–421.

4. A. The intrinsic and extrinsic pathways culminate in the common pathway for coagulation cascade, and this is where thrombin is formed. A prothrombinase complex comprises the Xa activating factor II (prothrombin) into factor IIa (thrombin). Thrombin then cleaves fibrinogen into fibrin monomers, which ultimately form in to cross-linked fibrin; additionally, factors V, VIII, and XI are activated, thereby initiating both arms of the coagulation cascade via positive feedback. Thrombin generation is the key step in regulating coagulation homeostasis. Prothrombin is inactive until converted into thrombin.

SUGGESTED READING

Slaughter T. Coagulation. In: Miller R et al., eds. *Miller's Anesthesia*. 7th ed. Philadelphia, PA: Churchill Livingston Elsevier; 2010:1769–1770.

5. C. The term *thrombin* is synonymous with *factor II*, which allows the reader to isolate the factor numerals likely involved in the answer. See Figure 28.1 for a review of the intrinsic and extrinsic pathways. Thrombin is part of the common pathway. Factor IIIa is not part of the coagulation cascade. Factor XIIa is part of the intrinsic pathway. C is the correct answer.

SUGGESTED READING

Slaughter T. Coagulation. In: Miller R et al., eds. *Miller's Anesthesia*. 7th ed. Philadelphia, PA: Churchill Livingston Elsevier; 2010:1769–1770.

29.

THE ENDOCRINE SYSTEM

Heather McFarland

The endocrine system plays a vital role in managing and maintaining homeostasis. It is vital in production, storage, and use of energy as well as development and growth. The feedback loops and regulatory mechanisms help to promote balance in the endocrine organs. This system of organs, hormones, and mechanisms all work together to maintain stability throughout the body upon exposure to stressors.

HYPOTHALAMUS

The hypothalamus and pituitary function together as regulatory bodies for the endocrine system and its various hormones. The hypothalamus sits near the corpus callosum and regulates the pituitary through hormones such as thyrotropin-releasing hormone (TRH), growth-hormone-releasing hormone (GHRH), prolactin-releasing hormone (PRH), gonadotropin-releasing hormone (GRH), and corticotropin-releasing hormone (CRH). Control of the hypothalamus secretion is complex and occurs from neuronal and chemical influences.[1]

PITUITARY

The pituitary gland sits in the sella turica below the base of the brain. There are two main lobes of the pituitary, each with a distinct role. The anterior pituitary, or the adenohypophysis, produces and secretes numerous hormones: prolactin, growth hormone (GH), luteinizing hormone (LH), follicle-stimulating hormone (FSH), thyroid-stimulating hormone (TSH), melanocyte-stimulating hormone (MSH), and adrenocorticotrophic hormone (ACTH). The posterior lobe, or the neurohypophysis, stores and secretes just two hormones: vasopressin (ADH) and oxytocin. These hormones are both produced in the hypothalamus and transported for storage and secretion upon triggering in the posterior lobe of the pituitary gland. The main function of ADH is to maintain extracellular fluid volume and plasma osmolality, whereas oxytocin functions to elicit contractions of the uterus and trigger mammary (breast milk) secretion.[1]

THYROID

The thyroid gland is a bilobar gland joined by an isthmus consisting of two main cell types, follicular and parafollicular cells. The gland sits anterior to the trachea, and the isthmus is located just below the cricoid cartilage. A pair of parathyroid glands is located posteriorly to each lobe. The thyroid gland is innervated by both the adrenergic and cholinergic nervous systems. Actions of thyroid hormones are influential in regulating cellular metabolism throughout the body. The thyroid contains about 90% of total the total iodine in the body.[2]

The primary source of iodine is exogenous, which is then reduced to iodide in the gastrointestinal (GI) tract and absorbed into the bloodstream. From the bloodstream, iodide trapping occurs; this means the iodide is actively transported to the follicular cells, where it is converted to the oxidized form and combined with tyrosine residues, making monoiodotyrosine and diiodotyrosine. These then combine by thyroid peroxidase to T3 (*tri*iodothyronone) and T4 (thyroxine), and they are then stored in the gland until needed (mnemonic: "*tri*" for T'3'). Regulation and release of these hormones is controlled by the hypothalamus, pituitary, and thyroid in a feedback system. Thyrotropin-releasing hormone is released by the hypothalamus triggering a release of TSH from the anterior pituitary. This then triggers the thyroid gland to produce and release T3 and T4. There is a negative feedback loop produced from excess T4 on the hypothalamus and pituitary glands. As T3 and T4 are released, they bind to three major proteins: thyroxine-binding globulin, prealbumin, and albumin.[2] The half-life of circulating T4 is approximately 6–7 days, whereas the half life of T3 is 24–30 hours.[1]

Triiodothyronone is the active form, which is formed from deiodination of T4.

PARATHYROID

The parathyroid consists of four glandular-type tissues that sit posteriorly to the thyroid gland. There are two types of cells in the parathyroid gland, oxyphil cells and chief cells. There is no known function for oxyphil cells. Chief cells produce parathyroid hormone (PTH), which is regulated by serum-ionized Ca^{2+} concentration. There are numerous other influences on PTH secretion, which include phosphate, magnesium, and catecholamine levels. The effects of PTH on Ca^{2+} regulation take place through bone resorption, renal Ca^{2+} resorption, and indirectly through 1,25-dihydroxyvitamin D.

ADRENAL

Sitting atop the kidneys are the adrenal glands. There are two main regions of the glands—the medulla and the cortex (Figure 29.1). The medulla constitutes a smaller portion of the adrenals than the cortex. The medulla is derived embryologically and is a specialized portion of the sympathetic nervous system (think of the medulla as being from the "medulla" of the brain; it is an extension of the nervous system) (Figure 29.2). It produces and secretes epinephrine and norepinephrine. These catecholamines are stored in the chromaffin cells and released upon sympathetic nervous system activation. The cortex makes up the majority of the mass of the adrenals. It is responsible for producing and secreting three hormones. The precursor to these hormones is endogenous and dietary cholesterol. The three hormones include glucocorticoids, mineralocorticoids, and androgens, which are essential in regulating a prolonged response to stress and are produced in different zones of the cortex. The zona glomerulosa produces mineralocorticoids, the zona fasciculata produces glucocorticoids, and the zona reticularis produces glucocorticoids and androgens.

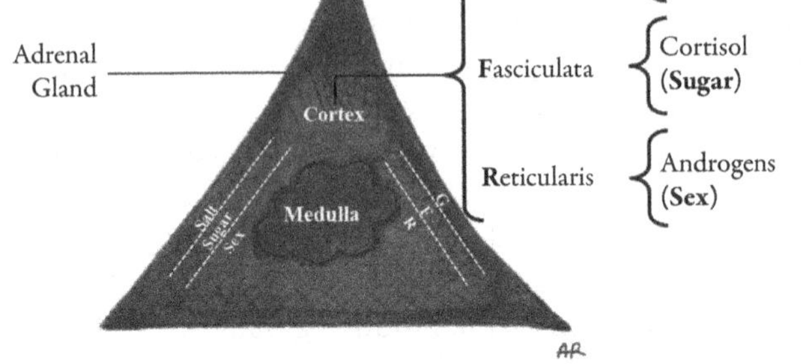

Figure 29.1 Adrenal gland.

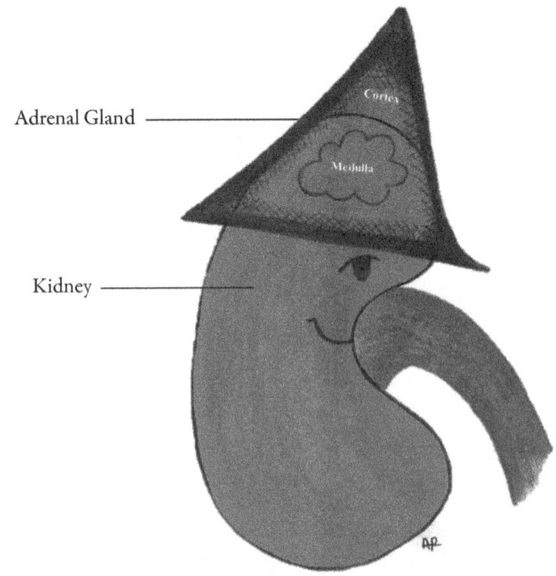

Figure 29.2 Adrenal gland "mnemonic" image reflecting functions of the cortex and medulla.

GLUCOCORTICOIDS

Cortisol is produced in the cortex under the feedback loop of ACTH released from the pituitary, which is under direction of CRH secreted from the hypothalamus. Cortisol has numerous effects on carbohydrate, protein, and fatty acid metabolism as well as mitigating the inflammatory process and bone formation. Glucocorticoids affect carbohydrate metabolism by enhancing gluconeogenesis, elevating blood glucose, and promoting hepatic glycogen synthesis.[1] They affect protein metabolism by degradation of muscle tissue and a negative nitrogen balance. The anti-inflammatory process is mitigated by stabilizing lysosomes, reducing the leukocyte response to local inflammation, and enhancing capillary integrity. The daily production of endogenous cortisol is approximately 20 mg, but can increase in stress responses up to 150–300 mg.[1] The feedback loop producing endogenous cortisol is influenced by the sleep-wake cycle, stress, and high glucocorticoid levels.

MINERALOCORTICOIDS

Aldosterone is produced in the cortex in the zona glomerulosa. It is regulated by the renin-angiotensin system and in turn is responsible for regulating fluid status as well as potassium levels. The juxtaglomerular apparatus is triggered to produced renin when it senses low perfusion pressure and vasoconstriction. The renin then converts angiotensin to angiotensin I, which is then converted to angiotensin II in the lungs by angiotensin-converting enzyme (ACE). Angiontensin II triggers the cortex to produce aldosterone. Aldosterone then acts on the kidneys to conserve sodium at the expense of excreting potassium; consequently the body retains fluid secondary to the increased serum sodium level.

ANDROGENS

Dehydroepiandrosterone (DHEA) and androstenedione are the androgens produced by the adrenals. In men, the testes produce testosterone, making the contribution from the adrenals insignificant. In women, the adrenals are the only contributing gland to androgen production, and malfunction with production can lead to masculinization in females.

PANCREAS

The pancreas sits posterior to the stomach in the periotoneum. It serves both an endocrine and exocrine purpose. The exocrine role is served mostly in the GI system where digestive enzymes are produced to break down carbohydrates, proteins, and fats. The endocrine role is to regulate plasma glucose levels. There are three types of cells that make up the pancreas: alpha, beta, and delta cells. Alpha cells produce glucagon, which promotes glycogenolysis, gluconeogenesis, ketogenesis, and increased cAMP levels. Beta cells produce insulin, which decreases plasma glucose by promoting glucose oxidation and glycogen formation. It inhibits lipolysis, increases protein synthesis in muscles, and decreases cAMP. Delta cells produce somatostatin, which in turn causes parietal cells to decrease secretion of gastric acid and decrease gastric emptying. Its net effect is to impede digestion by inhibiting production of gastrin, cholecystokinin, motlin, and histamine.

METABOLISM

Energy can neither be created nor destroyed according to the laws of thermodynamics. The human body must rely on chemical reactions within its own systems to release the energy needed to power the body; this is called metabolism. There are two main categories of metabolism. *Catabolism* is a breaking down and release of energy, and *anabolism* is when energy is used to build up the body. There are three sources that provide the fuel to convert into energy: carbohydrates, proteins, and lipids. The energy provided by these fuels is measured in kilocalories per gram. The basic metabolic rate (BMR) is the amount of energy the body expends at rest and provides sufficient energy for organ function. There are various formulas for calculating BMR, with the most common being the Harris-Benedict equation.

$$\text{For men: BMR} = 66 + (13.7 \times \text{wt in kg}) + (5 \times \text{ht in cm}) - (6.76 \times \text{age in years})$$

$$\text{For women: BMR} = 655 + (9.6 \times \text{wt in kg}) + (1.8 \times \text{ht in cm}) - (4.7 \times \text{age in years})$$

Direct and indirect calorimetry are alternative means to measure BMR. The basic metabolic rate is increased in many situations, including sepsis, burns, stress, increased thyroid activity, increased lean body mass, and fever.

When discussing the conversion of carbohydrates, proteins, and fats into energy, the reactions not only produce ATP for energy but also produce water and carbon dioxide. The respiratory quotient (RQ) is the ratio of oxygen consumed (numerator) to carbon dioxide eliminated (denominator) in a steady state. This ratio is affected by the type of substrate used to produce energy. A carbohydrate-rich diet will have an RQ = 1, proteins = 0.82, and fats = 0.7. In times of homeostasis, the body RQ = 0.8 (meaning that there is normally more CO_2 produced than O_2 consumed). In contrast, with stress on the body, the breakdown will shift to protein and fat with an RQ = 0.6 to 0.7.

CARBOHYDRATES

Carbohydrates are divided into two groups: simple and complex. Simple carbohydrates are absorbed directly into the bloodstream, whereas complex carbohydrates are broken down by digestive enzymes prior to absorption. The regulator of this carbohydrate metabolism is the liver. Production or consumption of glucose from carbohydrates is influenced by many factors, including glucose concentration, insulin, catecholamines, and glucagon.[3] Production of glucose is inversely related to production of glycogen, meaning in the anabolic state glucose is stored as glycogen and in a catabolic state glycogen is turned to glucose and is released into the bloodstream. In the catabolic state glucose can be produced through glycogenolysis; if glycogen stores are depleted gluconeogenesis is used to produce glucose. Gluconeogenesis is dependent on lactate, fatty acids, and amino acids and is mediated through glucagon, catecholamines, and insulin. Glucagon is a hormone excreted by the pancreas and is released during hypoglycemia or as a response to stress via epinephrine (as a result, sometimes glucagon is used to treat hypoglycemia instead of using dextrose). It works by cyclic adenosine monophosphate (cAMP) to promote gluconeogenesis, glycogenolysis, and lypolysis. In contrast, insulin is an *anabolic* hormone secreted by the pancreas. It promotes absorption of glucose into tissues from the bloodstream, where it can be stored for energy through glycogen and fatty acid synthesis.

REFERENCES

1. Schwartz J, Rosenbaum S. Anesthesia and the endocrine system. In: Barash P, Cullen B, Stoelting R. *Clinical Anesthesia*. 5th ed. Philadelphia, PA: Lippincott Williams & Wilkins; 2006.
2. Hines R, Marschall K. *Stoelting's Anesthesia and Co-Existing Disease*. 5th ed. Philadelphia, PA: Saunders; 2008.
3. Mushlin P, Gelman S. Hepatic physiology and pathophysiology. In: Miller R. *Miller's Anesthesia*. 7th ed. Philadelphia, PA: Elsevier; 2010:420.

FURTHER READING

Hyman S, Furman W. Nutritional and gastrointestinal disease. In: Miller R, Pardo M. *Basics of Anesthesia*. 6th ed. Philadelphia, PA: Elsevier; 2011.

QUESTIONS

1. Methods used to measure basal metabolic rate in a septic patient include:
   A. Urine catecholamines
   B. Indirect calorimetry
   C. Harris-Benedict equation
   D. Caloric spirometry
   E. Cellular intropy

2. All of the following characteristics describe the functions of glucagon EXCEPT:
   A. Glycogenolysis
   B. Gluconeogenesis
   C. Part of the stress response
   D. Produced by alpha cells

3. Which of the following diets would MOST increase carbon dioxide production?
   A. High fat
   B. High protein
   C. High elemental ion
   D. High carbohydrate

4. Which of the following factors most effects serum cortisol?
   A. Aldosterone
   B. Sleep-wake cycle
   C. Hypoandrogenism
   D. Cyclic adenosine monophosphate

5. Which of the following hormones provides negative feedback to the hypothalamus in order to regulate the secretion of thyroid-stimulating hormone (TSH)?
   A. Thyroxine
   B. Triiodothyronone
   C. Thyrotropin-releasing hormone
   D. Diiodotyrosine

ANSWERS

1. B. Indirect calorimetry directly measures metabolic demand and is commonly used in the critical care setting in order to determine oxygen consumption and carbon dioxide production (recall, this is used in the alveolar gas equation as well). The Harris-Benedict equation is used to provide an estimation of basal metabolic rate, however it can yield erroneous results in the setting of physiologic perturbations, such as sepsis, trauma, and so forth. Urine catecholamines may be used to assess for a pheochromocystoma or other adrenergic tumor, but is not useful for measuring basal metabolic rate. Options E and D are fictional and therefore distractors.
2. C. Glucagon is a pancreatic hormone that responds to epinephrine secretion (as part of the stress response), leading to an increase in glucose levels. As such, glucagon can be used instead of dextrose in the treatment of hypoglycemia. Glycogenolysis liberates glucose from its polysaccharide structure. Gluconeogenesis is the formation of glucose. Alpha cells produce glucagon, whereas beta cells produce insulin.
3. D. A high-carbohydrate diet results in the highest amount of CO_2 production per O_2 consumption. A carbohydrate-rich diet will have a RQ = 1, proteins = 0.82, and fats = 0.7. In times of homeostasis, the body RQ = 0.8. Increased CO_2 production can result in increased work of breathing and, therefore, increased rates of prolonged respiratory failure.
4. B. The sleep-wake cycle (thereby directly affecting ACTH) can affect cortisol levels. Aldosterone is a mineralocorticoid and is not related to glucocorticoid regulation. Hypoandrogenism refers to the levels of sex hormones. Cyclic adenosine monophosphate is a second messenger that is important in several biologic signals and processes. It is not specific to cortisol regulation.
5. A. "Tri"iodothyronone is the technical term for T3, and thyroxine is the technical name for T4. T4 provides feedback to the hypothalamus in order to regulate TSH secretion. Iodide trapping occurs from the bloodstream and is converted to the oxidized form and combined with tyrosine residues, making monoiodotyrosine and diiodotyrosine (chemical precursors, in effect). These then combine by thyroid peroxidase to make T3 and T4.

30.

NEUROMUSCULAR DISEASES AND DISORDERS

Ranu R. Jain

INTRODUCTION

The term *neuromuscular disorder* is broad and includes different syndromes and diseases that affect the function of the skeletal muscles, which may not be acquired or genetically determined. Diseases of the motor neurons are common in children. These diseases can have an effect at the level of the central nervous system (CNS), peripheral nerves, neuromuscular junction, or muscle fiber and may be associated with systemic problems and as a result have abnormal responses to the anesthetic agents.

MUSCULAR DYSTROPHY

The term *muscular dystrophy* refers to a group of genetic disorders causing progressive degeneration of skeletal muscle without any abnormality of the motor neuron.

DUCHENNE'S MUSCULAR DYSTROPHY

Duchenne's muscular dystrophy (DMD) is an X-linked recessive condition affecting 1 in 3500 male births. The onset of symptoms is usually around the age of 4 years, with delayed motor milestones, proximal muscle weakness, and Gower's sign. Pseudohypertrophy of the calves is common. During the teenage years, immobility is followed by development of skeletal deformities such as scoliosis. Patients with DMD frequently have delayed gastric emptying, which may predispose them to regurgitation and aspiration. Respiratory failure is common due to intercostal muscle weakness and scoliosis. Cardiomyopathy is also common.

Patients with DMD may require anesthesia for treatment of scoliosis or relief of contractures. The preoperative assessment should include thorough evaluation of cardiac and respiratory function.

The main concerns during anesthesia are the use of muscle relaxants and postoperative respiratory dysfunction. There are reports of cardiac arrest in patients with DMD undergoing anesthesia without any preexisting cardiac disease. The cardiac arrest is frequently due to hyperkalemia due to rhabdomyolysis. The use of succinylcholine and other malignant-hyperthermia-triggering agents, including inhaled agents such as halothane, should be avoided in patients with DMD. There is increased sensitivity to nondepolarizing agents.

BECKER MUSCULAR DYSTROPHY

Becker muscular dystrophy (BMD) is caused by a mutation in the dystrophin gene, the same gene that causes DMD and codes for the production of dystrophin, located on the X-chromosome. Becker muscular dystrophy occurs in about 1/18,450 live male births.

The clinical picture is similar to DMD. The symptoms appear late, and the progression is slow. Patients with BMD manufacture less than normal amounts of dystrophin protein that is smaller in size. Patients have enlarged calf muscles and waddling gait.

MYOTONIC DYSTROPHY

Myotonic dystrophy is an autosomal dominant disorder with an incidence of approximately 1:8000 and a male predominance. It is due to abnormal expansions of repeated areas of genes. There are two forms of myotonic dystrophy: Type I (98% of cases, with an onset in late adulthood) and Type II (2% of cases). Myotonic dystrophy is characterized by cardiac conduction defects, progressive muscle weakness, and delayed muscle relaxation. Association between myotonic dystrophy and malignant hyperthermia has been suggested but not confirmed.

Succinylcholine can cause a prolonged contracture and cardiac arrest from hyperkalemia, and nondepolarizing neuromuscular blocking agents have been used in reduced doses for patients with myotonic dystrophy. Regional anesthesia is the preferred technique for these patients.

Hypothermia and shivering may precipitate a myotonic crisis. Additionally, there may be worsening of symptoms in obstetric patients with increased chances of failure of uterine contraction that may lead to premature labor and postpartum hemorrhage.

SPINAL MUSCULAR ATROPHY

Spinal muscular atrophy (SMA) is among the most typical types of neurological diseases. Spinal muscular atrophy is characterized by degeneration of motor neurons, resulting in progressive muscle atrophy or wasting and weakness. Is an inherited condition and it does not affect the sensory nerves or the intellectual capacity of the patient. Spinal muscular atrophy affects about 1/6,000 to 1/10,000 people. The disease is in more than 95% of cases caused by a homozygous deletion in the survival motor neuron gene 1 (SMN1)

SMA Type 1—infantile SMA, or Werdnig-Hoffmann disease. Onset of symptoms occurs before 6 months of age. It is associated with severe neurological disease.

SMA Type 2—these patients are less symptomatic during early infancy, but the symptoms become more severe around the age of 2 to 3 years, with onset occurring between 6 and 18 months.

SMA Type 3—this is the least severe, with late onset of neurological symptoms around the age of 17 to 18 years. The patients have muscular weakness of the shoulders and legs. The loss of full-length functioning SMN protein leads to a degeneration of anterior spinal motor neurons, which causes muscle weakness.

Anesthetic risks for SMA patients include the following:

Airway: Tracheal intubation can be difficult.

Respiration: Infants with SMA I almost always need postoperative respiratory support. Patients with SMA II sometimes need support, while SMA III patients seldom need support. Opioids should be titrated carefully.

Circulation: Circulatory problems during anesthesia are rare.

Anesthetic drugs—Neuromuscular blockers: Patients with SMA may display increased sensitivity to and prolonged effect of nondepolarizing neuromuscular blockers. Intubation without muscle relaxation should be considered, and succinylcholine should be avoided.

Anesthetic techniques: All types of anesthetic technique have been used. Although none is absolutely contraindicated, none is perfect: anesthesia must be individualized.

The perioperative risks can be considerable and are mainly related to the respiratory system, from respiratory failure to difficult/impossible intubation. Perioperative care can be provided for children with SMA safely and effectively with total intravenous or inhaled anesthetics along with the judicious use of opioids to improve patient comfort without increased morbidity.

MULTIPLE SCLEROSIS

Multiple sclerosis (MS) is a demyelinating disease of the CNS with sparing of the peripheral nerves. The symptoms may last for a few days or for weeks, followed by remission. The most common manifestations of the disease include optic neuritis, gait disturbances, limb paresthesias, urinary incontinence, muscle rigidity, autonomic dysfunction, and restrictive lung disease due to kyphoscoliosis. Treatment with the corticosteroids may shorten the duration or severity of MS attacks. There is no definitive cure for MS, and patients with MS may present for any type of surgery. The preoperative assessment should include a detailed examination and documentation of neurological impairment. Premedication with diazepam may be beneficial as it relieves spasticity. Hyperkalemia may manifest with succinylcholine due to an increased number of extrajunctional acetylcholine receptors in wheelchair-bound patients and should be avoided. The response to nondepolarizing muscle relaxants can be variable, as patients with MS can be sensitive or resistant.

The use of neuraxial anesthesia in patients with MS is controversial, though epidural anesthesia and regional nerve blocks appear to be safe. Lumbar puncture has not been shown to be harmful in MS. Postoperative exacerbations of MS have been attributed to spinal anesthesia, most likely due to the neurotoxicity of the local anesthetic. An epidural anesthetic can be a combination of local anesthetic and opioids in order to reduce the concentration of local anesthetic. The duration of epidural infusions should be limited to minimize exposure of the nerve roots to local anesthetic. The intraoperative monitoring required will depend on the nature/extent of the surgery and the comorbidities of the patient. Patients with autonomic dysfunction may require invasive hemodynamic monitoring. Neuromuscular function should be closely monitored. Postoperative decline in neurologic functions has been reported in patients with MS. Finally, as platelet aggregation is increased in MS, thromboembolic precautions should be taken to reduce the risk of deep vein thrombosis.

AMYOTROPHIC LATERAL SCLEROSIS

Amyotrophic lateral sclerosis (ALS, Lou Gehrig's disease) is the most common adult motor neuron disease, with an annual incidence in the United States of 1–2:100,000, with a lifetime risk of approximately 1:2000. Approximately 5% to 10% of ALS cases are genetically determined; the remainder can be sporadic in origin. The onset of disease in ALS is between the fourth and seventh decades of life. It is a neurodegenerative disorder of the motor neurons, causing progressive weakness and muscular atrophy leading to paralysis. While ALS is not accompanied by cognitive impairment or sensory loss, dementia and sensory abnormalities may manifest. Respiratory failure may lead to death within a few years of diagnosis. Motor neuron loss occurs in the ventral horns of the spinal cord, the motor cortex, and most brain stem motor nuclei. Upper motor neuron findings include clonus and hyperreflexia; lower motor neuron signs include atrophy, weakness, and fasciculations. Amyotrophic lateral sclerosis is often confused with postpoliomyelitis syndrome, multifocal motor neuropathy with or without conduction block, endocrinopathies (especially hyperparathyroid or hyperthyroid states), lead intoxication, infections, and paraneoplastic syndromes.

MYASTHENIA GRAVIS

Myasthenia gravis (MG) is an autoimmune disease with an annual incidence of 0.25–2:100,000, with a substantially increased age-related frequency in those over 60 years of age. There are antibodies to the receptors of nicotinic acetylcholine receptors at the neuromuscular junction. Commonly, presentation is *weakness with exertion.* The weakness can affect ocular and bulbar muscles or respiratory function or may be generalized muscle weakness, which may lead to aspiration and respiratory failure. Up to 10% of patients with MG may have other autoimmune diseases like hypothyroidism, rheumatoid arthritis, systemic lupus erythematosus (SLE), and anemias, which may complicate their clinical manifestation and treatment.

Osserman and Genkins have classified MG as follows:

Class I—ocular myasthenia only, with ptosis and diplopia

Class IIA—generalized moderate weakness

Class IIB—generalized moderate weakness and/or bulbar dysfunction

Class III—acute fulminating presentation and/or respiratory dysfunction

Class IV—late severe generalized

The treatment of MG has three principles: (1) Enhance neuromuscular transmission with cholinesterase inhibitors and decrease the circulating antibodies by using plasmapheresis; (2) Use immunosuppressive therapy with either corticosteroids or azathioprine; (3) Use four to eight plasma exchanges over 1 to 2 weeks. The reduced plasma esterases diminish the metabolism of drugs such as succinylcholine, mivacurium, and remifentanil. Patients with MG may commonly present for a variety of surgeries, including obstetric procedures and, most commonly, thymectomy. Thymectomy may induce remission of the disease. A large thymoma may cause tracheal compression; therefore, the flow volume loops and chest/neck CT scan should be done in the preoperative period. Patients with MG may have cardiac conduction abnormalities, so cardiac assessment is also indicated in the preoperative period. The respiratory and bulbar function of the patient should be evaluated in the preop period. There should be no evidence of upper or lower respiratory tract infection, in order to reduce the risk of perioperative infection. Premedication of myasthenic patients with sedative drugs is not advised because of the potential for respiratory decompensation. For intraoperative management, all of the common intravenous agents (propofol, thiopental, or etomidate) are used for induction; maintenance is commonly achieved with either an intravenous agent or a volatile agent.

The use of neuromuscular blocking agents in patients with MG requires a thorough understanding of their different effects. Patients with MG have been shown to be relatively more resistant to succinylcholine than controls, with an ED95 of 2.6 times the normal. This is attributed to functional blockade of the acetylcholine receptors by antibodies, requiring higher doses of succinylcholine to overcome the blockade.

The reduced number of acetylcholine receptors at the neuromuscular junction makes patients with MG exquisitely sensitive to nondepolarizing neuromuscular blocking. Drugs that may accentuate the weakness in patients with MG include magnesium sulfate, aminoglycosides, vancomycin, quinidine, procainamide, narcotics, furosemide, dantrolene, beta blockers, and calcium channel blockers. Excessive doses of reversal agents may precipitate a cholinergic crisis, characterized by muscle weakness, bradycardia, increased secretions, and gut motility. Regional anesthesia should be used in these patients, and the doses of local anesthetics (especially esters) should be reduced in patients receiving anticholinesterase drugs. Even the use of high doses of amide local anesthetics can exacerbate symptoms. Neuraxial anesthesia should be carried out with care to avoid a high level of blockade and subsequent muscular weakness.

The course of MG during pregnancy is variable, although postpartum exacerbations are common. Regional anesthesia is ideal for analgesia during labor, but with attention paid to the level of block and avoidance of ester-type local anesthetics such as chloroprocaine. Preterm labor is more common in patients with MG. Magnesium sulfate given for preeclampsia may exacerbate weakness in MG. The antibody to the acetylcholine receptor crosses the placenta, and the newborn infant may develop neonatal MG, which usually resolves within a few weeks. The two main postoperative issues are the need for mechanical ventilation and the treatment of pain. Postoperative pain may be difficult to manage because of an apparent sensitivity of these patients to respiratory depressive side effects of narcotics and sedatives. The use of regional anesthesia for postoperative pain relief has been described, with patients experiencing no increase in respiratory depression and improved postoperative forced vital capacity.

EATON-LAMBERT SYNDROME

Eaton-Lambert syndrome (ELS) is a rare disorder due to defective release of acetylcholine at the presynaptic terminal. The disease presents with muscle weakness and hyporeflexia; ocular or bulbar muscles are rarely affected. Muscle strength improves with activity; autonomic dysfunction symptoms like dry mouth, dry skin, orthostatic hypotension, and bladder and bowel dysfunction are also manifested; these symptoms most often affect older males. An association between small-cell lung carcinoma and ELS is also reported. Nerve weakness is not improved by anticholinesterase but can be treated with 3,4-diaminopyridine, which increases transmitter release. These patients are sensitive to both depolarizing and nondepolarizing neuromuscular agents.

GUILLAIN-BARRÉ SYNDROME

Guillain-Barré syndrome (GBS) is an acute inflammatory demyelinating polyradiculopathy that is the most common cause of acute neuromuscular weakness. Frequently, there is a history of preceding infection of the upper respiratory or gastrointestinal tract. The classic clinical presentation is ascending symmetrical motor weakness, which plateaus within 28 days. Patients may also experience autonomic dysfunction and muscle pain. Diagnosis is by exclusion of other causes of weakness (such as MG) and nerve conduction studies, which reveal findings consistent with demyelination and superimposed axonal degeneration.

The treatment of GBS is mainly supportive, although plasmapheresis has been shown to be effective.

Intravenous immunoglobulin is also frequently administered; this may be superior to plasmapheresis, although the relapse rate is higher. Low concentrations of local anesthetics may be administered via epidural or peripheral nerve catheters to decrease pain without altering muscle strength. If the intercostal muscles are affected, the patient may require intubation if there is significant tachypnea, decrease in vital capacity < 15mL/kg, and hypoxemia. Patients may exhibit abnormal responses to neuromuscular blockers. The up-regulation of acetylcholine receptors leads to proliferation of extrajunctional receptors and a hyperkalemic response to succinylcholine, which has been reported to occur even after clinical resolution of symptoms. Resistance to nondepolarizing drugs has also been demonstrated, although in this case the patient subsequently developed an increased sensitivity to vecuronium. The course of the disease is self-limiting, with an excellent prognosis.

MALIGNANT HYPERTHERMIA

Malignant hyperthermia (MH) is inherited as an autosomal dominant trait with an unknown exact incidence, though studies reveal that MH may complicate 1:100,000 surgeries in adults and about 1:30,000 in children. The incidence depends on the concentration of MH families in a given geographic area. High-incidence areas in the United States include Wisconsin, Nebraska, West Virginia, and Michigan. However, the prevalence of genetic change that predisposes to MH is much higher. Malignant hyperthermia results from the excessive release of calcium from the sarcoplasmic reticulum in skeletal muscle cells in response to a triggering anesthetic agent. This calcium influx into the cell cytoplasm leads to an increase in oxidative phosphorylation and subsequent prominent rise in the cellular metabolic rate. If there is any doubt about MH susceptibility, the patient should be managed by a nontriggering anesthetic technique. Malignant hyperthermia is characterized by a rapid increase in aerobic and anaerobic metabolism—the body temperature may exceed 43°C (109.4°F)—along with tachycardia, muscle rigidity, and increased muscle permeability to potassium, calcium, and sodium. In MH, excessive release of myoglobulin from the muscle results in myoglobinuria. Trismus or masseter muscle spasm that occurs during induction may be indicative of MH. Malignant hyperthermia may occur in patients without a known muscle disease, and there is increased risk of MH in patients with multiple congenital musculoskeletal abnormalities, isolated congenital hip dislocation, central core disease, and in patients with DMD or BMD.

The clinical picture of MH may be confused with postanesthetic rhabdomyolysis after muscular stress, toxic reaction to drugs, intra or postoperative thyroid storm, or neuroleptic malignant syndrome (in which block of central dopaminergic pathways is precipitated by psychoactive drugs like haloperidol and phenothiazines). Malignant hyperthermia episodes can be prevented in susceptible patients by using nontriggering anesthesia and avoiding succinylcholine and all the inhalational agents except nitrous oxide. Propofol, all narcotics, thiopental, and nondepolarizing muscle relaxants are considered safe to use in patients with MH.

If MH is diagnosed, the anesthesia team should call the MH Hotline: 1-800-644-9737 (or outside the United States: 001-209-417-3722). Dantrolene is the drug of choice for treating MH. It decreases calcium release from the sarcoplasmic reticulum without altering calcium reuptake. The current formulation of dantrolene is packaged as a lyophilized yellow powder in 20-mg vials, with 3 g mannitol and enough base to maintain pH at 9.5 (this makes it more soluble in water for administration). Because of these physical properties, warming water also speeds dissolution. Once dissolved, the solution turns an orange color. Because datrolene is highly alkaline, it should be injected into large vein when given. The acute episode of MH is treated symptomatically. Intravenous dantrolene (2 to 10 mg/kg every 5 minutes) and continuous monitoring of end-tidal carbon dioxide levels, blood oxygen saturation, and core body temperature are required. The patient should be actively cooled by cold isotonic saline for IV infusion and for gastric, peritoneal, or rectal irrigation. Urinary output should be maintained to flush the excess myoglobin through the renal system.

SPINA BIFIDA

Myelomeningocele (most severe), meningocele (mild form), and occluta (least severe) are the three most common forms of spina bifida. Spina bifida results in the improper closure or rupture of the neural tube during development, manifested as an open spine, muscle imbalance, spasticity, hip and knee fractures, and paraplegia. Intrauterine repair of the myelomeningocele is now offered to mothers with significantly reduced morbidity for the fetus when successful.

SPINAL CORD INJURY

The spinal cord injury can be divided into the acute phase and chronic states. The cervical cord is often associated with head injury, with altered consciousness requiring tracheal intubation. These patients may require fiber-optic intubation, in order to minimize distraction of the cervical spine. Respiratory insufficiency may also ensue, since intercostal muscle paralysis can decrease alveolar ventilation by up to 60%. Pulmonary edema may occur due to the autonomic discharge causing hypertension and bradycardia; this is manifested as vasoconstriction and increased cardiac afterload, leading to left ventricular failure, leading to pulmonary edema. This is seen in up to 50% of cases of spinal cord injury.

In patients with lesions above T4, the sympathetic outflow is interrupted, with resulting vasodilation and bradycardia. As such, overly aggressive fluid resuscitation may further worsen pulmonary edema. Invasive hemodynamic monitoring may be needed if multiple associated traumatic injuries are noted. Respiratory and cardiovascular stability is essential for these patients, as hypotension and hypoxia may further worsen any spinal cord injury. These patients can become poikilothermic (adapting to their ambient temperature, like an insect or a pebble) below the level of the spinal cord injury—they are unable to maintain body temperature because of an interruption between peripheral temperature sensors and the hypothalamus, resulting in an inability to shiver and blocked peripheral vasoconstriction reflexes. Hyperkalemia resulting in cardiac arrest can manifest in patients following administration of succinylcholine, due to an increase in the number of postsynaptic receptors resulting from an up-regulation in response to decreased exposure to acetylcholine. The onset of this hyperkalemic response occurs within a week of injury, and possibly sooner. Although succinylcholine is considered safe to administer within the first 24 hours after injury, it is best to avoid after 48 hours of injury. This hypersensitivity has been reported up to 6 months after injury.

Autonomic hyperreflexia is also a challenge in paraplegic patients. There is massive reflex sympathetic discharge that occurs in patients with spinal cord lesions above the T4-T6 that is not seen in patients with spinal cord lesions below T10. Autonomic hyperreflexia is elicited by distention of a viscus or a surgical stimulus. Afferent impulses to the cord below the lesion cause a mass sympathetic response, resulting in vasoconstriction and hypertension. This is unique because the sympathetic activity resulting from pain, and so forth, is not opposed by the parasympathetic system. Most of the body's blood is restricted above the lesion, with associated hypertension and flushing (see Figure 20.1). In more technical terms, baroreceptor reflexes result in bradycardia and vasodilation above the lesion and the hypertensive response can result in cardiac ischemia, cerebral hemorrhage, and retinal hemorrhage. Either general or regional anesthesia can be used in these patients, but no technique is absolutely free of potential response by the patient. Autonomic hyperreflexia has even been described in patients undergoing extracorporeal shockwave lithotripsy for renal calculi, a common problem in patients with spinal cord injuries, despite the use of a spinal anesthetic, though an inadequate block may have been the culprit in these patients. Spinal or epidural opiates may also be administered to avoid the degree of sympathetic blockade associated with the use of local anesthetics. Although cord injury above T6 results in painless labor, the uterine contractions may precipitate autonomic hyperreflexia.

CRITICAL ILLNESS POLYNEUROPATHY

Neuromuscular dysfunction in intensive care unit patients with nonneurological illness is termed critical illness polyneuropathy (CIP). It is characterized by muscle weakness, difficulty in weaning from mechanical ventilation, and prolonged rehabilitation. There are other coexistent factors, such as prolonged use of neuromuscular blocking agents, electrolyte disorders, use of aminoglycoside antibiotics, and renal failure. The electrophysiological studies exhibit fibrillation potentials and positive sharp waves consistent with axonal polyneuropathy. Immobility also can lead to an up-regulation of acetylcholine receptors, and the administration of depolarizing neuromuscular blocking drugs can lead to hyperkalemia and cardiac arrest.

The treatment is supportive therapy.

MITOCHONDRIAL DISORDERS

Mitochondrial respiratory chain diseases frequently present to the neurologist with CNS and/or neuromuscular symptoms. Accurate diagnosis and management rely on a team approach including multidisciplinary clinical assessment, muscle histochemistry, mitochondrial respiratory chain enzymology, and genetics. Most adult-onset phenotypes are associated with mitochondrial DNA (mtDNA) mutations. Whole-genome mtDNA sequencing is increasingly available for clinical use. Recently, nuclear genes, especially POLG and MFN2, have been shown to be important in adult presentations of mitochondrial disorders. Curative therapy is available for only a small proportion of cases, but it is especially important not to miss primary coenzyme Q_{10} deficiency. Treatment of all the mitochondrial disorders is supportive and symptomatic. Coenzyme Q_{10}, creatine, carnitine, and vitamins are often used. Supportive therapy in a multidisciplinary environment is essential for all patients and families with genetic mitochondrial respiratory chain diseases.

ANESTHETIC PEARLS

PREOPERATIVE PLANNING

Neuromuscular diseases may be undiagnosed in pediatric patients, or the symptoms may not have been noticed, so a detailed history and exam is essential in this patient population.

ANESTHETIC CONCERNS

- In general a "stress free" anesthetic is beneficial due to limited respiratory and cardiovascular reserve of the myopathic patient. Patients may be extremely sensitive to the respiratory depressant effects of drugs. Surgery under regional anesthesia should be encouraged to avoid the adverse effects of general anesthesia and narcotics if possible.
- A thorough preoperative examination of the patients airway is recommended patient may be difficult to mask ventilate or intubate. If the patient is not cooperative then the anesthesiologist should have a back up planning to manage a difficult airway.
- Choice of anesthetic induction method, inhalation or intravenous, should be according to the individual patient concerns.
- Neuromuscular blockers have unpredictable effects. Succinylcholine may produce hyperkalemia leading to cardiac arrest. Nondepolarizing blockers may have unpredictably prolonged effects.
- Evans myopathy, King Denborough syndrome, and central core disease have been shown to have association with MH.

POSTOPERATIVE CONCERNS

Patients require close observation in the postoperative period due to the risk of gastrointestinal dysfunction, aspiration, and postoperative respiratory depression after general anesthesia.

In all pediatric anesthetics, especially when the patient has signs of a neuromuscular disorder, capnography and minute ventilation and core temperature should be documented. Serum electrolytes and urine myoglobin should be checked, as this would provide documentation that this myopathic individual has not suffered complications of anesthesia.

REFERENCES

1. Barash P, Cullen B, Stoelting R. *Clinical Anesthesia*. 5th ed. Philadelphia, PA: Lippincott Williams & Wilkins; 2006.
2. Davis P, Cladis F, Motoyama E. *Smith's Anesthesia for Infants and Children*. 8th ed. Philadelphia, PA: Mosby; 2011.
3. Cote C, Lerman J, Anderson B. *A Practice of Anesthesia for Infants and Children*. 5th ed. Philadelphia, PA: Elsevier Saunders; 2013:1053.
4. Hachenberg T, Schneemilch C. Anesthesia in neurologic and psychiatric diseases: is there a "best anesthesia" for certain diseases? *Curr Opin Anaesthesiol*. 2014;27(4):394–402.
5. McLeod M, Creighton R. Anesthesia for pediatric neurological and neuromuscular diseases. *J Child Neurol*. 1986;1:189.
6. Briggs E, Kirsch J. Anesthetic implications of neuromuscular disease. *J Anesth*. 2003;17(3):177–185.

QUESTIONS

1. Which of the following disorders is not associated with malignant hyperthermia?
   A. Central core disease
   B. King-Denborough syndrome
   C. Multi-mini core disease
   D. Eaton Lambert syndrome

2. Which of the following statements is true regarding the anesthetic management of a patient with muscular dystrophy (MD)?
   A. Succinylcholine should be avoided
   B. Administration of volatile anesthetics is contraindicated
   C. There is no risk of respiratory depression
   D. A larger dose of nondepolarizing muscle relaxants will be needed

3. All of the following describe the formulation of dantrolene available for clinical use EXCEPT:
    A. Highly acidic
    B. Contains mannitol
    C. Best mixed in cold water
    D. Rapidly dissolvable
    E. Turns yellow once dissolved

4. You are called to intubate a 16-year-old patient who presents with newly diagnosed myasthenia gravis (MG) and is admitted to the intensive care unit for respiratory support. Which of the following BEST describes the degree of the patient's disease according to the Osserman and Genkins classification?
    A. Class I
    B. Class IIA
    C. Class IIB
    D. Class III
    E. Class IV

ANSWERS

1. D. All of the remaining disorders have a demonstrated association with malignant hyperthermia. Eaton Lambert syndrome is characterized by a defective release of acetylcholine at the presynaptic terminal and does not have intrinsic muscle cell pathophysiology.

FURTHER READING

Barash P, Cullen B, Stoelting R. *Clinical Anesthesia*. 6th ed. Philadelphia, PA: Lippincott Williams & Wilkins; 2006: 600–601.

2. A. Succinylcholine is contraindicated in muscular dystrophy (MD) patients secondary to ectopic increase in extrajunctional nicotinic acetylcholine receptors, activation of which can cause potentially lethal hyperkalemia, muscle fiber swelling, and rhabdomyolysis. Volatile anesthetics are contraindicated in MD, as a lack of membrane stabilizing protein in combination with another destabilizing agent (volatile anesthetic) may also result in rhabdomyolysis and hyperkalemia. As a result, the anesthesia machine should be purged and a totally intravenous anesthetic (TIVA) planned. The respiratory depressant effects of all anesthetic drugs are enhanced in MD patients, and as such short-acting/rapidly metabolized drugs are more ideal. There have been case reports demonstrating increased sensitivity to nondepolarizing neuromuscular blocking agents in MD, and as such an increased dosing requirement would not be expected.

FURTHER READING

Barash P, Cullen B, Stoelting R. *Clinical Anesthesia*. 6th ed. Philadelphia, PA: Lippincott Williams & Wilkins; 2009:516.

3. A. Native dantrolene is quite insoluble in water, and the current formulation packaged has 3 g mannitol and enough base to maintain pH at 9.5 (more basic in order to maximize dissolution). Warming water speeds dissolution, but dantrolene is not rapidly dissolvable. Once dissolved, the solution turns orange and should be injected into a large vein.

FURTHER READING

Barash P, Cullen B, Stoelting R. *Clinical Anesthesia*. 6th ed. Philadelphia, PA: Lippincott Williams & Wilkins; 2009:606–607.

4. D. Osserman and Genkins have classified myasthenia gravis as follows:

    Class I—ocular myasthenia only, with ptosis and diplopia

    Class IIA—generalized moderate weakness

    Class IIB—generalized moderate weakness and/or bulbar dysfunction, no respiratory involvement

    Class III—acute fulminating presentation and/or respiratory dysfunction

    Class IV—late severe generalized

For an acute fulminating MG, aggressive therapy with plasma exchange and immunosuppressives would be more likely.

FURTHER READING

Barash P, Cullen B, Stoelting R. *Clinical Anesthesia*. 6th ed. Philadelphia, PA: Lippincott Williams & Wilkins; 2009:1064.

31.

SPECIAL PROBLEMS OR ISSUES IN ANESTHESIOLOGY

Cheryl Gore and Imelda Tjia

PHYSICIAN IMPAIRMENT OR DISABILITY

As physicians, we have a duty to our patients to provide great care. Part of providing great medical care is ensuring that we, as physicians, are in the best possible shape to provide that care. There are several things that can impair or cause disability in the physician, including substance abuse, fatigue, aging, and visual and auditory impairment. As physicians, it is important to recognize these problems and seek help before patients are harmed.

SUBSTANCE ABUSE

Substance abuse can range from medications prescribed to physicians, such as narcotics for pain relief, to over-the-counter substances such as alcohol, to taking drugs from the workplace such as fentanyl or propofol. The anesthesiologist has a ready supply of drugs, many of which have a very high abuse potential. Because of the ready availability of opiates and other drugs with abuse potential, anesthesia personnel find themselves at a higher risk of drug misuse. Among anesthesia personnel, opioid abuse remains the primary form of addiction, with fentanyl and sufentanil being the primary drugs abused. Other forms of addiction in the anesthesiologist, such as alcohol and street drugs, show a rate similar to that of the general population. Some data show that anesthesia physicians have a higher rate of abuse than others, but later studies showed rates very similar to other specialties. The theories behind the abuse are many and are not examined in depth in this chapter. It is worthwhile to mention that the causes include exposure theory, genetics of the physician, biochemical makeup of the physician, and psychiatric disorders.[1]

Recognition of the impaired physician can be difficult. Denial of the problem by the physician and by those surrounding the physician may make the diagnosis of impairment even more difficult. Bryson and Silverstein describe particular signs to look for[1]:

- Withdrawal from family, friends, and leisure activities
- Mood swings, with periods of depression alternating with periods of euphoria
- Increased episodes of anger, irritability, and hostility
- Spending more time at the hospital, even when off duty
- Volunteering for extra call
- Refusing relief for lunch or coffee breaks
- Requesting frequent bathroom breaks
- Signing out increasing amounts of narcotics or quantities inappropriate for the given case
- Weight loss and pale skin

Addicted physicians will go to extremes to feed their need for their drug of choice. Charting drugs not given, not giving opioids at all to patients, raiding the sharps box for leftover narcotics, and documenting large doses of opioids given to patients when only small amounts were given are only some of the ways the addicted physician maintains the habit.

It is the responsibility of each institution and/or individual that recognizes an impaired physician to report them to the appropriate agency, otherwise, those individuals may be penalized as well.

Which agency to report the impaired physician to depends on local, state, and federal regulations. Obviously the state medical board and the National Practitioner Data Base must be notified of any actions taken against an impaired physician. Criminal charges may also be brought against the physician for diversion of controlled substances by state, local, and federal authorities. The state medical board may decide to revoke or simply suspend the physician's license. Many states have rehabilitation programs designed to help the physician reenter the workforce. Each state deals differently with impaired physicians. The state of Texas has a Texas Physician Health Program. It provides a confidential program to serve physicians affected by substance use disorders, physical illnesses and impairment, and/or psychiatric conditions. Education based on the physician's specific needs is given, along with recognition and support in diagnosis and treatment.[2]

The American Board of Anesthesiology requires that each physician have an unrestricted license to practice medicine in at least one state. Their official statement regarding rehabilitation programs and board licensure is that as long as the medical board of that state allows the physician to practice, the ABA will allow the physician to practice.[1]

Once diagnosed, the impaired physician should start in therapy, which could include inpatient treatment, group therapy (such as Alcoholics Anonymous or Narcotics Anonymous), individual therapy, and when appropriate, admission into a halfway house. Naltrexone is a mu receptor antagonist and can be an adjunctive therapy in the impaired physician along with therapy. Naltrexone is known to reduce the cravings for alcohol and narcotics. Frequent monitoring of the physician with urine drug screens or blood drug samples keep the physician accountable for recovery.[1]

The recovery rate for physicians is excellent, with one study in the New Jersey PHP reporting 83.8% over a 9-year period.[3]

FATIGUE

The issue of fatigue is a very important topic. This issue is of definite significance during residency training. The Accreditation Council for Graduate Medical Education (ACGME), has set forth very specific guidelines for the amount of hours that a resident can be at work to reduce the issue of fatigue among residents. Part of the review that the ACGME performs is a Clinical Learning Environment Review (CLER), which includes duty hour oversight, fatigue management, and mitigation. This review looks at how the institution keeps track of duty hours, designs procedures to manage fatigue, and educates faculty members and residents in how to recognize the signs and symptoms of fatigue. Duty hours are currently limited to 80 hours per week but do not include time spent away from the institution in preparation for cases for the next day or reading for cases for the next day. Unfortunately, however, no such guidelines exist for practicing physicians after training. Fatigue can be a very real problem in the workplace for the physician. The signs of fatigue are physical as well as mental. The physician may experience a sense of listlessness, weakness, or tiredness. He or she may notice a lack of ability to concentrate mentally and may feel sleepy. Although sleepiness is a part of fatigue, fatigue is a more chronic condition.[4]

According to Medilexicon's medical dictionary, fatigue is:

> That state, following a period of mental or bodily activity, characterized by a lessened capacity or motivation for work and reduced efficiency of accomplishment, usually accompanied by a feeling of weariness, sleepiness, irritability, or loss of ambition; may also supervene when, from any cause, energy expenditure outstrips restorative processes and may be confined to a single organ.

The key phrase is "when ... energy expenditure outstrips restorative processes."[4] This process occurs frequently in the medical profession. Having a balanced work-life relationship is imperative to maintaining physical and mental abilities that are necessary for our jobs as physicians. While it can be challenging to take time for ourselves, if we continue to burn the candle at both ends, it will be not only ourselves but also our patients who suffer because we are not at our best.

Ways to combat fatigue are many, but most recommend ruling out any health issues that may be causing the fatigue. Even though work may be quite busy, there may be something else contributing to the fatigue. Exercise and, in particular, yoga seem to help with the feeling of tiredness and lethargy. The obvious is getting plenty of sleep. That can be difficult with certain schedules, but setting a regular sleep routine and sticking with it when the physician is not on call can be helpful. Drinking plenty of water, eating healthy (specifically omega-3s), eating more small frequent meals, shedding extra weight, and keeping cognizant of your own daily energy pattern will help combat the fatigue that can plague physicians through their career.[5]

AGING

All anesthesiologists will experience the symptoms of aging in some capacity. Some of the problems with aging are not real issues in the workplace. A minor ache here or there in a joint will not impair a physician to the point that they are unable to perform his or her job. However, some symptoms of aging might. Loss of cognitive function can happen slowly, and the inability to adequately care for a patient may be insidious, leaving the physician wondering when the loss of memory is something major or something minor.

Changes associated with aging include eye issues such as presbyopia, cataracts, glaucoma, and macular degeneration. These will impair the physician's ability to practice medicine if not recognized and treated. Presbycusis, or hearing loss, occurs as well and is an insidious process. This development is related to loss of receptors in the inner ear. As an anesthesiologist, we rely on our sense of hearing to observe the patient under anesthesia. Listening to the monitors—for the sound of the pulse oximeter, the rate of the pulse, and alarms on the anesthesia machine—is paramount in anesthesia. Hearing aids can assist the anesthesiologist to overcome this disability and continue to practice.[5]

A noticeable decrease in muscle strength and tone can occur during the aging process, leading to a decrease in stamina. Since the profession of medicine can be quite taxing, as physicians get older and experience the decrease in stamina, it may become harder to fulfill full-time duties. Exercise and strength training can offset some of this decrease in muscle strength and may increase stamina for the physician.[6]

Memory loss and cognitive dysfunction can occur during the process of aging. Complex cognitive skills decline with the aging process and can be one of the more detrimental aspects of aging in the anesthesiologist. While a momentary lapse of memory about where you left your eyeglasses may be explained away by normal forgetfulness, having difficulty learning and retaining information may be the beginning signs of Alzheimer's. Information processing does age as we age, and multitasking can be a problem, however, in cognitive function, there is variability.[6] Overall, if someone starts to have difficult with episodic memory, it may be time to be evaluated by a professional to rule out any organic dysfunction.

VISUAL AND AUDITORY IMPAIRMENT

While some might think this falls solely under the category of symptoms of aging, visual and auditory impairment can happen at any age for a variety of different reasons. Physicians can experience trauma, side effects from medications, genetic predisposition, and, yes, also the symptoms of the aging process that can all lead to visual and auditory impairment. Maintaining regular eye and, where necessary, hearing exams is paramount. It is important to seek out medical assistance whenever a problem arises. Preventive health maintenance can go a long way to keep more serious eye or hearing problems from occurring. As anesthesiologists, we rely heavily on our eyes and ears to care for our patients. It would be very difficult to do our job without good eyesight or adequate hearing. Since there are aids to assist the physician to maintain their eyesight and hearing, it is the physician's responsibility to seek out help to fulfill their obligations to their patients.

AMERICAN DISABILITIES ACT

The Americans with Disabilities Act of 1990 (ADA) prohibits discrimination and ensures equal opportunity for persons with disabilities in employment, state and local government services, public accommodations, commercial facilities, and transportation. It also mandates the establishment of TDD/telephone relay services.[6]

The ADA ensures that those persons with disabilities are accommodated in the workforce. Those with disabilities also have an avenue to pursue fair and equal treatment among their peers in the workplace despite their disabilities.

There are two parts to being disabled, physical and mental. Physical impairment can include, but is not limited to, any medical condition, disfigurement, and loss of any part of the body system including neurological, musculoskeletal, respiratory, cardiovascular, digestive, immune, and endocrine. Mental impairment can include but is not limited to psychological and mental disorders, encompassing intellectual disability, learning disabilities, and organic brain syndrome (Disabilities Guidebook, 2014).

ETHICS, PRACTICE MANAGEMENT, AND MEDICOLEGAL ISSUES

ETHICS

Merriam-Webster, 2014, defines ethics as "an area of study that deals with ideas about what is good and bad behavior: a branch of philosophy dealing with what is morally right or wrong."

Morals may vary with different cultures, religions, and/or nationalities. Ethics involves choices. It is important to make the right choice despite the fact that there may be difficult consequences to bear. For instance, choosing to inform the team and the patient that an antibiotic was given to the patient even though the patient was allergic to that antibiotic is important. Making the medical error can harm the patient, so the team and the patient need to be informed. The physician who made the mistake, however, must report the mistake to the quality assurance program at the institution and face possible repercussions. We all know what the right choice is. Ethics in the workplace is choosing the "right" or moral choice, even though other options may be more attractive.[8]

How do you make sure your decisions are ethical? Bush lists a series of questions that may assist in that conclusion.[8]

1. *How would you define the problem if you stood on the other side of the fence?*
2. *What is your intention in making this decision?*
3. *Whom could your decision or action injure?*
4. *Are you confident that your position will be as valid over a long period of time as it seems now?*
5. *Could you disclose without qualm your decision or action to your boss, your CEO, the board of directors, your family, society as a whole?*

We must always respect patients and their rights. Additionally, the anesthesiologist should not compromise his or her integrity.

PRACTICE MANAGEMENT

Practice management is defined as "Business management of medical and dental practices that may include capital financing, utilization management, and arrangement of capitation agreements with other parties."[9] The ACGME requires training programs to provide some didactic classes in practice management at the present time. Most training programs are now offering classes to assist residents in their knowledge of administrative infrastructure, business, and the management of the anesthesia office. It is important to understand these issues to ensure efficiency in the office and maximize reimbursement. The American Society of Anesthesiology (ASA) has a wide array of practice-management materials available on their website, www.asahq.org. These include coding and billing, practice management course offerings, and information on Medicare as well as interpretive guidelines, informational templates, and practice management news.[9] The ASA also offers a Practice Management Conference each spring to help individuals with their practice. The conference includes reviews of past practice management guidelines and recent updates on administrative and financial topics.

MEDICOLEGAL ISSUES

It is important to understand how medicine and law interact. It is imperative that the physician be aware of how to appropriately address potential errors. There are five components to consider regarding the legal aspects of medicine: consent, prescribing, confidentiality, record keeping, and probity.

Obtaining consent from a patient is a very basic and important job of the physician. The physician must be aware of the risks involved with the procedure and must relay the risks and benefits to the patient in the most judicious way. This may involve taking time to explain to the patient the risks and benefits in layman's terms and obtaining interpreters when necessary. In the end, the patient must have a minimal working knowledge of what is about to happen to them and the risks and benefits involved with the procedure.

Prescribing medicine is fraught with problems. It is the responsibility of the physician to be aware of the allergies of the patient, other drugs the patient may be taking, and special considerations based on the patients' age and coexisting diseases. Double-checking the patient's name and allergy and current drug list will go a long way to eliminate any medical error. In the hospital, the anesthesiologist has very little secondary checks before the medication reaches the patient. They must be ever vigilant in making sure that the patient's allergies are checked, along with the patient's medication list and disease list.

The core of the Health Information Healthcare Insurance Portability and Accountability Act (HIPAA) is maintaining the confidentiality of the patient's health information. It is the responsibility of the physician anesthesiologist to comply with the rules and regulation of HIPAA. Each physician must be careful when riding elevators, congregating in the lunchroom, or being in public areas to maintain conversation that does not disclose personal information about their patients. Sharing information between physicians when necessary for patient care is acceptable, but idle chat must be curtailed for the confidentiality of the patient.

Record keeping is paramount in anesthesia. From documenting conversations with the patient to describing the patient's airway and any difficulties that may have occurred, it is imperative that the anesthesiologist document thoroughly. Such complete records aid in future patient care and also provide insight and clarity for any potential questions or issues that may arise in the future.

Probity is the practice of being trustworthy and honest regarding signing documents, forms, and reports. Physicians are responsible for documentation on patient's charts, and it is essential to document honestly and truthfully. It may also be necessary to document information that the patient may not want to be documented; however, physicians have a legal and professional obligation to society at large to report anything that may negatively impact the public.[10]

PROFESSIONALISM AND LICENSURE

Professionalism encourages high-quality work, respects individuals and the community, and emphasizes the value of others.[11]

All practicing physicians must maintain licensure. Each state governs its own rules and regulations regarding licensure. However, maintaining a license requires honesty, trustworthiness, and moral character. Self-reporting on licensure forms is one of the primary ways that licensing boards discover issues that may interfere with the granting of the license to that physician. Without honest self-reporting, the boards will have to rely on background checks each year to find out discrepancies. The National Practitioner Data Bank (NPDB) is one entity that licensing boards use to maintain up-to-date information on the physician. The NPDB is a federal organization that "is primarily an alert or flagging system intended to facilitate a comprehensive review of the professional credentials of health care practitioners."[12] The NPDB evaluates medical malpractice claims, DEA registration infractions, licensure adverse actions, and unfavorable actions by federal agencies and healthcare plans.

ADVANCE DIRECTIVES/ DO NOT RESUSCITATE ORDERS: SUSPENDED ORDERS

Advance directives enable people to express their desires about treatment in the event of incapacitation. The Patient Self-Determination Act (PSDA) of 1990 increased their use. Healthcare institutions (hospitals, nursing homes, hospice programs) inform patients of two different types: (1) living wills and (2) healthcare proxies. With a living will, patients are able to decide in advance the extent of care they would like to receive in certain situations.[13] However, because it is difficult to predict certain situations, some people prefer to use a healthcare proxy; this is a surrogate decision maker designated to make decisions regarding healthcare when a patient loses decision-making abilities.[13] It is important for the surrogate to understand the patient's preferences. In most cases, the combination of a living will and healthcare proxy is best for carrying out a patient's wishes.

Patients have a right to refuse treatment and resuscitation efforts in critical situations by implementing "Do Not Resuscitate" (DNR) orders. "A decision not to resuscitate is considered for a variety of reasons: a request by a patient or family; advanced age of the patient; poor prognosis; severe brain damage; extreme suffering or disability in a chronically or terminally ill patient."[14] Should DNR orders be honored in the operating room (OR)? Patients may wish that DNR orders continue in the operating room for the fear of being in a worse condition after surviving resuscitation in the OR or may feel that death under anesthesia would be a peaceful end.[15] However, surgeons and anesthesiologists may feel restrained from correcting complications that may occur in the OR. Physicians "feel compelled to do all in their power to correct the situation."[15] Many believe that DNR orders should be suspended while the patient is in the OR. Patients who agree to surgery also agree to other interventions such as anesthesia. Anesthesia can induce apnea or hemodynamic instability, which can then be reversed with assisted ventilation, tracheal intubation, or cardiovascular medicines, which are maneuvers that may be viewed as resuscitative in nature.[16]

The clinical dilemma of honoring or suspending DNR orders prompts an in-depth discussion with the patient and the physician prior to going to the OR. It is important that the physician has a very clear understanding of the patient's goals and wishes. If the patient agrees to suspension of DNR orders, the degree of suspension must be fully understood by the healthcare team. Aside from "full suspension" of DNR orders, patients can agree to procedure-directed DNR orders or goal-directed DNR orders. Procedure-directed DNR orders require that the caregiver and patient anticipate various situations and the well-defined course of action the patient wishes the caregiver to follow in those situations. In the case of goal-directed DNR orders, the physician must have a clear understanding of the patient's goals, values, and preferences. Less focus is placed on the technical details of resuscitation.[16] The physician will have a set of guidelines to follow. The caregiver will possess flexibility to fulfill the patient's wishes.

Discussions with the patient serve two purposes: legal and ethical. One hospital has been sued for "negligence and battery related to the performance of CPR on a patient with DNR orders."[17] Ethically, the physician has a moral obligation to respect the patient's autonomy. Patients' goals and preferences can only be understood by having discussions with the patient. Caregivers must understand the patient's wishes. The patient's primary caregivers may have a complete understanding of the details of the DNR orders; however, it is the responsibility of all caregivers to have that complete knowledge. Intraoperative caregivers should communicate with the primary caregivers to avoid misinterpretations of patients' goals and wishes.

PATIENT PRIVACY

Physicians have an obligation to keep patient's medical information private and confidential. When patients trust that their physician will maintain details of their medical history confidential, patients will readily disclose details about their medical history necessary for appropriate treatment. Moreover, patients must also be confident that no one else will have access to their medical records without their authorization.

The Standards for Privacy of Individually Identifiable Health Information (Privacy Rule) establishes a set of national standards for the protection of certain health information. The US Department of Health and Human Services (HHS) issued the Privacy Rule to implement the requirement of the Health Insurance Portability and Accountability Act of 1996 (HIPAA).[18] The law enables people to have health insurance and protects the confidentiality and security of healthcare information while controlling the healthcare industry's administrative costs.[19] The patient's medical record is protected and cannot be lawfully disclosed without the patient's written authorization "outside the context of treatment."[20]

Privacy protection is extended to a patient's information in electronic, written, or oral form. The protected health information (PHI) secured by HIPAA includes the information healthcare providers have entered in the patient's chart, conversations that have transpired between healthcare providers, names, dates, telephone numbers, social security and medical record numbers, disease, diagnosis, procedures, or prognosis in any medium (files, voicemail, e-mail, fax, or verbal communications). Healthcare providers (doctors, nurses, pharmacies, hospitals), healthcare clearinghouses (physician and hospital billing services), and governmental health plans (Medicare and Medicaid programs) must comply with the HIPPA law.[19] If disclosure of PHI is for the purposes of treatment, payments, or operations, or is mandated by law, the patient's authorization is not necessary. Conversely, if the PHI is for other purposes, the patient must grant authorization.[20]

Also, HIPAA specifies that the patient has the following rights:

1. The patient must receive a notice of the privacy practices of any healthcare provider, healthcare clearinghouse, or health plan.
2. Patients also have the right to see their PHI and request that errors in their records are corrected.
3. Patients have a right to see a list of disclosures that have been made of their PHI.
4. Patients can request special treatment to their PHI.
5. Patients can request confidential communications.
6. Patients have a right to complain.

A patient also has the right to submit a complaint concerning improper disclosure of PHI or concerns about the provider's compliance with privacy policies.[19]

INFORMED CONSENT

Prior to the delivery of anesthesia care, the anesthesia provider must discuss the anesthetic plan, including the risks and the benefits of the anesthetic, and obtain permission from the patient. Informed consent is permission granted with the knowledge of the possible consequences.[21] Consent given by the patient means that the patient has a complete understanding of the risks, benefits, and alternatives. Consent is a process that protects the patient's autonomy, which is the "patient's capacity to think, decide and protect his own interests."[22] Given this information, the patient has the right to consent or refuse treatment. Informed consent requires honest disclosure of medical information to the patient.[23] However, circumstances may exist that limit a patient's autonomy. The patient may be a child or suffer mental illness and may require a parent or legal guardian to grant consent.

The consent process for anesthesia should stimulate a discussion between the anesthesia provider and the patient about the options the patient may have and the associated risks and benefits. This process provides an opportunity for the anesthesiologist and the patient (and/or guardian) to establish a relationship. A "majority of patients wish to meet the anesthesiologist preoperatively for both information and opinion. The caregiver's opinions are biased in favor of the patient's best medical interests."[22] The anesthesiologist should offer an opinion about different options as well as the advantages and disadvantages of those options. The anesthesiologist must help patients understand the reasons for various recommendations. The patient will then be able to make well-informed decisions. Anesthesiologists take an approach blending the two extremes of autonomy and paternalism—obtaining consent while developing a relationship, providing honest, comprehensible information, listening to patient's concerns, and adjusting the proposed treatment plan accordingly.[21]

It is imperative that a discussion for anesthesia care occurs separately from the surgical discussion. In some institutions, consent for anesthesia is implied when a patient agrees to proceed with surgical intervention. However, a surgeon is not qualified to discuss the risks of anesthesia. "A separate consent for anesthesia is needed and should prompt a discussion with patients about their treatment options. Anesthesia is associated with its own risks and consequences separate from surgery."[22] When a patient gives informed consent to anesthesia care, he should understand that the consent does not release the anesthesia provider from liability. Written consent simply indicates that a discussion regarding the risks and benefits of anesthesia care occurred.

PATIENT SAFETY—MEDICATION ERRORS: ASSESSMENT AND PREVENTION

Anesthesiologists are in a very unique position regarding medication management. Anesthesia providers decide, order, prepare, and administer the medications. "They are the only health care providers responsible for the entire medication delivery chain (order, preparation, transport, administer, record, and monitor outcomes). The rapid-paced nature of care in the operating room frequently precludes pre-administration double-checks commonly in place in other parts of the hospital."[24] All facets of medication management in the perioperative period are under the direct control of the anesthesia providers. A medication error is defined as "any error involving the prescribing, ordering, selection or administration of a medication."[25] The risk of medication errors increases as the number of administered drugs increases. A survey of anesthesiologists regarding medical errors revealed that most anesthesiologists experience at least one actual or potential medication error while in clinical practice. Most errors did not result in harm to the patient. The most common medication error was a "syringe swap," involving the administration of a muscle relaxant when an anticholinesterase was intended.[26] However, anesthesia providers continue to strive to understand the root cause of medication errors to ultimately prevent the errors from occurring.

Interventions include educating and raising awareness of the risk of medication errors, emphasizing labeling compliance, developing a national reporting program for drug errors, and identifying other effective strategies to reduce the incidence of medication errors.[25] Although it may seem that individual practitioners are to blame for medication errors, safeguards can be implemented into the medication delivery system to help prevent errors.

Recommended system improvements include using color-coded labels, optimizing the legibility of the labels (font, size, color, and information included), and organizing the drug drawers and workspace by separating similar-appearing medication vials. Standardizing syringe sizes for certain medications and using prefilled syringes prepared under quality-assured conditions are other measures that promote safer drug administration practices. Double-checking the ampules as the drug is being prepared and drawn up and rechecking the label prior to the administration of the drug by a second person or a barcode reader are additional safety measures. Using automated medication-dispensing systems with single-issue drawers and barcode scanners could further increase the safety of medication dispensing.[25,27] Anesthesiologists know that safe management of medication is an important training topic, and recognize the importance of training residents in safeguards that should be used when administering medications. Clearly from the reported events of medication errors, training alone is insufficient. Additional processes and tools should be explored to enhance medication safety in the OR.

DISCLOSURE OF ERROR TO PATIENTS

In 1999, a report by the Institute of Medicine (IOM), *To Err Is Human*, revealed that adverse medical events as the cause of death exceeds the number of injuries resulting from automobile injuries.[28] Three distinctive events are discussed here:

1. A "serious event" is defined as an event, occurrence, or situation involving the clinical care of a patient in a medical facility that results in death or compromises patient safety and results in an unanticipated injury requiring the delivery of additional healthcare services to the patient.[29]
2. An "adverse event" is an unintentional, definable injury that was the result of medical management and not a disease process.[29]
3. A "medical error" is the failure of a planned action to be completed as intended, or the use of the wrong plan to achieve an aim.[29]

Although it may be difficult, physicians have a duty to fully inform patients and families of such events. Failure to disclose errors could undermine the trust between a physician and patient.

Healthcare organizations have quality improvement programs that encourage error reporting. The philosophy of improvement programs is to understand the causes of error. In most instances, the occurrence of adverse events is due to the combination of errors committed by an individual and flaws in the healthcare delivery system. In the patient safety movement, organizations are moving from the "blame and shame" response toward a "high reliability response that confronts, reports and learns from the error."[30] By analyzing the causes for errors, changes can be made in the healthcare system that will prevent individual errors from reaching and possibly harming the patient.

When explaining a medical error, the physician must consider several aspects of the disclosure, and should explain the events in an objective and narrative way in a timely fashion to avoid the appearance of a cover-up. Avoiding speaking defensively and evasively may help to strengthen the physician and patient relationship.[31] Patients want basic information of the event and an apology. There are two different types of apologies: an apology of sympathy and an apology of responsibility.[32] Some states consider an apology as evidence of liability. In those situations, physicians must weigh the risks and benefits with hospital administrators, risk managers, and hospital attorneys prior to issuing an apology. Patients are reassured by remorse and efforts to rectify the harm. It is also important to convey that measures will be taken to rectify the harm and to prevent future recurrences.[31]

Ethically, failing to disclose errors prevents a patient from knowing about critical incidents and could undermine public trust in medicine.[31] Disclosing a medical error to the patient allows the patient to receive adequate treatment to mitigate the effects resulting from the mistake. Legally, physicians have a duty to inform patients of medical errors. Some studies have suggested that disclosure of a mistake may decrease the likelihood of legal liability. Information may even strengthen the physician-patient relationship, and a lawsuit may not result. However, the physician may have greater troubles if the patient pursues legal action and the physician did not disclose the error.[31] Physicians should consult with hospital representatives and risk-management or departmental supervisors when uncertain how to disclose and discuss medical errors with a patient.

REFERENCES

1. Bryson E, Silverstein J. Addiction and substance abuse in anesthesiology. *Anesthesiology*. 2008;109:905–917.
2. Texas Physician Health Program. Texas Medical Board website. http://www.tmb.state.tx.us/page/TXPHP. Accessed April 30, 2014.
3. Brett J. Dealing With the Impaired Physician. American Academy of Family Practice Physicians website. http://www.aafp.org/afp/2009/1101/p1007.html. Published November 1, 2009. Accessed April 30, 2014.
4. What Is Fatigue? What Causes Fatigue? Medical News Today website. http://www.medicalnewstoday.com/articles/248002.php. Published January 1, 2012. Accessed April 29, 2014.
5. 9 Ways to Get Your Energy Back. WebMD website. http://www.webmd.com/balance/features/get-energy-back. Accessed April 29, 2014.

6. Is This Normal Aging or Not? http://www.webmd.com/healthy-aging/features/normal-aging-changes-and-symptoms. Accessed April 30, 2014.
7. The Americans With Disabilities Act of 1990 and Revised ADA Regulations Implementing Title II and Title III. United States Department of Justice Civil Rights Division website. http://www.ada.gov/2010_regs.htm. Accessed March 5, 2014.
8. Work-Place Ethics. Central Michigan University website. http://www.chsbs.cmich.edu/leader_model/development/media/Targeted%20Lessons/workplace_ethics.htm. Accessed April 30, 2014.
9. Practice Management. American Society of Anesthesiologists website. https://www.asahq.org/For-Members/Practice-Management.aspx. Accessed January 1, 2014.
10. Davies M, Barclay I, Bown S. Avoiding easy mistakes: Five medicolegal hazards for junior doctors. Medical Protection Society website.http://www.medicalprotection.org/uk/booklets/medicolegal-hazards. Published July 1, 2012. Accessed May 2, 2014.
11. Gracious Professionalism. FIRST (For Inspiration and Recognition of Science and Technology) website. http://www.usfirst.org/abou-tus/gracious-professionalism. Accessed May 5, 2014.
12. About Us. The Data Bank National Practitioner. http://www.npdb.hrsa.gov/topNavigation/aboutUs.jsp. Accessed May 5, 2014.
13. Advance Care Directives. MedlinePlus U.S. National Library of Medicine:NIH Natioanl Institutues of Health website. http://www.nlm.nih.gov/medlineplus/ency/patientinstructions/00472.htm. Accessed May 1,2014.
14. Miles S, Cranford R, Schultz A. The Do-Not-Resuscitate Order in a teaching hospital. *Ann Intern Med.* 1982;96:660–664.
15. Walker R. DNR in the OR: Resuscitation as an operative risk. *JAMA.* 1991;266(17):2407–2412.
16. Truog R, Waisel B, Burns J. DNR in the OR. *Anesthesiology.* 1999;90:289–295.
17. Truog R. Do not resuscitate orders during anesthesia and surgery. *Anesthesiology.* 1991;74:606–608.
18. Health Information Privacy. Department of Health and Human Services website. http://www.hhs.gov/ocr/privacy. Accessed April 28, 2014.
19. What Is HIPAA? Tennessee Department of Health website. https://health.state.tn.us/hipaa. Accessed April 28, 2014.
20. Annas G. HIPAA Regulations: a new era of medical-record privacy? *N Engl J Med.* 2003;348:1486–1490.
21. Habiba M. Examining consent within the patient-doctor relationship. *J Med Ethics.* 200;26:183–187.
22. White S. Clinical Ethics: Consent for anaesthesia. *J Med Ethics.* 2004;30:286–290.
23. Miller R, ed. *Miller's Anesthesia.* 7th ed. Philadelphia, PA: Elsevier; 2010.
24. A *Wake Up Safe* Patient Safety Alert: Decreasing the Risks of Intravenous Medication Errors. Wake Up Safe website. http://wakeupsafe.org/intravenousmederrors2.iphtml. Accessed April 28, 2014.
25. Merry A, Anderson B. Medication errors: new approaches to prevention. *Pediatr Anesth.* 2011;21:743–753.
26. Orser B, Chen R, Yee D. Medication errors in anesthetic practice: a survey of 687 practitioners. *Can J Anaesth.* 2001;48:139–146.
27. Stabile M, Webster CS, Merry AF. Medication administration in anesthesia: Time for a paradigm shift. Anesthesia Patient Safety Foundation website. http://www.apsf.org/newsletters/html/2007/fall/02_medical_administration.htm.
28. Blendon R, DesRoche C. Views of practicing physicians and the public on medical errors. *N Engl J Med.* 2002;347(24):1933–1940.
29. Liebman C, Hyman C. A Mediation skills model to manage disclosure of errors and adverse events to patients. *Health Aff.* 2004;23(4):22–32.
30. Espin S, Levinson W, Regehr G, Baker G, Lingard L. Error or "act of God"? A study of patients' and operating room team members' perceptions of error definition, reporting, and disclosure. *Surgery.* 2006;139(1):6–14.
31. Hebert P, Levin A, Robertson G. Bioethics for clinicians: 23. Disclosure of medical error. *Can Med Assoc J.* 2001;164(4):509–512.
32. Kaira J, Massey K, Mulla A. Disclosure of medical error: policies and practice. *J R Soc Med.* 2005;98:307–309.
33. Barash P, Cullen B, Stoelting R, Cahalan M, Stock M. *Clinical Anesthesia.* 7th ed. Philadelphia, PA: Lippincott Williams & Wilkins; 2013:4683–4793.
34. Barash P, Cullen B, Stoelting R, Cahalan M, Stock M. *Clinical Anesthesia.* 7th ed. Philadelphia, PA: Lippincott Williams & Wilkins; 2013:4745.
35. Barash P, Cullen B, Stoelting R, Cahalan M, Stock M. *Clinical Anesthesia.* 7th ed. Philadelphia, PA: Lippincott Williams & Wilkins; 2013:4821.

FURTHER READING

Accreditation Council for Graduate Medical Education website. http://acgme.org/acgmeweb/Portals/0/PDFs/ab_ACGME PoliciesProcedures.pdf. Published January 1, 2014. Accessed April 29, 2014.

Avoiding Easy Mistakes: Five Medicolegal Hazards for Junior Doctors. Medical Protection Society website. http://www.medicalprotection.org/uk/booklets/medicolegal-hazards. Accessed April 29, 2014.

Disabilities Guidebook: Who Has a Disability under the ADA? Illinois Legal Aid Online website. http://www.illinoislegalaid.org/index.cfm?fuseaction=home.dsp_content&contentID=167. Accessed April 30, 2014.

Ethics. Merriam-Webster website. http://www.merriam-webster.com/dictionary/ethic. Accessed March 5, 2014.

Practice Management Definition. Reference MD website. http://www.reference.md/files/D020/mD020399.html. Published June 6, 2012. Accessed April 29, 2014.

Professionalism. Merriam-Webster Dictionary website. http://www.merriam-webster.com/dictionary/professionalism. Published January 1,2014. Accessed May 5, 2014.

QUESTIONS

1. Agencies that may be required by law to be informed of any disciplinary actions taken against an impaired physician include all of the following EXCEPT:
   A. National Practitioner Data Base
   B. State Medical Board
   C. Hospital Medical Board
   D. Chairman of the physician's department
   E. Coworker of the physician

2. Signs of the abusing physician include all of the following EXCEPT:
   A. Spending more time at the hospital, even when off duty
   B. Volunteering for extra call
   C. Requesting less call and an increase in vacation time
   D. Refusing relief for lunch or coffee breaks
   E. Signing out increasing amounts of narcotics or quantities inappropriate for the given case

3. One of the primary aspects of aging that affects the older anesthesiologist is:
   A. Complex cognitive skills reduction
   B. Joint aches
   C. Weight gain
   D. Cardiac disease
   E. Respiratory disease

4. What is the core of HIPAA, the Health Information Healthcare Insurance Portability and Accountability Act?
   A. Portability
   B. Confidentiality
   C. Insurance
   D. Data
   E. Liability

5. The National Practitioner Data Bank (NPDB) is one avenue that licensing boards use to maintain up-to-date information on the physician. Information that may be kept in the NPDB includes all EXCEPT:
   A. Medical malpractice claims
   B. Incidents of substance abuse
   C. Suspension of licensure
   D. Recent hours worked at job
   E. Limitation of a physician's license

6. Under the Health Insurance Portability and Accountability Act (HIPAA) of 1996, patients have the following rights EXCEPT:
   A. The patient must receive notices of privacy practices of any healthcare provider, healthcare clearinghouse, or health plan.
   B. Healthcare providers cannot disclose a patient's PHI (treatment, payments, operations, or other information mandated by law) without the patient's authorization.
   C. Patients have a right to complain.
   D. Patients have the right to see their PHI and request corrections to errors in their records.
   E. Patients can request confidential communications.

7. The following steps should be taken to prevent medication errors:
   A. Investigate the cause for the medication error and sanction the physician who committed the error.
   B. Address the error by simply increasing training for physicians.
   C. Implement interventions such as educating and raising awareness of medication errors in combination with systematic strategies such as using color-coded labels and the double-check system.
   D. Keep adverse drug events confidential.
   E. Avoid the use of technology for drug dispensing because of possible malfunction.

8. When a serious adverse event occurs:
   A. Patients must be told of the event in an honest and objective fashion.
   B. Apologies must never be issued, because it is admission of liability.
   C. It is acceptable to wait several days to disclose the serious adverse event to allow the physician time to speak with risk management.
   D. It is acceptable to forgo disclosing the event to the family if the event will be reported to the institution's quality improvement program.
   E. It is most likely due to the failure of one individual.

9. Regarding informed consent for anesthesia, all of the following are correct EXCEPT:
   A. Provides an opportunity for the anesthesiologist and the patient to establish a relationship
   B. Gives the patient an opportunity to obtain information and the anesthesiologist's opinion
   C. Is implied when a patient consents for surgery
   D. Anesthesiologists combine two extremes of autonomy and paternalism when discussing the anesthetic with patients
   E. Does not release the anesthesia provider from liability

ANSWERS

1. E. While having the partners of an impaired physician aware of the disease state and abusing potential of the physician may be helpful, it is not required by law. The agencies in this question, namely, the National Practitioner Data Base, State Medical Board, Hospital Medical Board, and chairman of the physician's department, are required to be informed of any disciplinary action taken against an impaired physician.[33]
2. C. Physicians who are abusing drugs would aim to spend more time in the hospital not less time. Most of the time the impaired physician will want to spend more time on call, frequently show up off duty, and refuse relief for lunch or coffee breaks. The impaired physician can also be seen signing out increased amount of narcotics inappropriate for the case or the patient.[34]
3. A. While all of these may represent the signs of aging, the anesthesiologist's ability to complete complex cognitive skills can severely affect his or her practice. Changes in the CNS include decrease in brain weight and a decrease in neuronal density. Also, a lack of ability to learn new tasks can be one of the signs of the aging physicians. The other answers to this question can definitely be signs of aging, but do not impact the anesthesiologist as much as complex cognitive skills reduction.[35]

4. B. All of these are aspects of the HIPAA, the Health Information Healthcare Insurance Portability and Accountability Act. However, the primary core concern of HIPAA is confidentiality or protecting the patient's health information. All patients' charts must be locked away and secure. Any identifying markers, such as names on operating room boards, must be sufficiently veiled so as not to give away information that is not necessary to care for the patient.

FURTHER READING

Barash P, Cullen B, Stoelting R, Cahalan M, Stock M. *Clinical Anesthesia*. 7th ed. Philadelphia, PA: Lippincott Williams & Wilkins; 2013:3220–3247.

5. D. Duty hours of a physician are not kept at the NPDB, however, medical malpractice claims, incidents of substance abuse, and suspension or limitations of a physician's license are all part of the data bank.

FURTHER READING

Barash P, Cullen B, Stoelting R, Cahalan M, Stock M. *Clinical Anesthesia*. 7th ed. Philadelphia, PA: Lippincott Williams & Wilkins; 2013:2133–2140.

6. B. Healthcare providers can disclose a patient's PHI if the information deals with treatment, payment, and operations or if the information is mandated by law. Also, HIPAA requires that healthcare providers (doctors, nurses, pharmacies, hospitals), healthcare clearinghouses (physician and hospital billing services), and governmental health plans (Medicare and Medicaid programs) comply. In other situations, patient authorization is necessary for disclosure. Further, HIPAA specifies that the patient has the following rights:

    1. The patient must receive a notice of the privacy practices of any healthcare provider, healthcare clearinghouse, or health plan.
    2. Patients also have the right to see their PHI and request that errors in their records be corrected.
    3. Patients have a right to see a list of disclosures that have been made of their PHI.
    4. Patients can request special treatment of their PHI.
    5. Patients can request confidential communications.
    6. Patients have a right to complain.

FURTHER READING

What is HIPAA? https://health.state.tn.us/hipaa.

7. C. Anesthesia providers are responsible for the entire delivery chain of medications. The possibility for errors increases as the number of drugs administered increases. In the event of a medication error, it is usually due to a combination of individual error and system flaws. In addition to increasing education and awareness of medication errors, implementing system changes (i.e., color-coded labels, standardized preparations/prefilled syringes, bar-coding system, automated medication dispensing systems, double-check system) will help to reduce and prevent medication errors.

FURTHER READING

1. Merry AF, Anderson BJ. Medication errors: new approaches to prevention. *Pediatr Anesth*. 2011;21:743–753.
2. Stabile M, Webster CS, Merry AF. Medication Administration in Anesthesia: Time for a Paradigm Shift. http://www.apsf.org/newsletters/html/2007/fall/02_medical_administration.htm.

8. A. In the event of a medical error, disclosure is important. The event should be discussed in an objective and narrative manner in a timely fashion. An apology can be helpful, however, it may be evidence of liability in some states. Reporting events to an institution's quality improvement program, will be helpful in the analysis of those events. Adverse events usually result from individual and system failures. By analyzing events, system changes may be implemented to prevent future adverse events. Although the event is reported to the quality program, the event should also be disclosed to the patient.

FURTHERING READING

Hebert PC, Levin AV, Robertson G. Bioethics for clinicians: 23. Disclosure of medical error. *Can Med Assoc J*. 2001;164(4):509–512.
Kair J, Massey KL, Mulla A. Disclosure of medical error: policies and practice. *J R Soc Med*. 2005;98:307–309.

9. C. Anesthesia consent must be obtained by the anesthesia provider, because anesthesia has risks and effects separate from surgery. Informed consent for surgery does not imply consent for anesthesia. The consent process for anesthesia should stimulate a discussion between the anesthesia provider and the patient about the options the patient may have and the associated risks and benefits. This process provides an opportunity for the anesthesiologist and the patient (and/or guardian) to establish a relationship. A "majority of patients wish to meet the anesthesiologist preoperatively for both information and opinion." Anesthesiologists take an approach blending the two extremes of autonomy and paternalism—obtaining consent while developing a relationship, providing honest, comprehensible information, listening to

patient's concerns, and adjusting the proposed treatment plan accordingly. A patient giving informed consent to anesthesia care should understand that the consent does not release the anesthesia provider from liability.

FURTHER READING

Habiba MA. Examining consent within the patient-doctor relationship. *J Med Ethics*. 200;26:183–187.

White SM. Clinical ethics: consent for anaesthesia. *J Med Ethics*. 2004;30:286.

SECTION VI

PROFESSIONAL CHALLENGES

32.

ANESTHESIA, ORGANIZED MEDICINE, AND HEALTHCARE POLICY

Sherif Zaafran and George W. Williams

INTRODUCTION

> Politics is the science of who gets what in the setting of finite resources.
>
> Author Unknown

Becoming a physician is a straightforward process. You study hard in high school and college. After a grueling set of MCAT testing and interviews, you earn a spot in medical school, spend your 4 years, graduate, go through residency training, and finally start a practice. So long as you know how to treat a patient, and you are well trained in your specialty, there is nothing else you need to worry about.

This perspective smacks into reality the moment the residency is completed and medical practice begins. The reality is, there are an infinite number of forces out there that affect how we practice. These forces include the rules that govern how we practice, how we are compensated for our work, who dictates our practice structure, who attempts to compete with us (whether appropriately or inappropriately), and so forth. One learns early on that unless we understand and play an integral part in this process, we run the risk of being a bystander in the care of our patients. This affects not only the practice of medicine in general but also specifically the practice of our specialty, anesthesiology. The narrative should be that as consultants, no one understands how to deliver care in the safest way possible to our patients better than us, so naturally we should be the ones writing the rules. But the right to do so is not a given. This chapter discusses the different entities that play a role in healthcare policy and how we as physicians and anesthesiologists can navigate the process in a way that empowers us to play an integral role in affecting policy for delivering care to our patients.

There are different types of players that affect the healthcare policy that we as physicians operate under—federal agencies, state agencies, and organized medicine. At the federal level, the US Department of Health and Human Services is the principal agency involved in federal regulation. Federal regulation is one of the basic tools government uses to carry out public policy. Federal agencies create regulations (also known as "rules") when Congress provides the authority to do so. For example, if Congress passed a law that all medical students should wear a short white coat, a federal agency would be responsible for defining how short is "short," what font any name embroidery should be, how many pockets are acceptable, and so forth. In effect, regulations can be as important as the legislation itself. At the state level, individual states have varying legislative and regulatory structures that manage and implement both federal and state policy. In Texas, for example, the Texas Health and Human Services Commission oversees the Texas health and human services system. And the Texas Department of Insurance governs and regulates the provision of private health insurance to patients in Texas. Finally, organized medicine comprises organizations for medical professionals that play an important role as entities that advocate on our behalf as both general physicians and anesthesiologists in particular. Professional medical organizations also interact with government agencies in formulating regulation. All these entities form the backbone for the rules and regulations that we operate under. Affecting the process requires an understanding of the role that each type of entity plays and the processes through which rules come about.

FEDERAL AGENCIES

As stated above, the principal federal agency affecting healthcare regulation is the US Department of Health and Human Services. Each fall and spring, the Department publishes a list of all regulations under development or review, called the Regulatory Agenda. In the fall, the Department also publishes a Regulatory Plan, which summarizes priorities for the coming year. Laws that govern this Department come from several different sources:

- Affordable Care Act—The Department uses regulations and guidance to implement parts of the Affordable Care Act that deal with private and public health insurance.
- Health Insurance Portability and Accountability Act (HIPAA)—HIPAA provides protections for personal health information and gives patients a variety of rights.
- Health Information Technology—The Health Information Technology for Economic and Clinical Health (HITECH) Act provides the Department with the authority to write regulations and guidance to support development of a nationwide health information technology infrastructure.
- Laws regarding health insurance—The McCarran-Ferguson Act provides that even though the insuring or provision of healthcare may be national in scope, the regulation of insurance is left to the states. Likewise, the Health Maintenance Organization (HMO) Act provides that HMOs or health service plans are regulated by the states. As a result of these two federal statutes, much of the task of health insurance regulation is left to the states. A few key examples of how the task of insurance regulation can be complex:
  - The private group plans (or fully insured plans) purchased from insurance carriers by employers as a benefit for employees are usually overseen by the insurance commissioner or department of insurance in each state.
  - Self-funded plans (or self-insured plans) are health plans that employers or unions create just for their employees and their families. They are overseen by the US Department of Labor's Employee Benefits Security Administration.
  - Individual plans sold through the health insurance marketplaces are regulated by a marketplace board in every state. This state board oversees the function of the marketplace and the plans sold within it.
  - Managed care plans are regulated by several state and federal agencies.
  - Medigap policies (Medicare Supplement Insurance policies) are regulated by federal agencies, as well as some state laws.
  - Medicaid is a joint program that is controlled by the state health department and the federal Centers for Medicare and Medicaid Services.
  - Medicare is run by the federal Centers for Medicare and Medicaid Services.
  - TRICARE is overseen by the US Department of Defense.
  - The Veteran's Health Care system (including CHAMPVA) is regulated by the US Department of Veteran's Affairs.

All of these sources have different effects. For example, the Medicare Conditions of Participation, Conditions for Coverage, and Requirements are sets of requirements for acceptable quality in the operation of healthcare entities. There is a set of conditions for each type of provider or supplier subject to certification. In addition to each condition there is a group of related quality standards, with the condition or requirements characterizing the quality or result of operations to which all the standards are directed. In the case of anesthesia, these are the rules saying what type of anesthesia care model is considered safe by Medicare's standards. A state survey agency ascertains whether and how each standard is met. The interpretive guidelines merely define or explain the relevant statute and regulations and do not impose any requirements that are not otherwise specifically written in a statute or regulation. Each provider type (e.g., physician, anesthesiologist assistant, nurse anesthetist) is surveyed in accordance with the appropriate protocols based on the substantive requirements in the regulations to determine whether a citation is appropriate. While an institution may fail to comply with one or more of the subsidiary standards during any given survey, it cannot participate in Medicare unless it meets each and every condition or attains substantial compliance with requirements. Most hospitals would not be able to remain solvent while not participating in Medicare, and as a result, any rules set by Medicare are generally universally adopted.

STATE GOVERNMENTS

Every state is unique in the way it administers services related to the provision of healthcare, and as such, it is not possible to fully prepare the reader for what they may encounter in different parts of the country. In order to ease the explanation of the variances between states, we discuss two large states, Texas and Ohio. Texas has a smaller government infrastructure when compared with Ohio, most notably in that the legislature in Texas meets every 2 years for a period of about 6 months, whereas in Ohio, the legislature is continually available. On the executive/agency side, the Texas Health and Human Services Commission oversees the Texas Health and Human Services System, which is composed of five agencies: the Health and Human Services Commission (which encompasses Medicaid, Medicaid, Children's Health Insurance Program, and Food Stamps, among others), the Department of Aging and Disability

Services (which provides long-term care for elderly or disabled), the Department of State Health Services (which licenses facilities), the Department of Assistive and Rehabilitative Services (which facilitates independent living arrangements), and the Department of Family and Protective Services. This is in contrast to the state of Ohio, where services are provided by the Ohio Department of Health (encompassing several functions, including licensing of facilities, public health, and long-term care coordination), the Department of Medicaid (solely created to administrate Medicaid), and Job and Family Services (Food Stamps and Adult Protective Services). Clearly, there are enormous differences in how different states are structured and function. This means that each state offers an opportunity to achieve radically different policies than could be achieved nationally. From a strategy perspective, it would be easier and less detectable for an organization to achieve policy change on a state-by-state basis than on a national basis. This is the provision that CMS has in place to allow for individual States to opt out of nurse anesthetist supervision.

Sometimes disputes are decided in the state court system. It should be noted that in many states judges are elected (both in Texas and Ohio) instead of being appointed, as occurs in the US Supreme Court. This should be a consideration, as the judge deciding a case that affects patient care and/or the practice of medicine may be subject to the pressures associated with any public official who has to garner support (or money) to be reelected.

ORGANIZED MEDICINE

The term organized medicine refers to the professional organizations that advocate for and pursue policy goals on behalf of their members, medical professionals.

AMERICAN MEDICAL ASSOCIATION

The American Medical Association (AMA) is a professional physicians' organization (founded in 1847). Its goals are to protect the interests of American physicians, advance public health, and support the growth of medical science. The AMA investigates alleged cases of medical quackery; engages in medical research on drugs, foods, cosmetics, and other substances; and sponsors health education programs. The organization also approves in-hospital doctor training programs; it was largely responsible for the upgrading of American medical education in the early 20th century. Other functions include monitoring professional ethics and supervising continuing medical education for physicians.

Structurally, the AMA functions as a federation. Representatives from medical societies in all states and many counties, from medical specialty organizations, and from federal health organizations (including branches of the military) constitute the AMA house of delegates. The house of delegates reviews resolutions from these member organizations, decides on policy for the AMA, and provides direction for AMA programs. Thus, the AMA both represents and is responsive to the "house of medicine." Because of this relationship, the AMA works to build consensus among both medical societies and specialty societies as it promotes its public health agenda. With almost 300,000 members, the AMA maintains a stewardship for ensuring both the standards of the profession and for promoting the health of the nation.

Whether one agrees with every policy or position the AMA holds, from the public's (and most legislators') perspective, the AMA is the only representative body that can speak for all physicians in the country at one time. Therefore, lack of participation in the AMA weakens the collective voice of physicians in the halls of government nationwide. If one desires a change in the AMA's stance on pressing issues of the day, it is important to become more engaged in the AMA, not less.

AMERICAN SOCIETY OF ANESTHESIOLOGISTS

The American Society of Anesthesiologists (ASA) is an educational, research, and scientific association of physicians organized to raise the standards of the medical practice of anesthesiology and to improve patient care. In 2012, the ASA had a membership of 48,000 national and international members and had more than 100 full-time employees. The ASA is governed by its house of delegates. The house of delegates is composed of ASA delegates and directors (designated by geographic distribution), ASA officers, all past presidents, the editor-in-chief of the journal, the chairs of all sections, the chair of the ASA delegation to the American Medical Association house of delegates, each member of the Resident Component Governing Council not to exceed five members, and a nonvoting member of the Medical Student component. The house of delegates meets each year during the society's annual meeting. During the interim between the meetings of the house of delegates, the ASA board of directors exercises authority to manage the business and financial affairs of the Society, and superintends and directs the publication and distribution of all official documents, journals, and reports consistent with policies of the house of delegates. The board of directors meets three times each year. The Society also has many special committees. In addition, 55 component societies work to implement and complement the Society's goals at the community level. There are many educational products provided by the ASA specifically for anesthesiologists that would be difficult to obtain otherwise. This serves the interests of anesthesiologists seeking to meet the continuing education needs of various states around the country.

POLITICAL ACTION COMMITTEES

Each of the entities above has a political action committee (PAC) component that serves as the advocacy arm of each of the organization. They are AMPAC and ASAPAC, with similar state PACs as well. These entities communicate with legislators at the state and federal level regarding issues that are important to the practice of medicine and anesthesiology and that will lead to better care for the patients that we take care of on a daily basis. In effect, a PAC is an IRS/Federal Election Commission–recognized bank account that solely serves the purpose of contributing to political candidates supportive to the issues of medicine. There are PACs for lawyers, nurses, teachers, and other professional groups for similar purposes. Organizational dues alone are not adequate to support the functions of political advocacy for many reasons, including some tax laws. Figure 32.1 clearly demonstrates the contribution/effect relationship of PAC participation. In the 1990's the elimination of supervision of nurse anesthetists by anesthesiologists was initially discussed and there was a sudden increase in anesthesia related PAC contributions, but this increased participation was too late to affect the outcome (even with outcomes literature sanctioned and requested by Medicare that suggested that physician supervision is warranted). Following this time frame, more PAC contributions allowed more effective communication on anesthesiology issues, which was associated with a badly needed and long overdue RVU update for anesthesiology services. Finally, ASAPAC's increased contributions were associated with repeal of the Teaching Rule (which should have been called the teaching penalty). This was a Medicare rule that cut payments to teaching anesthesiologists in half (50%) if they had two residents caring for two Medicare patients. This rule was clearly harmful to anesthesiology programs and forced several residencies to close. Following its repeal, there were more anesthesiology residencies to meet the increased need for anesthesiologists.

DISCUSSION

The practice of medicine involves a complex interplay of rules and regulations promulgated by a variety of different entities at the federal and the state level. The ability to affect the process requires an understanding of the process in all its complexities. Thankfully, organized medicine—particularly the ASA and related state organizations that represent the interests of anesthesiology—has the framework and the expertise that can play that pivotal role in all areas that affect our profession. This also requires an understanding that being medically or logically correct does not translate into policy that serves the interests of patients or physicians. As a group, anesthesiologists are one among many voices competing for the attention of those who write the rules and legislation affecting us. What raises our voices above all of the others is a combination of vigilance, relationships, tact, leadership, compromise, and always remembering to put the interests of our patients first and foremost.

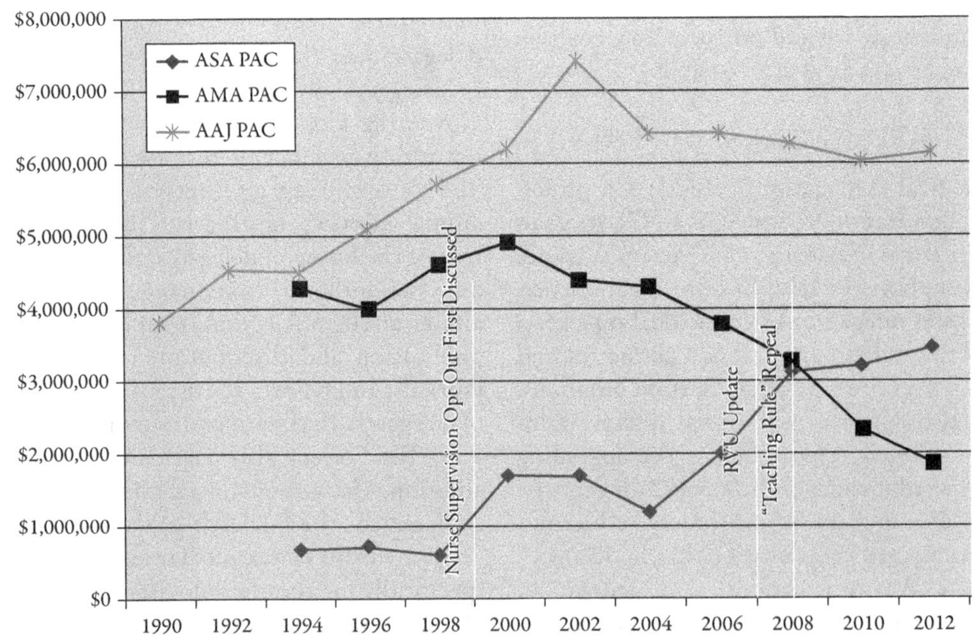

Figure 32.1 PAC contribution data listed by organization as documented by the Federal Election Commission and www.opensecrets.org. Image created by George Williams, MD.

ADVOCACY

The first step in any attempt to affect rules that govern us is to develop relationships with those who legislate policy. We are one stakeholder in a sea of many who seek to have their voice heard. The PAC components of organized medicine serve to further that purpose. The practice of medicine and the practice of anesthesiology require a concerted effort on our part to educate our legislators on how we can best serve our patients. The advantage we have is that practically every county has a hospital, and every hospital has physicians and, in most instances, anesthesiologists. The exception is rural areas. In our grassroots efforts, we aim to identify physicians who can develop a relationship with legislators in their district and serve as the expert for those legislators when it comes to healthcare policy. These relationships are developed over time. It takes supporting legislators during their election efforts and communicating with them on a constant basis as a constituent in their district. Supporting candidates for political office is expensive, but when we fail to financially support legislators we risk losing an important voice at the state level.

The second step in advocacy is helping to write legislation that furthers our goals in providing better and safer care for our patients. For example, in Texas (the chapter author's state), we have succeeded at multiple levels in securing legislation that ensures patients know the difference between a physician and a nonphysician, allows us to negotiate for fair payments for our services with insurance carriers, provides rules ensuring the safe provision of anesthesia in office-based settings, and more. This important and crucial role helps our legislators, as we identify for them ways to ensure a fair playing field and ultimately better care for our patients.

The third step in advocacy is helping prevent passage of legislation that does not serve the best interests of our patients. This is why communicating with our legislators and educating them is an important and crucial role in advocacy.

The fourth step is developing alliances with other stakeholders, as it serves the interests of helping us provide better care for our patients. The larger the coalition of stakeholders we are able to build, the stronger chance we have of securing the rules we need to take care of our patients.

Advocacy takes many forms. For example, the Health Resources and Services Administration (HRSA) is funding a Nursing Workforce Development program via grants from HHS. The Nurse Anesthetist Traineeship funded 81 nurse anesthetist education programs in 2012 in the amount of $2.3 million to provide traineeships to licensed registered nurses enrolled as full-time students in a master's or doctoral nurse anesthesia program. Traineeships were intended to pay all or part of the costs of the tuition, books, and fees, and the reasonable living expenses (stipends) of the individual during the period for which the traineeship is provided. This is an example of effective advocacy on the part of nurse anesthesia education. This is in contrast to the inadequate funding of graduate medical education (GME) positions for physicians (even though more GME funding has been advocated by the American Association of Medical Colleges), as there are more medical school graduates than funded GME positions in the setting of a physician shortage. Advocacy, or the lack thereof, has already affected (in one way or another) each member of the anesthesia care team that may be reading this chapter.

So suppose you have helped to pass legislation that you feel will serve the best interest of your patients. Now you can rest easy. Absolutely not! Legislation is only the first step, and one of the biggest hurdles to overcome is the translation of legislation into rules and regulations. After legislation is passed, it is referred to the appropriate agency. For healthcare or insurance issues at the state level the agency can vary, as mentioned above. Once legislation is referred to these agencies, public hearings are held to hear public comment from stakeholders. Different stakeholders will typically testify and try to ensure that the rules are written in a way that is slanted in their favor. It is extremely important that our organized specialty societies closely monitor these public hearings and testify when appropriate to ensure that our interests and the interests of our patients are best served. This requires time and organization.

Both advocacy and rule writing also play an important role at the federal level, especially with the relevant agencies mentioned earlier in the chapter. It is clear that involvement in writing the rules for our profession is a crucial component of our practice. It is the least taught skill in medical school and residency training, but it is arguably the most impactful, as it has a tremendous effect on how we are able to deliver care. In contrast, nearly every allied health provider is instructed for a semester or longer on how to advocate effectively. The inclusion of advocacy training is required by the ACGME under the core competency of professionalism, however most residency programs lack any structured education on this topic. Discussion in the literature is currently raising this issue.[1]

VOTING

As basic as it sounds, voting is one of the most important forms of advocacy that we can undertake. This should be done not only because it is your civic duty but also because it is the most important thing to policy makers. Whether or not *you* voted is a matter of public record; most politicians have access to public databases that indicate individual voting patterns. This is commonly why there are potholes in the "bad" side of town (or the side of town less likely to vote). In the setting of finite resources, the average politician will likely focus on the population who will actually show up to the polls and keep them in office. As a case in point, it is difficult to walk into a legislator's office and ask for their support for more GME when one look into a public database indicates that you have not voted in the last 8 years. In fact, a commonly applied definition of a likely voter is someone who has voted in *any* election in the preceding 6 years. Most physicians are *not* likely voters. In fact, physicians are less likely to vote that anyone in the general population.[2] This must improve if we are to most effectively advocate for our patients.

The content of this chapter is included in the ABA content outline, but its content is pertinent to every practicing anesthesiologist. We have barely scratched the surface of advocacy issues in this chapter. It is the hope of the authors that readers will be more motivated now to be involved in the protection of patients and the profession by becoming engaged in advocacy.

REFERENCES

1. Croft D, et al. Perspective: is it time for advocacy training in medical education? *Acad Med.* 2012;87(9):1165–1170.
2. Grande D, et al. Do doctors vote? *Society of General Internal Medicine.* 2007;22:585–589.

INDEX

Page numbers followed by *f, t,* or *b* indicate figures, tables, or boxes, respectively.